Fifth International Visual Field Symposium

Documenta Ophthalmologica
Proceedings Series volume 35

Editor H. E. Henkes

1983 **Dr W. JUNK PUBLISHERS**
a member of the KLUWER ACADEMIC PUBLISHERS GROUP
THE HAGUE / BOSTON / LANCASTER

Fifth International Visual Field Symposium

Sacramento, October 20–23, 1982

Edited by E. L. Greve and A. Heijl

1983 **Dr W. JUNK PUBLISHERS**
a member of the KLUWER ACADEMIC PUBLISHERS GROUP
THE HAGUE / BOSTON / LANCASTER

Distributors

for the United States and Canada: Kluwer Boston, Inc., 190 Old Derby Street, Hingham, MA 02043, USA
for all other countries: Kluwer Academic Publishers Group, Distribution Center, P.O.Box 322, 3300 AH Dordrecht, The Netherlands

Library of Congress Cataloging in Publication Data

```
International Visual Field Symposium (5th : 1982 :
   Sacramento, Calif.)
   Fifth International Visual Field Symposium, Sacra-
mento, October 20-23, 1982.

   (Documenta ophthalmologica. Proceedings series ;
v. 35)
   1. Perimetry--Congresses.  2. Visual fields--Con-
gresses.  3. Glaucoma--Diagnosis--Congresses.  I. Greve,
Erik L.  II. Heijl, A. (Anders)  III. Title.  IV. Series.
[DNLM: 1. Glaucoma--Congresses.  2. Perimetry--Congresses.
3. Visual fields--Congresses.  4. Visual disorders--Con-
gresses.  W3 DO637 v.35 / WW 145 I61 1982f]
RE79.P4I56  1982      617.7'0754      83-6200
```

ISBN-13: 978-94-009-7274-2   e-ISBN-13: 978-94-009-7272-8
DOI: 10.1007/978-94-009-7272-8

Copyright

DEDICATION

These proceedings are dedicated to Dr Louise L. Sloan and Professor Gaetan Jayle, who were both honorary members of the International Perimetric Society.

INTRODUCTION

The 5th International Visual Field Symposium of the International Perimetric Society was held on October 20–23, 1982, in Sacramento, California, before the joint meeting of the International Congress of Ophthalmology and the American Academy of Ophthalmology. A majority of the members of the International Perimetric Society took part in the meeting together with many guests.

The topics of the symposium were: *glaucoma*: correlation between the visual field and the optic disc; the visual field in low-tension glaucoma; *neuro-ophthalmology* and *ergo-perimetry*. Apart from this there were many papers on *automated perimetry* and general topics.

The papers concerning the correlation of optic disc and visual field dealt with several aspects: peripapillary atrophy, defects in the retinal nerve fiber layer, fluorescein angiography and the characteristics of the glaucomatous excavation itself. New and interesting findings were presented showing that the careful, detailed observation of the disc and peripapillary area is rewarding.

The visual fields in low-tension glaucoma were studied extensively by four groups. Various approaches to the problem have led to some differences in results, which were extensively discussed.

In the general glaucoma session the visual fatigue phenomenon was discussed extensively; apparently conflicting results were demonstrated regarding the stability of contrast threshold measurements during one and the same test session in glaucoma.

The relationship between the visual field and the performance at the working place was considered in the session on ergo-perimetry.

The neuro-ophthalmology session paid special attention to psycho-physical and electrophysiological tests, other than perimetry, for the detection of early damage.

Automated perimetry is a field of research that shows rapid progress. On the one hand new perimeters have appeared on the market, on the other hand, refinements of existing strategies have been reported.

This new and flourishing method of examination has also been used as a tool for the investigation of many other perimetric problems. It is becoming more and more obvious that advanced automatic perimetry cannot be used as an everyday help in clinical routine, but may also assist us in collecting scientific data in a more objective and unbiassed way than before. Examples of this type of usage were the analysis of short- and long-term fluctuation in measured thresholds, the dependence of thresholds upon the length of the test session and computerized analysis of hemianopic defects. Further exciting developments are expected to be reported during the next meeting of the IPS, when automated perimetry will again be one of the major topics.

A wide variety of subjects was discussed in the general topics session. Part of the sessions have given rise to interesting discussions. They have been printed here as far as possible.

We want to express the gratitude of our society to Drs Keltner and Johnson who spent a lot of time and energy in organizing this symposium. Their efforts resulted in an interesting and valuable symposium with a very pleasant social program. We also want to thank Mrs Els Mutsaerts, the staff of the secretariat in Malmö, and Mr Wil Peters, and all authors for their kind co-operation. After this meeting we are looking forward to the tenth anniversary of the IPS with its 6th International Visual Field Symposium at Santa Margherita Ligure on the Mediterranean coast in May 1984.

Erik Greve
Anders Heijl

CONTENTS

Glaucoma: Visual field and low-tension glaucoma

Glaucoma: General

Ergo-perimetry

Neuro-ophthalmology

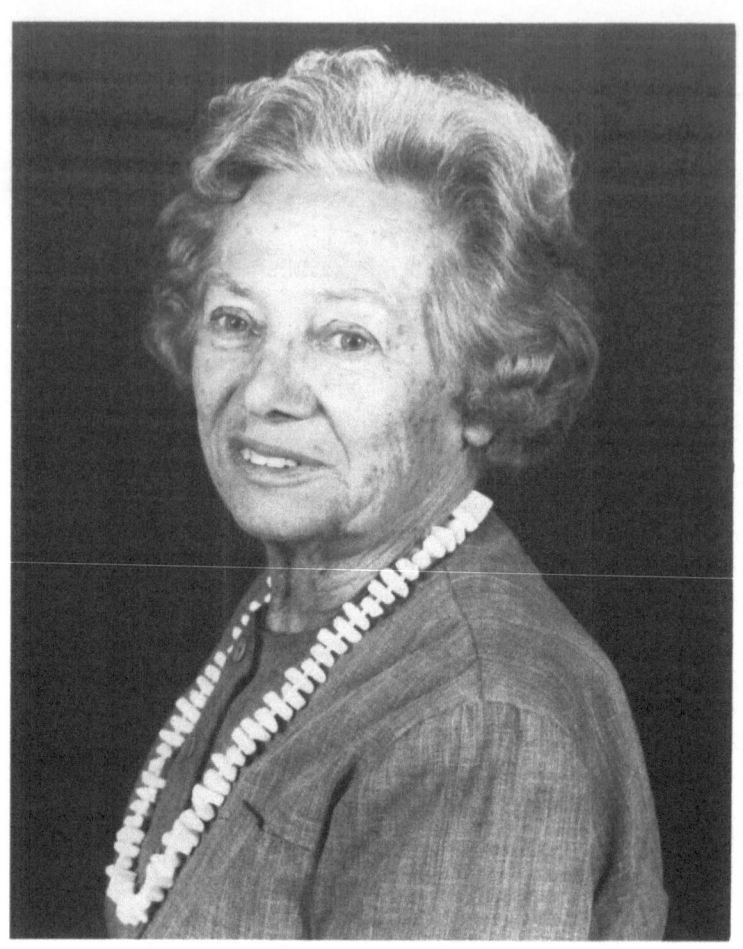

LOUISE L. SLOAN – AN APPRECIATION

Visual scientists and clinicians the world over were recently saddened to hear of the death of Louise L. Sloan. Dr Sloan was truly a pioneer, not only in the basic research fields of visual psychophysics and physiological optics, but also in the application of these fields to the diagnosis and treatment of visual disorders. In a career that spanned more than half a century, she made fundamental contributions in such diverse areas as perimetry, visual acuity, color vision, binocular vision and optical aids for the visually impaired.

Dr Sloan was born on May 31, 1898, in Baltimore, Maryland. She received her Ph.D. degree in Experimental Psychology from Bryn Mawr College in Pennsylvania in 1926 and remained there as an instructor until 1928. She then worked for a year as a research assistant in the Department of Ophthalmology, Harvard University, before being invited by her professors, Clarence Ferree and Gertrude Rand, to work as an instructor of Physiological Optics at the Wilmer Institute, Johns Hopkins University. With the exception of a three-year period during World War II, when she worked as a scientist for the Air Force, she remained at the Wilmer Institute for the rest of her working life. In 1963 she was appointed Associate Professor Emeritus of Ophthalmology, but continued in her position as Director of the Laboratory of Physiological Optics until her retirement in 1973. Despite a long, debilitating illness, she continued to pursue her investigations until her death in early 1982.

Dr Sloan was a dedicated professor and a hardworking scholar and investigator. In 1971 the Optical Society of America awarded her the Tillyer Medal for her many distinguished accomplishments in the field of vision. The 33rd Scientific Meeting of the Wilmer Residents Association and a 1981 Interdisciplinary Symposium for Vision Scientists and Clinicians were dedicated to her. Dr Sloan served on the Committee on Vision of the National Research Council, the Vision Study Section for the National Institutes of Health, and the American Committee on Optics and Visual Physiology. She was also a member of the Editorial Advisory Boards of *Vision Research* and *Experimental Eye Research*.

Dr Sloan authored or co-authored more than 100 scientific articles. Although we will highlight only her work in perimetry here, she also made equally important contributions to at least a half-dozen other research areas. Early in her career, Dr Sloan published several investigations on visual field defects in glaucoma. In 1936, together with Dr Frank B. Walsh, she reported the clinical characteristics of idiopathic flat detachment of the macula (central serous retinopathy). In that article she described the technique of determining the minimum light thresholds at different eccentricities on a visual field meridian. This test is now known as static profile perimetry. Some of her other important contributions in perimetry were: threshold gradients of the rods and cones in dark-adapted and light-adapted eyes; area and luminance of the test target as variables in projection perimetry; and perimetric techniques for detecting selective impairment of cone function. In addition, she played a major role in the creation of the First Interprofessional Standard for Visual Field Testing, published by the National Academy of Sciences.

For Dr Sloan, visual science was never an end in itself, but rather a tool to be used to help those in need. Her lifetime of dedicated service leaves not only ophthalmology and visual science, but also countless visually handicapped people greatly in her debt. Colleagues, friends, students and patients alike will miss her boundless enthusiasm, stimulating companionship, and kind counsel and encouragement. In appreciation, vision scientists will forever honor the pioneering contributions of Louise L. Sloan.

Roberto N. Sunga, M.D.
Bruce Drum, Ph.D.
Department of Ophthalmology
George Washington University Medical Center
Washington, D.C. 20037
U.S.A.

SELECTED BIBLIOGRAPHY

1. Ferree, C. E., Rand, G. and Sloan, L. L. Sensitive methods for the detection of Bjerrum and other scotomas. Arch. Ophthalmol. 5(2): 224–60 (1931).
2. Sloan, L. L. The paracentral field in early glaucoma. Arch. Ophthalmol. 5(4): 601–22 (1931).
3. Ferree, C. E., Rand, G. and Sloan, L. L. Roenne's nasal step as studied with stimuli of different visibilities. Arch. Ophthalmol. 6(6): 877–900 (1931).
4. Ferree, C. E., Rand, G. and Sloan, L. L. Selected cases showing the advantages of a combined tangent screen and perimeter. Arch. Ophthalmol. 10(3): 166–84 (1933).
5. Walsh, F. B. and Sloan, L. L. Idiopathic flat detachment of the macula. Am. J. Ophthalmol. 19(3): 195–208 (1936).
6. Sloan, L. L. and Woods, A. C. Perimetric studies in syphilitic optic neuropathies. Arch. Ophthalmol. 20(3): 201–53 (1938).
7. Sloan, L. L. Instruments and technics for the clinical testing of light sense. III. An apparatus for studying regional differences in light sense. Arch. Ophthalmol. 22(3): 233–51 (1939).
8. Sloan, L. L. Light sense in pigmentary degeneration of retina. Arch. Ophthalmol. 28(4): 613–31 (1942).
9. Sloan, L. L. Rate of dark adaptation and regional threshold gradient of the dark-adapted eye: Physiologic and clinical studies. Am. J. Ophthalmol. 30(6): 705–20 (1947).
10. Sloan, L. L. The threshold gradients of the rods and the cones: In the dark-adapted and in the partially light-adapted eye. Am. J. Ophthalmol. 33(7): 1077–89 (1950).
11. Sloan, L. L. Area and luminance of test object as variables in examination of the visual field by projection perimetry. Vision Res. 1(1/2): 121–38 (1961).

12. Sunga, R. N. and Sloan, L. L. Pigmentary degeneration of the retina: Early diagnosis and natural history. Invest Ophthalmol. 6(3): 309–25 (1967).
13. Sloan, L. L. The Tubinger perimeter of Harms and Aulhorn. Recommended procedures and supplementary equipment. Arch. Ophthalmol. 86(6): 612–22 (1971).

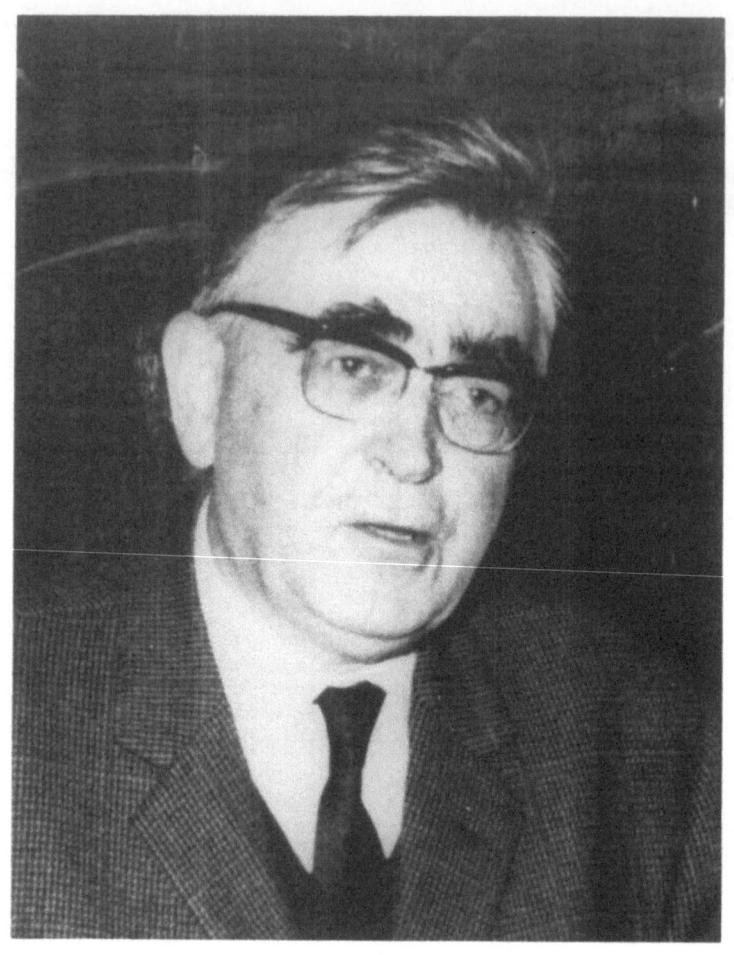

GAETAN JAYLE, 1903–1982

Le professeur Jayle s'est éteint cette année après une très longue, très douloureuse et très cruelle maladie. L'école d'ophtalmologie de Marseille a perdu en lui son chef incontesté, et l'ophtalmologie française un de ses guides les plus écoutés dans le domaine de l'exploration fonctionnelle.

Gaetan Jayle est né en 1903 d'une famille médicale, originaire d'Auvergne. Il a fait ses études à Montpellier où il a été nommé interne en 1928. Il s'y est orienté vers l'anatomie sous la direction du Professeur Delmas. Nommé prosecteur en 1928, il a passé l'agrégation d'anatomie en 1933 et fut nommé la même année à Marseille. Il y enseigna l'anatomie aux côtés du Professeur Corsy titulaire de la chaire et du Professeur Agrégé Salmon chef de Travaux. Mais il était attiré par l'ophtalmologie. Après un internat chez Villard, il entra dans le service du Professeur Aubaret où il occupa rapidement les fonctions d'agrégé. En 1942 il lui succéda à l'Hôtel Dieu; et c'est en 1974 qu'il occupa le nouveau service d'ophtalmologie de l'Hôpital de la Timone.

Le Professeur Jayle a été profondément marqué par cette carrière qui le faisait appartenir à deux disciplines. Elle explique ses orientations. Fondamentaliste d'une part, il était profondément clinicien de l'autre. Anatomiste, il souhaitait compléter et comprendre l'étude des structures par la physiologie, qui les anime et les transcende, d'où sa prédilection pour le perfectionnement des explorations fonctionnelles, qui sont une application pratique de la physiologie.

Ses premiers travaux sont donc d'anatomie mais d'une anatomie devant beaucoup aux disciplines neurophysiologiques. Ils ont porté sur le système nerveux végétatif et sa description originale du pneumogastrique est aujourd'hui classique. L'anatomie est mère de la chirurgie, on retrouve donc sous sa plume des techniques nouvelles concernant les opérations de la cataracte, du décollement de la rétine, et la kératoplastie.

La physiologie le hantait, il s'est appliqué à la biochimie du cristallin et de l'humeur aqueuse avec Derrien et Ourgaud démontrant que les lois de Derrien s'appliquent mieux aux équilibres ioniques du Cl, du Na et du K que les lois antérieures plus classiques et donnant des résultats peu explicables.

Avec son frère Max Jayle il a mené des recherches immunologiques générales qu'il a appliquées à la pathologie oculaire (importance de l'haptoglobinémie et des séromucoïdes dans les infections où elle est un indice sûr).

L'endocrinologie l'a longuement arrêté avec les problèmes de la sénescence.

L'oeil est un organe privilégié dans ce sens mais au delà des problèmes de la presbytie, il restait à décrire les transformations anatomiques et physiologiques sous l'influence de l'âge.

Beaucoup de descriptions maintenant classiques des cristalloïdes antérieures et postérieures, du jaunissement du cristallin, de la fibrillation du vitré, des stades prémonitoires de la dégénérescence sénile lui sont dûs et là encore le professeur Jayle s'est attaché à mettre en parallèle altérations anatomiques et fonctionnelles. Ce travail a fait l'objet d'un rapport au Congrès International de 1962.

L'ouvrage dans lequel il s'est révélé au mieux sous ses deux aspects est son livre sur les mouvements conjugués des globes oculaires et les mystagmus paru en 1941. Après y avoir rappelé les conceptions classiques de Grasset et de Landouzy, il passe au crible de la critique les acquisitions modernes sur les voies oculogyres aux étages cortico-sous-cortical, optostrié, tronculaire et supranucléaire. Il décrit les mouvements conjugués et classe les nystagmus en spontanés ou vestibulaires et en provoqués d'origine visuelle. Ce livre oublié est un admirable travail de synthèse dont seul était capable un esprit maniant avec élégance les deux disciplines anatomiques et physiologiques.

Tous ces travaux sont certes admirables mais le grand titre de gloire du professeur Jayle est et restera l'impulsion incomparable qu'il a donnée en France aux examens d'exploration fonctionnelle visuelle. Ses travaux et ceux qu'il a entrepris avec l'admirable équipe composée de Aubert, Bérard, Boyer, Saraco, Vola, sont nombreux.

Isolons de suite l'électrologie. Technique neuve, elle souffrait du fatras de connaissances patiemment accumulées, non coordonnées et parfois contradictoires. G. Jayle a d'emblée reconnu qu'il fallait explorer l'électrorétinogramme dans des conditions d'adaptation différentes et codifiées. Il enregistra d'abord sous adaptation à la lumière des stimulations rouges et blanches puis au cours de l'adaptation à l'obscurité. Il pratique en somme un examen dynamique selon son expression. Il semble aussi avoir été un des premiers à confronter l'électrorétinogramme et les potentiels évoqués. De ces idées est sorti l'admirable description du syndrome maculaire photopique qui a fait l'objet de la thèse de l'une des ses filles. Ce syndrome est encore aujourd'hui celui qui est le mieux caractérisé en électrorétinographie clinique et suffirait à lui seul à la réputation du professeur Jayle.

Il ne devait cependant pas mépriser les investigations moins objectives dérivées de la psychophysique. La clef de ses travaux se trouve dans le remarquable rapport qu'il fit devant la Société Francaise d'Ophtalmologie en 1951 sur la vision nocturne. Il y affirme d'emblée que son étude se présente sous deux aspects celui des seuils lumineux bruts ou absolus, tels qu'ils sont inscrits dans la courbe globale d'adaptation lumineuse, celui plus topographique et localisé du champ visuel nocturne. Il démontre qu'en dehors des avitaminoses bien connues de la pathologie générale, l'inscription de la courbe d'adaptation possède une grande importance non seulement dans le glaucome et la rétinite pigmentaire mais dans quantité d'autres maladies. Il lui reconnaît une place de choix parmi les investigations tant sur le plan physiopathologique que diagnostique, pronostique ou thérapeutique. La partie originale du rapport tient dans la description de trois domaines d'adaptation photopique, mésopique, scotopique, diurne, crépusculaire, et nocturne, et à la place qu'il a donné au mésopique. Certes, le domaine mésopique avait été pressenti avant lui, mais il est le premier à lui attribuer sa véritable importance non seulement dans l'exploration fonctionnelle mais aussi dans la vie quotidienne. Notre existence en effet se déroule rarement dans une ambiance scotopique. Les éclairages modernes peuplent notre nuit qui est ainsi devenue mésopique. Il a défini les limites de ce domaine et en a exploré les possibilités pathologiques et physiologiques.

En 1958 il a ainsi décrit un rapport entre l'acuité visuelle mésopique et l'acuité visuelle photopique connu depuis sous le nom de quotient de Jayle:

$$Q = \frac{\text{A.V. mésop.}}{\text{A.V. photop.}}$$

La moyenne de ce rapport est de 7/10 pour les sujets jeunes et tombe à 5/10 pour les sujets de plus de 60 ans.

Les remarquables travaux sur la campimétrie qui ont suivi paraissent prendre leur source précisément dans cette étude préliminaire de l'adaptation.

Le Professeur Jayle s'est d'abord doté d'un instrument de recherche remarquable qu'il a construit avec Blet, 'l'explorateur universel du sens lumineux.' Vaste coupole de 1 mètre de diamètre dans l'hémisphère de laquelle il pouvait projeter toutes les variétés de tests imaginables mais avec une grande précision photométrique, colorimétrique, et temporelle. Il avait ainsi en mains l'outil nécessaire à une périmétrie cinétique et statique. Il s'est alors livré à des études très poussées sur les différents méridiens et parallèles du champ, tentant de réaliser une anthropométrie fonctionnelle parallèle à l'anthropométrie anatomique. Très rapidement il s'est rendu compte que le champ strictement diurne ne répond pas au dynamisme de la fonction visuelle sans cesse changeante avec l'adaptation lumineuse. Il a voulu que la campimétrie soit à la fois diurne, crépusculaire, et nocturne pour s'apercevoir bientôt de l'exaltation des conséquences sensorielles des déficits en adaptation mésopique.

Une campimétrie plus simple fut alors conçue, plus à la portée du clinicien et qui s'avère d'une manipulation clinique commode et rapide.

Dans le même esprit il créa ce qu'il appela le 'check up' périmétrique qui consiste en une recherche rapide des seuils en dix points privilégiés du champ central et moyen. Cette recherche de dépistage permet par sa rapidité de ne pas laisser passer un syndrome campimétrique dans nos consultations toujours obérées par le temps, mais elle est surtout annonciatrice de ce qui viendra plus tard, du campimètre de Friedman par exemple, ou des techniques simplifiées d'Armaly.

Au point de vue théorique son travail a surtout consisté à confronter les isoptères mésopiques et photopiques et à décrire les niveaux d'adaptation et les qualités photométriques des tests nécessaires à obtenir le même tracé à la même excentricité dans les deux circonstances.

Ces recherches lui ont valu de présider le premier symposium international de périmétrie réuni à Marseille à l'occasion du Congrès mondial d'ophtalmologie de 1974.

Son oeuvre peut se résumer en quelques mots. Alliant une forte culture anatomique à une pensée profondément physiologique il fut le pionnier des explorations visuelles fonctionnelles modernes. Son nom s'attache aux méthodes d'examen électrorétinographiques cliniques qu'il a créées. Il a donné à l'étude de l'adaptation et du champ visuel la précision photométrique qui y était jusqu'à présent inconnue et a dégagé l'importance de la vision mésopique de la gamme des états diurnes et nocturnes. N'est ce pas assez pour que son nom reste dans la liste de ceux qui ont marqué notre génération? Plus une oeuvre est grande plus elle se laisse facilement cerner en quelques mots.

A. Dubois Poulsen
Ancien Professeur agrégé à la Faculté de Médecine
Ophtalmologiste Honoraire des Quinze-vingts
14, Rue de Remusat
Paris, XVI
France

CORRELATION OF THE PERIPAPILLARY ANATOMY WITH THE DISC DAMAGE AND FIELD ABNORMALITIES IN GLAUCOMA

DOUGLAS R. ANDERSON

(Miami, Florida, U.S.A.)

Key words. Optic disc, cupping, excavation, glaucoma, visual field loss, peripapillary cresent, peripapillary halo.

ABSTRACT

The thesis of this presentation is that the conformation of the peripapillary tissues helps determine how susceptible a particular disc is to pressure-induced damage, and also which portion of the disc (and field) will be most affected. The evidence comes from the clinical records of 108 patients seen at the Bascom Palmer Eye Institute.

INTRODUCTION

Intending to correlate the type and locations of glaucomatous disc excavation with the type and location of visual field loss, I collected for several months examples of glaucomatous field loss from patients who provided a reliable field examination and whose optic discs had been photographed in the course of clinical consultation or care rendered by me or one of my associates. I was not very selective, but collected as many cases as possible until I had obtained a variety that represented both early and late cases, diffuse and localized field loss, peripheral and paracentral field defects, and typical and less typical cases. After 108 cases had been assembled, I began to review the disc photographs that corresponded to the field diagrams.

OBSERVATIONS

Low-tension glaucoma vs. ocular hypertension

I noticed that a rather conspicuous peripapillary crescent or halo* typified cases of low-tension glaucoma (Figs. 1 & 2). In contrast, a crescent was not

*The term 'halo' has been used by various authors to mean either a thin border of sclera visible around the disc or an area of uncovered choroidal tissue next to the disc. In this paper I am using the term in the latter sense.

Greve, E. L., Heijl, A. (eds.) Fifth International Visual Field Symposium.
©1983 Dr W. Junk Publishers, The Hague/Boston/Lancaster.

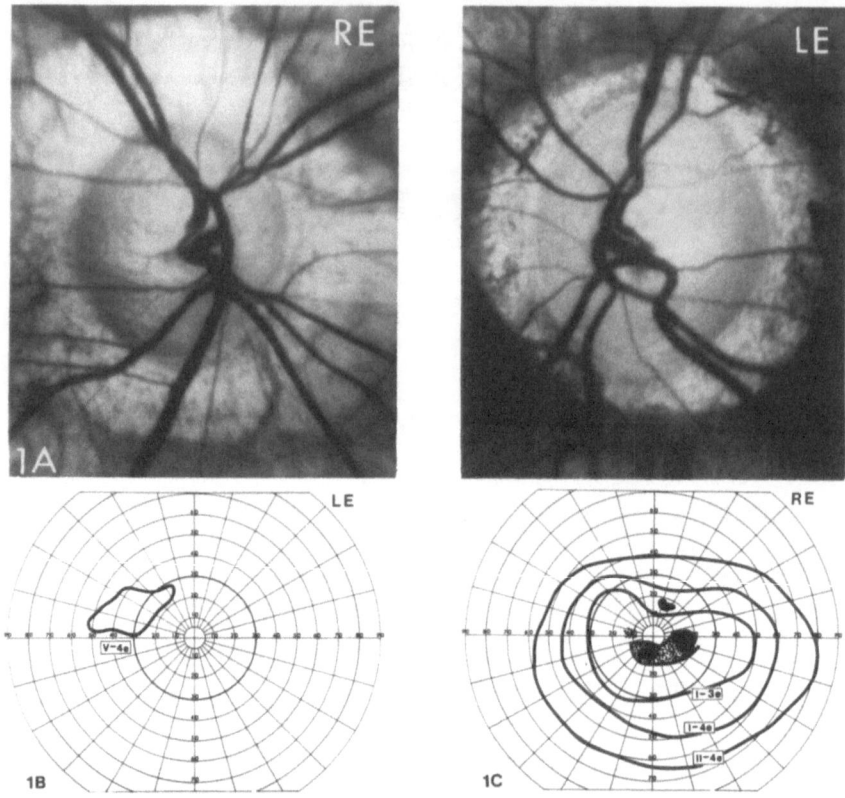

Fig. 1. Discs and fields of a 47-year old myopic (−3.25, −4.25) man with 'low-tension glaucoma'. Only after repeated measurements were the pressures ever found to be abnormal, ranging from 8−20 mm Hg in the right eye to 11−24 mm Hg in the left (A − discs of the right and left eyes; B − visual field of the left eye; C − visual field of the right eye).

prominent around the resistent disc that occurs in 'ocular hypertension', by which I mean cases of elevated intraocular pressure with neither recognized disc damage nor recognized field loss (Fig. 3). It is as if the disc may be more susceptible to damage (producing low tension glaucoma) when the boundaries of the peripapillary tissues do not coincide with each other and the disc edge; and contrariwise that the disc is more resistant to damage when there is good alignment of the tissue layers.

Open-angle glaucoma

Of course, correct alignment is not an absolute protection, and disc damage certainly can occur. Therefore, there are cases of open-angle glaucoma without a peripapillary crescent or halo. My impression from the series collected is that when disc damage occurs in the presence of correctly aligned peripapillary layers, it has seemingly taken a substantial pressure elevation to produce

2

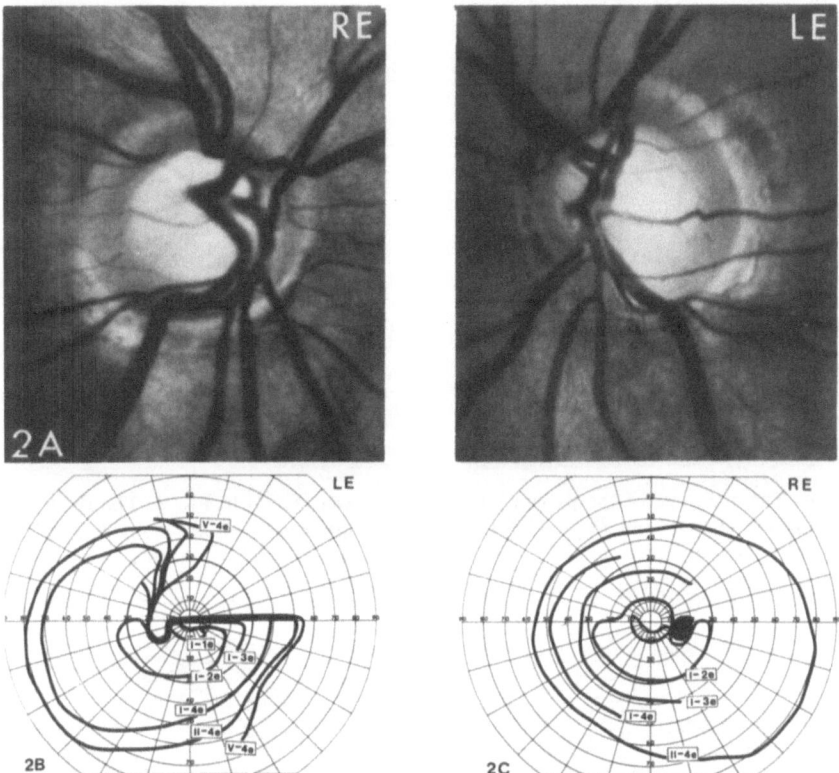

Fig. 2. Discs and fields of a 56-year old woman with 'low-tension glaucoma'. The peri-papillary tissues are irregularly arranged at the inferior temporal margins of the discs. There is cupping toward the inferior pole of the disc and a superior nasal visual field loss, more marked in the left eye (A — discs of the right and left eyes; B — visual field of the left eye; C — visual field of the right eye).

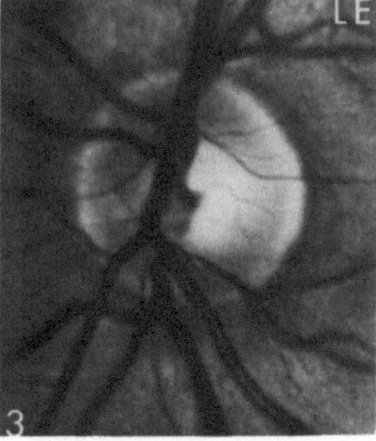

Fig. 3. Left optic disc that has withstood a pressure typically between 25 and 28 for twelve years. The pressure was 21 mm Hg at the lowest and 32 at the highest.

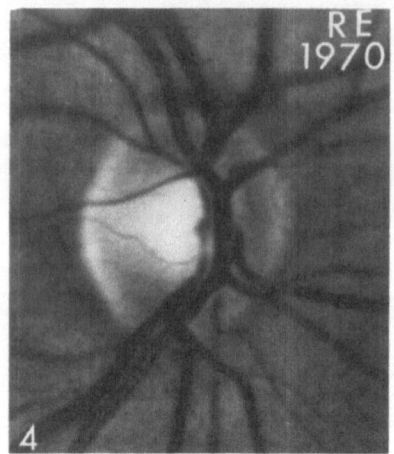 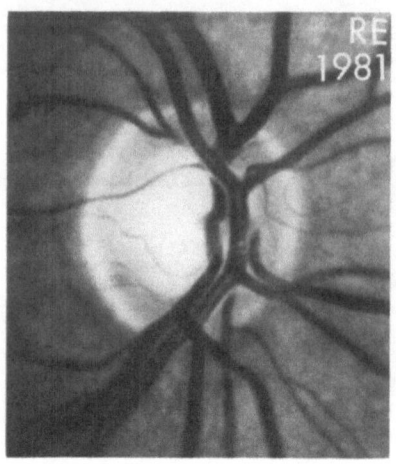

Fig. 4. The right eye of the patient whose left eye was shown in Fig. 3. The right eye pressure has ranged from 28 to 44 for twelve years and shows progressive change (A – 1970; B – 1981).

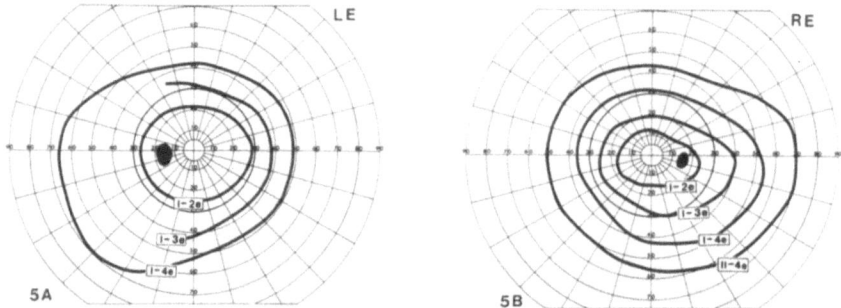

Fig. 5. Visual fields in 1981 of the right and left eye of the patient whose discs are shown in Figs. 3 & 4. The disc of the right eye shows a generalized depression compared to the left, particularly on the nasal side (A – field of left eye; B – field of right eye).

the damage (Fig. 4). This contrasts with low-tension glaucoma, in which damage occurs at normal intraocular pressures.

It also seemed characteristic of cases with normally aligned peripapillary tissues that the initial pressure-induced enlargment of the excavation occurs concentrically, representing tissue damage diffusely throughout the disc. In keeping with this (Fig. 5), the field loss was often a mild and non-specific generalized depression (contraction of all isopters). Ultimately, as seen in examples of late stages, the tissue loss is somewhat more profound at the poles of the disc. At this stage, arcuate defects are noted in the field, but the visual threshold is also distinctly abnormal outside the arcuate region because there has already occurred considerable loss of tissue in all other sectors of the disc as well (Fig. 6).

There were also cases of open-angle glaucoma in the presence of a peripapillary crescent. In such cases, the tissue damage is often more distinctly

4

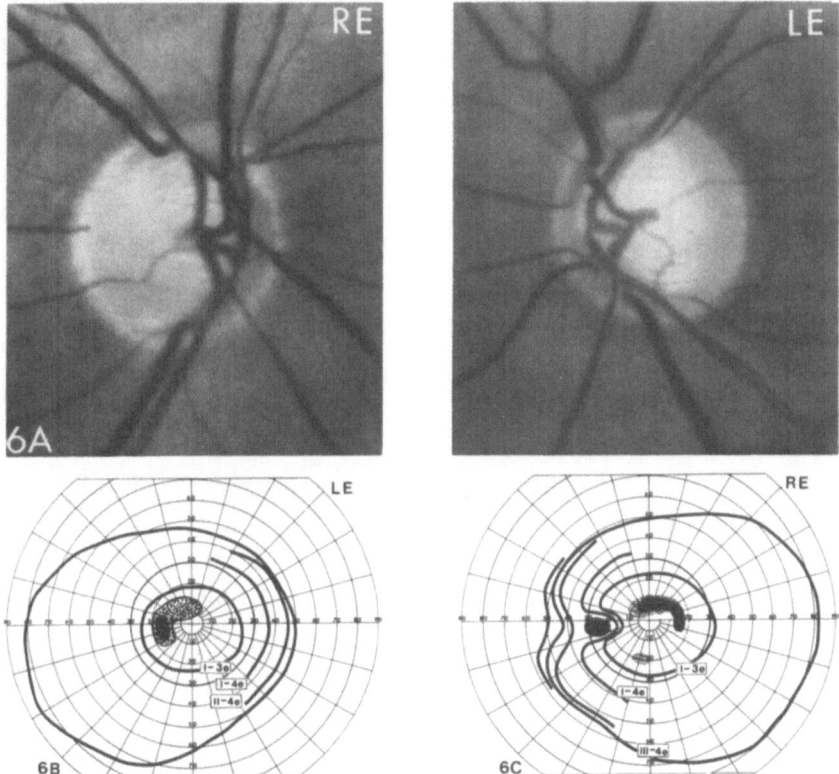

Fig. 6. Chronic open angle glaucoma with pressures in the mod 20's, typically a bit higher in the right eye. There is a generalized enlargment of the cup and a generalized depression of the field (note the inward position of the 13e and 14e isopters), but in this late stage also producing nerve fiber bundle defects, especially in the more advanced right eye (A – discs of the right and left eye; B – field of the left eye; C – field of the right eye).

localized, with a corresponding localized field loss in keeping with the distribution of the affected nerve fiber bundles. For example, there might be a typical upper arcuate and a peripheral upper nasal field defect associated with cupping adjacent to a slight crescent around the inferior temporal disc margin, reflecting the usual slightly tilted insertion of the optic nerve.

The correlation between the crescent, the excavation, and the field loss is particularly striking in cases in which the two eyes of an individual are dissimilar (Figs. 7, 8, 9). In such cases, the asymmetry between the two eyes in the location and degree of cupping (and field loss) is related to the disc configuration. Some examples have a very localized tissue loss that produces a striking notch resembling a pit at the disc margin. Such cases have a very dense arcuate field defect extending all the way from the blind spot to the nasal periphery. Often the pressure elevation is not very marked. It is as if the crescent had made one region of the disc disproportionately more susceptible to the pressure elevation, causing a very localized excavation and a discreet field loss.

5

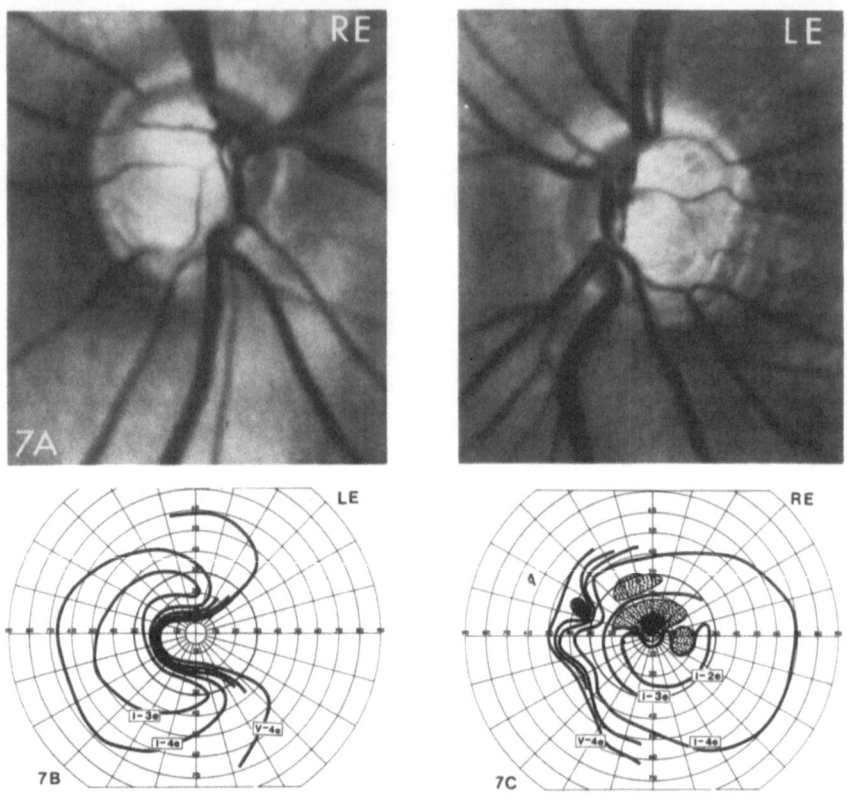

Fig. 7. Chronic open angle glaucoma with mildly elevated intraocular pressure. The inferior margin of the disc of the right eye has a small conical crescent (not well seen in the photograph) associated with an upper nerve fiber bundle defect. The cresent of the left eye is located at the temporal margin of the disc, and is associated with early involvement of the central field (A – discs of the right and left eyes; B – field of the left eye; C – field of the right eye).

DISCUSSION

Primrose (7, 8, 9) has reported a very high prevalence of peripapillary crescents and halos in glaucoma. Wilensky and Kolber (10) have shown peripapillary atrophic changes to be more common in patients with glaucoma than in a control group of normals and ocular hypertensives. Laatikainen (4) noted that a deficient peripapillary choriocapillary system was common in glaucoma, particularly of the low-tension variety. Peripapillary crescents and halos have also been mentioned from time to time by other authors, and it has been thought that these are either a senile change or are acquired along with the cupping as a result of the elevated intraocular pressure.

However, the halos and crescents observed in this study are generally in keeping with the shape and tilt of the optic disc configuration, and I wonder if they might be congenital or at least have a congenital basis. For example,

6

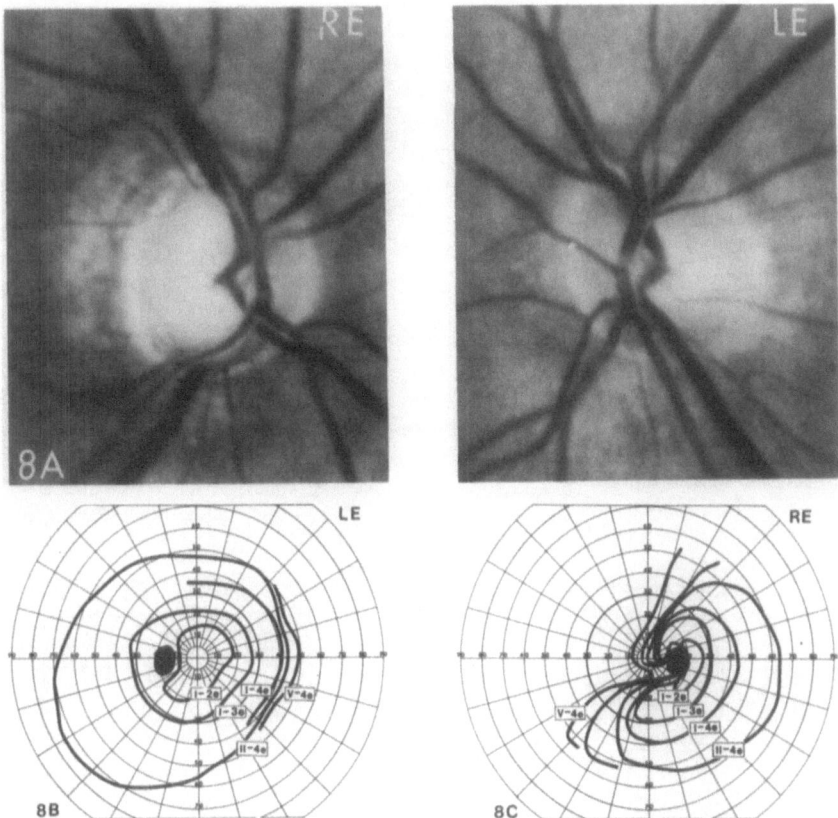

Fig. 8. A case of unilateral low-tension glaucoma. The right eye shows disruption of the peripapillary tissues temporaly, excavation of the disc, and visual field loss. The intra-ocular pressure is equal in the two eyes, and within the normal range (A – right and left discs; B – field of the left eye; C – field of the right eye).

a congential crescent may mark a sector that is anatomically weak and suscep-tible to damage from intraocular pressure. An underlying congential basis for a crescent would not preclude that it might enlarge or evolve, as does myopic chorioretinal atrophy – with the abnormality appearing at congenitally weak locations determined by the anatomical tilt of the disc insertion.

There are two possible explanations for the apparent association of cres-cents with glaucoma. The first is that the peripapillary atrophy may occur *along with* the localized disc damage as a pressure-indiced acquired change in a location that is susceptible because of its anatomic configuration. However, it should be noted that pathologic excavation and crescents (or halos) may each be seen without the company of the other. Total cupping of the disc can occur without producing a peripapillary halo at all, and halo formation – if acquired – does not necessarily preceed or accompany the cupping. On the other hand, crescent formation is not necessarily a late event, but can certainly preceed cupping. I have found one example of localized progressive cupping documented in a region of a non-changing crescent.

7

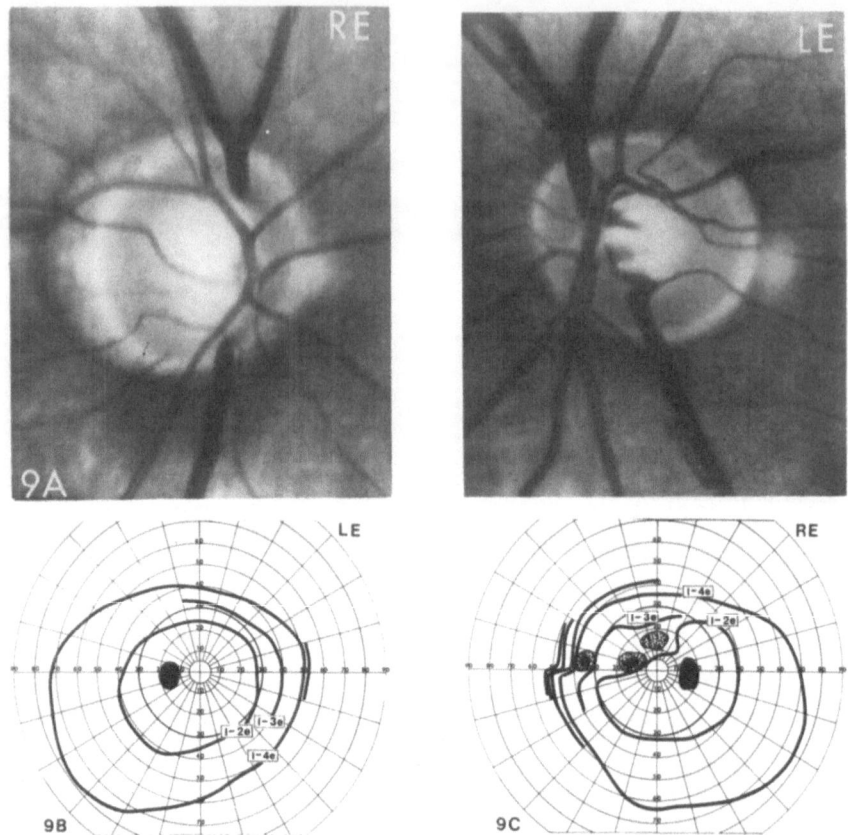

Fig. 9. Pigmentary glaucoma with *equal* elevation of intraocular pressure in the two eyes. The right eye, with the peripapillary crescent, has cupping and field loss, while the left eye does not. However, the location of the cupping, which is predominantly inferior, does not precisely coincide with the location of the crescent (A – discs of the right and left eyes; B – field of the left eye; C – field of the right eye).

The second explanation could be that misalignment of the peripapillary tissue layers is congenital and makes the disc more susceptible to the effects of intraocular pressure. This would explain the high prevalence of crescents and halos in glaucoma – a group selected for scrutiny by virtue of having disc damage in response to elevated intraocular pressure.

Could it be that the presence of a peripapillary crescent or halo may participate in determining the susceptibility to damage from elevated intraocular pressure and in facilitating the occurrence of low-tension glaucoma? Could the location of the peripapillary abnormality govern which region of a particular disc is most susceptible to damage? One can't help wondering if the peripapillary crescent of myopia is what accounts for the recently reported association of myopia with an increased risk of glaucomatous damage (2, 5, 6). Perhaps a temporal crescent also accounts for the early involvement of fixation that seems more frequent in myopia (1, 3).

Obviously, there are more factors involved than just the presence or absence of a crescent and the level of intraocular pressure. Not everyone with a halo

8

or crescent has low-tension glaucoma, or even has glaucomatous damage if they develop elevated intraocular pressure. The point is, however, that perhaps the peripapillary configuration is one of the factors in the formula for damage.

It should also be noted that crescents are not all alike, and the several tissue layers can overlap in a variety of combinations. The edges of the pigment epithelial and choriocapillaris layers are not easily identified. The details of the variations may be important, because sometimes cupping is more prominent near one portion of the crescent than in another (Fig. 9).

I want to be the first to point out that the present evidence is preliminary. The present observations simply suggest an association of glaucomatous damage and peripapillary anatomy. Both the association and the implications must be tested by more rigorously controlled observations. Until such data is obtained, it may be premature to speculate by what pathophysiologic mechanism the anatomic misalignment of peripapillary tissues might enhance the susceptibility to pressure.

ACKNOWLEDGEMENT

Mrs Rosalie K. Allely provided invaluable assistance in assembling the field diagrams and disc photographs for review. Barbara French and E. Barry Davis prepared the illustrations.

This work was supported in part by The National Glaucoma Research Program of The American Health Assistance Foundation, Washington, D.C.

REFERENCES

1. Carroll, F. D. and Forbes, M. Centrocaecal scotomas due to glaucoma. Tr. Am. Acad. Ophthal & Otolaryngol. 72:643–648 (1968).
2. Daubs, J. and Crick, R.P. Effect of refractive error on the risk of ocular hypertension and open-angle glaucoma. Trans. Ophthalmol. Soc. U.K.: 121–126 (1981).
3. Greve, E. L. and Furuno, F. Myopia and glaucoma. Albrecht von Graefes Arch. Klin. Exp. Ophthalmol. 213:33–41 (1980).
4. Laatikainen, L. Fluorescein angiographic studies of the peripapillary and perilimbal regions in simple, capsular and low-tension glaucoma. Acta Ophthalmol, Suppleementum 111 (1981).
5. Perkins, E. S. and Phelps, C. D. Open angle glaucoma, ocular hypertension, low-tension glaucoma, and refraction. Arch. Ophthalmol. 100:1464–1467 (1982).
6. Phelps, C. D. Effect of myopia on prognosis in treated primary open-angle glaucoma. Am. J. Ophthalmol. 93:622–628 (1982).
7. Primrose, J. Clinical Review of glaucomatous discs. In Cant, J. S.: The Optic Nerve. London. Henry Kimpton Pub., pp. 311–316 (1972).
8. Primrose, J. Early signs of the glaucomatous disc. Brit. J. Ophthalmol. 55:820–825 (1971).
9. Primrose, J. The incidence of the peripapillary halo glaucomatosus. Trans. Ophthalmol. Soc. U.K. 89:585–587 (1969).

10. Wilensky, J. T. and Kolber, A. E. Peripapillary changes in glaucoma. Am. J. Ophthalmol. 81:341–345 (1976).

Author's address:
Dr D. R. Anderson
Bascom Palmer Eye Institute
Department of Ophthalmology
University of Miami School of Medicine
P.O. Box 016880, Miami, FL 33101
U.S.A.

THE FIRST OBSERVABLE GLAUCOMA CHANGES AFTER AN OPTIC DISC HAEMORRHAGE

P. JUHANI AIRAKSINEN

(Oulu, Finland)

Key words. Disc haemorrhage, early glaucoma, nerve fibres, optic disc, visual fields.

ABSTRACT

29 ocular hypertensive patients with an optic disc haemorrhage, normal optic discs and normal visual fields were followed up in this partly retrospective study up to 14 (mean 5.2) years. During this time early glaucoma damage developed in 11 patients (12 eyes). Retinal nerve fibre layer (RNFL) photographs revealed a nerve fibre loss in 10 of the 12 cases (83%) but accurate cup–disc ratio measurements showed measurable optic disc changes in only half of the pathologic cases. Routine visual field examinations showed field loss only in one of the 12 eyes at the time the first structural damage was observed. During follow-up field loss was recorded in 4 more eyes but 7 eyes showed normal fields in spite of RNFL defects. RNFL photography seems to be a useful examination method for detection of early glaucoma damage.

INTRODUCTION

The purpose of this study was to record the first observable structural and functional glaucoma changes that developed after optic disc haemorrhages in ocular hypertensive eyes which otherwise showed no other pathology.

MATERIAL AND METHODS

In a material of more than 1500 patients with manifest and suspect glaucoma whose optic discs had been photographed repeatedly during a follow-up of 1 to 12 years there were 90 patients who showed a typical splinter haemorrhage of the optic nerve head (1). At the time when the haemorrhage occurred 25 of these 90 patients had normal optic discs, normal central visual fields examined with a Friedmann visual field analyser and normal peripheral fields examined with a Goldmann perimeter (V/4 target). Four patients with this criteria were included later and thus a total of 29 patients (30 eyes) participated in this study. There were 9 men and 20 women aged 47 to 82 (mean 63) years. Their total follow-up time was 1 to 14 (mean 5.2) years and during this time their optic discs with the surrounding retinal nerve fibre layer (RNFL) were photographed 2 to 7 (mean 3.2) times.

Optic disc stereophotographs were taken with a Zeiss fundus camera and Allen stereo separator with a green filter on black-and-white film. During the past 2 years RNFL photographs were additionally taken with a Canon CF-6OZ wide angle fundus camera and a monochromatic, blue filter. Photographic techniques have been described in detail in (1) and (3). For quantitation of optic cup enlargement, reflecting the narrowing of the neural rim, we used cup–disc ratio measurements. The stereophotographs were available as 20 times enlarged black-and-white paper prints. In these prints the disc diameter is 30 to 35 mm. For calculation of the horizontal and vertical cup–disc ratios we measured the respective cup and disc diameters with a millimetre ruler in a stereoviewer. An accuracy of better than 1 mm in the measurement of the cup diameter could not be achieved. A cup diameter increase of 1 mm in the photographs (corresponding to about 50 μm on the disc) results in a cup–disc ratio increase of approximately 0.03. Therefore only a cup–disc ratio increase of more than 0.03 can be regarded as an acquired change.

In the majority of cases the patients' visual fields were examined every six months with a Friedmann analyser. On the last visit of this study they were additionally examined with combined kinetic and static perimetry with a Goldmann perimeter in a routine manner the perimetrist not knowing whether the patient had pathologic changes or not. In selected cases manual static profile perimetry was performed in standard meridians 45°–225° and 135°–315°.

RESULTS

The results are summarised in Table 1. During the observation period 11 patients (12 eyes) developed glaucomatous changes. The horizontal cup–disc ratio increased more than 0.03 in four patients (cases 2–5 in Table 1) and the vertical cup–disc ratio in five patients (cases 1–4 and 11). In all the other cases the change of both horizontal and vertical cup–disc ratios was 0.03 or less. Observation of the RNFL photographs revealed a sector-shaped nerve fibre defect in 10 eyes of 9 patients (cases 3–11). In all but one case the RNFL defect developed at the same location where the preceding haemorrhage had been observed. Both disc and RNFL changes were visible in the first photographs taken on the average 20 months after the bleeding. It is, however, not possible to tell how soon the defects had developed after the haemorrhage since the patients are routinely photographed once every one to two years.

At the time when the first structural changes were observed pathologic central visual fields were recorded in one patient only (case 11). During the follow-up the fields were examined twice a year and glaucomatous changes developed in 4 more patients 11 to 26 (mean 15) months after the disc or RNFL changes had been found. The remaining 7 cases revealed no field

12

Table 1. Results of the 12 eyes which developed glaucomatous changes after an optic disc haemorrhage.

Case No.	Increase of vertical or horizontal cup–disc ratio of more than 0.03	Presence of a retinal nerve fibre layer defect	Development of a visual field defect
1	+	–	–
2	+	?	–
3	+	+	+
4	+	+	+
5	+	+	+
6	–	+	+
7 OD	–	+	–
OS	–	+	–
8	–	+	–
9	–	+	–
10	–	+	–
11	+	+	+

damage even at the last visit 6 to 55 (mean 21) months after the anatomic changes had been observed although their fields were additionally examined with combined kinetic and static Goldmann perimetry.

DISCUSSION

RNFL and optic disc

A majority of the methods that have been developed for quantitative assessment of the optic disc are at present not suitable for routine clinical use partly because their sensitivity has not been clearly established. Evaluation of cup–disc ratio, however, is easy to perform and it is a widely used method in the follow-up of glaucomatous patients. Because cup–disc ratio determination is usually made with an opthalmoscope the reproducibility of the results is not good; particularly inter-individual estimates show astonishingly high variation (8). With some practice an accuracy of ±0.1 may be achieved (7).

With the present method high accuracy (0.03) could be achieved by observation of enlarged black-and-white stereophotographs. This resolution is of the same order as was reported for the electronic subtraction method (4). The results show, however, that even this sensitivity is not high enough for detection of optic disc changes when measurements are made only in one or two fixed meridians since in 50% of the cases there was a visible nerve fibre loss which did not result in a measurable change of the neural rim configuration (Table 1). Furthermore Fig. 1 shows that if vertical and horizontal cup–disc ratios had been observed separately, detection rate for disc observation would have been even smaller. If, however, we had not looked at the optic disc at all but evaluated only the RNFL we would have detected 83% of the pathologic cases. Combined evaluation of RNFL and vertical cup–disc ratio would have been the best solution since it would have revealed all the 12 eyes with early glaucoma changes after an optic disc haemorrhage.

13

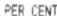

```
                  10      20      30      40      50      60      70      80      90
        ---------+---------+---------+---------+---------+---------+---------+---------+---------+

CDRh    HHHHHHHHHHHHHHHHHHHHHHHHHHHHHH 33 %

CDRv    HHHHHHHHHHHHHHHHHHHHHHHHHHHHHHHHHHHHHHH 42 %

RNFL    HHHHHHHHHHHHHHHHHHHHHHHHHHHHHHHHHHHHHHHHHHHHHHHHHHHHHHHHHHHHHHHHHHHHHHHHHHHHH 83 %


        ---------+---------+---------+---------+---------+---------+---------+---------+---------+
```

Fig. 1. Percentages of true positives by different criteria.

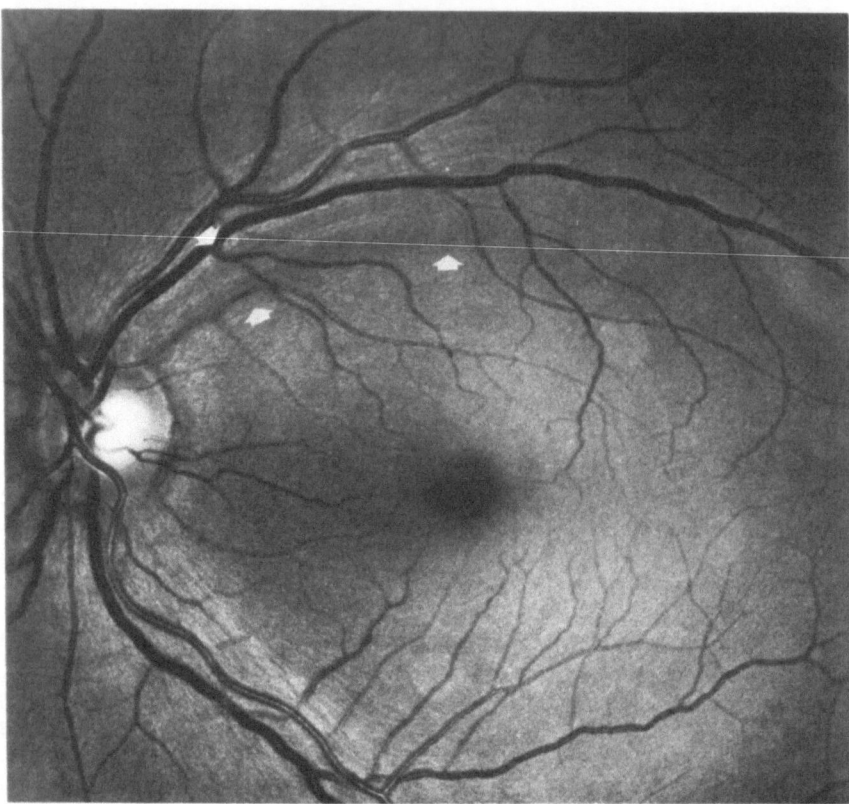

Fig. 2. A sector-shaped retinal nerve fibre layer (RNFL) defect (arrows) has developed in association with a disc haemorrhage. Stereoscopic observation showed that the defect is located in the deeper retinal layers and in its upper part as well as closer to the disc the defect is covered by more superficial fibres. In spite of the fibre loss the neural rim has remained unchanged.

The results of this study indicate that after a discrete but observable nerve fibre loss in association with a disc haemorrhage the neural rim of the optic nerve head does not necessarily become narrower or the change is so small that it cannot be detected with cup—disc measurements in the meridians

14

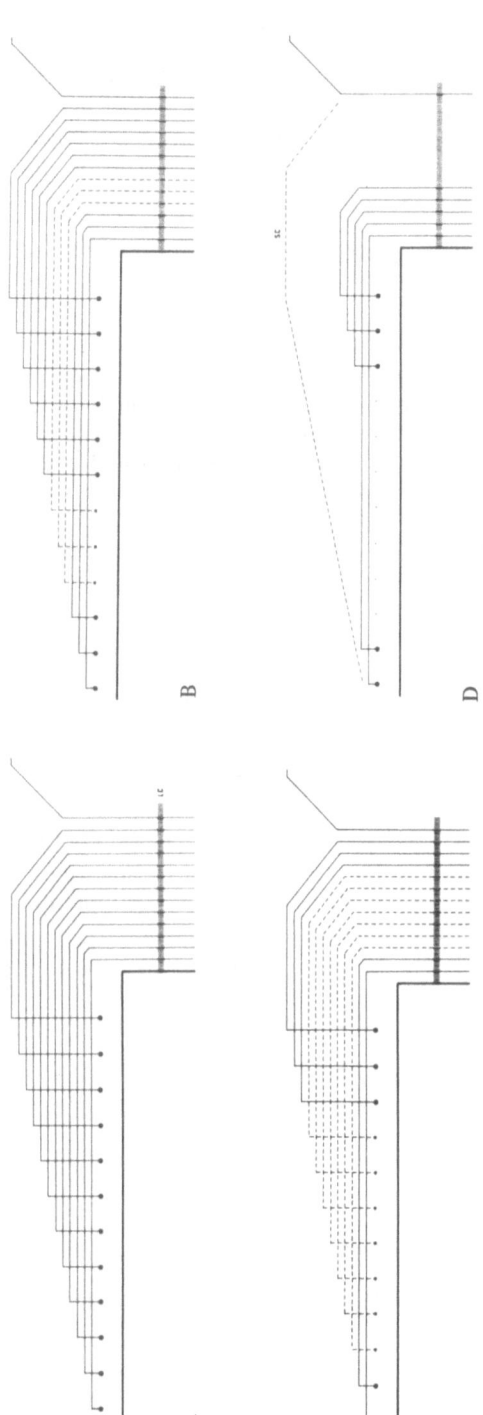

Fig. 3. Schematic representation of hypothetical mode of progression of very early glaucoma changes in the retinal nerve fibre layer (RNFL) and anterior optic nerve head.

A. Retinal nerve fibres (solid lines) are arranged so that more peripherally originating fibres are situated deep in the retina and they are covered by an increasing number of more proximal fibres closer to the optic nerve head. Fibres with a peripheral origin lie peripherally in the optic nerve head while more proximal fibres are located more axially (GC = ganglion cells, LC = lamina cribrosa). (The drawing is based on studies by Radius & Anderson (10) and by Minckler(9).)

B. Broken lines indicate degenerated nerve fibres in the deeper retinal layers. Peripherally a defect of these fibres is more or less denuded but closer to the disc an increasing number of more proximally originating fibres rise to the superficial layers to cover the defect and form an apparently normal neural rim configuration, leaving the defect in the depth. At this early stage damage might be modest enough not to affect neural rim appearance but particularly in case of a focal fibre loss the defective area is clearly outlined in the retina and can be photographed there.

C. Disease progression causes degeneration of a larger number of axons.

D. When a larger number of axons have been lost the normal neural rim configuration can no longer be maintained and the remaining structures collapse resulting in a neural rim notching in case of focal fibre loss or in concentric cup enlargement in case of diffuse fibre loss (SC = surface contour of the original RNFL).

15

chosen by us. Similar findings have been reported also in other forms of glaucoma with no evidence of disc haemorrhages (6). In the present study there were three cases with particularly good picture quality. Stereoscopic observation showed that the nerve fibre defect was situated in the deeper retinal layers and closer to the optic disc it was covered by more superficial fibres (Fig. 2). This may give an explanation to the unchanged neural rim configuration in the early glaucoma cases (Fig. 3A–D).

RNFL and visual field

In the present study routine visual field examinations were not very helpful in detecting the first glaucoma damage. In fact there was a visual field defect in only one of 10 eyes with observable RNFL defect and during subsequent follow-up field defects were recorded in four more eyes although more recently a modified Armaly-Drance method was used (2). In studies which compare examination methods the results depend largely on examination strategies and quality of equipment. In the present study visual fields were examined with conventional and commonly used methods in a routine manner so that the perimetrist was not aware of the patients' other ocular findings. As it was felt that our present perimetric equipment does not compare well with the photographic techniques, a need for more detailed study with automatic threshold perimeters was evident. Results of that study are reported elsewhere in this proceedings (5).

The fact that carefully performed conventional routine perimetry failed to show field loss in so many cases and that detailed stereoscopic optic disc observation failed to reveal early structural changes in half of the cases suggests that observation of the RNFL with improved examination techniques (3) can be very useful for detection of early glaucoma damage and may reveal changes in the retina prior to their appearance in the disc and visual field. It must be emphasized, however, that in the present study we included only patients with an optic disc haemorrhage and it is not clear to what extent these results are applicable to all glaucoma patients.

ACKNOWLEDGEMENT

This study was supported by the Emil Aaltonen Foundation.

REFERENCES

1. Airaksinen, P. J., E. Mustonen and H. I. Alanko. Optic disc haemorrhages. An analysis of stereophotographs and clinical data of 112 patients. Arch. Ophthalmol. 99:1795–1801 (1981).
2. Airaksinen, P. J., E. Mustonen and H. I. Alanko. Optic disc haemorrhages precede retinal nerve fibre layer defects in ocular hypertension. Acta Ophthalmol. 59:627–641 (1981).
3. Airaksinen, P. J., H. Nieminen and E. Mustonen. Retinal nerve fibre layer photography with a wide angle fundus camera. Acta Ophthalmol. 60:362–368 (1982).

4. Alanko, H. I. and P. J. Airaksinen. Sensitivity of the electronic subtraction method in evaluation of simulated optic disc changes. Acta Ophthalmol. 60:293–300 (1982).
5. Heijl, A. and P. J. Airaksinen. Correlation between computerized perimetry and retinal nerve fibre layer photography after optic disc haemorrhage. Doc. Ophthalmol. Proc. Series 35:19–25 (1983).
6. Iwata, K., K. Nanba and H. Abe. Die beginnende Fundusveränderung infolge rezidivierender kleiner Krisen beim Posner-Schlossman-Syndrom – ein Modell fur das Glaucoma Simplex. Klin. Monatsbl. Augenheilk. 180:20–26 (1982).
7. Leydhecker, W., G. K. Krieglstein and E. v. Collani. Observer variation in applanation tonometry and estimation of the cup–disc ratio. In: G. K. Krieglstein and W. Leydhecker (eds.): Glaucoma Update. Springer, Berlin, Heidelberg, New York, pp. 101–111 (1979).
8. Lichter, P. R. Variability of expert observers in evaluating the optic disc. Trans. Am. Ophthalmol. Soc. 74:532–572 (1976).
9. Minckler, D. S. The organization of nerve fiber bundle in the primate optic nerve head. Arch. Ophthalmol. 98:1630–1636 (1980).
10. Radius, R. L. and D. R. Anderson. The course of axons through the retina and optic nerve head. Arch. Ophthalmol. 97:1154–1158 (1979).

Author's address:
Dr P. J. Airaksinen
Dept. of Ophthalmology
University of Oulu
SF-90220 Oulu 22
Finland

CORRELATION BETWEEN COMPUTERIZED PERIMETRY
AND RETINAL NERVE FIBRE LAYER PHOTOGRAPHY
AFTER OPTIC DISC HAEMORRHAGE

ANDERS HEIJL and P. JUHANI AIRAKSINEN

(Malmö, Sweden/Oulu, Finland)

Key words. Retinal nerve fibre layer, automatic perimetry, glaucoma, optic disc haemorrhage.

ABSTRACT

Earlier studies have shown that in early glaucoma retinal nerve fibre layer RNFL defects often exist in cases where manual and semi-automatic perimetry give normal results (e.g. Airaksinen (1)). In the present study automatic perimetry including high-resolution profile perimetry was performed in patients with documented disc haemorrhages with and without RNFL defects. Automatic perimetry on the Competer revealed field defects in nine out of ten eyes with RNFL defects and normal manual and semi-automatic fields, but extensive automatic profile perimetry aimed at areas with photographically documented RNFL defects was necessary in order to find defects in two of these cases. A field defect was also found in one of five cases without photographic RNFL defects.

Visual field defects thus seem to occur in a higher proportion of cases with RNFL defects than previously thought, but they can be very subtle and hard to find. Automatic perimetry and RNFL photography complement each other in the early detection of glaucomatous damage.

INTRODUCTION

The techniques of retinal nerve fibre layer (RNFL) photography have improved during the past few years and at the same time a number of studies have appeared indicating that RNFL defects may be present in early glaucomatous cases with normal visual fields (2, 9, 11, 12).

It is somewhat unexpected not to be able to document any visual field loss in association with RNFL defects, since particularly a sector-shaped RNFL defect represents a clearly outlined anatomic loss of neural tissue that ought to go along with deterioration of function. All studies mentioned above were performed with manual perimetry on the Goldmann perimeter or screening on the Friedmann Visual Field Analyser. This is why it was considered

Greve, E. L., Heijl, A. (eds.) Fifth International Visual Field Symposium.
©1983 Dr W. Junk Publishers, The Hague/Boston/Lancaster.

indicated to examine patients who had shown disc haemorrhages and normal routine fields with modern high-quality computerized perimetry.

MATERIAL

Fifteen eyes of 13 patients were studied. They all fulfilled the following criteria:

a. Photographically documented optic disc haemorrhage.
b. Normal test results on screening with the Friedmann analyser and conventional kinetic and static testing on the Goldmann perimeter (a detailed description of the perimetric techniques is given in Ref. 2).
c. Clear enough media to permit good quality retinal nerve fibre photography.

The material was subdivided into two groups:

1. Ten eyes with RNFL defects. Five of these came from the material presented by Airaksinen in this volume (1) and were all patients with normal fields and RNFL defects in that material.
2. Five eyes without RNFL defects of those patients in the same study who had not developed any pathological changes.

All the patients underwent a careful clinical opthalmological examination including wide-angle black-and-white RNFL photography with the Canon CF-60Z fundus camera and optic disc stereophotography in order to have fresh, enlarged photographs available by the time of the computerized visual field testing which followed 6 to 14 days later. The photographic methods have been described in detail before (3, 4).

The visual field testing was performed with the Competer automatic computerized perimeter (8) which in addition to the original standard 64 test-point central pattern was equipped for static profile perimetry (6). Threshold measuring test protocols were used both for the central pattern (test logic I in Ref. 5) and the static profile perimetry.

Stimulus presentation time was usually 0.25 sec, background luminosity 1 cd/m^2. All subjects were corrected for ametropia and near.

The automatic fields were interpreted as previously described (6, 7). Pathologic or suspect areas in the central patterns were further examined with profile perimetry. In cases where extensive testing was necessary the patients were allowed to rest between tests which were sometimes spread out over two days. If in patients with RNFL defects the central pattern was normal and gave no clue as to the location of the defect, the RNFL photographs were used to guide us further in the perimetric testing. The eccentricity of the defect was measured, its most probable meridians were estimated and subsequently tested with profile perimetry with 1° resolution.

Patients without RNFL defects were subjected to automatic perimetry in the central pattern plus profile perimetry in the standard meridians 45°–225° and 135°–315°.

Width and location of visual field defects determined by profile perimetry were compared to width and location of the corresponding RNFL defects in the wide-angle photographs. The scale for the measurements was obtained by performing profile perimetry in the horizontal meridian through the blind spot. The distance from the blind spot to the foveola was related to the corresponding distance measured from the wide-angle photographs. Usually 1 mm in the photograph corresponded to 15 minutes of arc in the visual field.

RESULTS

In group 1 (patients with RNFL defect) the central pattern test localized a visual field defect in seven of the ten eyes. In the remaining three cases the central patterns were normal when examined twice. In these cases the use of profile perimetry, directed by the RNFL photographs identified field defects in two more cases (Figs. 1 & 2), while in one case no field loss could be found in spite of extensive testing.

In four cases of group 1 quality of photographs was good enough to allow observation of the course of the RNFL defects to a retinal area far away from the disc where the ganglion cells of the degenerated fibres were located. The width of this area and its distance from fixation correlated well with respective measurements from visual fields recorded with static profile perimetry.

In group 2 (patients without RNFL defects) both the central pattern and the static profiles were normal in four of the five cases. The fifth patient had a slightly suspect area in the upper nasal field in the central pattern test. Profile perimetry showed a reproducible relative defect in the 165° meridian. This eye had a fresh splinter haemorrhage of the optic disc inferotemporally at the same location as four years earlier.

DISCUSSION

In the majority of eyes with a RNFL defect the automatic perimetry was able to locate a corresponding visual field defect despite the fact that routine perimetry had failed to do so. However, in two cases where the defect had been misssed by the Friedmann analyser and Goldmann perimeter they were missed also by the central pattern of the Competer and it was only through extensive automatic profile perimetry assisted by RNFL photographs that visual field defects corresponding to the nerve fibre loss could be identified. One of the defects (Fig. 1) was a narrow but dense arcuate scotoma which probably curved between the test points of the central pattern; the other was a rather small, shallow defect which could easily have been missed also with profile perimetry had the meridians been chosen arbitrarily (Fig. 2). It is not realistic to assume that any type of clinical perimetry — automatic or manual — would be able to identify such field defects with some degree of certainty. That this is true also when using automatic perimetry on some other instrument, was demonstrated when eleven of the eyes of this study five months later were examined with an Octopus 2000 using standard programme #31. This test missed defects to the same extent as the Competer central pattern. It is evident from this study, however, that good quaity wide-angle RNFL

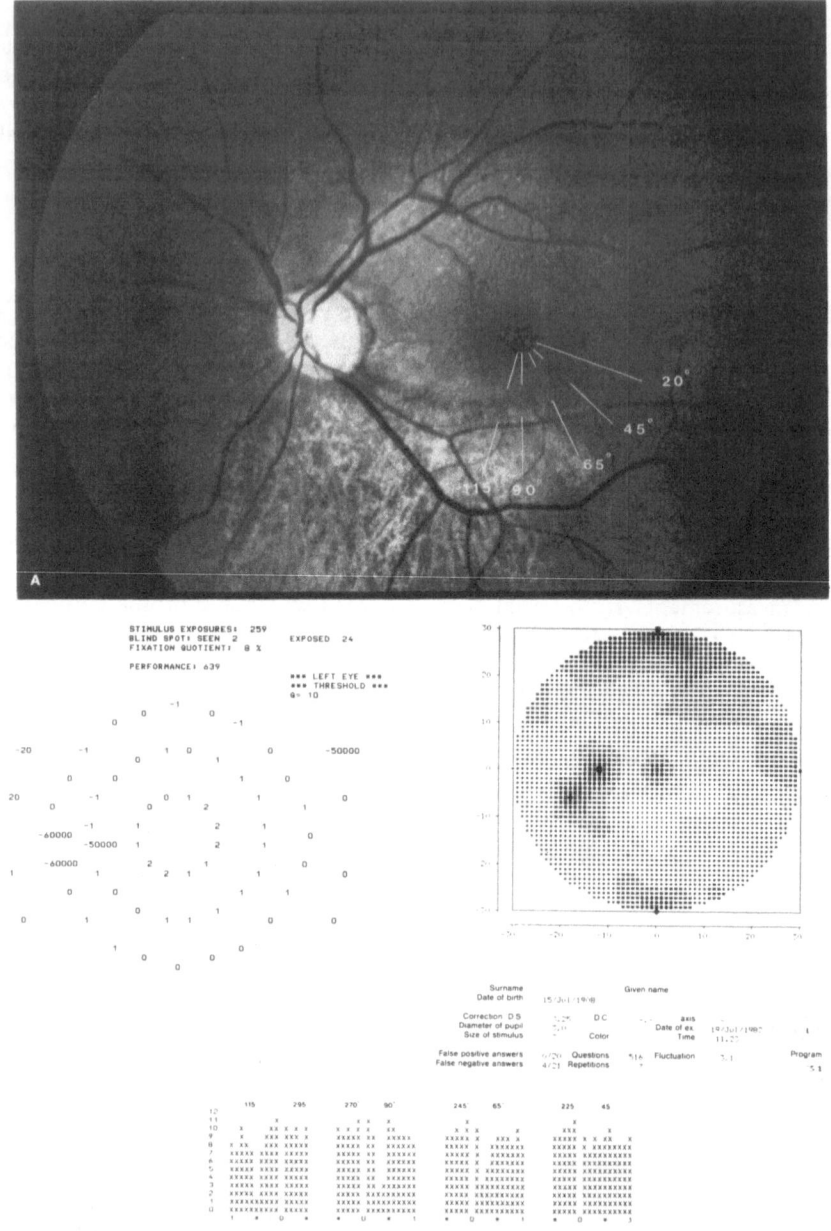

Fig. 1. RNFL photograph from a 74-year old woman showing a narrow, inferior RNFL defect curving centrally from the disc margin (a). This lesion was not visible ophthalmoscopically or with a fundus lens. The Competer (b) and Octopus (c) central patterns show no corresponding field loss, but static profile perimetry performed in the meridians indicated in (a) demonstrated a very narrow but deep arcuate scotoma close to fixation (d). The point of fixation has not been tested in the profiles. Each intensity step on the *y*-axis of the profiles corresponds to 0.3 log units. This case shows that diagnosis with the help of RNFL photography is not limited to younger patients, but is possible also in older individuals even with somewhat turbid optic media.

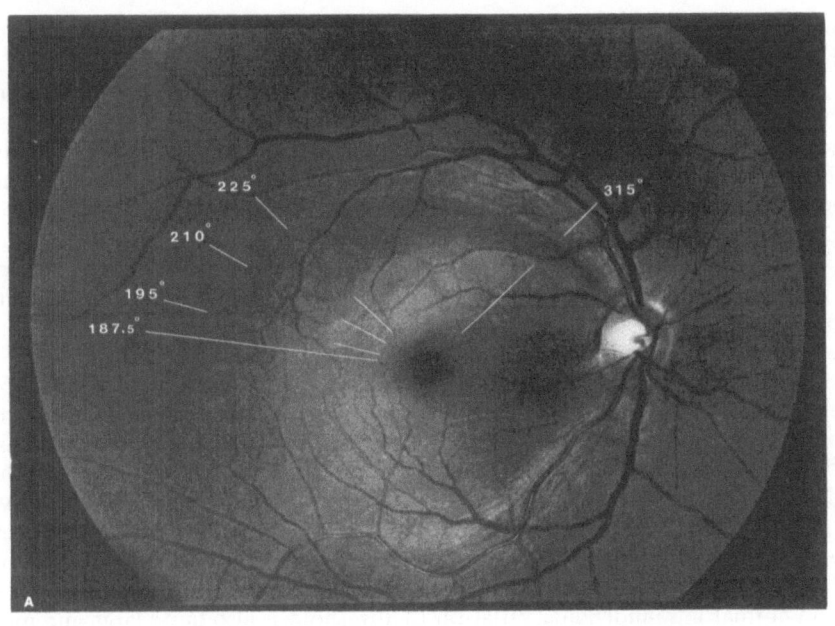

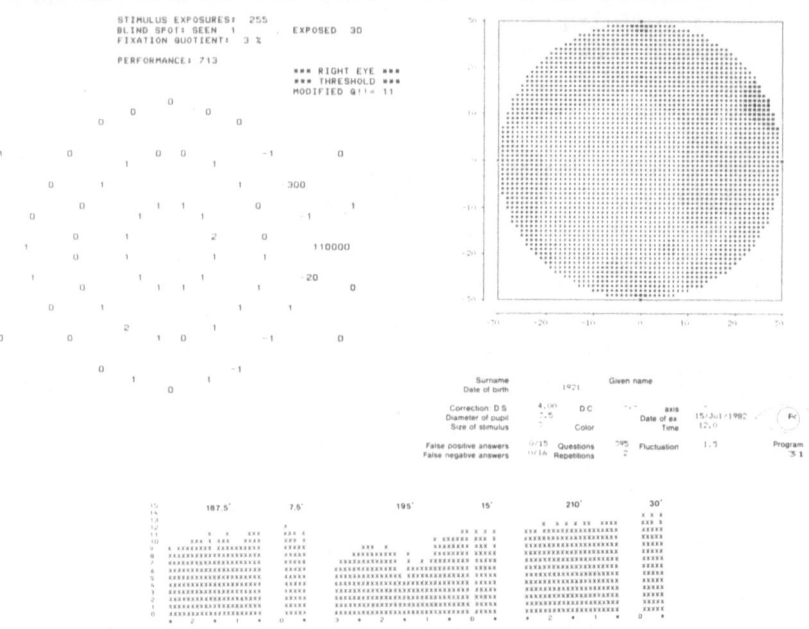

Fig. 2. RNFL photograph (a) showing a sector-shaped RNFL defect superotemporally. Measured from the photograph the peripheral end of this defect is situated between 9° and 16° from fixation approximately 15° above the horizontal meridian. The Competer (b) and Octopus (c) central patterns show no corresponding field loss, but when profile perimetry was performed in the meridians indicated in (a) a shallow but reproducible defect was revealed in the 195° meridian (d). The points between 1° and 4° in the 187.5° and 210° meridians have not been tested.

23

photographs are useful in very early cases since they can be used to direct high resolution perimetry.

Many cases with RNFL defects show visual field defects even with conventional perimetry. Such eyes were excluded from the present study and yet it was possible to detect field loss in all but one of ten cases with RNFL defects. Therefore the conclusion might be drawn that visual field defects are present in a higher percentage of patients with glaucomatous RNFL defects than was previously thought. However, also this investigation showed that there is no perfect correspondence between visual field and nerve fibre layer; in one case the visual field was normal in spite of a RNFL defect and in another the opposite was true – the RNFL was normal while a reproducible field defect was found.

In the first of these two cases the quality of the photographs was good enough for localization of the pathologic retinal ganglion cell area of the narrow and incomplete but sharply delineated RNFL defect. Yet no visual field changes could be found. Since there seemed to be fibres left in the defective area this might be due to overlapping of remaining retinal receptive fields. On the other hand very small field defects can be hard to identify even with the most sensitive perimetric techniques – the slightest shift of fixation can make the stimulus or part of it fall on an adjacent and functioning area. The normal intra-individual variation of threshold is also quite large and may mask small negative deviations of sensitivity.

The second of these two cases had a shallow and wide field defect but no RNFL defect could be identified in spite of high picture quality allowing stereoscopic comparisons between different retinal areas. Quigley and Addicks recently reported that loss of nerve fibres would not be detected clinically in primate eyes, until there is thinning of the RNFL of about 50% or more (10). It may thus be possible that this patient had clinically undetectable, diffuse nerve fibre loss which is difficult to document photographically. Another possibility would be that the axons while still alive had suffered some damage making them permanently or intermittently non-functioning.

As was shown in this study automatic perimetry and RNFL photography can be usefully combined for detection of early glaucomatous damage. Whether the present results, obtained in patients with disc haemorrhages, are valid also in patients with glaucoma without haemorrhages remains open, but if haemorrhage is a sine qua non in early glaucoma the present results should have broad applicability.

ACKNOWLEDGEMENTS

This study was supported by the Järnhardt Foundation (Dr Heijl) and the Emil Aaltonen Foundation and the Rasmussen Foundation (Dr Airaksinen).

REFERENCES

1. Airaksinen, P. J. The first observable glaucoma changes after an optic disc haemorrhage. Doc. Ophthalmol. Proc. Series 35:11–17 (1983).

24

2. Airaksinen, P. J., Mustonen, E. and Alanko, H. I. Optic disc haemorrhages precede retinal nerve fibre layer defects in ocular hypertension. Acta Ophthalmol. 59:627–641 (1981).
3. Airaksinen, P. J., Mustonen, E. and Alanko, H. I. Optic disc haemorrhages – An analysis of stereophotographs and clinical data of 112 patients. Arch. Ophthalmol. 99:1795–1801 (1981).
4. Airaksinen, P. J., Nieminen, H. and Mustonen, E. Retinal nerve fibre layer photography with a wide angle fundus camera. Acta Ophthalmol. 60:362–368 (1982).
5. Heijl, A. Computer test logics for automatic perimetry. Acta Ophthalmol. 55:837–853 (1977).
6. Heijl, A and Drance, S. M. Computerized profile perimetry in glaucoma. Arch. Ophthalmol. 98:2199–2201 (1980).
7. Heijl, A., Drance, S. M. and Douglas, G. R. Automatic perimetry (Competer). Ability to detect early glaucomatous field defects. Arch. Ophthalmol. 98:1560–1563 (1980).
8. Heijl, A. and Krakau, C. E. T. An automatic perimeter for glaucoma visual field screening and control. Construction and clinical cases. Albrecht von Graefes Arch. Klin. Exp. Ophthalmol. 197:13–23 (1975).
9. Iwata, K., Nanba, K. and Abe, H. Typical slit-like retinal nerve fiber layer defect and corresponding scotoma. Acta Soc. Ophthalmol. Japa. 85:1791–1803 (1981).
10. Quigley, H. A. and Addicks, E. M. Quantitative studies of retinal nerve fiber layer defects. Arch. Ophthalmol. 100:807–814 (1982).
11. Quigley, H. A., Miller, N. R. and George, T. R. Clinical evaluation of nerve fiber layer atrophy as indicator of glaucomatous optic nerve damage. Arch. Ophthalmol. 98:1564–1571 (1980).
12. Sommer, A., Miller, N. R., Pollack, I., Maumenee, A. E. and George, T. The nerve fiber layer in the diagnosis of glaucoma. Arch. Ophthalmol. 95:2149–56 (1977).

Authors' address:
Dr A. Heijl
Dept. of Ophthalmology
University of Lund
Malmö General Hosptial
S-214 01 Malmö
Sweden

Dr P. J. Airaksinen
Dept. of Ophthalmology
University of Oulu
SF-90220 Oulu 22
Finland

KINETIC QUANTITATIVE PERIMETRY OF RETINAL NERVE FIBER LAYER DEFECTS IN GLAUCOMA BY FUNDUS PHOTO-PERIMETER

TETSURO OGAWA, FUMIO FURUNO, AKIRA SEKI
TADASHI MIYAMOTO and YASUO OHTA
(Tokyo, Japan)

Key words. Fundus photo-perimeter, nerve fiber layer defect, glaucomatous visual field defect, nerve fiber bundle defect.

ABSTRACT

We compared the clinical appearance of retinal nerve fiber layer defects (RNFLDs) and retinal sensitivity as measured with the fundus photo-perimeter. If RNFLDs were observed, corresponding visual field defects were present but the sensitivity within a given field is not recognizable from the appearance of the RNFLDs. The functional impairment caused by the nerve fiber damage was not limited to the RNFLD but extended to the normally appearing retina in the vicinity of the RNFLDs. All cases (5 eyes) with discernible RNFLDs were found in low-tension glaucoma cases, but most of the cases in which the RNFLDs were difficult, or impossible, to evaluate tended to be primary open-angle glaucoma cases. This may suggest that in low-tension glaucoma and primary open-angle glaucoma the processes of optic nerve fiber impairment on the disc are different.

INTRODUCTION

Glaucomatous visual field changes result from the impairment of nerve fiber bundles at the optic nerve head, and reflect the distribution of damaged nerve fiber bundles (2). Typical glaucomatous visual field changes such as isolated paracentral scotomas, nasal steps, arcuate scotomas and sector-shaped defects are included in the category of nerve fiber bundle defect (1).

Hoyt et al. (3, 4) reported that it is possible to observe retinal nerve fiber alterations in the peripapillary area by ophthalmoscopy in glaucoma, especially with red-free light, and that the appearance of retinal nerve fiber layer defects (RNFLDs) correlate well with the visual field defects. However, it is difficult to determine the exact retinal eccentricity corresponding to the test target position on the field chart using a conventional perimeter. This problem has been solved by a recently developed fundus photo-perimeter (FPP) (6, 7) by which it is now not only possible to see the correct test target position on the retina directly via a TV monitor but also to simultaneously record visual field testing results by fundus photography.

To elucidate the relationship of RNFLD to visual field defects more clearly, the authors performed quantitative kinetic perimetry by the FPP in glaucoma cases with both discernible and indiscernible RNFLDs.

SUBJECTS AND METHODS

Kinetic perimetry with the FPP was performed on 5 eyes in 4 glaucoma cases with arcuate scotomas and in which distinct RNFLDs were observed. The FPP procedure was also performed on 7 eyes in other glaucoma cases which also showed arcuate scotomas but in which ophthalmoscopy revealed no, or indistinct RNFLDs. The areas of retinal nerve fiber layer corresponding to visual field defects were examined with magnified red-free photographs. Perimetry with the FPP was performed under the following conditions: background luminance 10 asb, test target size 6.4 minutes.

RESULTS

1. Cases which showed discernible retinal nerve fiber layer defects

Case 1: 55-year old male, low-tension glaucoma.

Wedge shaped RNFLDs were observed as dark bands in both retinas. In the left eye, the RNFLD connected to the disc at 4 to 6 o'clock, while the macular side border of RNFLD was traceable as far as the temporal side of the fovea, but the external border gradually disappeared about 2 disc diameters from the disc (Fig. 1, upper left figure). In the right eye, the border of the RNFLD was also traceable near the fovea, but the external border was more indiscernible than that of the left eye (Fig. 2, upper left figure).

The visual field of the left eye showed an arcuate scotoma resembling the RNFLD in shape. The 45° and 135° profile perimetry disclosed a deep defect coinciding with the arcuate scotoma and small wedge-shaped defects (Fig. 1, bottom figure). The right eye showed an arcuate defect and a nasal step (Fig. 2, bottom figure).

The upper left figures of Figs. 1 and 2 show the results of kinetic perimetry with the FPP. Target luminances were 1000, 10, 3.2 asb and 1.6 asb for the left eye (Fig. 1, upper right figure) and 1000, 32 asb and 5.0 asb for the right eye (Fig. 2, upper right figure).

In both eyes the 1000 asb isopters revealed arcuate defects equivalent to the RNFLDs. The 10, 3.2 asb isopters in the left eye and the 5 asb isopter in the right eye disclosed nasal steps. The nasal steps did not coincide with the RNFLD borders but slightly deviated to the macular side.

Case 2: 55-year old male, low-tension glaucoma.

The macular side border of the RNFLD was traceable for about two disc diameters from 8 o'clock on the disc, but its external border was obscure.

28

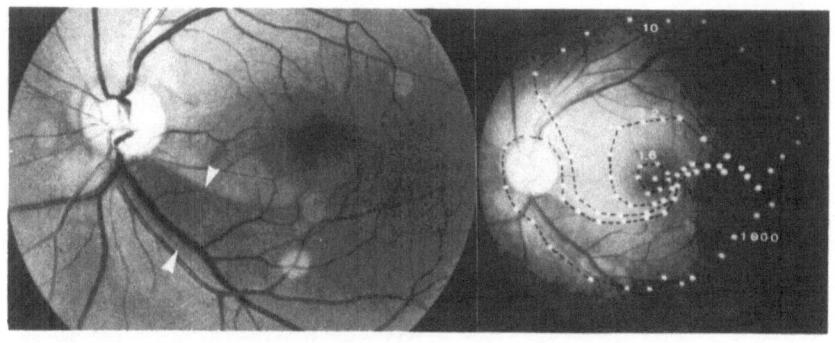

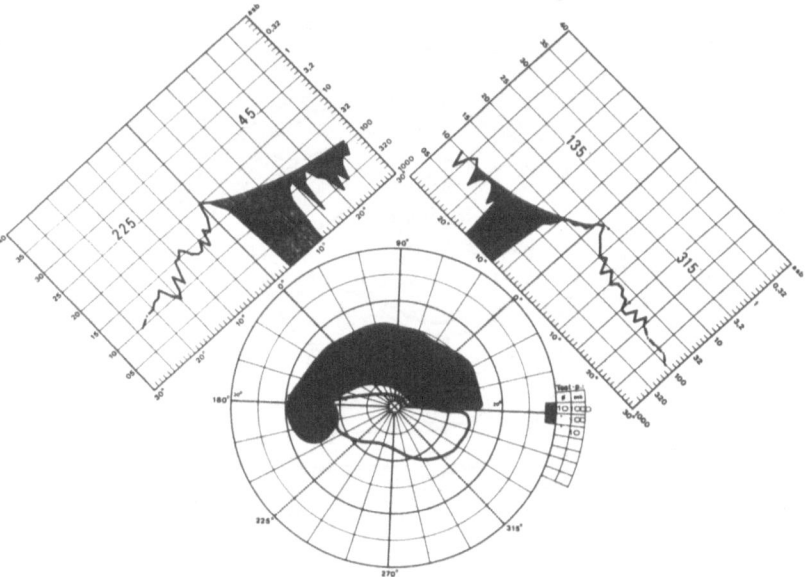

Fig. 1. Case 1, left eye. Upper left figure: wedge-shaped RNFLD was observed as dark band. Upper right figure: kinetic perimetry with the FPP, 1000 asb isopter showed an arcuate defect equivalent to the RNFLD. Bottom figure: the visual field had an arcuate scotoma resembling the RNFLD in shape.

The inferior arcuate vessels stood out more clearly than vessels in other areas (Fig. 3, upper left figure). In the upper nasal field the arcuate scotoma had broken through (Fig. 3, bottom figure). Kinetic perimetry with the FPP at a luminance of 1000 asb disclosed an arcuate defect connected to the disc which coincided with the macular side border of the RNFLD. The 3.2 asb isopter disclosed a nasal step which deviated to the macular side (Fig. 3, upper right figure).

Case 3: 54-year old male, low-tension glaucoma.

Two wide wedge-shaped RNFLDs were observed on the upper and lower half of the retina (Fig. 4, upper left figure). An altitudinal defect and an

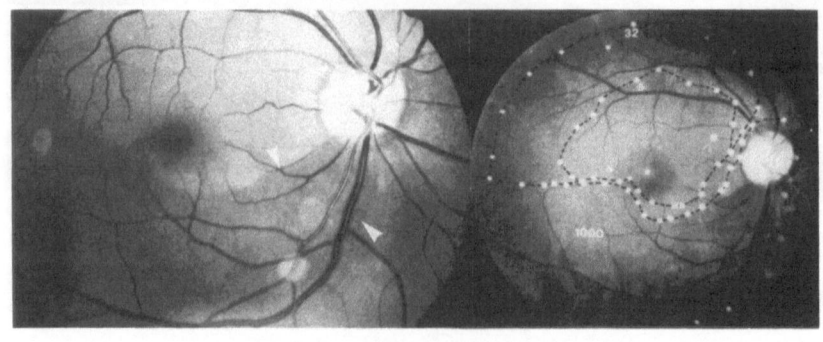

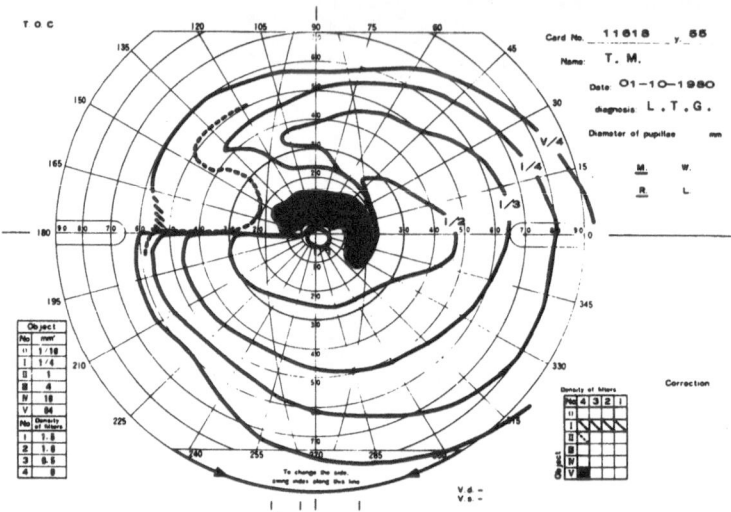

Fig. 2. Case 1, right eye. Upper left figure: wedge-shaped RNFLD was observed. Upper right figure: 1000 asb isopter showed acuate defect equivalent to the RNFLD. Bottom figure: the visual field had an arcuate defect and nasal step.

arcuate defect were recognized in the upper and lower fields, respectively (Fig. 4, upper left figure). The FPP procedure disclosed double arcuate defects which were detected by the 1000 asb isopter in the lower half retina and the 32, 10 asb isopters in the upper half of retina. These results agreed with the RNFLD borders. The arcuate defect in the upper half of the retina contained a scotoma in the distal portion of the RNFLD (Fig. 4, bottom figure).

2. Cases which showed indiscernible retinal nerve fiber layer defects

In our experience, glaucoma with discernible RNFLDs is far less frequent than glaucoma without discernible RNFLDs. Therefore, we also performed kinetic perimetry with the FPP on 7 eyes in 5 other glaucoma cases which showed arcuate defects but had indiscernible RNFLDs. Measurement with

30

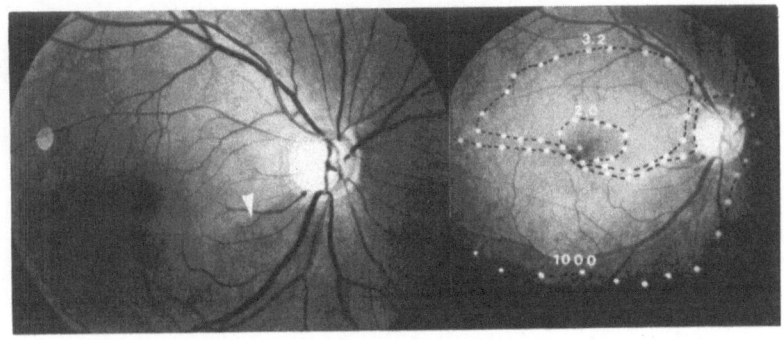

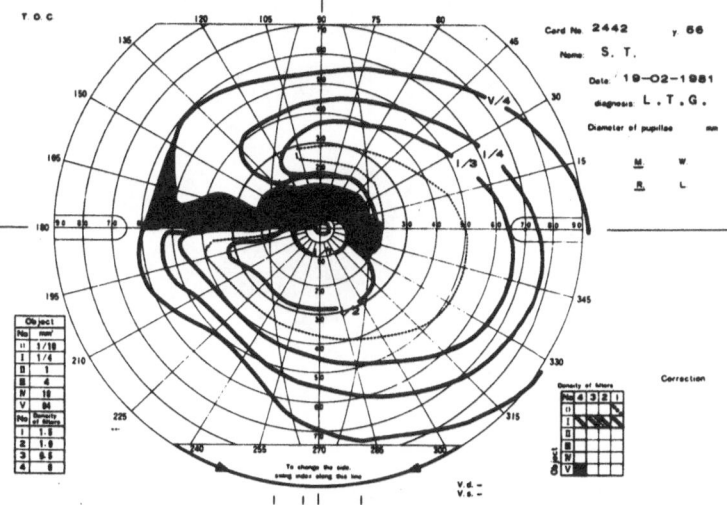

Fig. 3. Case 2, Upper left figure: magnified red-free photography. Upper right figure: kinetic perimetry with the FPP. Bottom figure: perimetry with the Goldmann perimeter.

the FPP yielded isopters similar to those obtained by the Goldmann perimeter (GP) in all cases. Magnified red-free photographs of the retina corresponding to the visual field defects with the FPP suggested RNFLDs, but the borders were not defined. A representative case is described below.

Case 4: 62-year old female, low-tension glaucoma.

Kinetic results with GP showed I/3 arcuate scotoma on the superior Bjerrum area within which I/4 paracentral scotomas were measured (Fig. 5, bottom figure). The FPP with a target luminance of 1000 asb disclosed an arcuate scotoma (Fig. 5, upper right figure). The retina corresponding to the arcuate scotoma lacked the striations of nerve fiber bundles which indicated RNFLD, but the borders of the RNFLD were obscure (Fig. 5, upper left figure).

31

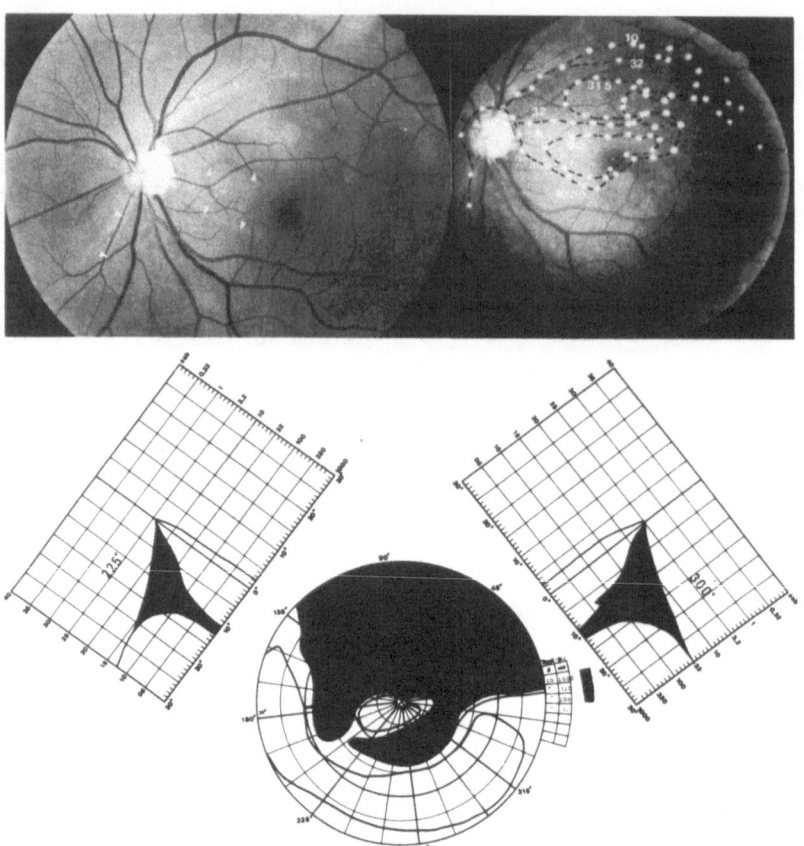

Fig. 4. Case 3, Upper left figure: two wide wedge-shaped RNFLDs were observed on the upper and lower half of the retina. Upper right figure: FPP kinetic perimetry. Bottom figure: altitudinal defect in the upper half field and arcuate defect in the lower half field.

COMMENTS AND DISCUSSION

Hoyt et al (4) described the characteristics of field defects corresponding to RNFLDS as follows: (1) every visible RNFLD has an analogue in the visual field; (2) the size of the field defect will equal or exceed the area predicted from the size of the RNFLD; (3) the densest portion of the field defect will lie further from the blind spot than would be predicted ophthalmoscopically from the distance between the RNFLD and the optic disc.

It is difficult, however to determine the exact retinal location corresponding to the test target position of the field chart using a conventional projection perimeter. Recently new types of perimeters have been developed and applied clinically. These permit observation of the correct position of the test target on the retina through a TV monitor and retinal sensitivity measurement. Mizogami et al. (5) first applied this type of perimeter to juvenile glaucoma

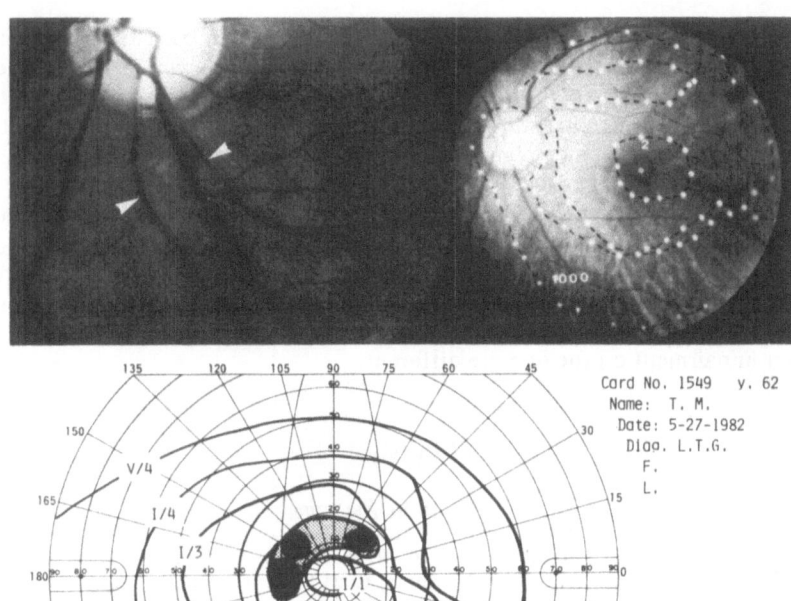

Fig. 5. Case 4, Upper left figure: magnified red-free photograph. Upper right figure: kinetic perimetry with the FPP. Bottom figure: results of perimetry with GP.

cases with slit-like RNFLDs. Spot-like scotoma was detected in agreement with RNFLD, but visual field changes corresponding to the slit-like defects could not be measured. Thus the relationship between RNFLDs visible as dark bands and the visual field changes was not clear.

In the present cases, advanced RNFLDs were observed. On perimetry with the FPP, arcuate defects equivalent to the borders of the RNFLDs were detected, indicating the presence and location of visual field defects. Visual field changes beyond the border of RNFLD were also detected with lower luminance targets, which indicated that the RNFLD border did not always coincide with the border of the visual field changes. This also suggested the presence of fine distribution of damaged nerve fibers in normally appearing retina in the vicinity of RNFLD. A nucleus of the arcuate defect was revealed in the RNFLD in case 3, suggesting that visual sensitivity could not be evaluated on the basis of RNFLD.

On the other hand, 7 eyes in 5 other glaucoma cases, which showed arcuate defects had no discernible RNFLD corresponding to the visual field defects. Therefore glaucoma with arcuate defects did not always show a visible

33

RNFLD corresponding to the field defect. Quigley et al. (8) reported that 84% of glaucoma with field loss showed RNFLD in which 5% had local atrophy and 95% had diffuse atrophy. Diffuse atrophy can be difficult to distinguish from normal nerve fiber bundles. Also the condition of optical media and the degree of pigmentation of pigment epithelium may influence the visibility of nerve fiber bundles. These factors probably account for the difficulty in recognizing RNFLDs in all glaucoma cases with arcuate defects.

All cases which had discernible RNFLDs were found in low-tension glaucoma and indiscernible RNFLDs showed a tendency to appear in primary open-angle glaucoma cases in this study. This may suggest that in low-tension glaucoma and primary open-angle glaucoma the processes of optic nerve fiber impairment on the disc are different.

REFERENCES

1. Drance, S. M. Visual field defects in glaucoma. In: Symposium on Glaucoma, pp. 190–208. C. V. Mosby Co., St. Louis (1975).
2. Harrington, D. O. The Visual Fields. C. V. Mosby Co., St. Louis (1976).
3. Hoyt, W. F., Sclicke, B. and Eckelhoff, R. J. Fundoscopic appearance of a nerve-fibre-bundle defect. Brit. J. Ophthalmol. 56:577–583 (1972).
4. Hoyt, W. F., Frisen, L. and Nowman, N. M. Fundoscopy of nerve fiber layer defects in glaucoma. Invest. Ophthalmol. 12:814–829 (1973).
5. Mizokami, K., Tagami, Y. and Isayama, Y. The reversibility of visual field defects in the juvenile glaucoma cases. Doc. Ophthalmol. Proc. Series 19: 241–246 (1979).
6. Ohta, Y., Miyamoto, T. and Harasawa, K. Experimental fundus photo-perimeter and its application, Doc. Ophthalmol. Proc. Series 19: 351–358 (1979).
7. Ohta, Y., Tomonaga, M., Miyamoto, T. and Harasawa, K. Visual field studies with fundus photo-perimeter in postchiasmatic lesions. Doc. Ophthalmol. Proc. Series 26: 119–126 (1981).
8. Quigley, H. A., Miller, N. R. and George, T. Clinical evaluation of nerve fiber layer atrophy as an indicator of glaucomatous optic nerve damage. Arch. Ophthalmol. 98:1564–1571 (1980).

Authors' address:
Dept. of Ophthalmology
Tokyo Medical College Hospital
6-7-1 Nishi-shinjuku Shinjuku-ku
Tokyo Japan 160

THE RELATION BETWEEN EXCAVATION AND VISUAL FIELD IN GLAUCOMA PATIENTS WITH HIGH AND WITH LOW INTRAOCULAR PRESSURES

ERIK L. GREVE and H. CAROLINE GEIJSSEN

(Amsterdam, The Netherlands)

Key words. Glaucoma, excavation, visual field, low-tension glaucoma.

ABSTRACT

One group of relatively young patients with high intraocular pressures (IOP) (> 40 mm Hg) and glaucomatous visual field defects, and two groups of relatively old patients with low IOP (low-tension glaucoma) and glaucomatous visual field defects were examined. The differences of the appearance of the optic disc and the disc—visual field relationship is described. The patients with high-tension glaucoma have a large and steep excavation with comparatively small glaucomatous visual field defects. The patients with senile sclerotic low-tension glaucoma (SSLTG) have a pale, sloping disc with a moth-eaten aspect. The visual field is large with respect to the cup—disc ratio at the laminar level. The patients with focal ischemic glaucoma had a local excavation in the vertical meridian. The visual field is large with respect to the horizontal laminar cup—disc ratio. It was demonstrated that subgroups of open-angle glaucoma can be identified. The possible consequences for their pathogenic mechanism are discussed.

INTRODUCTION

Primary open-angle glaucoma (POAG) can be defined as a disease of the optic disc with excavation and with typical visual field defects irrespective of the level of the intraocular pressure (IOP). Glaucomatous excavation and visual field defects can be found with an IOP as low as 10 mm Hg and as high as 60 mm Hg in patients with open angles. Between those extremes the whole range of IOP can be found.

Are there recognizable differences in the POAG with low IOP and high IOP? We had the impression that a different type of excavation could be found in these two groups and that the relation between excavation and visual field was different.

We therefore investigated the excavation and visual fields in two groups with glaucomatous visual field defects at each end of the IOP spectrum.

Greve, E. L., Heijl, A. (eds.) Fifth International Visual Field Symposium.
©1983 Dr W. Junk Publishers, The Hague/Boston/Lancaster.

IOP: the IOP criteria were based on applanation measurements in diurnal and, if necessary, nocturnal IOP curves. A patient was classified in the group of low IOP if the highest IOP did not exceed 26 mm Hg (the average IOP in the low IOP groups was about 17 mm Hg; see results). In the age group above 65 years up to 9% of a population (framingham study) has an IOP of 22 mm Hg or more without visual field defects. About 4% has an IOP of 25 mm Hg ore more.

A patient was classified in the group of high IOP if the highest IOP was 40 mm Hg or more.

It could be argued that an IOP limit of 26 mm Hg is too high for low-tension glaucoma. For the purpose of this investigation it is not important because the limits of 26 mm Hg and 40 mm Hg, respectively, seem far enough apart to separate two different IOP groups.

Angle: all patients had open angles.

Refraction: myopic refractions of more than 6 diopters were excluded. This was done because myopic glaucoma has a type of disc and distribution of the visual field defect that is different from non-myopic glaucoma (4).

Visual field: the visual field examination was done with a modified Visual Field Analyser (Amsterdam front plate) and kinetic and static perimetry with the Tübingen perimeter. Most patients had several visual field examinations and were followed for many years.

Classification of visual field defects: a proposed classification of glaucomatous visual field defects (GVFD) (Fig. 1):
Stage O—I: relative small GVFD with an intensity of 0.6 log unit up to 1.0 log unit.
   I: small GVFD with an intensity of more than 1.0 log unit up to maximum luminance.
  II: incomplete nerve fiber bundle defect (NFBD = arcuate defect) for maximal luminance.
 III: complete (from blind spot to nasal horizontal meridian) NFBD for maximal luminance or incomplete (II) NFBD with nasal breakthrough.
  IV: complete NFBD for maximal luminance with nasal breakthrough involving less than one quadrant.
   V: complete NFBD for maximal luminance with nasal breakthrough involving more than one quadrant. Two stage V defects in the upper and lower half of the visual field from a central and temporal island.
  VI: temporal island.

Optic disc: the evaluation of the optic disc has often given rise to differences of opinion. Intra- and inter-observer differences occur frequently (7).

36

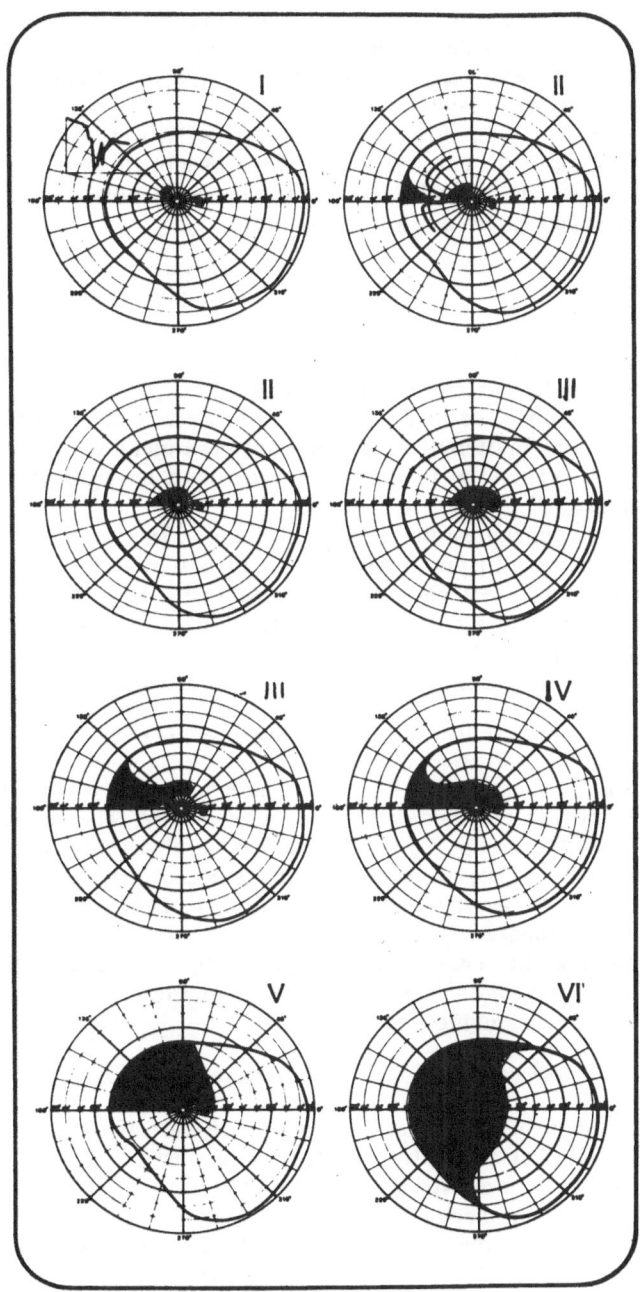

Fig. 1. Classification of visual field defects.

We evaluated the horizontal and vertical cup–disc ratio (CDR) *at two levels*: at the retinal level (CDRR) and at the level of the lamina cribrosa

37

(CDRL). The cup size at the retinal level was considered to be determined by a depression relative to the retinal level. The cup size at the cribrosa level was determined by the visible lamina cribrosa. Of all patients stereophotographs were available in addition to drawings made after evaluation with the fundus contact lens in mydriasis. The two-level CDR was compared with the stage of the visual field. The relation between visual field stage and CDR was expressed in a visual field/CDR quotient. The peripapillary atrophy (PPA) was measured and expressed in a PPA/disc ratio.

RESULTS

The *high-tension glaucoma* group had a mean age of 52 years. There were 20 eyes of 11 patients. In many of these eyes gonioscopic findings of late congenital glaucoma could be found: anterior iris insertion, large numbers of iris processus with obscuration of the scleral spur, prominent Schwalbes line. The mean IOP was 37 mm Hg. In this group we found no signs of retinal and choroid sclerosis.

We found no general cardiovascular risk factors. In short: a healthy group of relatively young glaucoma patients with high IOP and signs of late congenital glaucoma. These high-tension patients had a large CDR both at the retinal and at the laminar level, both in the horizontal and in the vertical meridian (Fig. 2a).

The low-tension glaucoma group consisted of two subgroups.

1. Senile sclerotic low-tension glaucoma (SSLTG)

This group has a mean age of 82 years. There were 22 eyes of 11 patients. The angles showed no abnormalities on gonioscopy. The mean IOP was 18 mm Hg. In this group eight patients had cardiovascular disease which required treatment. They were called SSLTG because they could be *identified as a group* by the presence of extensive retinal and choroidal sclerosis and peripapillary choroidal atrophy.

The excavation was characterized (Fig. 2b) by a large cup—disc ratio at the retinal level and a moderate CDR at the laminar level (Table 1). The optic disc tissue had a pale and moth-eaten aspect.

2. Focal ischemic low-tension glaucoma (FILTG)

The average age of this group was 72 years. There were 29 eyes of 15 patients. The average IOP was 17 mm Hg. The angles showed no abnormalities. The term 'focal ischemic' is derived from Spaeth (12). Four patients had choroidal sclerosis. Eight patients had cardiovascular disease. This group is characterized by local excavation of the neural tissue rim, located in the vertical meridian. It also implies that apart from the focal damage the rim is in reasonable shape as far as contour and color is concerned.

Thus, the two groups of LTG patients could be identified on the basis of the appearance of the optic disc and peripapillary area and the presence of a GVFD.

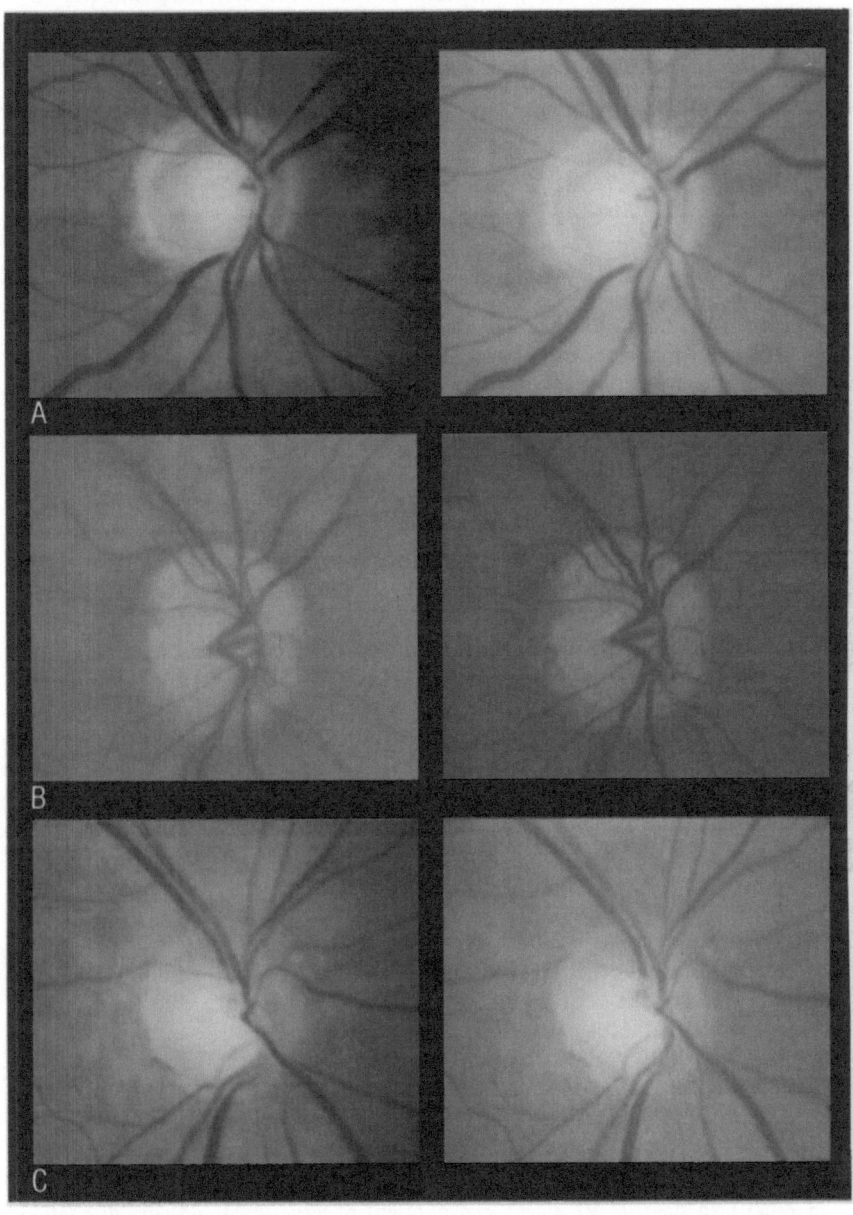

Fig. 2. a) Stereo photograph of an optic disc of a patient with high-tension glaucoma (HTG); b) Stereo photograph of an optic disc of a patient with senile sclerotic low-tension glaucoma (SSLTG); c) Stereo photograph of an optic disc of a patient with focal ischemic low-tension glaucoma (FILTG).

Table 1. Horizontal (CDRR →) cup–disc ratio at the retinal level, horizontal (CDRL →) cup–disc ratio at the laminar level, vertical (CDRR ↑) cup–disc ratio at the retinal level, vertical cup–disc ratio (CDRL ↑) at the laminar level and mean visual field stage (in VF-stage) for each of the three glaucoma groups.

HTG	CDRR →	CDRL →	CDRR ↑	CDRL ↑	M̄ VD stage
HTG	0.8	0.7	0.9	0.8	2.4
SSLTG	0.8	0.3	0.9	0.5	2.75
FILTG	0.6	0.5	0.8	0.8	2.3

The HTG patients were selected on the basis of their IOP and age and the presence of a GVFD.

Table 1 shows the CDR at the retinal and laminar levels of the three groups. The difference between the groups is clear. The HTG group has a large and steep excavation in all directions. The SSLTG group has a sloping excavation slighlty larger in vertical direction. The FILTG group has a larger vertical CDR than horizontal CDR. The CDR is approximately of the same size at the retinal and at the laminar level.

The mean visual field stages in the three groups are comparable in size.

Table 2 shows the relation between mean visual field stage and laminar CDR both in horizontal and vertical direction, and the visual field/CDRL quotient. The visual field/CDRL quotient is twice as much for SSLTG as for HTG and FILTG.

It means that in SSLTG one finds a comparable large visual field defect and a small laminar CDR. It furthermore shows that the visual field/CDRL quotient is comparable in horizontal and vertical direction for the HTG group.

In both LTG groups the visual field/CDR quotient is higher in vertical direction. Again the overall visual field/CDRL quotient is higher in the SSLTG group as compared to the FILTG group.

DISCUSSION

The main purpose of this paper is to show that different types of POAG can be identified on other characteristics than IOP. In our opinion it is not realistic to reserve the term POAG only for those patients who have an IOP above the statistical limit and/or low C-values.

In Bristol, 1980, at the occasion of the first symposium of the European Glaucoma Society, we have already described the preliminary results of an investigation of HTG and LTG. We then emphasized the difference in visual

Table 2. Combined horizontal and vertical cup–dis ratio at the laminar level (CDRL ↳), mean visual field stage (M̄ VF stage), and quotient of visual field and cup–disc ratio at the laminar level for combined horizontal-vertical and horizontal and vertical respectively.

	CDRL ↳	M̄ VF stage	VF/CDRL ↳	VF/CDRL →	VF/CDRL ↑
HTG	0.75	2.40	3.2	3.4	3.0
SSLTG	0.40	2.75	6.9	9.2	5.5
FILTG	0.65	2.30	3.5	4.6	2.9

field — disc relation in these two groups. In a separate article the special distribution of visual field defects in myopic glaucoma was demonstrated (4). In this paper and in a second paper in this volume (6) we describe a group which we called *senile sclerotic low-tension glaucoma* (SSLTG). This group can be identified on the basis of the typical appearance of the optic disc and peripapillary area. The same type of disc can be found (in a slightly earlier stage) without demonstrable visual field defects. This has been called the 'Senile Exkavation' in the older German literature (2, 11).

We suggest that the histopathological basis for this LTG group can be found in the older German literature and in more recent work on age changes of the optic nerve (1, 3, 5, 13). These studies described findings in the optic disc of old people without known glaucomatous disease that closely resemble those found in glaucoma and could give an explanation both for the aspect of the excavation and for the visual field defects. There is a great individual diversity in age changes of the optic nerve. Changes similar to those in glaucoma may occur in a diffuse manner or with a vertical polar localization. They are accompanied by severe arteriosclerotic changes of the posterior ciliary arteries and the small centripetal arteries of the optic nerve. The asymmetry between the two eyes that is often found in these cases may point to the involvement of local factors. Senile peripapillary choroidal atrophy likewise has been reported long ago.

We added a second LTG group called focal ischemic glaucoma. The term 'focal ischemic' was used because the authors believed the underlying pathogenic mechanism to be vascular. This type of LTG has been reported earlier (8, 12). In both groups it is unlikely that the IOP is the exclusive damaging factor and other factors, possibly micro-vascular, may play an important part.

We demonstrated that there is a difference in the aspect of the optic disc in the three glaucoma groups. The cup—disc ratio at two levels has been used in an attempt to objectivate the typical appearance of the disc at opthalmoscopy. The cup—disc ratio is only one part of the description of several types of discs. Furthermore we demonstrated that there is a difference in the relation between visual field size and excavation in the three groups (see summary Table 3).

Thus, it is possible to create subgroups in the large group of POAG patients on the basis of disc and visual field evaluation. So far we have separated four 'subgroups': young HTG, myopic glaucoma, SSLTG and FILTG. Other subgroups and combinations of these groups will exist.

One could speculate that the large excavation and comparatively small visual field defects of the HTG group is mainly caused by direct action of the IOP (9, 10). This group of young HTG has been selected to exclude vascular disease.

Table 3. Summary presentation of the findings. For abbreviations see Tables 1 & 2. For explanation see text.

				VF/CDRL
HTG	CDRR ≈ CDRL	CDR ↑≈ CDR →	VF/CDRL ↑≈ VF/CDRL →	3.2
SSLTG	CDRR > CDRL	CDR ↑≳ CDR →	VF/CDRL ↑< VF/CDRL →	6.9
FILTG	CDRR ≈ CDRL	CDR ↑> CDR →	VF/CDRL ↑< VF/CDRL →	3.5

Similarly one could speculate that the typical pale, moth-eaten sloping excavation of the SSLTG group is caused by senile atrophy with or without an additional effect of IOP on perfusion pressure. The damage in focal ischemic glaucoma has already been attributed to focal ischemia.

A last speculation could be that a high visual field/CDRL quotient points in the direction of senile optic atrophy.

Finally the fact that the SSLTG group and especially the pre-defect or early defect stage of this group has not been identified earlier, may be due to the referral pattern òf many glaucoma clinics. The SSLTG patients were found in a general opthalmological practice where early detection was done by an experience glaucomatologist. In the glaucoma clinic only the late stages were found. These late stages do not show the characteristics of the optic disc and visual field—disc relation as well.

REFERENCES

1. Brownstein, S., Front, R. L., Zimmerman, L. E. and Murphy, S. B. Non-glaucomatous cavernous degeneration of the optic nerve. Arch. Opthalmol. 98:354 (1980).
2. Der Augenartzt: Band V, Thieme, Leipzig, p. 756 (1963).
3. Dolman, C. L., McCormick, Q. and Drance, S. M. Aging of the optic nerve. Arch. Ophthalmol. 98:2053 (1980).
4. Furuno, F. and Greve, E. L. Myopia and glaucoma. Albrecht von Graefes Arch. Klin. Exp. Ophthalmol. 213: 33 (1980).
5. Giarelli, L., Melato, M. and Campos, E. Fourteen cases of cavernous degeneration of the optic nerve. Ophthalmologica 174: 316 (1977).
6. Greve, E. L. and Geijssen, H. C. Comparison of glaucomatous visual field defects in patients with high and with low intraocular pressures. Doc. Ophthalmol. Proc. Series 35:101–105 (1983).
7. Lichter, P. R. Variability of expert observers in evaluating the optic disc. Trans. Am. Ophthalmol. Soc. 74:532 (1976).
8. Lichter, P. R. and Henderson, J. W. Optic nerve infraction. Am. J. Ophthalmol. 85:302 (1978).
9. Quigley, H. A. and Addicks, E. M. Regional differences in the structure of the lamina cribrosa and their relation to glaucomatous optic nerve damage. Arch. Ophthalmol. 99:137 (1981).
10. Quigley, H. A., Addicks, E. M., Green, W. R. and Maumenee, A. E. Optic nerve damage in human glaucoma. Arch. Opthalmol. 99:635 (1981).
11. Sachsenweger, R. Altern und Auge. Ein Handbuch der Gerontologie und Geriatrie des menschlichen Sehorgans. Thieme, Leipzig, p. 263 (1971).
12. Spaeth, G. L. Low tension glaucoma: its diagnosis and management. Doc. Ophthmol. Proc. Series 22:263 (1979).
13. Vrabec, F. Age changes of the human optic nerve head. Albrecht von Graefes Arch. Klin. Exp. Ophthalmol. 202:231 (1977).

Authors' addresses:
Dr E. L. Greve
Glaucoma and Visual Field Dept.
Eye clinic of the University of Amsterdam
Academic Medical Center
Meibergdreef 8, 1105 AZ Amsterdam
The Netherlands

H. C. Geijssen
Dept. of Ophthalmology
Sint Lucas Hospital
Jan Tooropstraat 164, 1061 AE Amsterdam
The Netherlands

COMPUTER-GENERATED DISPLAY FOR THREE-DIMENSIONAL STATIC PERIMETRY: CORRELATION OF OPTIC DISC CHANGES WITH GLAUCOMATOUS DEFECTS

WILLIAM M. HART, JR. and ALLAN E. KOLKER

(St. Louis, Missouri, U.S.A.)

Key words. Perimetry, glaucoma, scotoma, computer, optic disc.

ABSTRACT

Contiguous area (3D) threshold static perimetry was used to examine limited areas of the visual fields of selected patients with known or suspected glaucoma. Patients with previously normal visual fields were selected on the basis of ophthalmoscopic evidence of optic disc pathology, or on the basis of transient or newly acquired visual field defects detected by kinetic perimetry. Shallow depressions in the Bjerrum region adjacent to the blind spot were demonstrable by this technique in patients whose visual fields were apparently normal by conventional techniques of perimetry. Defects that appeared transient by kinetic perimetry remained demonstrable by 3D threshold static perimetry. The findings support the concept of a critical phase in the evolution of glaucomatous visual field defects, and demonstrate the superiority of threshold static perimetry for detection of this phase.

INTRODUCTION

Numerous investigators have studied the natural history of early glaucomatous visual field defects (2, 4, 6, 9, 10). In a retrospective study we have described the temporal characteristics of the onset and development of glaucomatous visual field defects in a group of 98 eyes (10). A common phenomenon within this group was found to be a fluctuating course in which initial defects were transient. The transient course was not related to coincident fluctuations in intraocular pressure. We have since evaluated the sensitivity of 3D threshold static perimetry in the detection of these defects at a time when they are inapparent by conventional perimetric techniques.

METHODS

Patients were chosen by several different criteria. All were being followed with known or suspected primary open angle glaucoma. Patients were selected

Greve, E. L., Heijl, A. (eds.) Fifth International Visual Field Symposium.
©*1983 Dr W. Junk Publishers, The Hague/Boston/Lancaster.*

whose visual fields by conventional kinetic perimetry had shown recent development of a transient visual field defect in the Bjerrum region or a newly acquired nasal step. Patients were also selected who had recent onset of optic disc pathology. Normal subjects were selected within age-matched groups for comparative examinations.

Three-dimensional threshold static perimetry and subsequent display of the resultant visual field surfaces were carried out as previously described (11). Selection of the area of the visual field for examination was based on the known density distribution of earliest defects (10). This area in the Bjerrum region covered a quadrant 20 degrees on each side, with one corner located at the point of fixation. Quadrants were chosen for examination based on the results of kinetic perimetry, or on the basis of optic disc pathology. Thus, an inferior nasal step suggested examination of the inferotemporal quadrant, while a notch at the inferior pole of the optic disc directed attention to the superotemporal quadrant.

RESULTS

Twenty-three patients were examined. All but one had defects demonstrable by 3D threshold static perimetry. Fourteen were found by kinetic perimetry to have manifest defects, and one had no detectable defects by either techniqe. Five had defects which were detectable by 3D static perimetry, where kinetic perimetry had failed to detect any abnormality. The final 3 showed only blind spot enlargement or baring of the blind spot by kinetic perimetry, but were found to have focal defects by the 3D technique. Among the 14 patients with manifest defects by kinetic perimetry, 2 had defects that consisted of nasal steps alone. Examination of these subjects by 3D static perimetry, demonstrated the presence of shallow depressions in the Bjerrum region which had not been detected by kinetic perimetry.

In normal subjects the Bjerrum region has a sloping contour, falling away from the point of fixation and the margin of the blind spot. Figure 1 illustrates the results for the inferotemporal Bjerrum region of a right eye, and the superotemporal Bjerrum region of a left eye. Surface images of the superotemporal region, when viewed from the 225 degree meridian and at 20 degrees of elevation, are seen from a tangential aspect. Rotation of the 3D surface, so that it is viewed from the 45 degree meridian, allows a more advantageous inspection of its surface (Fig. 2). Minor undulations in the surface reflect the uncertainty inherent in careful manual threshold examinations. This level of noise has been found to approximate 3 dB (9). We have therefore accepted as a defect any depression of 4 decibels, involving 2 or more adjacent locations, or any depression of 5 decibels or more.

Two cases will be summarized. The first illustrates the presence of a stable defect by 3D perimetry, when the same defect was only transiently demonstrable by kinetic perimetry. A 32-year old man had intraocular pressures varying between 20 and 30 mm Hg, and had asymmetry of the optic disc cups. The cup in the right eye appeared significantly larger than that in the left, and a notch was evident at the inferior pole of the disc in the right eye.

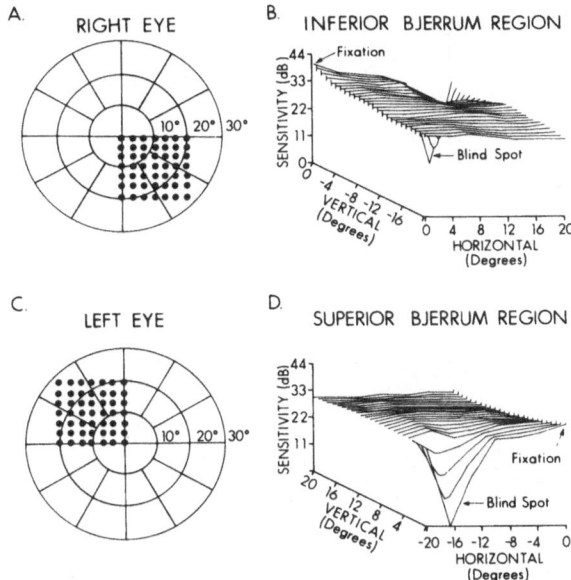

Fig. 1. 3D static perimetry in normal eyes. A: test object pattern covering inferior Bjerrum region; B: resulting 3D visual field surface seen from 225 degree meridian and 20 degrees of elevation; C: test object pattern for examining superior Bjerrum region; D: resulting 3D visual field surface (same orientation as in B).

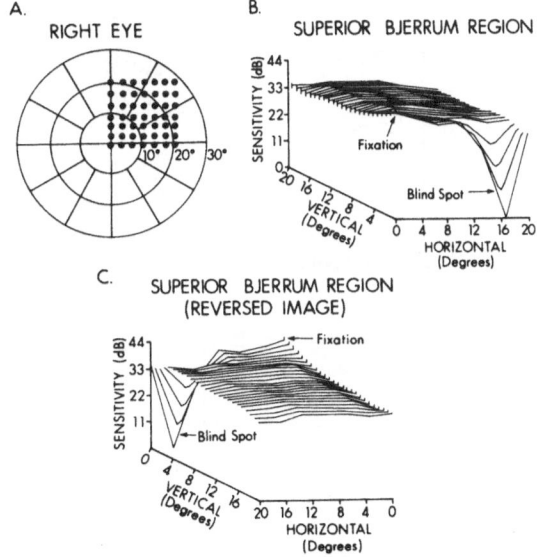

Fig. 2. 3D static perimetry of the superior Bjerrum region in a normal right eye. A: test object pattern covering superotemporal quadrant; B: 3D visual field surface viewed from 225 degree meridian and 20 degrees of elevation (surface from this aspect is seen tangentially); C: 180 degree reversal of image shows visual field surface as seen from 45 degree meridian. A more perpendicular view of the visual field surface in the Bjerrum region is obtained.

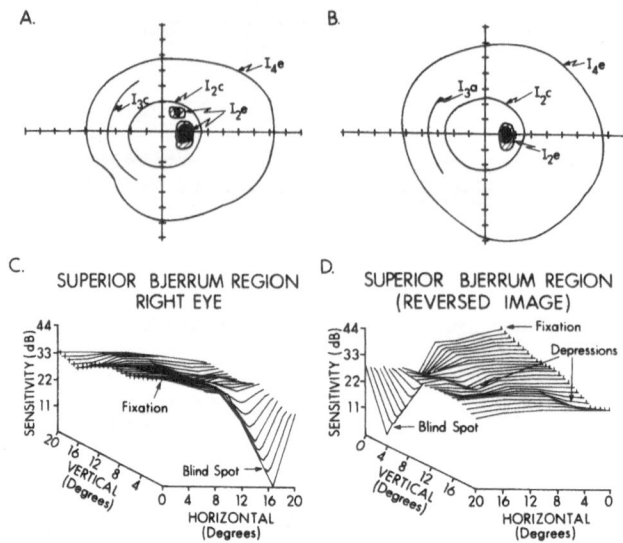

Fig. 3. Visual field of right eye, Case 1. A: kinetic perimetry demonstrated small, shallow defect in superior Bjerrum region of a right eye in January 1982; B: kinetic perimetry showed apparently normal visual field in March 1982; C: superior Bjerrum region of 3D visual field surface in right eye; D: reversed image (same surface as in C), showed two areas of depression.

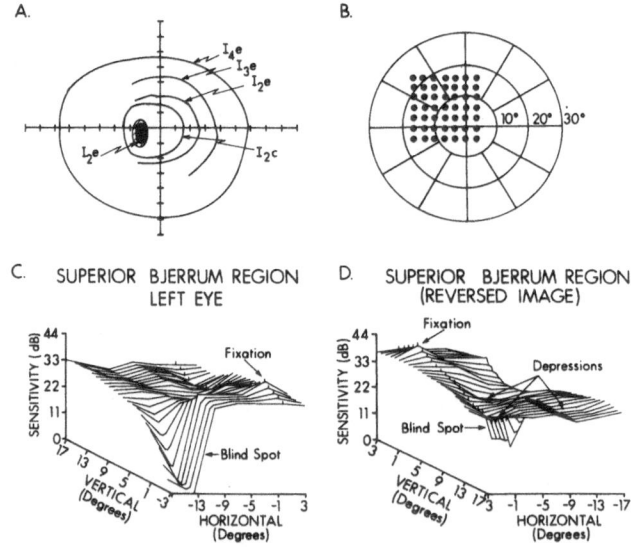

Fig. 4. Visual field, Case 2. A: kinetic perimetry of left eye demonstrated apparently normal pattern; B: test object pattern used to examine superotemporal Bjerrum region; C: resulting 3D visual field surface; D. image of same surface, following 180 degree rotation.

In January of 1982 a small, relative scotoma was detected in the superior Bjerrum region of the right eye adjacent to the blind spot (Fig. 3A). In March of 1982 re-examination of this region by kinetic perimetry failed to demonstrate the presence of the defect (Fig. 3B). Three-dimensional static perimetry of the superotemporal quadrant in the right eye (Figs. 3C & D) demonstrated multiple shallow depressions adjacent to the superior pole of the blind spot.

The second case showed the presence of a shallow depression in the Bjerrum region in the absence of a demonstrable defect by kinetic perimetry. The patient was a 65-year old woman with a longstanding history of elevated intraocular pressure, normal visual fields, and intraocular pressures varying between 25 and 35 in both eyes. Examination of the discs showed asymmetric, pathologic cupping, the left disc being more extensively involved at its inferior pole. Attention was therefore directed to the superior Bjerrum region in the left eye where 3D static perimetry (Fig. 4) demonstrated a shallow depression of the visual field. This was 6 decibels deep at one location, and 5 decibels deep at 2 other locations in the superior Bjerrum region.

DISCUSSION

Our work and that of others has supported the concept of a critical phase in the development of glaucomatous visual field defects (4, 9, 10, 8). The earliest defects detectable by kinetic perimetry are frequently shallow and transient (10, 18), and are most commonly found in the superior Bjerrum region. Over the past 15 years there have been numerous improvements in perimetric techniques for following the development of visual field defects in primary open-angle glaucoma. It has been determined that static perimetry is more sensitive than kinetic perimetry for the detection of shallow defects in the visual field surface (7, 3, 17). Careful prospective evaluation with conventional perimetry has shown that initial defects are often transient. Such defects are characteristically shallow, are located within the Bjerrum region, and follow a predictable course of progression in which they reappear at the same location and at a greater depth (10). Case 1 illustrates that while defects may appear to be transient by kinetic perimetry, they can be stably detected by threshold static perimetry.

Since kinetic and suprathreshold static perimetry are less sensitive than threshold techniques for detection of defects, it follows that if we use them as a criterion for detection we will miss patients with early glaucoma, who have otherwise apparently normal visual fields. The presence of optic disc pathology, however, solves much of the selection problem for us. Multivariate analysis of risk factors for the development of glaucomatous visual field loss has ranked optic disc pathology high in the order of importance (12). Other studies have demonstrated that optic disc pathology, including asymmetry or the presence of notching (16); baring of a circumlinear vessel (15); and surface haemorrhages on the optic disc (1, 5), are important morphological markers for incipient disease. Case 2 illustrates this principle. Although the patient had no demonstrable visual field defect by kinetic or suprathreshold static perimetry, the presence of pathologic cupping of the disc provided a convenient criterion by which to select the patient for more extensive evaluation of the visual field.

The advent of machine-automated techniques of threshold static perimetry have more recently provided us, for the first time, with the capacity to critically explore contiguous areas of the visual field most likely to contain relatively small and shallow glaucomatous visual field defects (14, 13). All such defects are likely to be expressed within 20 degrees of fixation even when the initial defect by kinetic perimetry may be expressed only as a nasal step. Thus, a logical strategy for threshold static visual field evaluation in suspected glaucoma should include: 1) selection of patients based on a combination of multiple factors, including ophthalmoscopic evidence of pathologic change in the optic disc (with or without elevated intraocular pressure); 2) the use of test object patterns for automated contiguous area threshold static perimetry covering the central 20 degrees of the visual field; and 3) use of a weighted distribution of test object locations that matches the probability distribution of initial glaucomatous visual field defects.

ACKNOWLEDGEMENT

This work was supported by grant No. EY-02044 from the National Eye Institute.

REFERENCES

1. Airaksinen, P. J., Mustonen, E. and Alanko, H. I. Optic disc haemorrhages precede retinal nerve fibre layer defects in ocular hypertension. Acta Ophthalmol. 59:627–641 (1981).
2. Armaly, M. F. Visual field defects in early open angle glaucoma. Tr. Am. Ophthamol. Soc. 69:147–162 (1971).
3. Armaly, M.F. Selective perimetry for glaucomatous defects in ocular hypertension. Arch. Ophthalmol. 87:518–524 (1972).
4. Aulhorn, E. and Harms, H. Early visual field defects in glaucoma. In: Glaucoma, Symp. Tutzing Castle 1966. Leydhecker, W. (ed.), pp. 151–186, Karger, Basel/New York (1967).
5. Bengtsson, B., Holmin, C. and Krakau, C. E. T. Disc haemorrhage and glaucoma. Acta Ophthalmol. 59: 1–14 (1981).
6. Drance, S. M. The early field defects in Glaucoma. Invest. Ophthalmol. 8: 84–91 (1969).
7. Drance, S. M., Wheeler, C. and Pattullo, M. The use of static perimetry in the early detection of glaucoma. Can. J. Ophthalmol. 2:249–258 (1967).
8. Furuno, F. and Matsuo, H. Early stage progression in glaucomatous visual field changes. Doc. Ophthalmol. Proc. Series 19:247–253 (1978).
9. Greve, E. L., Furuno, F. and Verduin, W. M. A critical phase in the development of glaucomatous visual field defects. Doc. Ophthalmol. Proc. Series 19: 127–136 (1978).
10. Hart, W. M., Jr. and Becker, B. The onset and evolution of glaucomatous visual field defects. Ophthalmology 89:268–279 (1982).
11. Hart, W. M., Jr. and Hartz, R. K. Computer-generated display for three-dimensional static perimetry. Arch. Ophthalmol. 100:312–318 (1982).
12. Hart, W. M., Jr., Yablonski, M., Kass, M. A. and Becker, B. Multivariate analysis of the risk of glaucomatous visual field loss. Arch. Ophthalmol. 97:1455–1458 (1979).

48

13. Heijl, A. and Drance, S. M. A clinical comparison of three computerized automatic perimeters in the detection of glaucoma defects. Doc. Ophthalmol. Proc. Series 26:43—48 (1981).
14. Heijl, A., Drance, S. M. and Douglas, G. R. Automatic perimetry (COMPETER). Ability to detect early glaucomatous field defects. Arch. Ophthalmol. 98:1560—1563 (1980).
15. Herschler, J. and Osher, R. H. Baring of the circumlinear vessel. An early sign of optic nerve damage. Arch. Ophthalmol. 98:865—869 (1980).
16. Pederson, J. E. and Anderson, D. R. The mode of progressive disc cupping in ocular hypertension and glaucoma. Arch. Ophthalmol. 98:490—495 (1980).
17. Portney, G. L. and Krohn, M. A. The limitations of kinetic perimetry in early scotoma detection. Ophthalmology 85:287—293 (1978).
18. Werner, E. B. and Drance, S. M. Early visual field disturbances in glaucoma. Arch. Ophthalmol. 95:1173—1175 (1977).

Authors' address:
Dept. of Ophthalmology
Washington University School of Medicine
St. Louis, MO 63110
U.S.A.

CORRELATION BETWEEN THE STEREOGRAPHIC SHAPE OF THE OCULAR FUNDUS AND THE VISUAL FIELD IN GLAUCOMATOUS EYES

HAJIME NAKATANI and NORIHITO SUZUKI

(Osaka, Japan)

Key words. Stereoscopical measurement of ocular fundus, retinal excavation.

ABSTRACT

Vertical and equidistant parallel grating lines were projected onto the ocular fundus from the right side and the fundus was photographed in a routine manner. By means of analyzing the phase shift of the grating images on the ocular fundus, it became possible to measure the ocular fundus stereoscopically and quantitatively. In glaucomatous eyes with visual field changes, the excavation started in the retinal area and the corresponding visual field was damaged. We conclude that the glaucomatous visual field changes are due to degeneration of retinal ganglion cells and/or nerve fibers and the papillary changes are secondary to the results of nerve degeneration in the retina.

INTRODUCTION

We have been intending to develop a clinical method for measurement of the papillary excavation stereographically and quantitatively. Four years ago, at the International Symposium on Glaucoma in Japan, we reported that profiles of the ocular fundus were obtained by analyzing the grating images on the ocular fundus. Using this method, we showed that if the diameter of glaucomatous papillary excavation became larger and its depth deep enough its shape was transformed from a triangle to a trapezoid (3).

Because many profiles of an ocular fundus were obtained by analyzing grating images, the stereographic configuration of the ocular fundus were made by reconstruction of these profiles.

In the present report, we attempted to study the correlation between the stereographic configuration of the ocular fundus and the glaucomatous visual field referring to papillary excavation. Our results showed some doubt about the previous theory that glaucomatous visual field changes are due to primary disc changes.

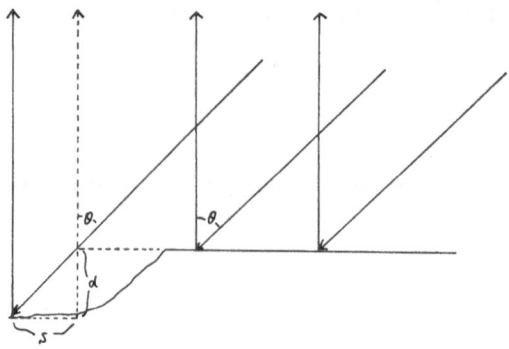

Fig. 1. The principle of the measurement of papillary excavation. $d \times \theta = s$.

METHOD

We used the idea that Holm and Krakau reported (1). Vertical and equidistant parallel grating lines were projected onto the ocular fundus from the right side, and the fundus was photographed in a routine manner. The angle between the incidence of the gratings and that of the fundus camera was 0.1 radian. Where the surface of the ocular fundus is in one level, the grating images on it should be straight. On the other hand, where the surface of the ocular fundus is not in one level, the grating images on it should be distorted, and a phase shift of grating images takes place (Fig. 1). For example, when depth is d, phase shift is s and angle is θ, we have the following relationships, $s = d \times \theta$; $d = s/\theta$ (Fig. 1). In the same manner, by means of analyzing the phase shift of all grating images on the ocular fundus, we were able to obtain profiles of the ocular fundus, and the stereographic configuration of the ocular fundus by reconstructing these profiles.

CLINICAL RESULTS

Case 1: 30-year old man with normal left eye.

The ocular fundus of this case showed no abnormalities ophthalmoscopically. Figure 2 demonstrates the ocular fundus with the grating images. Analyzing all these grating images on the ocular fundus and reconstructing these profiles, we were able to obtain a stereographic configuration of the papillary and the retinal surface. The physiologic excavation was located in the central area of the papilla and was cone-shaped. The rim of the papilla and the retina were in the same level (Fig. 3).

Case 2: 57-year old man with glaucomatous right eye with the visual field as shown in Fig. 4.

The papillary excavation of this case was not clear ophthalmoscopically.

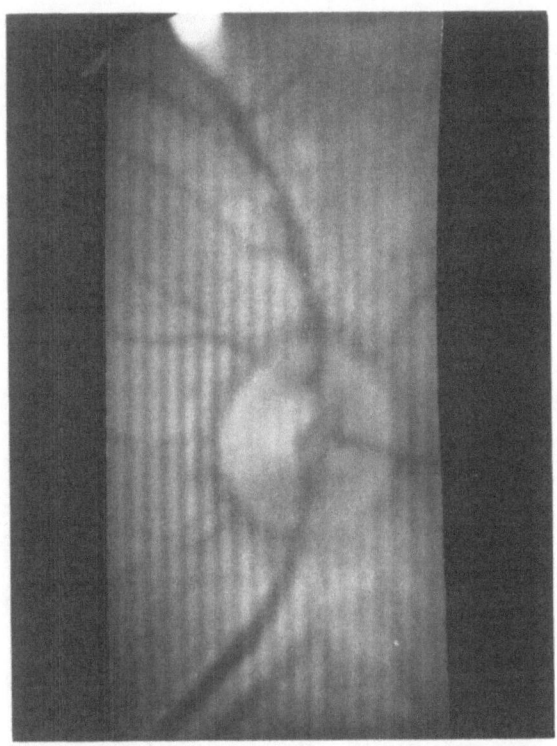

Fig. 2. The grating images on the retinal and papillary surface of case 1 (normal eye).

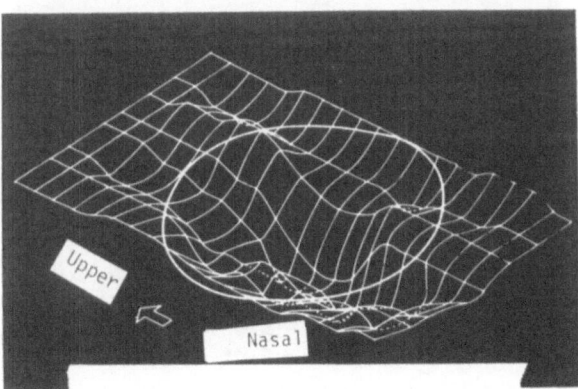

Fig. 3. Stereographic shape of retinal and papillary surface of case 1 (normal eye). Circle shows papilla-retina border.

Analyzing the grating images on the ocular fundus (Fig. 5), we were able to obtain a stereographic configuration of the papillary and retinal surface. The reconstructed retinal surface was not smooth but wrinkled. The excavation

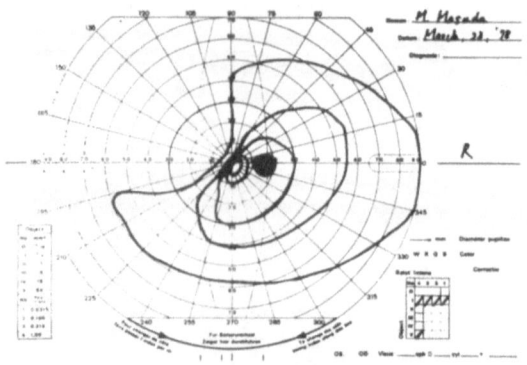

Fig. 4. The visual field of case 2.

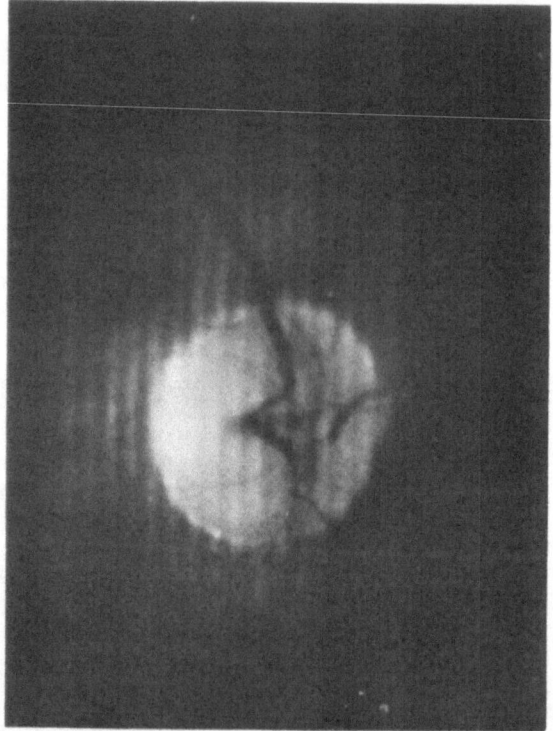

Fig. 5. The grating images on the retinal and papillary surface of case 2 (glaucomatous eye).

started in the retinal area and the corresponding visual field was damaged (Fig. 6).

Case 3: 45-year old woman with glaucomatous left eye with visual field as shown in Fig. 7.

54

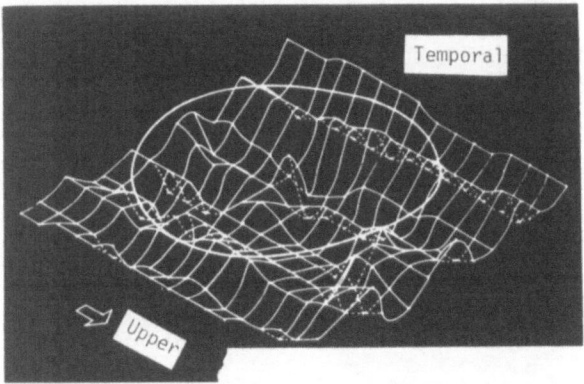

Fig. 6. Stereographic shape of retinal and papillary surface of case 2.

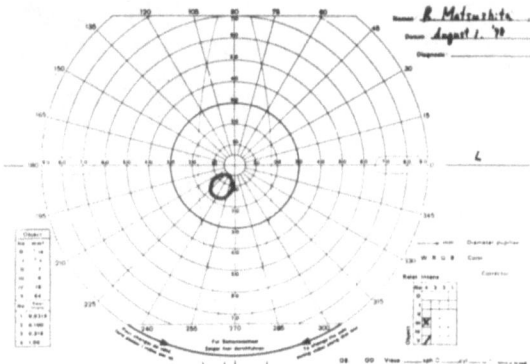

Fig. 7. The visual field of case 4.

Analyzing the grating images on the ocular fundus (Fig. 8), we were able to obtain the reconstruction of a stereographic configuration of the papillary and retinal surface (Fig. 9). In this case, distinct retinal excavation was observed with the rim of the papilla extensively destroyed. However, the upper nasal rim and the corresponding visual field remained unchanged.

DISCUSSION

Though there have been many theories regarding the cause of glaucomatous visual field defects, the theory that glaucomatous visual field defects are due to retrograde neural damage has been generally accepted. Following this theory, the disc damage due to increased intraocular pressure is incurred and primary visual field change is incurred, while the degeneration of ganglion cells and nerve fibers in the retina are secondary changes. When the disc is damaged first, the visual field changes of glaucoma should take place anywhere with the same probability. As a matter of fact, however, in the early stage of glaucoma, visual field changes exist in the peripapillary area.

55

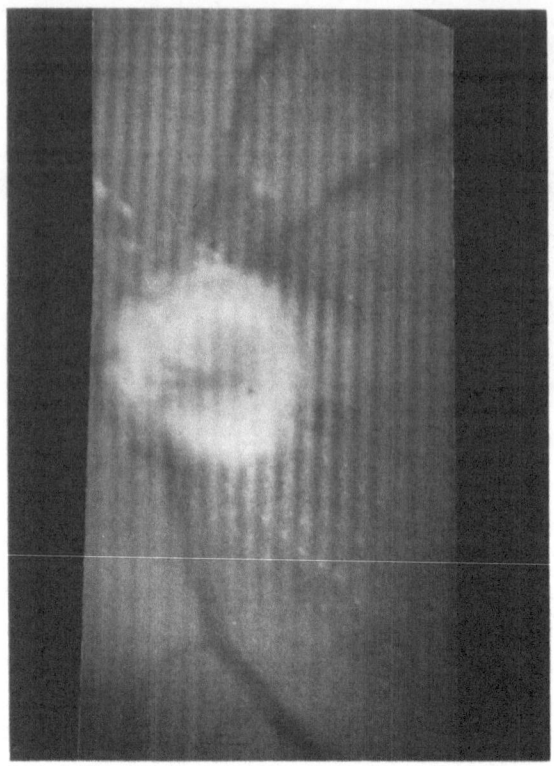

Fig. 8. The grating image on the retinal and papillary surface of case 3 (glaucomatous eye).

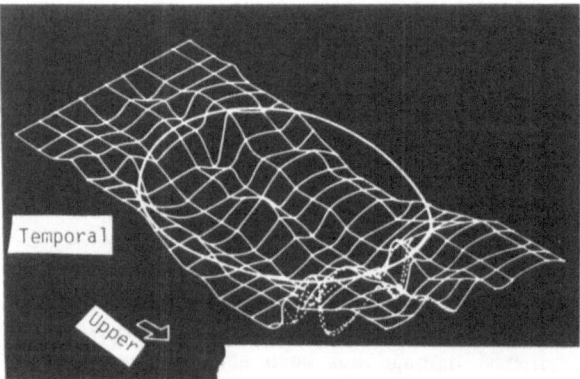

Fig. 9. Stereographic shape of retinal and papillary surface of case 3.

Matsumoto reported that the scleral deformation according to increased intraocular pressure, measured by laser holographic interferometry, was largest near the noptic nerve (Figs. 10, 11) (2). Following this report, it is reasonable

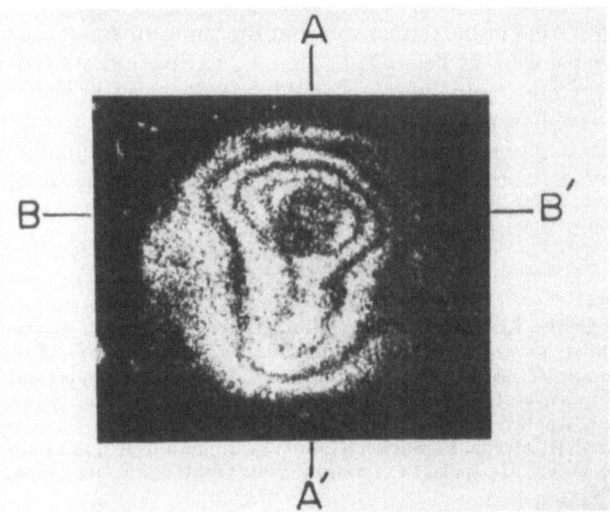

Fig. 10. Fringes of laser holographic interference pattern caused by increased IOP (2).

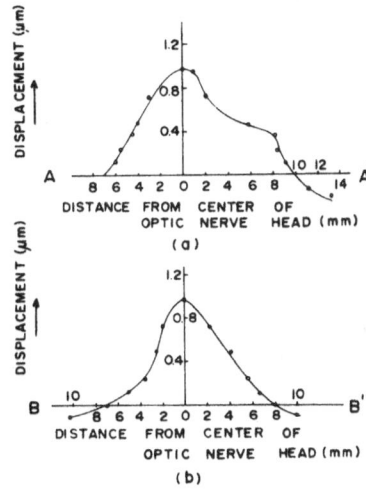

Fig. 11. Relative displacement of the sclera by increased IOP (2).

that the early change of glaucomatous visual field occurs near Mariott's spot. Accordingly one explanation of Matsumoto's report is the possibility that the glaucomatous visual field changes should be due to primary nerve degeneration in the retina.

In our results, the reconstructed retinal surface of the normal eye was smooth. The papillary excavation was located in the central area and was cone-shaped. At that time the rim of the papilla and the peripapillary retina were in the same level. The reconstructed retinal surface of the glaucomatous eye with visual field changes, on the other hand, was very wrinkled. The

57

excavation started in the retinal area and the smoothness of the corresponding rim of the papilla was destroyed. That is, excavation started in the retinal area and the corresponding visual field was damaged in glaucomatous eyes. Since we have never experienced that the area in undisturbed smoothness of reconstructed retina showed disturbance of the corresponding visual field, the destroyed smoothness was surely though to give some visual field defects.

REFERENCES

1. Holm, O. and Krakau, C. E. T. A photographic method for measuring the volume of papillary excavation. Ann. Ophthalmol. 1:327–332 (1969–1970).
2. Matsumoto, T., Nagata, R., Saishin, T. and Nakao, S. Measurement by holographic interferometry of the deformation of the eye accompanying changes in intraocular pressure. Applied Optics 17:3538–3539 (1978).
3. Nakatani, H., Maeda, K., Sumie, K., Suzuki, N., Satoh, H. and Yokozeki, S. A profile on the surface of papillary excavation. Folia Ophthalmol. Jap. 30:412–418 (1979).

Authors' addresses:
Hajime Nakatani
Dept. of Ophthalmology
Osaka University Medical School
Fukushima, Fukushimaku
Osaka 553
Japan

Norihito Suzuki
Dept. of Applied Physics
Osaka University
Faculty of Engineering
Yamadakami, Suitashi
Osaka 565
Japan

THE RELATIONSHIP BETWEEN A CIRCUMLINEAR VESSEL GAP AT THE NEURORETINAL RIM AND GLAUCOMATOUS VISUAL FIELD LOSS

GORDON BALAZSI and ELLIOT B. WERNER*

(Montreal, Quebec, Canada/Philadelphia, Pennsylvania, U.S.A.)

Key words. Glaucoma, ocular hypertension, optic disc, visual field.

ABSTRACT

We reviewed stereo disc photographs of 232 control, ocular hypertensive and glaucomatous patients to assess the value of baring of the circumlinear vessel of the optic nerve head as a sign of glaucomatous damage. We found a significant correlation between the presence of this sign and the diagnosis. The sign is rarely false positive. There is a 35% false negative rate in eyes with a circumlinear vessel and known glaucomatous visual field defects. However, the presence of a circumlinear vessel gap sign is generally associated with nerve head damage and always deserves further evaluation.

INTRODUCTION

Herschler and Osher (1) have recently described the circumlinear vessel of the optic nerve head. This blood vessel may be either an arteriole or a vein. It originates near, but not at the bifurcation of the central retinal vessels, runs along the margin of the optic cup and leaves the disc at its temporal margin to supply the macular area (Fig. 1). Since the location of this vessel defines the margin of the cup, when the cup enlarges in glaucoma, retinal or neurologic disease, a gap will appear between the margin of the damaged neuroretinal rim and this circumlinear vessel (Fig. 2). On the basis of their studies (1, 2), Herschler and Osher maintain that such a gap does not occur in normal eyes and is always a sign of optic nerve damage. In order to test this hypothesis, we reviewed a series of patients to see how well the presence of a circumlinear vessel gap was correlated with glaucomatous damage.

METHODS

We randomly selected 182 patients from the files of the glaucoma service of the Royal Victoria Hosptial. This population comprised 118 patients with

*To whom requests for offprints should be addressed.

Greve, E. L., Heijl, A. (eds.) Fifth International Visual Field Symposium.
©1983 Dr W. Junk Publishers, The Hague/Boston/Lancaster.

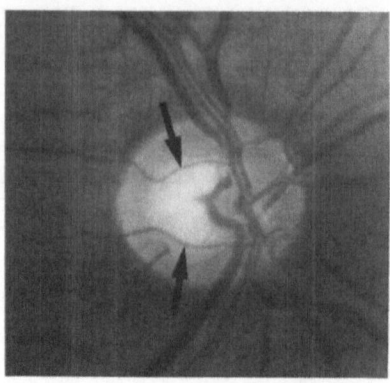

Fig. 1. Normal optic disc in right eye of 28-year old male control. Superior and inferior circumlinear vessels (arrows) closely follow the neuroretinal rim as they course temporally to supply the macular area.

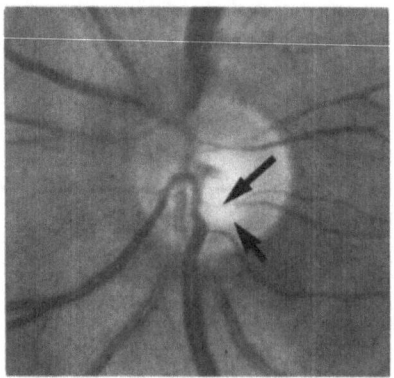

Fig. 2. Gap sign seen in left eye of 41-year old male glaucoma patient with a superior nerve fiber bundle visual field defect. A gap of pallor separates the inferior circumlinear vessel (long arrow) from the neuroretinal rim (short arrow).

persistently elevated ocular pressure but normal visual fields, 27 patients with elevated ocular pressures and a glaucomatous visual field defect in only one eye, and 37 patients with elevated pressures and field defects in both eyes. We also selected 50 normal individuals as controls. These were consecutively seen patients from the eye clinic presenting with minor superficial trauma, conjunctivitis, blepharitis, or small refractive errors. All controls had intra-ocular pressures less than 22, a visual acuity of 20/25 or better in each eye, normal visual fields, and no detectable intraocular or neurologic abnormality.

We reviewed the stereo disc photographs of all 464 eyes by shuffling the slides and presenting them randomly without reference to the diagnosis. We noted whether or not a circumlinear vessel was present, its location, and whether or not there was a gap between the vessel and the neuro-retinal rim. We then identified the patient on each slide and reviewed the diagnosis and visual field.

Table 1. Average age and intraocular pressure at time of initial examination in each group.

	No. of eyes	Mean age ± 1 standard deviation	Mean intraocular pressure ± 1 standard deviation
Controls	100	41.6 ± 15.5	16.3 ± 2.33
Elevated intraocular pressure normal visual fields both eyes	236	59.2 ± 14.6	27.3 ± 3.79
Elevated intraocular pressure uniocular visual field defect			
eye with no visual field defect	27	64.0 ± 15.0	26.6 ± 4.89
eye with visual field defect	27	64.0 ± 15.0	31.5 ± 6.79
Elevated intraocular pressure bilateral visual field defects	74	66.9 ± 14.0	29.0 ± 6.70

Table 2. Prevalence of a circumlinear vessel in the eyes of each study group. The prevalence data for a positive gap sign are indicated for those eyes which have a circumlinear vessel.

	No. of eyes	CLV present	Gap present
Controls	100	50 (50%)	3 (6%)
Elevated intraocular pressure normal visual fields both eyes	236	141 (60%)	30 (21%)
Elevated intraocular pressure uniocular visual field defect			
eye with no visual field defect	27	12 (44%)	8 (67%)
eye with visual field defect	27	16 (59%)	7 (44%)
Elevated intraocular pressure bilateral visual field defects	74	50 (68%)	36 (72%)
Total	464	269 (58%)	84 (31%)
Chi-square		$\chi^2 = 7.9$ N.S.	$\chi^2 = 73.6$ $p > 0.0001$

RESULTS

Table 1 shows the average age and intraocular pressure at the initial examination for each diagnostic category. The controls were significantly younger than each of the patient groups ($t = 8.36, p < 0.0001$).

Table 2 shows the prevalence of a circumlinear vessel in each diagnostic category and the prevalence of a gap in those eyes with a circumlinear vessel.

61

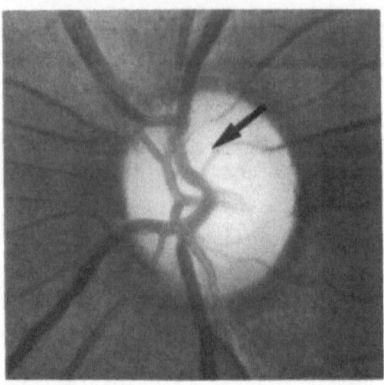

Fig. 3. Positive gap sign found in one of the 50 normal controls which had a circumlinear vessel. This patient is a 48-year old black female with intraocular pressures of 20 in both eyes and normal visual fields. This patient has a large cup/disc ratio for a normal patient and has a very small gap (arrow).

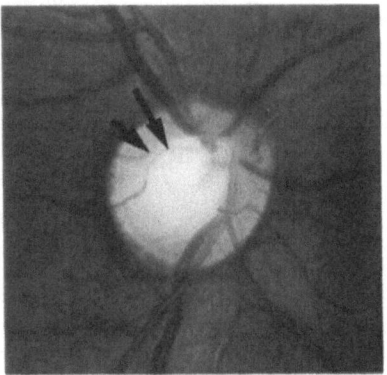

Fig. 4. Pseudogap sign. Careful observation reveals a small circumlinear vessel (small arrow) and no gap sign in right eye of 24-year old male control. The large vessel directly below it (large arrow) gave the initial impression of a positive gap sign.

There was no significant difference in prevalence of the presence of a vessel among the various groups. The differences in the prevalences of a gap in those eyes with a vessel were, however, significant.

DISCUSSION

The controls in our study were significantly younger than the patients. Although the effect of age on the size of the optic cup is a subject of some disagreement, most studies have not shown a clinically important effect of age alone on cup size (3–10). We felt, therefore, that the age differences in our sample would not affect the results.

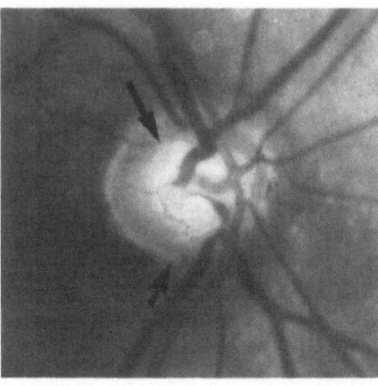

Fig. 5. False negative gap sign. A single superior circumlinear vessel (long arrow) in a patient with a superior nerve fiber bundle defect corresponding to a notch in the inferior neuroretinal rim (short arrow). The circumlinear vessel is thus not situated in the damaged area of the optic disc.

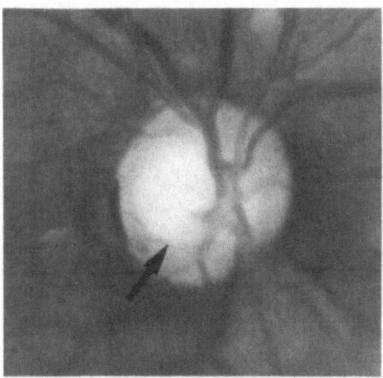

Fig. 6. False negative gap sign. A normal appearing circumlinear vessel at the inferior neuroretinal rim of an eye with an early superior nerve fiber bundle visual field defect (arrow).

Overall, 58% of the eyes in our study had a circumlinear vessel. This agrees well with the 64% prevalence reported by Herschler and Osher (1). The differences in the prevalences among the groups was not significant showing there was no correlation of the presence of a circumlinear vessel with glaucoma. There was, however, a strong correlation of the presence of a gap between a circumlinear vessel and the neuro-retinal rim with the diagnosis.

Of the 50 control eyes with a circumlinear vessel, we found a gap in only three for a false positive rate of 6%. One example is shown (Fig. 3).

In one of the controls, we found a vessel pattern which suggested the presence of a gap during the initial slide review. On close examination, however, this proved not to have a gap (Fig. 4). We call this the 'pseudogap' sign.

63

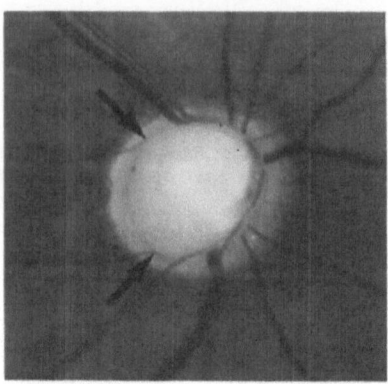

Fig. 7. False negative gap sign. Superior and inferior circumlinear vessels closely follow the neuroretinal rim (arrows) despite advanced glaucomatous optic disc cupping and visual field defects. The vessels seem to have receded with the cup.

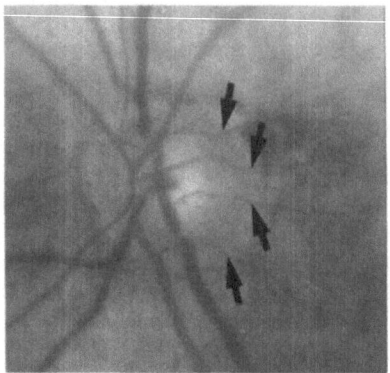

Fig. 8. False negative gap sign. In this patient with known glaucomatous visual field defects, it is unclear which vessels are circumlinear (arrows) and we were unable to assess their significance.

The prevalence of a gap sign in the patients with elevated intraocular pressure rises to 21%. This is significantly greater than the controls, but significantly less than the patients with established visual field defects. It would appear that any sample of so-called 'ocular hypertensives' contains an appreciable number of patients with early optic nerve damage, (1, 6, 11−13). Whether or not the presence of a gap sign can predict future visual field loss is a crucial question which will require a prospective study.

Of the 66 eyes with glaucomatous visual field defects, we found a circumlinear vessel gap in 43 or 65%, giving a false negative rate of 35%. On reviewing these 23 false negatives, we found that each disc fit one of four explanations for the absence of a gap. In nine cases, the circumlinear vessel was situated at an area on the disc not corresponding to the visual field defect (Fig. 5).

In five cases, a circumlinear vessel was associated with a small, very early visual field defect (Fig. 6). In eight cases of clearly advanced damage, the vessel gave the appearance of having receded with the cup (Fig. 7). In one case, the anatomy of the vessels was anomalous and we were confused as to which vessel was circumlinear (Fig. 8).

There is a strong statistical correlation between the presence of a circumlinear vessel gap sign and glaucomatous visual field defects. The sign may, however, be falsely negative in cases of very early field loss. There is also a significant prevalence of a gap sign in subjects with consistently elevated intraocular pressure and no visual field defect. The sign is rarely present in eyes which otherwise appear normal. Therefore, it seems safe to conclude that when present, a gap between a circumlinear vessel and the neuro-retinal rim is strong presumptive evidence of optic nerve damage and deserves further evaluation.

REFERENCES

1. Herschler, J. and Osher, R. H. Baring of the circumlinear vessel. An early sign of optic nerve damage. Arch. Ophthalmol. 98:865–869 (1980).
2. Osher, R. H. and Herschler, J. The significance of baring of the circumlinear vessel. Arch. Ophthalmol. 99: 817–818 (1981).
3. Snydacker, D. The normal optic disc. Am. J. Ophthalmol. 58: 958–964 (1964).
4. Armaly, M. F. Genetic determination of cup/disc ratio of the optic nerve. Arch. Ophthalmol. 78: 35–43 (1967).
5. Czechowicz-Janicka, K., Majewska, K., Przadka, L. et al. Surface and shape of the optic disc in healthy subjects in various age groups. Ophthalmologica (Basel) 174:261–265 (1977).
6. Leibowitz, H. M., Drueger, D. E., Maunder, L. R. et al. The Framingham Eye Study Monograph. Survey Ophthalmol. 24: Suppl:335–610 (1980).
7. Schwartz, B., Reinstein, N. M. and Lieberman, D. M. Pallor of the optic disc: Quantitative photographic evaluation. Arch. Ophthalmol. 89:278–286 (1973).
8. Schwartz, J. T., Reuling,F. H. and Garrison, R. J. Acquired cupping of the optic nerve head in normotensive eyes. Br. J. Ophthalmol. 59: 216–222 (1975).
9. Pickard, R. A method of recording disc alterations and a study of the growth of normal and abnormal disc cups. Br. J. Ophthalmol. 7: 81–90 (1923).
10. Pickard, R. The alteration in size of the normal optic disc cup. Br. J. Ophthalmol. 32:355–361 (1948).
11. Armaly, M. F. and Sayegh, R. E. The cup/disc ratio: The findings of tonometry and tonography in the normal eye. Arch. Ophthalmol. 82:191–196 (1969).
12. Becker, B. Cup/disc ratio and topical corticosteroid testing. Am. J. Ophthalmol. 70:681–686 (1970).
13. Werner, E. B., Saheb, N. and Thomas, D. Variability of static visual thresholds in patients with elevated IOPs. Arch. Ophthalmol. 100:1627–1631 (1982).

Authors' addresses:
Dr G. Balazsi,
Dept. of Ophthalmology
McGill University and Royal Victoria Hospital
Montreal, Quebec
Canada

Dr E. B. Werner
Scheie Eye Institute
51 North 39th Street
Philadelphia, PA 19104
U.S.A.

FLUORESCEIN ANGIOGRAPHIC DEFECTS OF THE OPTIC DISC IN GLAUCOMATOUS VISUAL FIELD LOSS

KATSUHIKO NANBA and BERNARD SCHWARTZ*

(Boston, Massachusetts, U.S.A.)

Key words. Absolute fluorescein filling defect, visual field loss, glaucoma, fluorescein angiography, optic disc.

ABSTRACT

The areas of absolute fluorescein filling defects of the optic discs of glaucoma patients and the areas of visual field, determined with the Goldmann perimeter, were measured by planimetry. There was a significant negative correlation between the percent areas of filling defects and the areas of the visual fields. With minimal field loss, the percent areas of filling defects were significantly greater in glaucoma patients than in comparable normal and ocular hypertensive patients. These observations support the concepts that fluorescein filling defects of the optic disc in patients with glaucoma, representing areas of ischemia, may both precede visual field loss and also are highly correlated with it.

INTRODUCTION

A number of studies have been done to evaluate the relationship between changes in the optic disc and changes in visual field that occur in patients with ocular hypertension and glaucoma (1, 2, 4, 6). These studies confirm that changes in the disc usually precede visual field changes in patients with early glaucoma.

Fluorescein angiography of the optic disc has shown that localized areas of filling defects or hypofluorescence occur in glaucomatous, ocular hypertensive, and normal eyes (5, 7). The filling defects are associated with the visual field loss in glaucoma (9, 10). The number and size of filling defects in the optic disc are greater in ocular hypertensive and glaucomatous individuals than in normal individuals (5, 7). A study of filling defects in the disc showed a high topographic correspondence with the site of the visual field loss and a qualitative relation between the area of the filling defect and the degree of visual field loss (3).

*To whom requests for offprints should be addressed.

Greve, E. L., Heijl, A. (eds.) Fifth International Visual Field Symposium.
©1983 Dr W. Junk Publishers, The Hague/Boston/Lancaster.

The purpose of this study was to characterize quantitatively the relationship between the area of a filling defect and the degree of visual field loss.

MATERIALS AND METHODS

Fluorescein angiograms of eyes from the following subject groups were analyzed: 74 eyes of 64 patients with glaucoma, 19 eyes of 19 ocular hypertensive individuals, and 22 eyes of 22 normal subjects. All of the individuals in each subject group were seen at New England Medical Center's Department of Ophthalmology.

Glaucomatous patients were those having ocular pressures equal to or greater than 21 mm Hg with typical glaucomatous optic disc and visual field changes.

The characteristics of the glaucoma population were as follows: forty-one patients were male and 33 were female. There were 57 whites and 17 non-whites. Of the glaucomatous eyes, all but five had a diagnosis of chronic open angle glaucoma. One eye had a diagnosis of chronic angle-closure glaucoma. Four had secondary open angle glaucoma. In two of these, the secondary glaucoma was attributable to blunt trauma, in one, to iritis, and in the fourth, to aphakic glaucoma.

Eighteen glaucomatous eyes had a paracentral scotoma; 26 had a paracentral scotoma and either a nasal or a temporal step; five had an arcuate scotoma; 14 had an arcuate scotoma, extending to the periphery; 11 had a field loss of one quadrant or more.

Ocular hypertensive subjects were those with ocular pressures equal to or greater than 21 mm Hg on at least two independent examinations, with normal visual fields, and either with or without glaucomatous optic discs. Normal subjects were those with no history of ocular trauma or inflammation, with ocular pressures less than 21 mm Hg on two or more occasions, and with normal visual fields.

All visual fields were determined with a Goldmann perimeter by static and kinetic perimetry. The area of each isopter was measured by planimetry with a compensating polar planimeter, excluding any defects.

The techniques used for fluorescein angiography of the optic disc and for reading the angiograms have been described previously (7). Only those filling defects that could be detected as areas that did not fill in the full arterial and venous phases of the angiogram were considered absolute filling defects and were selected for study. Informed consent was obtained from all patients and subjects undergoing fluorescein angiography.

The techniques for tracing the perimeters of absolute filling defects of the optic disc and for measuring their areas by planimetry have been described previously (3, 5). A planimetric measurement of the area of an absolute filling defect in an optic disc was expressed as a percentage of the area of the disc.

To determine the reproducibility of measurements of the areas of the visual fields by planimetry, the areas contained by the II-4-e isopter were measured on two independent occasions for 17 eyes with almost normal fields and for ten eyes with advanced field loss. The coefficients of variation

68

(standard deviation/mean × 100) for planimetry were 0.3% for the group with almost normal visual fields and 3.9% for the group with advanced visual field loss. To determine the reproducibility of the filling defects for the group with advanced field loss, we also traced and measured the filling defects on two occasions for 17 eyes with almost normal visual fields and for nine eyes with advanced field losses. The coefficient of variation for the group with almost normal visual fields was 5.3%. For the group with advanced visual field loss, the coefficient of variation was 2.1%.

For analysis when fluorescein angiograms were available for both right and left eyes of the same individual, only the eye with the greater area of visual field (i.e., the smaller visual field defect) was used. This determination was made independently for each isopter. Further, when an individual had a series of fluorescein angiograms, we selected only the angiogram that corresponded to the greatest area of visual field loss. This determination was also made independently for each isopter. Analyses were also done separately for only right or left eyes. A subject's visual field was usually tested at the same time the fluorescein angiogram was done, or within one to three weeks of the angiogram.

For statistical analyses the Mann-Whitney U test and the Spearman rank correlation were used for two-tailed tests (8). A p level of ≤0.05 was chosen as significant.

RESULTS

The relationships between the percentages of the area of a filling defect and the area of visual field for several isopters are shown in Figs 1 through 4, and the correlations are presented in Table 1. We found that the greater the area of a filling defect, the smaller the area of intact visual field.

Spearman correlation coefficients for the percent areas of filling defects are shown in Tables 1 and 2. The highest negative correlation was obtained in the II-4-e isopter (Tables 1 and 2). An analysis of the right and left eyes separately (Table 2) shows similar results to those found for samples consisting of both right and left eyes, but only one eye from each person.

When the frequency distribution of the filling defects in those glaucomatous patients with almost normal visual fields are compared with those showing more advanced field loss, the percent areas of the filling defects in the

Table 1. Spearman correlations (r_s) for percent area of filling defect vs area of visual field.[a]

Isopter	r_s	n	p
V-4-e	−0.5261	24	0.0083
III-4-e	−0.7052	21	0.0004
II-4-e	−0.8013	59	< 0.0001
I-4-e	−0.6013	21	0.0039
0-4-e	−0.4831	40	0.0016
0-3-e	−0.6240	19	0.0043

[a]Samples consist of right and left eyes, but only one eye for each person.

69

Table 2. Spearman correlations (r_s) for percent area of filling defect vs area of visual field for right (OD) and left (OS) eyes.

Isopter	OD			OS		
	r_s	n [a]	p	r_s	n [a]	p
V-4-e	−0.5000	13	0.0819	−0.3626	14	0.2026
III-4-e	−0.6818	11	0.0208	−0.6636	11	0.0260
II-4-e	−0.7957	39	<0.0001	−0.8634	33	<0.0001
I-4-e	−0.5874	12	0.0446	−0.7902	12	0.0022
0-4-e	−0.3019	26	0.1339	−0.8216	22	<0.0001
0-3-e	−0.5000	9	0.1705	−0.5385	12	0.0709

[a]Some individuals had both right and left eyes measured.

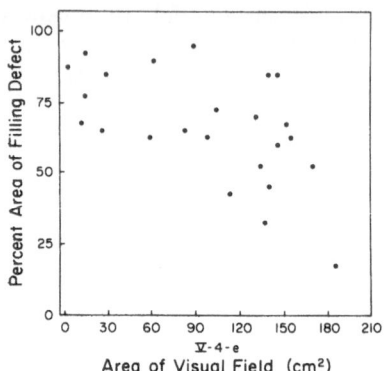

Fig. 1. The relationship between percent area of filling defect and area of intact visual field for the V-4-e isopter for glaucomatous eyes.

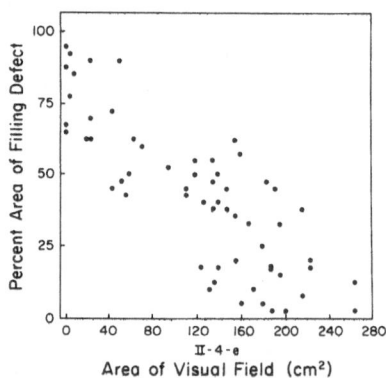

Fig. 2. The relationship between percent area of filling defect and area of intact visual field for the II-4-e isopter for glaucomatous eyes. Note scatter of areas of fluorescein defects at the level of 120 cm² to 220 cm² of the visual field.

discs of the eyes with almost normal fields are distributed over a wide range. This tendency is more obvious in the II-4-e and 0-4-e isopters than in other isopters (Figs. 2 and 4).

Figure 5 is a scatter plot showing percent area of filling defects for normal,

70

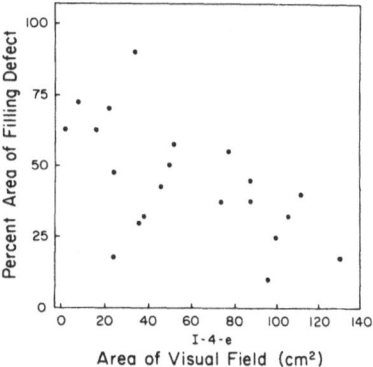

Fig. 3. The relationship between percent area of filling defect and area of intact visual field for the I-4-e for glaucomatous eyes.

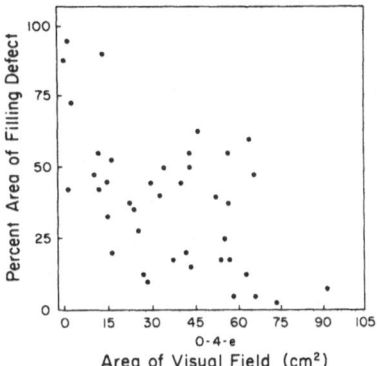

Fig. 4. The relationship between percent area of filling defect and area of intact visual field for the 0-4-e isopter for glaucomatous eyes. Note scatter of areas of fluorescein defects at the level of 37.50 cm² to 67.50 cm² area of the visual field.

ocular hypertensive, and glaucomatous patients with comparable areas of visual fields. To study the scatter of filling defects we chose glaucomatous patients whose visual fields (II-4-e isopter) were within the range of the mean area minus the standard deviation of normal subjects. For the normal group ($n = 29$) the mean plus or minus one standard deviation was 179 ± 23 cm². This sample consisted of the 22 normal individuals who were used in all other analyses in this study plus seven other normal individuals who were included in an attempt to obtain a better estimate of the mean area of the normal visual fields. For the ocular hypertensive group ($n = 19$) the mean of the area of the visual field plus or minus one standard deviation was 188 ± 18 cm². A glaucomatous group ($n = 22$) was selected whose visual field areas were comparable to the mean of the normal group minus one standard deviation that is greater than 156 cm². The mean area of visual field for this glaucomatous group plus or minus one standard deviation was 184 ± 29 cm². Mann-Whitney U tests were done for the II-4-e isopter only because this was

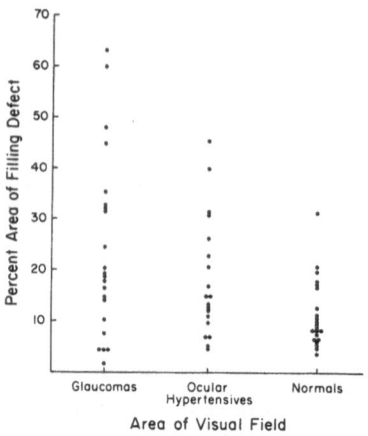

Fig. 5. Scatter plot of the percent area of filling defects vs the II-4-e isopter for glaucomatous, ocular hypertensive, and normal eyes.

a retrospective study and limited data for normal or ocular hypertensive subjects were available for the other isopters.

Mann-Whitney U testing revealed no significant differences in age between normal, ocular hypertensive, and glaucomatous subjects. There was a significant difference in the frequency distribution of the percent areas of filling defects in the II-4-e isopter for normal and chronic open angle glaucomatous subjects only (Mann-Whitney U = 141.5, p = 0.0183). A borderline significant difference was revealed in the percent areas of filling defects between normal and ocular hypertensive subjects (Mann-Whitney U = 135.0; p = 0.0530), but there was no significant difference between ocular hypertensives and open angle glaucoma subjects.

COMMENTS

The results of our study are consistent with the earlier finding of a negative correlation of the percent area of a filling defect with the area of visual field in glaucoma (3). The highest correlation is obtained for the II-4-e isopter. Comparisons between isopters are limited because our study was a retrospective one in which each patient was not tested for all isopters.

Our finding of a wide variation of percent areas of filling defects in the initial stage of field loss in glaucomatous patients indicates that the filling defects may precede the field loss (10). Our present study also confirms the finding that the frequency distribution of filling defects in glaucomatous patients is significantly greater than those for normal subjects even though the areas of the visual fields of the glaucomatous subjects may be within normal limits. Our finding of a borderline significant difference between normal and ocular hypertensive subjects supports the finding in a previous study of a greater area of fluorescein filling defects in ocular hypertensive eyes compared to normal eyes (5).

72

This study indicates that filling defects may precede visual field loss and that filling defects may increase in size as visual field loss progresses. These observations demonstrate that fluorescein angiography of the optic disc appears to be an important method for evaluating the vascular loss in the optic disc, especially in patients with ocular hypertension and early glaucoma.

ACKNOWLEDGEMENTS

Statistical analysis was done by Judith Barton, M.S., and editorial assistance was provided by Karen Mitzner, M.A.

This study was supported in part by a grant from Research to Prevent Blindness, Inc., New York, NY, and in part by a grant from the National Eye Institute of the National Institutes of Health, No. EY-00936.

REFERENCES

1. Armaly, M. F. The correlation between appearance of the optic cup and visual function. Trans. Am. Acad. Ophthalmol. Otolaryngol. 73:893–913 (1969).
2. Drance, S. M. Correlation of optic nerve and visual field defects in simple glaucoma. Trans. Ophthalmol. Soc. U.K. 95:288–296 (1975).
3. Fishbein, S. L. and Schwartz, B. Optic disc in glaucoma. Topography and extent of fluorescein filling defects. Arch. Ophthalmol. 95:1975–1979 (1977).
4. Hoskins, H. D., Jr and Gelber, E. C. Optic disc topography and visual field defects in patients with increased intraocular pressure. Am. J. Ophthalmol. 80: 284–290 (1975).
5. Loebl, M. and Schwartz, B. Fluorescein angiographic defects of the optic disc in ocular hypertension. Arch. Ophthalmol. 95:1980–1984 (1977).
6. Pederson, J. F. and Anderson, D. R. The mode of progressive disc cupping in ocular hypertension and glaucoma. Arch. Ophthalmol. 98:490–495 (1980).
7. Schwartz, B., Rieser, J. C. and Fishbein, S. L. Fluorescein angiographic defects of the optic disc in glaucoma. Arch. Ophthalmol. 95:1961–1974 (1977).
8. Siegel, S. Non-Parametric Statistics for the Behavioral Services. New York, McGraw-Hill, (1956).
9. Spaeth, G. L. Fluorescein angiography: Its contribution towards understanding the mechanisms of visual field loss in glaucoma. Trans. Am. Ophthalmol. Soc. 73:491–553 (1975).
10. Talusan, E. D., Schwartz, B. and Wilcox, L. M., Jr. Fluorescein angiography of the optic disc. A longitudinal follow-up study. Arch. Ophthalmol. 98:1577–1587 (1980).

Author's address:
Dr B. Schwartz
Dept. of Ophthalmology
New England Medical Center, Inc. and
Tufts University School of Medicine
171 Harrison Avenue
Boston, MA 02111
U.S.A.

CAPILLARY HYPERPERMEABILITY OF THE OPTIC DISC AND FUNCTIONAL EVOLUTION IN GLAUCOMA

F. CARDILLO PICCOLINO, P. CAPRIS and G. SELIS

(Genoa, Italy)

Key words. Optic disc, glaucoma, visual field, fluorescein angiography.

ABSTRACT

Perfusion defects of the optic disc are a very common angiographic finding in glaucoma and they were already correlated by many authors with visual field alterations. On the contrary a sectorial hyperfluorescence has not yet been regarded as a typical feature of glaucomatous optic disc. We observed it in one of 54 cases of ocular hypertension and in 14 of 35 cases of open angle glaucoma. Hyperfluorescence is secondary to the hyperpermeability of capillaries crossing hypossic areas of the disc and can be considered a consequence of tissue acidosis. Our investigations demonstrated that capillary hyperpermeability is a temporary finding and a sign of functional deterioration in the glaucomatous disease.

INTRODUCTION

Perfusion defects of the optic disc are a very common angiographic finding in glaucoma and they were already correlated with visual field alterations by many authors (3–5, 7). On the contrary, leakage of fluorescein has not yet been regarded as a typical feature of the glaucomatous disc. In this study we report our experience on comparison between perimetry and fluorescein angiography of the optic disc in ocular hypertension and glaucoma, correlated to both the hypofluorescence and hyperfluorescence alterations.

MATERIAL AND METHOD

Disc fluorescein angiography was performed in 54 eyes with chronic hypertension and in 35 eyes with open angle glaucoma. All cases had a follow-up time from 6 months to 2 years. Magnified disc images were examined to detect the following angiographic features: 1) absolute fluorescence defects persistent in all the angiographic series; 2) hyperfluorescence secondary to

Greve, E. L., Heijl, A. (eds.) Fifth International Visual Field Symposium.
©1983 Dr W. Junk Publishers, The Hague/Boston/Lancaster.

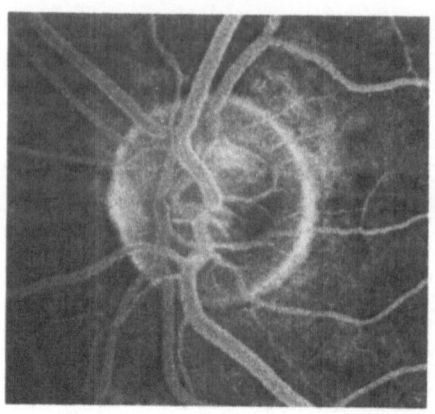

Fig. 1. Disc hyperfluorescence in a case of ocular hypertension.

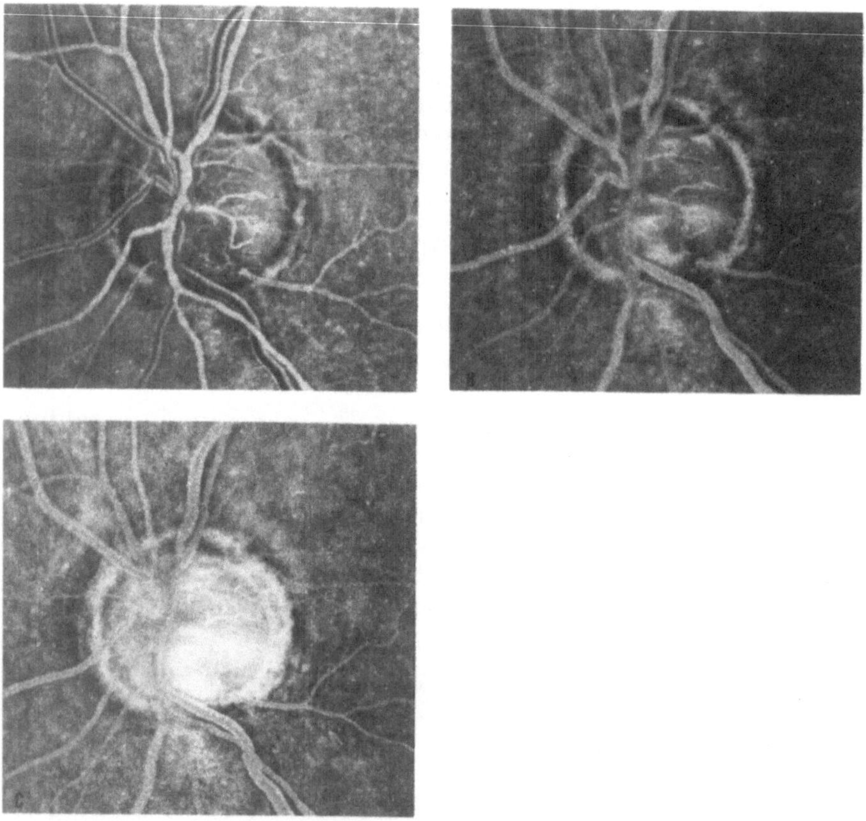

Fig. 2. Capillary leakage in a glaucomatous disc; (a, b, c): the angiographic series.

disc capillary hyperpermeability. Late peripapillary fluorescence, a common finding in normal conditions, was not considered in our study. The angiographic pattern of each case was correlated to the corresponding perimetric finding.

RESULTS

Disc areas of absolute hypofluorescence were present in 5 cases (9.2%) of ocular hypertension and in 33 cases (94.2%) of glaucoma. In ocular hypertension perfusion defects always included less than one disc sector. In glaucoma their extension exceeded one disc sector in 20 cases and involved the total disc area in 8 cases. Zones of hyperfluorescence were observed in 1 case (1.8%) of ocular hypertension (Fig. 1) and in 14 cases (40%) of glaucoma (Fig. 2, 3, 4). Fluorescein diffusion begun from the arterious-venous phase and increased in extension in the late phases. It was always located in areas of deep hypoperfusion of the papillary tissue. In 3 cases of glaucoma disc hyperfluorescence was no longer detectable after one year (Fig. 4), in 2 cases it reduced in extension after the same time. In glaucomatous patients visual field defects always corresponded to the disc areas of hypofluorescence. During the follow-up period further functional deteriorations appeared in 9 of the 14 cases (64%) with disc hyperfluorescence, (Fig. 5) and in 3 of the 21 cases (14%) without disc hyperfluorescence. The group with perimetric damage had frequently altered tension values. No modifications of either angiographic or perimetric findings were observed in cases of ocular hypertension.

DISCUSSION

The high percentage of absolute fluorescence defects in our cases of glaucoma is in agreement with previous observations (4, 7, 8).

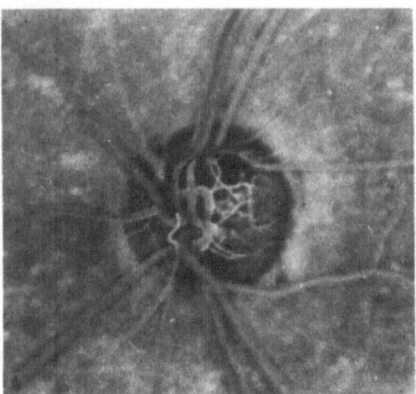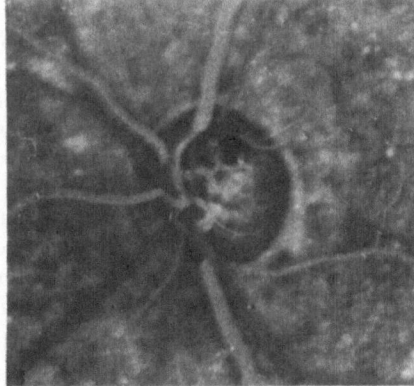

Fig. 3. Hyperpermeability of reticular capillaries crossing hypossic tissue.

77

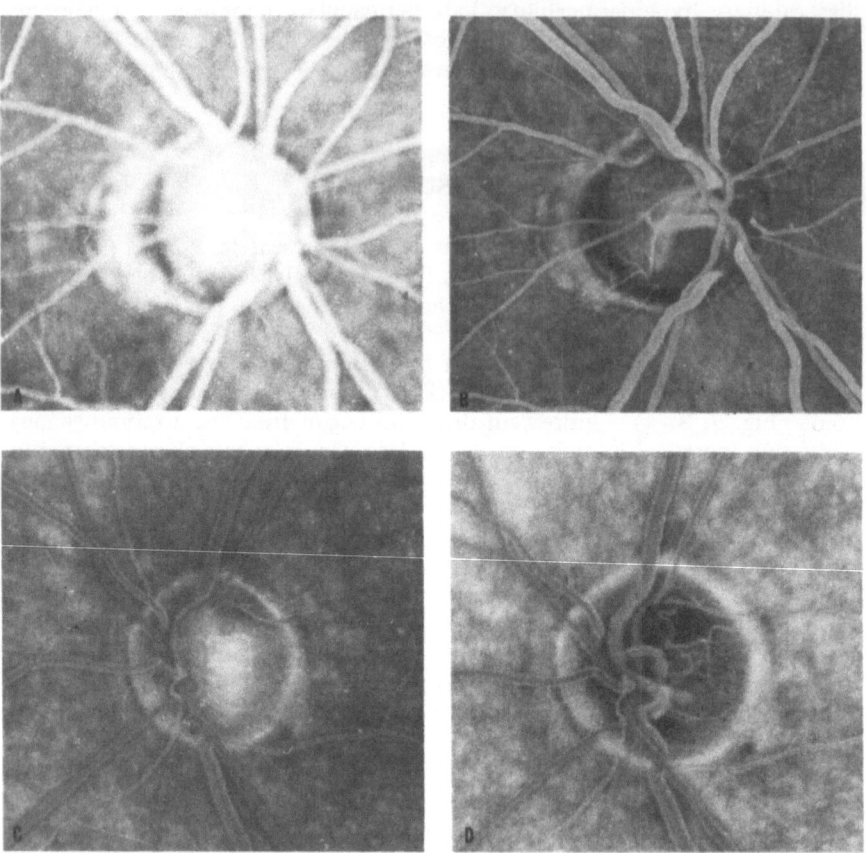

Fig. 4. Two cases of disc hyperfluorescence (a, c), disappeared after one year (b, d).

The hyperfluorescence disc areas are an evident sign of hypoperfusion and can be at present considered as a typical finding in glaucomatous disc. In our study a close relationship was always found between the size of hypoperfused areas and the extent of perimetric defects.

Absolute perfusion defects were also present in a few cases of ocular hypertension, which could support the vascular hypothesis of disc damage in glaucoma.

Late disc hyperfluorescence in glaucoma was previously reported by several authors (1, 2, 7–10) although with lower percentages than ours. This finding was explained as a staining of lamina cribrosa which is similar to the late peripapillary fluorescence observable in normal eyes (2).

In agreement with Tsukahara (10) we think that disc hyperfluorescence in glaucoma is due to the capillary hyperpermeability of the optic disc. In most of our cases the dye was observed leaking from capillaries of the prelaminar network.

78

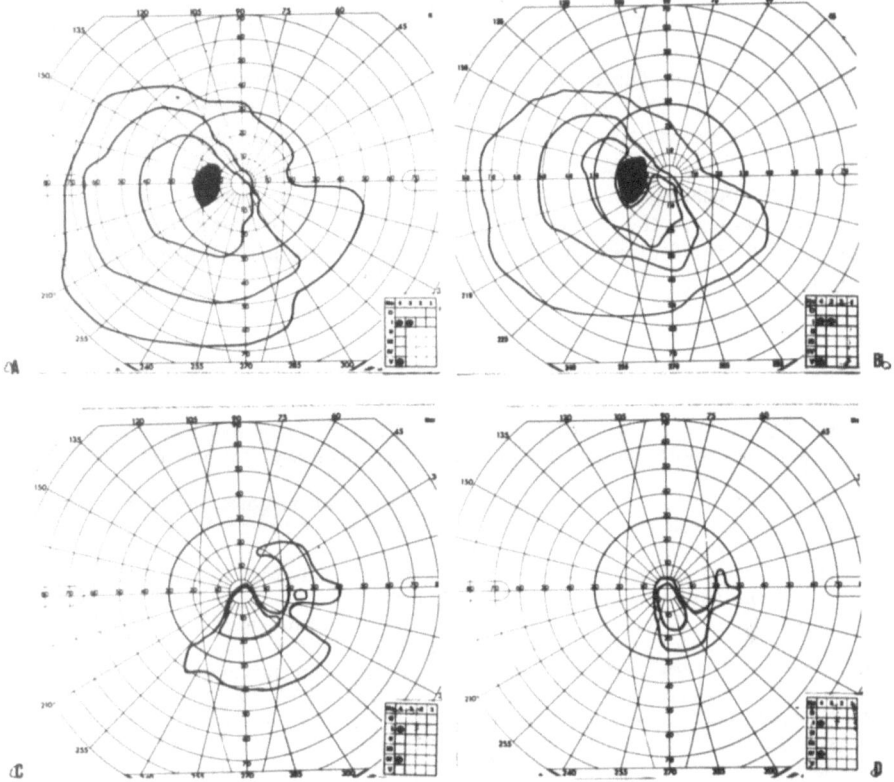

Fig. 5. Visual field deterioration in two cases of glaucoma with disc hyperfluorescence; (a, b): the case of Fig. 2; (c, d): the case of Fig. 4 (a, b).

The permeability alteration of these capillaries is not easy to explain. According to Tsukahara this finding cannot be correlated to a systemic vascular disease. We consider it of particular interest that in all cases of glaucoma the hyperpermeable vessels cross areas of hypoperfused tissue, or are located at their edges. Moreover a marked wall fluorescence is often limited to that vessel segment which runs across the ischemic area. Therefore vessel damage is in close relationship with the extension of the surrounding ischemic area and probably secondary to ischemia.

In the case of ocular hypertension with disc hyperfluorescence the hyperpermeable capillaries could mask a deep area of hypoperfusion.

A capillary leakage in the areas of ischemia has been already observed by Sonty and Schwartz in a fluorophotometric study on absolute perfusion defects in the optic disc (6).

In our opinion these capillary alterations are similar in nature to those observed in vessels crossing retinal ischemic areas and are probably due to the direct action of tissue acidosis in the hypossic areas. Retinal vessel hyperpermeability disappears after light coagulation of hypossic tissue. In the same way papillary leakage is a temporary finding as we observed in 5 cases. This means that the permeability changes disappear in both retinal and optic disc vessels as a consequence of tissue atrophy following tissue hypoxia.

Moreover, a high percentage of cases with disc hyperfluorescence had a progressive visual field reduction during the follow-up period. In the same group of eyes no variations in the size of disc perfusion defects have been observed.

By these considerations the detection of a capillary leakage in hypoperfused optic discs indicates the recent onset of circulatory disturbance in these cases. This could be the indirect sign of an evolving functional deterioration in the glaucomatous eye.

REFERENCES

1. Ben-Sira, I., Loebl, M., Schwartz, B. and Riva, C. E. In vivo measurements of diffusion of fluorescein into the human optic nerve tissue. Doc. Ophthalmol. Proc. 9:311–314 (1976).
2. Bonnet, M., Baserer, T. and Grange, J. D. Angiographie fluorescéinique de la paille dans l'hypertension oculaire et le glaucome. (Etude de 62 globes.) J. Fr. Ophtalmol. 2:239–246 (1979).
3. Hayreh, S. S. Pathogenesis of optic nerve damage and visual field defects in glaucoma. Doc. Ophthalmol. Proc. 22:89–109 (1980).
4. Oosterhuis, J. A. and Gortzak-Moorstein, N. Fluorescein angiography of the optic disc in glaucoma. Ophtalmologica 160:331–353 (1970).
5. Schwartz, B., Rieser, J. C. and Fisbein, S. L. Fluorescein angiographic defects of the optic disc in glaucoma. Arch. Ophthalmol. 95:1961–1974 (1977).
6. Sonty, S. and Schwartz B. Two-point fluorophotometry in the evaluation of glaucomatous optic disc. Arch. Ophthalmol. 98:1422–1426 (1980).
7. Spaeth, G. L. Fluorescein angiography: its contribution towards understanding the mechanism of visual loss in glaucoma. Trans. Am. Ophthalmol. Soc. 73:491–553 (1975).
8. Spaeth, G. L. The pathogenesis of nerve damage in glaucoma: contribution of fluorescein angiography. Grune & Stratton, New York (1977).
9. Talusan, E. D., Schwartz, B. and Wilcox, L. M. Fluorescein angiography of the optic disc. A longitudinal follow-up. Arch. Ophthalmol. 98:1579–1587 (1980).
10. Tsukahara, S. Hyperpermeable disc capillaries in glaucoma. Adv. Ophthalmol. 35:65–72 (1978).

Authors' address:
University Eye Clinic
Viale Benedetto XV, 5
16132 Genoa
Italy

OPTIC DISC CHANGES WITH THE PROGRESSION OF GLAUCOMATOUS VISUAL FIELD DAMAGE

KUNIYOSHI MIZOKAMI, KIYOSHI OKUBO and YOSHIMASA ISAYAMA

(Kobe, Japan)

Key words. Glaucoma, progression of visual field, cup size, fluorescein angiogram.

ABSTRACT

It is not clearly defined yet whether the early glaucomatous visual field damage originates in vasogenic or mechanical changes at the optic disc.

In the present study, we determined whether changes occur in fluorescein angiographic filling pattern and in cup size change with the development of new visual field damage. Our subjects comprised three ocular hypertensive and five primary open angle glaucoma patients.

For the purpose of exact determination of cupping changes to visual field correlation, we employed cup-to-disc area ratio (C/D.A.) at each side of the disc (upper and lower).

The change of cup size (C/D.A.) provided a direct correlation to newly developed visual field damage especially in early stage glaucoma, while angiographic filling defects could not provide a good correlation to visual field in ocular hypertension and early stage glaucoma.

From these results it would be surmised that. the fluorescein angiographic disc capillary dropout is a secondary event after nerve fiber loss has begun to occur.

INTRODUCTION

It is not clearly defined yet whether the early glaucomatous visual field damage originates in vasogenic or mechanical changes at the optic disc.

In a previous study (1, 2). we demonstrated that the fluorescein angiogram provides a good correlation of changes in the optic disc with visual field loss, but in recent studies, Quigley et al. (4) reported that histologically no selective damage to nerve head capillaries was seen in mildly damaged glaucoma specimens. While poor vascular supply may be an important step in the pathogenesis of glaucoma nerve damage, anterior disc capillary dropout might alternatively be a secondary event after nerve fiber loss has begun to occur.

Greve, E. L., Heijl, A. (eds.) Fifth International Visual Field Symposium.
©*1983 Dr W. Junk Publishers, The Hague/Boston/Lancaster.*

Table 1. Ocular hypertension.

| | Initial age | Sex | Follow-up period | Cup/disc area ratio (%) | | | |
| | | | | Initial | | End of follow-up | |
				upper	lower	upper	lower
Case 1	42	M	7 yrs. 8 mo.	47	51	50	55
Case 2	38	M	4 yrs. 10 mo.	24	30	27	34
Case 3	41	F	7 yrs. 7 mo.	40	35	38	34

The purpose of this study was to determine whether changes occur in fluorescein angiographic filling pattern and in cup size changes, with the development of new visual field damage.

By following up patients with serial disc fluorescein angiogram and stereoscopic disc photograph, we wish to make it clear which changes precede; the vascular changes or cup size change.

SUBJECTS AND METHODS

Our subjects comprised three patients with ocular hypertension and five primary open angle glaucoma patients in whom visual field defects developed during the course of their follow-up (Table 1). Follow-up periods were five to eight years. During the course all patients had received ocular medication to lower their IOP. The disc fluorescein angiograms and stereoscopic disc photographs of these subjects were carried out several times during each course. Visual fields were measured by Goldmann perimeter. The method for carrying out the fluorescein photogram and stereoscopic disc photograph has been reported previously (1). For exact determination of cup to field correlation disc photographs were positioned in a slide projector and were magnified by about 20 times, then disc and cup margins were traced on paper. The margin of the cup was given by a stereoscopic photograph.

Each disc tracing was divided into both an upper and lower half along the 180 degree meridian, and cup-to-disc area ratios (C/D.A.) at both sides were calculated using a planimeter.

The comparison of fluorescein angiogram was then followed by the side-by-side sequential projection taken on each date, comparing them phase by phase with particular attention to any difference in the filling pattern between the two angiograms.

RESULTS

Ocular hypertension (Case 1–3, Table 1)

In ocular hypertensive patients, we detect no clear changes in cup size (C/D.A.) (under 4%) and in angiographic filling pattern during the course of follow-up. In the first and second cases angiographic filling defects were clearly seen on

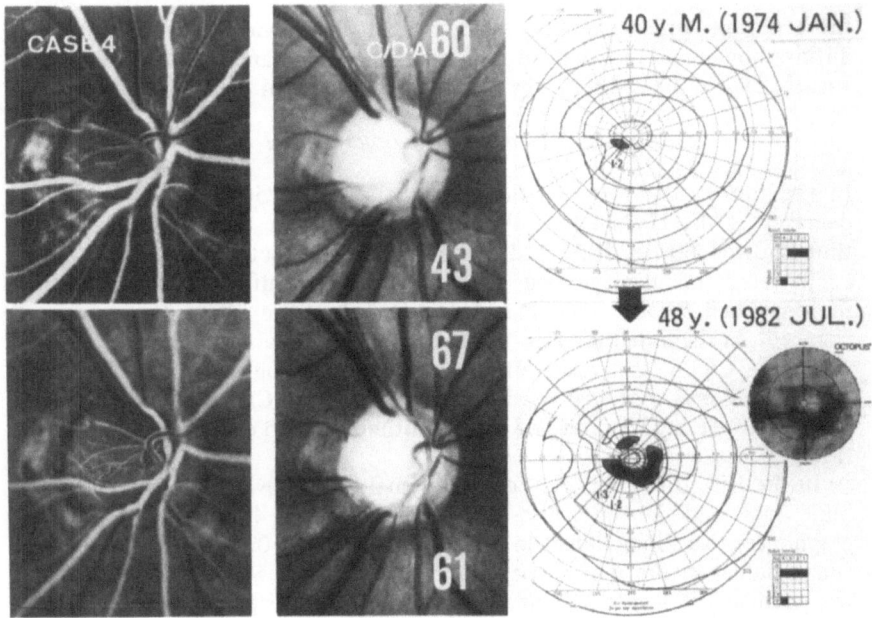

Fig. 1. Case 4, POAG.

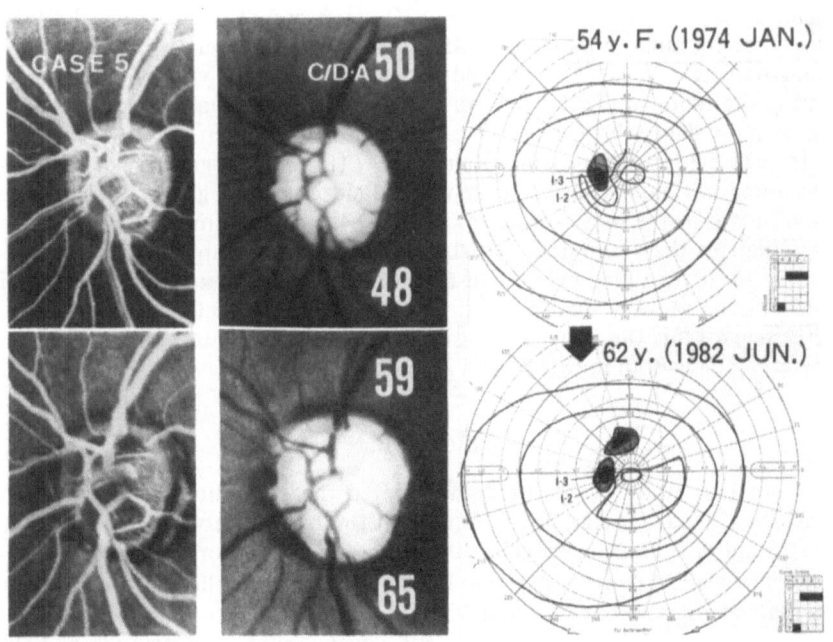

Fig. 2. Case 5, POAG.

the lower and upper part of disc cupping but no obvious changes were seen during the course. In the third case, no filling defect and no change was seen. Visual fields in these three cases remained normal until the end of follow-up.

Primary open angle glaucoma (Figs. 1 & 2).

In the fourth case (Fig. 1), the lower half of the visual field was already damaged at the beginning of this follow-up, and the upper half disc at this time showed 60% C/D.A. and absolute filling defect on angiogram. After eight years this damage had progressed with significant enlargement of scotoma, and C/D.A. was changed to 67% but the filling defect was unchanged. At the initial time the upper half of the visual field remained normal with 43% C/D.A. and relative filling defect on angiogram. After eight years newly developed scotomas were seen at this area and C/D.A. was significantly changed to 61% (an increase of 18%) but there was no change in angiographic filling defect.

In the fifth case (Fig. 2), the initial visual field showed enlargement of the blind spot, and the optic disc at that time showed 48% C/D.A. and angiographic relative filling defect in the lower part, and 50% C/D.A. and absolute filling defect in the upper disc. After eight years newly developed scotoma was seen at the upper half of the visual field. Corresponding with this progression of damage, C/D.A. was significantly changed to 65% (an increase of 17%) but angiographic relative filling defect was unchanged.

Until the end of the follow-up, the lower half of the visual field remained normal with angiographic absolute filling defect. While the C/D.A. was changed to 59% (an increase of 9%). Cases 6 and 7 were more advanced stage patients than cases 4 and 5. In their angiograms relative and absolute filling defects were clearly observed corresponding to the visual field damage. During the follow-up C/D.A.'s were changed with the visual field progression, but no more detectable changes were seen in the angiogram.

In case 5 (upper part of disc) and case 7 (lower), progression of cupping was noted without any change in visual field and angiogram. The last case (case 8) was in the most advanced stage. At the initial time of follow-up the lower part of the visual field had already completely disappeared with angiographic absolute filling defect and 69% C/D.A. The upper part of the visual field was moderately damaged with relative filling defect and 67% C/D.A. After seven years the visual field was slightly advanced, but no more changes were detectable both in C/D.A. and angiogram.

DISCUSSION

In a previous study (1, 2), we demonstrated that the fluorescein angiogram provides a good correlation of changes in the optic disc with glaucomatous visual field defects. Poor vascular supply may be an important step in pathogenesis of glaucoma nerve damage, but anterior disc capillary dropout might alternatively be a secondary event after fiber loss has begun to occur.

Talusan et al. (6) reported that the development of a new visual field defect is associated with angiographic changes of circulation of the optic disc.

In this study, especially in ocular hypertensive and early glaucomatous patients, angiographic filling defect could not provide a good correlation to newly developed visual field damage.

On the contrary, the second case showed reversed correlation between angiographic filling pattern and progression of visual field damage. The lower half of the visual field remained normal with absolute filling defect, but in the upper half newly developed scotoma was seen with no change relating to filling defect, while in the more advanced stage (cases 6, 7 and 8) angiographic filling defect provided a good correlation to their visual field damage, but development of new visual field defects were never associated with newly developed angiographic changes.

However, in our previous study (1, 2), the quantitative calculation of angiographic disc capillaries demonstrated statistically a significant difference between the normal and early glaucomatous optic disc which damage is not detected by Goldmann perimeter. In the early glaucomatous disc a mild diminishing of fluoresceins might occur.

So it might be suggested that visible changes in a filling defect by angiography indirectly reflect events more posteriorly at the actual site of the damage.

On the other hand, Pederson et al. (3) reported that progression of disc cupping often precedes visual field progression from elevated IOP and the mode of early progression is usually a generalized expansion of the cup.

For the purpose of exact determination of cupping changes to visual field correlation, we employed cup-to-disc area ratio (C/D.A.) at each side of the disc. In this determination we could make it clear that the cup size changes provide a direct correlation to newly developed visual field damage especially in early glaucomatous stage.

Furthermore, progression of disc cupping occasionally preceded the detection of visual field damage by Goldmann perimeter. Quigley et al. (4, 5) demonstrated that histologically definite diffuse loss of axons occur prior to reproducible visual field defects in some patients suspected of having glaucoma. The cup size enlargement prior to detection of visual field damage in our cases 5 and 7 might be an early glaucomatous stage that axons are being lost diffusely.

From these results, it would be surmised that the fluorescein angiographic disc capillary dropout is a secondary event after nerve fiber loss has begun to occur.

REFERENCES

1. Mizokami, K., Uchizono, H., Isayama, Y. and Yamanaka, A. Volume of the optic cup and fluorescein angiography in glaucoma. Acta Soc. Ophthalmol. Jap. 79:93–100 (1975).
2. Mizokami, K. and Uchizono, H. Optic disc changes in early glaucomatous eyes. Excerpta Medica, International Congress Series 450:1457–1461 (1978).
3. Pederson, J. E. and Anderson, D. R. The mode of progressive disc cupping in ocular hypertension and glaucoma. Arch. Ophthalmol. 98:490–495 (1980).
4. Quigley, H. A., Addicks, E. M., Green, W. R. and Maumenee, A. E. Optic nerve damage in human glaucoma. II. The site of injury and susceptibility to damage. Arch. Ophthalmol. 99:635–649 (1981).

5. Quigley, H. A., Addicks, E. M. and Green, W. R. Optic nerve damage in human glaucoma. III. Quantitative correlation of nerve fiber loss and visual field defect in glaucoma, ischemic neuropathy, papilledema, and toxic neuropathy. Arch. Ophthalmol. 100:135–146 (1982).
6. Talusan, E. D., Schwartz, B. and Willcox, L. M. Fluorescein angiography of the optic disc. A longitudinal follow-up study. Arch. Ophthalmol. 98:1579–1592 (1980).

Authors' address:
Dept. of Ophthalmology
School of Medicine
Kobe University
Kusunoki-cho, 7-chome, Chuo-ku
Kobe 650
Japan

OPTIC DISC ANALYSIS BY COMPUTERIZED IMAGE SUBTRACTION AND PERIMETRY

F. CARDILLO PICCOLINO, G. C. PARODI and F. BELTRAME

(Genoa, Italy)

Key words. Optic disc, glaucoma, visual field, image subtraction.

ABSTRACT

A computerized method of image subtraction was used to analyze the optic disc in 20 cases of open angle glaucoma. From the photographic and angiographic images of the optic disc a third image was obtained with a point by point subtraction of the density levels. The resulting image was displayed on a monitor and an arbitrary color scale clearly showed the areas where pallor and hypofluorescence overlap in the same papillary sector. The method allowed for the detection of 'critical areas' in the optic disc that showed a close correlation to the location of the perimetric defect.

INTRODUCTION

Pallor is a classic sign of optic disc damage in glaucoma. However its evaluation depends on many different factors:objectivity of the observer, kind of light used in fundus examination, contrast in color tonalities of the various anatomical elements in the papillary and peripapillary areas. Different colorimetric and densitometric techniques were previously used to obtain a quantitative and objective analysis of this parameter (1, 3, 5).

The angiographic features of the optic disc in glaucoma are also susceptible to different subjective interpretations. Perfusion defects generally are easily detectable, but in some cases the evaluation is uncertain because it is based on the comparison of minimal differences in optical densities.

Previously we used a computerized method of image equidensitometric elaboration to objectively evaluate disc pallor and fluorescein injection defects in glaucoma (6). We observed a close correlation between perimetric alterations and disc areas with concomitant pallor and hypofluorescence. In this study we propose a computerized system of image subtraction for a more direct detection of such pathological disc areas. We have previously introduced this method to quantify fluorescein diffusion in diabetic retinopathy (2).

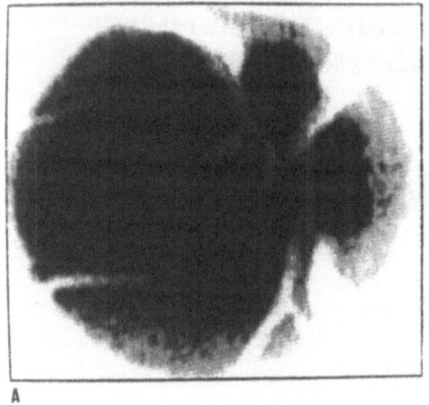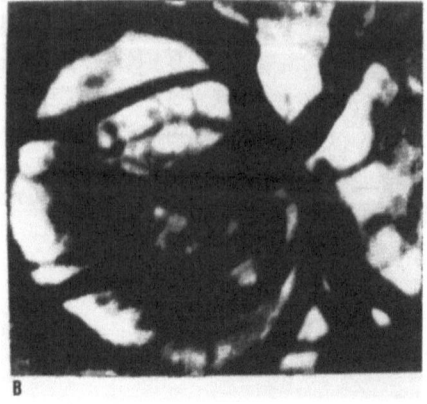

Fig. 1. The two disc images stored by the computer; (a) the photographic image; (b) the angiographic image.

MATERIALS AND METHODS

We used an automated image analyzer controlled by a minicomputer. After the storage of two images the system is programmed to obtain a third image which is the subtraction, point by point, of the density values of the two images.

The two images, taken by a TV camera, refer to red free light photogram and the angiogram in the early venous phase of the same optic disc (Figs. 1a, b).

The region of the image to be analyzed (the papillary area) is 'extracted' by using a 'window' programmable as to size and position. Properly chosen reference points allow alignment of the images. The selected sub-images are subtracted point by point, specifically the angiographic from the photographic one. A difference image is obtained in which the picture point with positive density difference are the only ones to be visualized. They are displayed according to a linear grey level scale corresponding to the subtraction computed values.

To enhance the results the system provides a pseudocolor transformation of the same image. Figure 2 shows the procedure used to match the pseudocolor scale to the grey scale. Chromatic tonalities ranging between red and white allow the distinction of picture point with different subtraction values.

We set our color-matching program so as to avoid the appearance of white color in ten normal cases which were tested. Therefore white areas could be obtained only if high difference values were present in the subtraction image. Such areas had to be the sign of superposition of pallor and deep hypofluorescence in the same district of the disc (Fig. 3a).

By this method we studied the optic disc in 20 cases of open angle glaucoma. Perimetric defects were present in only one visual field quadrant of each case. 15 of these cases had been previously studied by computerized equidensitometry (6).

88

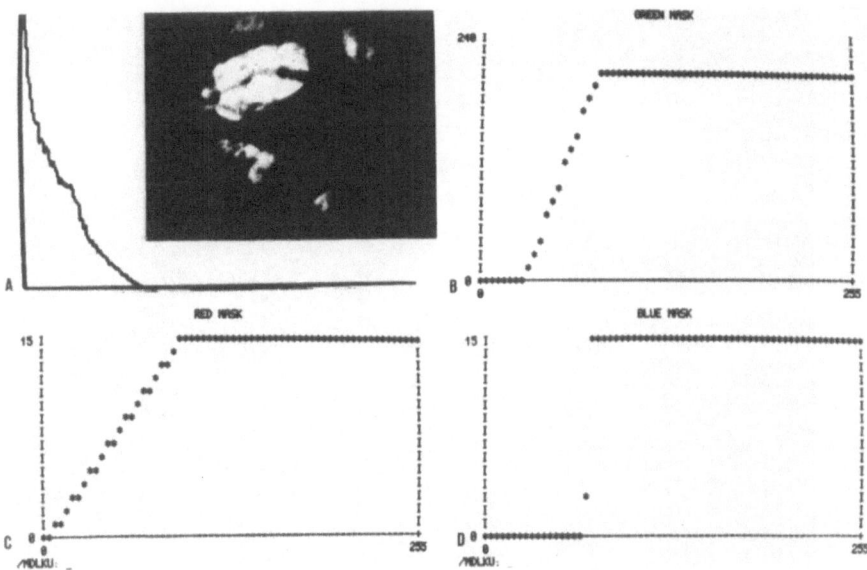

Fig. 2. (a) Disc subtraction image in grey scale; (b, c, d) green, red and blue intensities vs grey levels.

RESULTS AND CONSIDERATIONS

In all examined cases the disc subtraction image presented more or less wide areas with colors ranging between yellow and white. These areas with the highest values of the densitometric gradient revealed the concomitance of pallor and hypofluorescence in the same papillary sector. In each case the perimetric defects corresponded to the location of these areas on the optic disc (Fig. 3b). Therefore our method allows for the direct display of 'critical' zones of the disc probably due to a severe vascular disturbance. Detection of such areas can be considered as a significant index of the existence of a visual field defect in the corresponding sector.

The computerized image subtraction method is also able to assign a numerical value to the degree of disc damage. Since the major difference values correspond to the amjor degree of pallor and hypofluorescence, the optic disc damage could be quantitatively expressed with the quotient:

$$Q = \frac{\bar{d} \cdot \Sigma n_d}{\Sigma n_t}$$

where $\bar{d}$ is the mean subtraction value, n_d is the number of picture points in the difference image, n_t is the total number of points in the analyzed area.

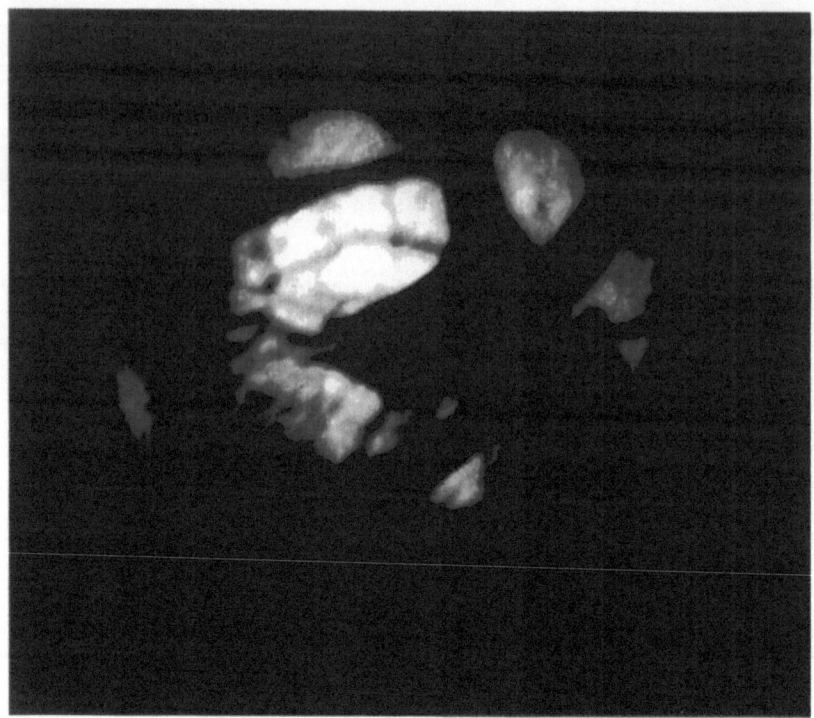

a

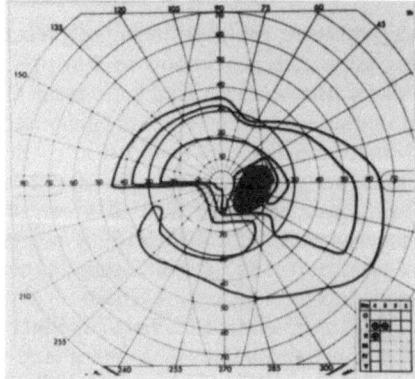

b

Fig. 3. (a) Subtraction image displayed in color scale corresponding to a glaucomatous disc; (b) visual field in the same case.

Detecting the 'critical' disc areas and measuring the papillary damage in large and longitudinal studies could probably allow us to obtain further information on the correlation between anatomical and functional damage in glaucoma.

90

ACKNOWLEDGEMENT

This study was supported by a grant from Consiglio Nazionale delle Ricerche, Roma, Italy.

REFERENCES

1. Berkowitz, J. S. and Balter, S. Pallor of the optic disc. Am. J. Ophthalmol. 69: 385–386 (1970).
2. Cardillo Piccolino, F., Beltrame, F. and Parodi, G. C. Valutazione quantitativa dell' edema retinico nella retinopatia diabetica: methodo computerizzato di sottrazione fluoroangiografica di fase. Boll. Oculist. 1–2:59–55 (1982).
3. Davies, E. W. G. Colorimetric measurement of the optic disc. Exp. Eye Res. 9: 106–113 (1970).
4. Drance, S. M. Correlation between optic disc changes and visual field defects in chronic open angle glaucoma. Trans. Am. Acad. Ophthalmol. Otolaryngol. 81: 224-226 (1976).
5. Rosenthal, A. R., Falconer, D. G. and Barret, P. Digital measurement of pallor disc ratio. Arch. Ophthalmol. 98:2027–2031 (1980).
6. Zingirian, M., Rolando, M. and Cardillo Piccolino, F. Relationship between fundus densitometric analysis and perimetry. Doc. Ophthalmol. Proc. Ser. 26:389–393 (1981).

Authors' address:
University Eye Clinic
Viale Benedetto XV, 5
16132 Genoa
Italy

DISCUSSIONS

Discussions of papers on fluorescein angiography of the optic disc.
1. 'Fluorescein angiographic defects of the optic disc in glaucomatous visual field loss', by K. Nanba and B. Schwartz.
2. 'Optic disc changes with the progression of glaucomatous visual field damage', by K. Mizokami, K. Okubo and Y. Isayama.
3. 'Capillary hyperpermeability of the optic disc and functional evolution in glaucoma', by F. Cardillo Piccolino, P. Capris and G. Selis.

S. S. Hayreh: In the literature there are a large number of fluorescein fundus angiographic studies on the optic disc in glaucoma and allied disorders, demonstrating circulatory disturbances in the disc. I would like to comment on the paper by Piccolino et al. about the staining of the optic disc in these eyes. We have investigated prospectively by fluorescein fundus angiography over one hundred eyes with ocular hypertension, open angle glaucoma and low-tension glaucoma. Our studies so far indicate that optic disc staining is seen in about a third of the open angle glaucoma cases and in about one sixth of those with low-tension glaucoma and those with ocular hypertension. Our findings indicate that this staining involves only a segment of the disc — mostly in the temporal region, and does not represent staining of the collagen of the lamina cribrosa. It showed no definite relationship to the intraocular pressure at the time the angiography was performed. We have found no evident factor showing a correlation with the late staining of the disc. Thus, the pathogenesis of segmental optic disc staining on fluorescein fundus angiography in ocular hypertension, open angle glaucoma and low-tension glaucoma remains unclear.

B. Schwartz: I wish to make several points regarding fluorescein angiography of the optic disc, based on our extensive experience of taking over one thousand fluorescein angiograms. First, one must determine whether the areas of disc hypofluorescence represent relative or absolute filling defects. The absolute defect persists throughout the entire fluorescein angiogram and is easier to read and detect than the relative defect which either fills slowly or incompletely during the cycle of the angiogram.

My comments will be limited to our observations on the absolute fluorescein filling defects. Absolute defects are seen in essentially all open angle glaucomatous patients with visual field loss (5). The fluorescein filling defect corresponds topographically with the site of the visual field defect (2). Furthermore, these filling defects are common in ocular hypertensive eyes and are significantly greater in area in ocular hypertensive eyes compared to normal eyes (3). In addition, on longitudinal follow-up of ocular hypertensive patients we have observed that, when a new visual field defect has occurred, a new filling defect can be detected in the optic disc (7). Furthermore, we have followed three ocular hypertensive patients whose optic discs showed fluorescein filling defects present at the corresponding topographic site of a future visual field defect.

We have also noticed and measured leakage of the disc vessels, as evidenced by the accumulation of fluorescein, particularly at the site of the fluorescein filling defect (1, 4). We have particularly studied these findings, using two-point fluorophotometry to analyze fluorescein filling in the area of the defect so that it can be readily compared to an adjacent area that has no filling defect (6).

Thus, our observations confirm Dr Piccolino's findings on sectorial hyperfluorescence of the optic disc in glaucoma. Furthermore, our observations indicate that in ocular hypertensive and glaucomatous eyes there are two main signs of vascular damage: 1) the area of hypofluorescence or the fluorescein filling defect; and 2) particularly at the sites of these defects, hyperfluorescence, representing leakage of the vessels.

REFERENCES

1. Ben-Sira, I., Loebl, M., Schwartz, B. and Riva, C. E. In vivo measurements of diffusion of fluorescein into the human optic nerve tissue. Doc. Ophthalmol. Proc. Series, International Symposium on Fluorescein Angiography 9:311−314 (1976).
2. Fishbein, S. and Schwartz, B. Optic disc in glaucoma: topography and extent of fluorescein filling defects. Arch. Ophthalmol. 95:1975−1979 (1977).
3. Loebl, M. and Schwartz, B. Fluorescein angiographic defects of the optic disc in ocular hypertension. Arch. Ophthalmol. 95:1980−1984 (1977).
4. Loebl, M., Schwartz, B. and Riva, C. E. Fluorescein diffusion in the optic disc in glaucoma. (Association for Research in Vision and Ophthalmology Abstract) Supplement to Invest. Ophthalmol. Vis. Sci., p. 31 (1977).
5. Schwartz, B., Rieser, J. C. and Fishbein, S. Fluorescein angiographic defects of the optic disc in glaucoma. Arch. Ophthalmol. 95:1961−1974 (1977).
6. Sonty, S. and Schwartz, B. Two-point fluorophotometry in the evaluation of the glaucomatous optic disc. Arch. Ophthalmol. 98:1422−1426 (1980).
7. Talusan, E. and Schwartz, B. Fluorescein angiography of the optic disc: a longitudinal follow-up study. Arch. Ophthalmol. 98:1579−1584 (1980).

Dr Ernest (on paper 3 only): Because of the absence of the blood-ocular barrier between the peripapillary choroid and the optic nerve, there is normally late fluorescein staining of the disc; did the authors examine the optic disc of their patients with stereofluorescein angiograms so that they were certain that the leakage was from superficial capillaries?

Discussion on 'The relationship between a circumlinear vessel gap at the neuroretinal rim and glaucomatous visual field loss', by G. Balaszi and E. B. Werner.

Michael A. Motolko: I would just like to make a few points concerning the usefulness of baring of a circumlinear vessel as a sign of early acquired damage at the optic disc. My comments are based on a study of over 300 stereophotographs performed by Sutter, Motolko and Phelps.

The first point is that there was a high degree of inter-observer variability in detecting the presence of a circumlinear vessel and in determining whether or not the vessel, if present, was bared. In our study, a preliminary learning trial was conducted in which 174 stereophotographs were examined independently by 3 observers and strict criteria for a circumlinear vessel and baring were defined. Then another group of 144 stereophotographs of glaucomatous, ocular hypertension and normal eyes were examined in a masked fashion, independently by the same 3 observers. Although in many eyes, baring of a circumlinear vessel was easily recognized, in other eyes, it was difficult for trained observers to agree. Despite a learning trial, the 3 observers disagreed about the presence or absence of a vessel in approximately 25% of eyes and when we all agreed a vessel was present, disagreed about whether or not it was bared in 25% of eyes. Thus in our hands, the sign suffered from poor inter-observer reproducibility.

Bared vessels (in the presence of a circumlinear vessel gap) were present in 73% of 22 glaucomatous eyes, 41% of 71 ocular hypertensive eyes and 14% of 51 normal eyes. Thus, my second point is that the sign may not be as specific for glaucoma as hoped. If our results can be extrapolated to the population at large, an eye with baring of a circumlinear vessel is more likely to be glaucomatous than if it did not have a bared vessel, but it is still several times more likely to be normal than to be glaucomatous, for the simple reason that glaucomatous eyes comprise less than 2% of the general population, whereas 14% of normal eyes may have a bared vessel.

An unsettling result of our study was the 41% prevalence of baring of the circumlinear vessel in our patients with ocular hypertension. This prevalence is close to the 65% prevalence of baring found by Herschler and Osher and implies that many of these eyes, which we have followed without treatment and which we have assumed were undamaged by high pressure, actually may have sustained early optic nerve damage.

However, during long-term follow-up (average 1.1 years) of 44 ocular hypertensive eyes with bared circumlinear vessels, only 3 developed visual field defects. We therefore conclude that baring of a circumlinear vessel is a difficult sign for trained observers to detect with certainty and, although present frequently in glaucoma, is of low specificity as a sign or predictor of glaucomatous damage.

Discussion on 'Correlation of the peripapillary anatomy with the disc damage and field abnormalities in glaucoma', by D. R. Anderson.

S. S. Hayreh: Dr Anderson has stressed the frequent presence of peripapillary crescent or halo in eyes with low-tension glaucoma, and postulated that this may represent a congenital abnormality making such an optic disc more vulnerable to damage than the one without such a crescent; he stated that the crescent may not be due to glaucoma. All the available evidence strongly suggests that this is not the case. I discussed the subject of peripapillary choroidal atrophy (i.e. peripapillary crescent or halo) in glaucoma in detail elsewhere (Hayreh, S. S. In 'Glaucoma. Conceptions of a disease', edited by K. Heilmann and K. T. Richardson. Thieme, Stuttgart, 1978, pp. 110–112). Such a change has been described by a large number of authors. For example, Primrose (Br. J. Ophthalmol. 55:820–825, 1971) found peripapillary halo in 94% of his glaucoma cases and found it was twice as likely to occur in glaucomatous eyes as in non-glaucomatous eyes. Also Wilensky et al. (Am. J. Ophthalmol. 81:341–345, 1976) found the halo significantly ($p < 0.01$) more in glaucomatous eyes than in non-glaucomatous eyes. On fluorescein fundus angiography a large number of investigators have shown peripapillary choroidal vascular filling defects in eyes with ocular hypertension, open angle glaucoma and low-tension glaucoma. Our studies in eyes with anterior ischemic optic neuropathy have shown that these eyes develop a similar peripapillary crescent or halo after the acute changes have resolved (Hayreh, S. S. Br. J. Ophthalmol. 58:964–980, 1964); thus suggesting that the peripapillary halo is an acquired ischemic lesion. All these observations indicate that the peripapillary crescent or halo seen in eyes with various types of glaucoma is an acquired lesion, secondary to peripapillary choroidal ischemia, and not a congenital lesion. Moreover, all eyes with peripapillary crescent, e.g., seen in myopes, do not invariably develop glaucomatous optic disc and visual field changes.

A COMPARATIVE STUDY OF VISUAL FIELDS OF PATIENTS WITH LOW-TENSION GLAUCOMA AND THOSE WITH CHRONIC SIMPLE GLAUCOMA

SUSAN ANDERTON and ROGER A. HITCHINGS

(London, England)

Key words. Profile, low-tension glaucoma, chronic simple glaucoma, visual field defect, cup/disc ratio.

ABSTRACT

30 eyes from a total of 26 patients with LTG were compared with 30 eyes of CSG patients. They were matched by age and distance vision.

The profile fields were compared and showed a greater number of defects occurring close to fixation in LTG while the degree of the slope was steeper in LTG. The cup/disc ratios were compared in some of the pairs and showed dissimilar ratios in certain cases.

INTRODUCTION

Low-tension glaucoma (LTG) is a condition consisting of an open angle, typical glaucomatous disc cupping, but pressures within the normal range as opposed to the higher pressures of chronic simple glaucoma (CSG).

The visual fields of these two groups appear to be typically glaucomatous but certain differences have been shown between the two as in Levene's detailed review of LTG in 1980 (1). He concluded that there were certain characteristics in LTG such as early dense defects extending to within 5° of fixation, sudden visual loss, early involvement of fixation, slow progression of the field and disproportion between marked disc changes and the field defect.

This initial study was undertaken to compare the visual profiles on the two groups of glaucoma. Low-tension glaucoma (LTG) and chronic simple glaucoma (CSG).

MATERIALS AND METHODS

Patients are included into the LTG clinic at the hospital on the following criteria: 1) glaucomatous cupping; 2) visual field defect; 3) 24 hour phasing showing intraocular pressure $\leqslant 21$; and 4) open angles.

For this investigation a total of 30 eyes from 23 patients were studied. The visual fields of these eyes were performed on the Goldmann perimeter using the Armaly-Drance method. This was followed by a profile of the field also performed on the Goldmann perimeter using the following meridians: 45°, 135°, 225° and 315°.

These fields were charted by the same technician throughout and they were repeated within a short period of time to verify the findings.

These fields were then matched up with similar fields of CSG patients by superimposing one upon the other and obtaining correspondence to within 5° at least 6 out of 8 points on the I4 isopter.

The patients were then matched for age to within 10 years and visual acuity not separated by over one line on the Snellens Chart.

Once these three criteria were matched the patient with CSG underwent kinetic and profile perimetry as for the LTG patient.

A note was made of the cup/disc ratio of each eye in both groups of patients wherever possible. The pupil size and the treatment the patient was on were also recorded.

RESULTS

The types of defects that occurred were put into one of five groups: 1) isolated scotoma; 2) nasal step; 3) arcuate; 4) nasal loss with arcuate; 5) altitudinal.

The greater number showed an arcuate defect and the rest were evenly distributed throughout the remaining four groups.

From the 30 pairs, 25 had a normal 'Hemi' field and the remaining five had various defects present in both hemispheres.

With reference to the profile perimetry only 14 pairs showed a normal 'Hemi' field.

To compare the degree of the slope of the defect it was assumed that the sensitivity was the same on the two halves of the normal profile. The start of the defect was identified by comparing with the normal slope. Then the number of degrees from the start of the slope to the absolute defect was measured.

This showed the mean extent of slope to be:

$$\text{LTG} = 2.43° \qquad \text{SD} = 1.87$$
$$\text{CSG} = 4.35° \qquad \text{SD} = 3.02$$
$$p < 0.05$$

The relationship of an absolute scotoma to fixation showed the following results:

	0–5°	6–10°	11–15° (degrees from fixation)
LTG	46	8	0
CSG	31	15	5

The cup/disc ratio was compared with 13 pairs of disc photographs and it was shown that not all of these were a similar ratio.

CONCLUSION

It has been shown (using profile perimetry) in the 30 matched pairs that absolute defects $\leqslant 5°$ from fixation are more common in LTG. Secondly the slope of the LTG field is significantly steeper than CSG field and not all patients with the same visual field defect had the same cup/disc ratio.

ACKNOWLEDGEMENTS

We wish to thank the Frost Foundation Fund for supporting Mrs Susan Anderton's sessions to make this study possible.
We thank Mrs Kay Mills for typing the paper.

REFERENCE

1. Levene, R. A. Low-tension glaucoma: A critical review and new material. Surv. Ophthalmol. 24:621 (1980).

COMPARISON OF GLAUCOMATOUS VISUAL FIELD DEFECTS IN PATIENTS WITH HIGH AND WITH LOW INTRAOCULAR PRESSURES

ERIK L. GREVE and H. CAROLINE GEIJSSEN

(Amsterdam, The Netherlands)

Key words. Glaucoma, visual field examination, low-tension glaucoma.

ABSTRACT

The type of visual field defect, the distance of the visual field defect to the center and the size of the defect in the upper and lower half of the visual field in three groups of glaucoma patients were compared. Group 1: 20 eyes of patients with high-tension ($\geqslant 40$ mm Hg) glaucoma (HTG); group 2: 22 eyes of patients with senile sclerotic low-tension glaucoma (SSLTG); group 3: 24 eyes of patients with focal ischemic low-tension glaucoma (FILTG). We found no difference in type of visual field defect nor in distance to the center. However, we did find a difference in the distribution of visual field defects over the lower and upper half of the visual field. In the HTG group the mean size of the visual field defect was approximately similar in the upper and lower half. In the SSLTG group the larger defect was more often found in the upper visual field half. In FILTG the localization of the larger defect was even more frequent in the upper half. Thus, it seems that the optic nerve has a different sensitivity distribution in different types of glaucoma.

INTRODUCTION

It is conceivable that the damage to the optic disc, caused primarily by a high intraocular pressure (IOP), may be of a different type or may have a different distribution than that caused by an other (e.g. microvascular) mechanism in the presence of a normal IOP. Different mechanisms may cause different visual field defects (7).

An example of a different distribution has been found in the location of visual field defects in myopic glaucoma (5).

It has already been demonstrated that the visual field in anterior ischemic optic neuropathy (AION), a disease related to glaucoma, has a different distribution of visual field defects (2, 3, 6, 8, 12, 13).

The definition of low-tension glaucoma (LTG) has been influenced by individual interpretations of statistical limits, the results of population studies and the mechanisms of glaucomatous damage. Several limits for IOP have been given. Requirements for C-values have similarly been given. It is not the purpose of this article to argue about what is and what is not LTG. However, if one wants to investigate the differences between so-called primary open angle glaucoma (POAG; IOP ⩾ 22 mm Hg) and so-called LTG (IOP < 22 mm Hg) one should realize that there is a gradual transition between the two artificially separated groups and that we have no means to differentiate the two groups in the transition zone.

This IOP transition zone may cover a large range of IOP values. If the mechanisms operating in high-tension glaucoma (HTG) and low-tension glaucoma (LTG) are different, a combination of these mechanisms may operate in the transition zone.

Therefore, it seems worthwhile to investigate glaucoma groups at each end of the IOP spectrum if one aims at separating visual field defects due to different damaging mechanisms.

We have investigated the type, location and extension of glaucomatous visual field defects in glaucoma patients at the end of the IOP spectrum: HTG and LTG.

METHODS

The criteria for IOP measurement, gonioscopy, refraction, visual field examination, including classification of glaucomatous visual field defects, and disc evaluation have been presented in a related article in this volume (7). In that same article the three groups of glaucoma patients have been described in detail. It concerns one group of HTG (20 eyes of 11 patients; and two groups of LTG: senile sclerotic LTG (SSLTG), 22 eyes of 11 patients, and focal ischemic LTG (FILTG), 24 eyes of 15 patients.

In these three groups we investigated: 1) type of visual field defect; 2) distance of the visual field defect to the center; and 3) size of the defects in the upper and lower half of the visual field.

RESULTS

We compared *characteristics* of the visual fields of stages 0–I (7) and I together and those of stages II and III (7) together for the three groups. We found no differences in the *intensity distribution* (homogeneity) of the defects.

The *distance to the center* of the visual field defects is presented in Table 1. There are no significant differences in the three glaucoma groups. Certainly the defects in the LTG group are not closer to the center than in the HTG group (9).

We found a difference in the *distribution of visual field defect* over the upper and lower half of the visual field.

The stage of the visual field of the upper and lower half respectively has been presented as a quotient. If the quotient is 1 the stages are similar in the

Table 1. Distance to the center of VF defects in three groups of glaucoma patients.

	HTG		SSLTG		FILTG	
	No.#	%	No.#	%	No.#	%
1–5	10	46	5	39	6	33
5–10	8	36	3	23	8	44
11–15	2	9	2	15	2	11
16–20	2	9	0	0	0	0
21–25	0	0	0	0	1	6
> 25	0	0	3	23	1	6

HTG = high-tension glaucoma.
SSLTG = senile sclerotic low-tension glaucoma.
FILTG = focal ischemic low-tension glaucoma.

two halves. Defects up to stage IV were included (7). In the HTG group the average quotient was 1.2; in the SSLTG group: 2.3; and in the FILTG group: 4.1. Thus, the stages of visual field defects were about equally distributed over the upper and lower half of the visual field in HTG. In SSLTG a 2.3 times larger stage visual field defect was found in the upper half. In FILTG the discrepancy between the visual field stage in upper and lower half of the visual field was even greater. The larger visual field defect was in the upper visual field half again. The quotient doubles from HTG to SSLTG to FILTG.

DISCUSSION

Levene (9) in his review of LTG stated that most investigators believe that the visual field defects in LTG and POAG are similar. He added that dense visual field defects close to fixation occurred more frequently in LTG than in POAG. Gramer et al. (6) stated that the preponderance of visual field defects LTG occurred in the inferonasal visual field. Several authors have found no differences in visual field defects in POAG and LTG (4, 10, 11, 12). In a related paper in this volume we have described differences in the appearance of the optic disc and disc—visual field relation in three groups of glaucoma patients: HTG, SSLTG and FILTG.

This study demonstrates that in addition to the above-mentioned factors the *distribution* of the visual field defects over the upper and lower halves of the visual field is different in the three groups.

All these factors argue in favour of different mechanisms of damage to the optic disc. It is striking that in FILTG the larger visual field defects are found much more often in the upper visual field half than in HTG. This may point to the fact that the lower half of the optic disc is more sensitive to a specific type of vascular damage. However, in AION the reverse is found: most of the defects reported were located in the lower half of the visual field (3, 6, 8, 12, 13). There is general agreement that the damage to the optic disc in AION is caused by acute obstruction of the blood supply in the short posterior ciliary arteries.

If the distribution of visual field defects in **AION** and **FILTG** is so different and if furthermore the aspect of the optic disc (excavation) is so different, the underlying damaging mechanisms are probably different.

The number of eyes in the HTG group and SSLTG group are not large enough to draw definite conclusions. However, if in HTG the damage is equally distributed over the upper and lower halves of the visual field one could argue that a high IOP affects the upper and lower halves of the optic disc in a similar, possibly mechanical, manner.

If a chronic microvascular component is involved, the lower half of the optic disc is more frequently affected than the upper half as in SSLTG and FILTG. In this theory FILTG is the purest form of LTG where IOP plays hardly any role as a damaging factor.

The fact that in some other studies no differences have been found between so-called POAG and so-called LTG may be due to the fact that there is a large overlap between those groups and that in many POAG patients microvascular factors are active.

To our knowledge the only other study where an attempt has been made to separate the extremes of the glaucoma spectrum and to exclude the overlap area is that of Phelps et al. (12).

REFERENCES

1. Anderton, S. and Hitchings, R. A comparative study of visual fields of patients with low-tension glaucoma and those with chronic simple glaucoma. Doc. Ophthalmol. Proc. Series 35:97–99 (1983).
2. Aulhorn, E. and Karmeyer, H. Frequency distribution in early glaucomatous visual field defects. Doc. Ophthalmol. Proc. Series 14:75–83 (1977).
3. Aulhorn, E. and Tanzil, M. Comparison of visual field defects in glaucoma and in acute anterior ischemic optic neuropathy. Doc. Ophthalmol. Proc. Series 19:73–79 (1979).
4. Drance, S. M. The visual field of low tension glaucoma and shock-induced neuropathy. Arch. Ophthalmol. 95:1359 (1977).
5. Furuno, F. and Greve, E. L. Myopia and glaucoma. Albrecht von Graefes Arch. Klin. Exp. Ophthalmol. 213:33 (1980).
6. Gramer, E., Mohammed, J. and Krieglstein, G. K. Der Ort von Gesichtsfeldausfällen bei Glaukoma Simplex, Glaukom ohne Hochdruck und ischemischen Neuropathie. Medikamentöse Glaukom Therapie, J. F. Bergmann Verlag, München, p. 115 (1982).
7. Greve, E. L. and Geijssen, H. C. The relation between excavation and visual field in glaucoma patients with high and with low intraocular pressures. Doc. Ophthalmol. Proc. Series 35:35–42 (1983).
8. Hayreh, S. S. and Podhajsky, P. Visual field defects in anterior ischemic optic neuropathy. Doc. Ophthalmol. Proc. Series 19:53–70 (1979).
9. Levene, R. Z. Low-tension glaucoma: A critical review and new material. Surv. Ophthalmol. 24:621–664 (1980).
10. Motolko, M., Drance, S. M. and Douglas, G. R. Visual field defects in low-tension glaucoma. Arch. Ophthalmol. 100:1074–1077 (1982).
11. Motolko, M., Drance, S. M. and Douglas, G. R. The visual field defects of low-tension glaucoma. Doc. Ophthalmol. Proc. Series 35:107–111 (1983).
12. Phelps, C. D., Hayreh, S. S. and Montague, P. R. Visual fields in low-tension glaucoma, primary open angle glaucoma, and anterior ischemic optic neuropathy. Doc. Ophthalmol. Proc. Series 35:113–124 (1983).

13. Reuscher, A., Chromek, B. and Kommerell, G. Gesichtsfeldausfälle bei der Apoplexia papillae. Klin. Mol. Augenheilk. 169:397 (1976).

Authors' addresses:
Dr E. L. Greve
Glaucoma and Visual Field Dept.
Eye Clinic of the University of Amsterdam
Academic Medical Center
Meibergdreef 8, 1105 AZ Amsterdam
The Netherlands

H. C. Geijssen
Dept. of Ophthalmology
Sint Lucas Hospital
Jan Tooropstraat 164, 1061 AE Amsterdam
The Netherlands

THE VISUAL FIELD DEFECTS OF LOW-TENSION GLAUCOMA

A comparison of the visual field defects in low-tension glaucoma with chronic open angle glaucoma

MICHAEL MOTOLKO, STEPHEN M. DRANCE*
and GORDON R. DOUGLAS
(Vancouver, British Columbia, Canada)

Key words. Visual field defects, chronic open angle glaucoma, low-tension glaucoma.

ABSTRACT

The visual fields of 160 low-tension glaucoma (LTG) eyes and 154 chronic open angle glaucoma (COAG) eyes were compared in patients with the same degree of optic nerve change. No differences in the qualitative or quantitative characteristics were found. The field defects in those LTG eyes in which a major hemodynamic crisis had occurred were not different from those in whom no crisis had been documented.

INTRODUCTION

As early as 1857 von Graefe described a condition characterized by glaucomatous change at the optic nerve without elevated intraocular pressure (1). The characteristics of the visual field defects of low-tension glaucoma (LTG) have been controversial. Levene (3) has carefully reviewed the LTG literature from 1857 to 1980, and has provided a comprehensive bibliography. He states that while many observers have shown no difference in the visual field defects of LTG compared with those of chronic open angle glaucoma (COAG) others have found a higher incidence of altitudinal field defects in LTG and yet some authors described defects close to fixation (less than 5 degrees) in LTG. In reviewing his own 32 cases of LTG as compared to 160 consecutive cases of COAG, 94% of the LTG cases had dense defects within 5° of fixation at the initial examination compared with only 20% among the glaucomas. His conclusion was that the fields of LTG and COAG are similar qualitatively but quantitatively the LTG patients have a higher frequency of dense defects close to fixation. The differences have more than academic interest as they have been used to postulate an essential difference between COAG and LTG (4).

In all previous studies the LTG patients and COAG patients have been

*To whom requests for offprints should be addressed.

Greve, E. L., Heijl, A. (eds.) Fifth International Visual Field Symposium.
©1983 Dr W. Junk Publishers, The Hague/Boston/Lancaster.

compared at different stages of the disease. Since elevated pressure is often the factor which arouses suspicion of COAG, many of these patients are found early in the course of their disease, even prior to any changes at the optic disc, and might therefore show differences in field defects compared with LTG patients, who become candidates for visual field studies only when the optic disc has developed definitive glaucomatous change. One would therefore expect such patients to be detected later and demonstrate denser defects in their visual fields.

The present study was undertaken to examine the characteristics of the visual field defects in LTG and to compare them with field defects in COAG patients with the same degree of optic disc cupping in order to ascertain whether qualitative or quantitative differences exist in the field defects between these 2 disease entities.

MATERIALS AND METHODS

One hundred and sixty eyes of 100 patients with LTG were identified. The criteria for inclusion in this group consisted of peak intraocular pressures less than 22 mm Hg found on diurnal tension curves, characteristic glaucomatous appearance of the optic nerve and pressure of glaucomatous field defects in the absence of local disc malformations, neurological and orbital pathology confirmed by X-rays, tomograms, and CT scans, where applicable. Abnormalities of outflow facility did not lead to exclusion from the study. The degree of optic nerve cupping was estimated by using the cup/disc ratio to the nearest 0.1 in both vertical and horizontal diameters.

The eyes of these patients were then compared with 154 eyes of 107 patients with COAG and with the same degree of optic nerve cupping. Within each cup size these 2 groups were randomly matched for age and sex.

The most recent visual field plotted statically and kinetically on the Tubingen perimeter was examined In a few cases only fields on the Goldmann perimeter were available but the depth of each scotoma was determined by static testing. The visual fields were examined both qualitatively and quantitatively. The following types of defects were identified:
1. paracentral scotomata
2. arcuate scotomata (superior or inferior),
3. arcuate scotomata (superior or inferior) which broke through to the periphery
4. altitudinal defects (superior or inferior)
5. isolated nasal steps (superior or inferior)
6. sector defects
7. end stage defects

Each defect was characterized by its maximal depth on static perimetry comparing the macular threshold of that eye in apostilbs with the threshold of the depth of the defect in apostilbs. The width of the scotomata and their distance from fixation were also recorded.

All patients had a neurovascular assessment by an internist with emphasis on the presence of systemic vascular abnormalities. The incidence of hemodynamic crises was determined for both groups. For purposes of the study a

108

hemodynamic crisis was defined as an acute blood loss requiring transfusion of 4 or more units of blood, or a significant hypotensive event which was symptomatic, in the absence of an acute blood loss. Myocardial infarction with arrhythmia fell into this latter group. Myocardial infarction alone was not considered a hemodynamic crisis for purposes of this study.

The visual field defects of the LTG patients who had suffered a hemodynamic crisis were also compared to those of LTG patients who had not suffered such a crisis.

RESULTS

The average of both groups of patients was 72 years. The LTG patients ranged in age from 34 to 92 while the age for the COAG group was 40 to 95. Data for best corrected acuity was also available for the 116 LTG eyes and 135 COAG eyes and showed a similar distribution but the LTG group showed a small shift to the left, suggesting a slightly better acuity within that group. This was not related to the use of miotics.

There was a remarkable similarity of the field defects between LTG and COAG (Table 1). The most common defect was a superior arcuate scotoma. A superior arcuate scotoma demonstrating a breakthrough was also quite common. Altitudinal defects as previously illustrated were uncommon (2%).

The quantitative characteristics of the scotomata were also identical in both groups (Table 2). One hundred and twenty-nine of 160 LTG eyes (81%) had scotomata within 5° of fixation and 120 of 154 (80%) of COAG eyes had similar defects. The presence of maximal luminosity scotomata (1000 Abs in depth) anywhere in the central field was very common in both groups (128 of 160 (80%) of LTG and 129 of 154 (80%) of COAG eyes). This demonstrates the severe degree of disturbance present in both groups at that stage of the disease.

The incidence of a hemodynamic crisis (as defined) was more common in

Table 1. Qualitative comparison of field defects in patients with COAG and LTG.

Field defect		LTG (160 eyes)	COAG (154 eyes)
paracentral		3 (2%)	2 (1.5%)
Arcuate	superior	94 (59%)	90 (58%)
	inferior	40 (25%)	37 (24%)
Altitudinal		3 (2%)	4 (2.5%)
Isolated nasal step	superior	5 (3%)	6 (4%)
	inferior	9 (5%)	6 (4%)
End stage		6 (3%)	8 (5%)

109

Table 2. Comparison of density and proximity of scotoma to fixation in patients with low-tension glaucoma and chronic open angle glaucoma.

Field defect characteristic	LTG (160 eyes)	COAG (154 eyes)
Within 5° of fixation	129 (81%)	120 (80%)
1000 Abs nucleus	128 (80%)	129 (80%)

Table 3. Comparison of qualitative field defects in LTG patients with and without preceding hemodynamic crisis.

Field defect		Crisis (56 eyes)	No crisis (74 eyes)
Paracentral		1 (1%)	1 (1%)
Arcuate	superior	38 (68%)	41 (55%)
	inferior	11 (20%)	21 (28%)
Altitudinal		2 (3%)	1 (1%)
Isolated nasal step		1 (1%)	7 (9%)
End stage		3 (5%)	3 (4%)

the LTG group. Crises occurred in 33 of 100 (33%) as compared to 12 of 107 (12%) in the COAG group. These differences were statistically significant ($p < 0.01$).

The field defects of the LTG eyes who had a hemodynamic crisis were compared with the fields of the LTG eyes without a crisis (Table 3). There was no difference in the type, severity, and distribution of field defects.

COMMENT

This study shows no difference in the qualitative or quantitative visual field defects of LTG and COAG eyes when matched for the degree of optic nerve cupping. Differences in field defects which have been reported previously might have been due to comparing eyes at different stages of each disease. The severity of the defects are marked, both in relation to depth of the scotomata (80% of cases had absolute scotoma in the central field) and in distance from fixation (80% of cases had scotoma within 5° of fixation). The early field defect of low-tension glaucoma is little known since such patients, in the absence of elevated intraocular pressure and yet only minimally suspicious discs would not undergo visual field testing except in population screening. The similar incidence in the 2 groups of isolated paracentral scotomata (2%) in the presence of suspicious glaucomatous cupping show that a small percentage of cases develop relatively little field loss in the presence of extensive tissue change.

The finding that 1/3 of LTG and 1/10 of severe COAG patients have suffered a significant hemodynamic crisis is probably of clinical importance (2).

The LTG patients who suffered a hemodynamic crisis demonstrated field defects similar to the LTG patients in whom no crisis occurred. Although a hemodynamic crisis is more common in LTG it is nevertheless associated with field defects similar in all respects to those in whom no crisis has occurred.

The study does not suggest that the field defects of COAG and LTG are fundamentally different and that they should be used as evidence for different pathogenic mechanisms. It was also of interest to see that those patients with a preceding hemodynamic crisis both in COAG and LTG also showed no essential differences in the field defect. If these patients do have a more sudden field defect with better prognosis it cannot be recognized from the field defect.

ACKNOWLEDGEMENTS

This study was supported by the Ontario Ministry of Health Fellowship Grant; supported in part by Medical Research Council of Canada Grant No. MT-1578; and supported in part by the E. A. Baker Foundation for Prevention of Blindness, Canadian National Institute for the Blind.

REFERENCES

1. Von Graefe, A. Über die Ridectomie bei Glaucom und über den glaucomatosen Prozess. Albrecht von Graefes Arch. Ophthalmol. 3:456–650 (1857).
2. Drance, S. M., Morgan, R. W. and Sweeney, V. P. Shock-induced optic neuropathy. A cause of non-progressive glaucoma. New Engl. J. Med. 288:392–395 (1973).
3. Levene, R. Z. Low-tension glaucoma: A critical review and new material. Surv. Ophthalmol. 24:621–664 (1980).
4. Burde, R. H. Glaucomatous cupping sine glaucoma. Surv. Ophthalmol. 25:383–390 (1981).

Authors' address:
Dept. of Ophthalmology
University of British Columbia
2577 Willow Street
Vancouver, B.C.
Canada V5Z 3N9

VISUAL FIELDS IN LOW-TENSION GLAUCOMA, PRIMARY OPEN ANGLE GLAUCOMA, AND ANTERIOR ISCHEMIC OPTIC NEUROPATHY

CHARLES D. PHELPS, SOHAN S. HAYREH
and PAUL R. MONTAGUE

(Iowa City, Iowa, U.S.A.)

Key words. Visual fields, computer, low-tension glaucoma, primary open angle glaucoma, anterior ischemic optic neuropathy.

ABSTRACT

We compared the type and location of visual field defects in 94 eyes with low-tension glaucoma, 225 eyes with primary open angle glaucoma, and 160 eyes with anterior ischemic optic neuropathy. The distribution of defects in two varieties of glaucoma were similar; both involved the upper half of the visual field more frequently, the lower half less frequently, and central vision much less frequently than did anterior ischemic optic neuropathy. These differences in distribution of field defects were independent of the severity of field loss and of patient age. The most frequent defects in both low-tension glaucoma and primary open angle glaucoma were superior nasal defects and superior arcuate scotomas; the most frequent defects in anterior ischemic optic neuropathy were inferior hemifield loss and central scotomas.

These findings suggest that the pathogenic mechanism for optic nerve damage in low-tension glaucoma resembles that of primary open angle glaucoma more than it resembles that of anterior ischemic optic neuropathy.

INTRODUCTION

Anterior ischemic optic neuropathy (AION), low-tension glaucoma (LTG), and primary open angle glaucoma (OAG) are common ocular disorders that have certain features in common. All three disorders cause characteristic nerve fiber bundle visual field defects. The loss of vision in each condition results from destruction of axons of the retinal ganglion cells at the optic nerve head. The cause of the optic nerve head damage in AION is acute ischemia. Ischemia, which is chronic rather than acute, may also be the cause of the nerve head damage in LTG and OAG, but here the evidence for an ischemic pathogenic mechanism is more indirect and less certain than in AION.

In the present study we examined the frequency with which various areas in the visual field become defective in AION, LTG, and OAG. If optic nerve head ischemia is a common pathogenic mechanism for AION, LTG, and OAG, and if acute ischemia and chronic ischemia damage the optic nerve in the same way, one might expect the various sectors of the optic nerve head to be damaged with similar frequencies and the patterns of visual field loss to be similar in the three conditions. However, previous investigators have found that although all three conditions cause qualitatively similar nerve fiber bundle visual field defects the distribution of the defects in the three disorders is quantitatively different. AION, for example, has been found to frequently affect the center of the visual field and to reduce visual acuity, (1, 2) while both LTG and OAG rarely cause loss of central vision unless the disease is far advanced. Differences have also been found by some investigators (3), and denied by others (4), between the visual fields in LTG and OAG. Levene, for example, suggests that LTG is more likely than OAG to involve fixation or to affect areas in the visual field close to fixation.

It is not clear from our review of previously published studies if the differences that have been observed between the visual fields of AION, LTG, and OAG are substantive or merely reflect differences in the severity of the visual loss when the diseases come to medical attention. Perhaps patients with AION and LTG become symptomatic only if they have large visual field defects that encroach upon fixation, whereas patients with small peripheral visual field defects from OAG are detected at an early asymptomatic stage when their intraocular pressure is found to be high on a routine measurement.

In this study we subdivided our patients into those with mild, moderate, and advanced visual field loss, as judged by the amount of the visual field involved in the absolute defect. This permitted us to compare patients with AION, LTG, and OAG who had similar amounts of visual field loss. We also used an identical detection strategy to test the visual fields in each of the three disorders.

MATERIAL AND METHOD

We included in our study 125 patients with AION, 59 patients with LTG, and 148 patients with OAG. Patients were included only if they were cooperative and reliable during visual field testing. Patients were excluded who had other diseases known to affect the visual field, including aphakia, cataract sufficient to reduce visual acuity to less than 20/40, retinal vein or artery occlusion, macular degeneration, retinal detachment, diabetic retinopathy, myopic chorioretinal degeneration, and drusen of the optic nerve head.

The patients with AION in one or both eyes had 1) a sudden loss of vision, 2) a pale swelling of all or part of the optic disc, often associated with disc haemorrhage, 3) a disc-related visual field defect, and 4) fluorescein angiographic evidence of optic disc hypoperfusion. We excluded patients in whom temporal arteritis had caused the AION, because the visual loss in these patients was usually massive and little visual field remained. We also excluded patients whom we had not examined soon after the onset while the disc was still edematous.

114

The patients with LTG had 1) a highest recorded intraocular pressure of 22 mm Hg or lower, 2) a normal appearance of the anterior segment of the eye when examined by slit lamp and gonioscopy, 3) glaucomatous cupping of the optic disc, and 4) visual field defects. These patients all had had numerous intraocular pressure measurements, including at least one series of six 'around-the-clock' measurements.

The patients with OAG were similar to those with LTG, but had a highest recorded intraocular pressure of 23 mm Hg or higher. For some parts of our data analysis we divided the OAG eyes into two groups: those with moderate intraocular pressure elevations (23 to 34 mm Hg), and those with marked pressure elevations (higher than 34 mm Hg). In four patients, one eye met the criteria for LTG and the other for OAG. In these cases, each eye was classified separately, was assigned an 'age', and was said to have 'bilateral' involvement for purposes of comparing patients between diagnostic categories.

We tested all visual fields on the Goldmann perimeter and used as our screening strategy Armaly's technique of 'selective perimetry' (5), modified to include additional suprathreshold static presentations in the temporal field and a mapping of the entire I-4e isopter by kinetic presentations at least every 15 meridional degrees (6) (Fig. 1). Although each detected field defect was then mapped with a number of stimuli of differing intensities, for this study we used the appearance of the defect as described with the I-4e stimulus to define its shape and location. We selected the I-4e stimulus for two reasons:

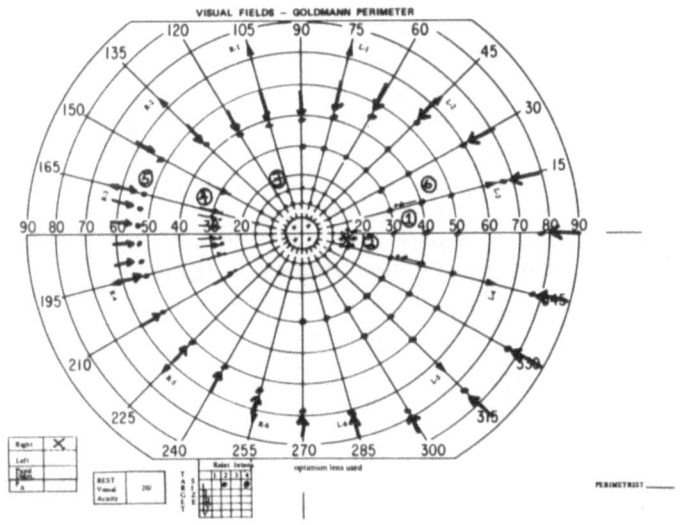

Fig. 1. The perimetric screening strategy used in this study. The stimulus that was threshold about 30 to 35 degrees temporally (Step 1) was used to plot the blind spot (Step 2), to explore the paracentral field with suprathreshold static presentations (Step 3) and to search for a central nasal step (Step 4). This stimulus varied from patient to patient, but most often was the I-2e. Then the I-4e stimulus was used to map the isopter, with special attention nasally (Step 5), and for suprathreshold static exploration of the temporal field (Step 6).

115

1) it is a standard stimulus in our clinic and is recorded on every visual field, and 2) it is the brightest, although not the largest, stimulus on the Goldmann perimeter. Thus we studied only absolute defects, or defects to maximum luminance.

For each patient we recorded the age, sex, diagnosis, eye (right and/or left), and highest intraocular pressure. We classified defects according to their location in the visual field (upper, lower, temporal, or a combination), distance in degrees from fixation, and morphologic type. The types of defects included peripheral nasal step ($\geqslant$ 30 degrees from fixation), large nasal defects that extended to within 30 degrees, paracentral scotoma, arcuate scotoma, hemifield loss (more than one quadrant defective in upper or lower hemifield), temporal sector-shaped scotoma, central scotoma (including cecocentral defects), and advanced defects such as central or temporal islands.

In eight eyes with AION, six eyes with LTG, and 21 eyes with OAG the visual field was so defective that no I-4e isopter could be recorded. These 35 eyes were not included in the frequency distribution part of the study. For the remaining eyes, we used a modification of the method of Aulhorn (7) to determine the frequency distribution. We made transparent overlays for each decade of patient age on which we drew the 'normal' I-4e isopter. We calculated the 'normal' isopter for each decade from the data of Zehnder-Albrecht (8). She had measured the I-4e isopter in 26 normal persons between the ages of 20 and 30 years and in 21 normal persons between the ages of 60 and 70 years. We assumed a linear isopter contracture with advancing age and calculated our 'normal' isopters for each decade by interpolating at each eccentricity between the means, less one standard deviation, of Zehnder-Albrecht's data for the third and seventh decades. We then placed the appropriate transparent overlay over each individual field plot as recorded on the standard Goldmann perimeter chart and, with the aid of a digitizing graphics tablet, entered into a computer each 'sector' on the visual field chart that was at least 50% defective. A 'sector' is the area bounded by two 15° meridional lines and two concentric circles on the field chart. The computer summated the number of times each sector was abnormal in each diagnostic group.

We tested differences in proportions for statistical significance with the Chi-square test, including Yates' discontinuity correction.

RESULTS

The average patient age (mean ± S.D.) was 60.8 ± 10.7 years for AION, 69.1 ± 11.4 years for LTG, and 64.6 ± 13.2 years for OAG. The proportion of patients who were women was 37% in AION, 73% in LTG, and 46% in OAG. This proportion was significantly higher in LTG than in AION ($\chi^2 = 19.47$, $p < 0.001$) or OAG ($\chi^2 = 6.70$, $p < 0.01$); the difference between AION and OAG was not significant at the 5% level of confidence.

Visual field defects were present in both eyes of 35 (28%) of the 125 patients with AION, 35 (59%) of the 59 patients with LTG, and 77 (52%) of the 148 patients with OAG. The differences between AION and either LTG and OAG in frequency of bilateral involvement were highly significant ($\chi^2 = 15.4$ and 15.2, respectively; $p < 0.001$).

Table 1. The location of visual field defects.

	AION (160 eyes) %	LTG (94 eyes) %	OAG (224 eyes) %
Upper field only	13.8	46.8	44.2
Lower field only	45.0	17.0	20.1
Upper and lower	23.1	30.9	34.4
Central scotoma only	13.8	1.1	0.4
Temporal scotoma only	4.4	4.3	0.9

The frequencies with which the upper, lower, central, and temporal parts of the visual field were defective are listed in Table 1. If the eyes with central scotoma as a sole defect are considered to have involvement of both the upper and lower hemifields, a defect was present in the lower hemifield in 131 (82%) of 160 eyes with AION, 46 (49%) of 94 eyes with LTG, and 123 (55%) of 224 eyes with OAG. The differences between AION and either LTG or OAG in frequency of lower hemifield defects were highly significant ($\chi^2 = 28.9$ and 29.1, respectively; $p < 0.001$). The small difference between LTG and OAG was not statistically significant. The upper half of the visual field contained a defect in 81 (51%) of 160 eyes with AION, 74 (79%) of 94 eyes with LTG, and 177 (79%) of 224 eyes with OAG. The differences between AION and either LTG or OAG in frequency of upper hemifield involvement were, again, highly significant ($\chi^2 = 18.5$ and 34.0, respectively; $p < 0.001$).

The OAG group included 143 eyes with a maximum intraocular pressure of 23 to 34 mm Hg, which will hereafter be deisgnated OAG (23–34) and 81 eyes with a maximum intraocular pressure greater than 34 mm Hg, which will be designated OAG (> 34). The frequency of upper hemifield involvement in the two OAG subgroups was similar (81% and 77%, respectively). The frequency of lower hemifield involvement was higher in OAG (> 34) than in OAG (23–34) (48% vs 67%, $\chi^2 = 6.4$, $p < 0.05$). As will be seen below, this difference was caused by the more extensive amount of average visual field loss in the higher pressure subgroup.

Central vision was impaired much more frequently in AION than in either LTG or OAG (Table 2). These differences were again highly significant ($\chi^2 = 29.1$ and 56.1, respectively; $p < 0.001$). The small differences between LTG and OAG in frequency of defects within either two or five degrees from fixation were not statistically significant.

Table 2. Proximity of nearest visual field defect to fixation.

Distance from fixation (in degrees)	AION (160 eyes) %	LTG (94 eyes) %	OAG (224 eyes) %
0	38.1	6.4	6.7
1–2	29.4	41.5	29.9
3–5	10.0	23.4	25.9
6–10	12.5	14.9	20.1
> 10	10.0	13.8	17.4

Table 3. Types of visual field defects (many eyes had more than one defect).

	AION (160 eyes) %	LTG (94 eyes) %	OAG (224 eyes) %
Superior			
nasal step, peripheral	4.4	11.7	6.3
nasal step, central	6.9	5.3	18.8
paracentral scotoma	4.4	11.7	13.8
arcuate scotoma	8.8	47.9	31.3
hemifield loss	5.6	5.3	7.1
Inferior			
nasal step, peripheral	8.1	6.4	2.2
nasal step, central	9.4	10.6	8.5
paracentral scotoma	5.6	10.6	9.4
arcuate scotoma	11.3	14.9	13.8
hemifield loss	29.4	2.1	7.1
Central scotoma	30.6	3.2	0.9
Temporal sector-shaped	14.4	4.3	4.5
Advanced defects	6.9	7.4	11.2

Table 4. The frequency of nasal steps.

	AION (160 eyes) %	LTG (94 eyes) %	OAG (224 eyes) %
Peripheral nasal steps			
with other defects	8.8	13.8	4.9
isolated	3.8	4.3	3.6
subtotal	12.5	18.1	8.5
Central nasal steps			
with other defects	12.5	8.5	21.9
isolated	3.8	7.4	5.4
subtotal	16.3	16.0	27.2
Total nasal steps	28.8	34.0	34.8

The types of visual field defects are shown in Table 3. The most common defects in AION were inferior hemifield loss (30%) and central scotoma (31%). The most common defects in both LTG and OAG were superior arcuate scotoma (48% and 36%, respectively) and superior nasal loss (18% and 28%, respectively). Horizontal steps in the nasal isopter, either peripheral or extending into the central 30 degree field, were encountered in about one third of the visual fields in all three disorders (Table 4). Some other more central defect usually accompanied the nasal step, but in 4% of the eyes with each disorder the only visual field defect was a peripheral nasal step that did not extend to within 30 degrees of fixation.

The computer-generated frequency distribution plots showed no differences between right and left eyes in any of the diagnostic categories, and for the

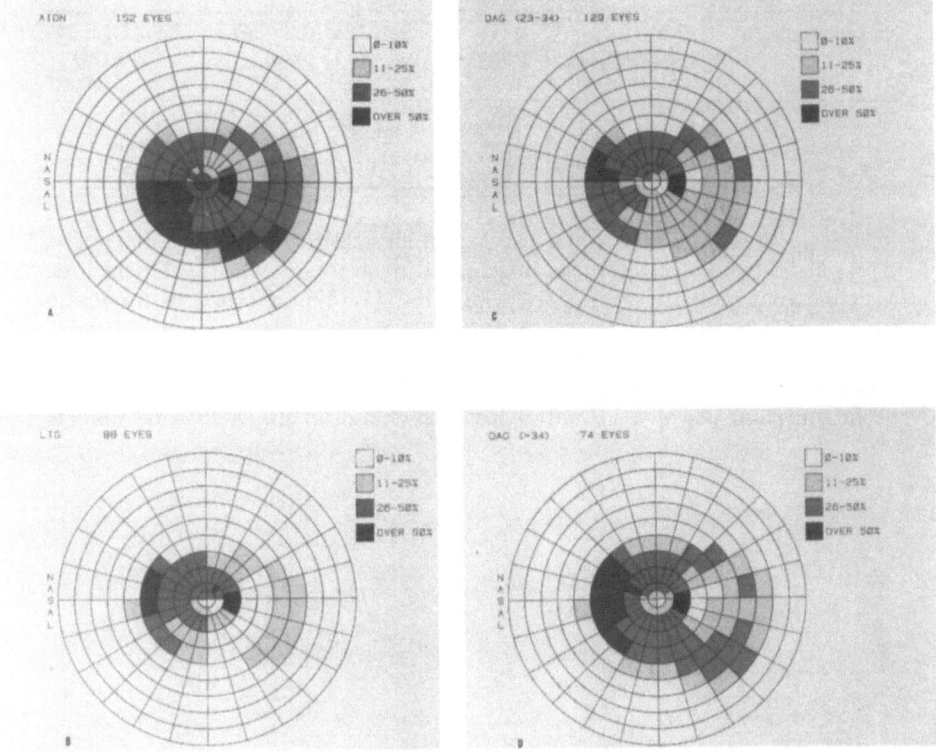

Fig. 2. Frequency distribution of visual field defects in all eyes; (A) anterior ischemic optic neuropathy; (B) low-tension glaucoma; (C) primary open angle glaucoma (maximum intraocular pressure 22–34 mm Hg); (D) primary open angle glaucoma (maximum intraocular pressure greater than 34 mm Hg).

remainder of the analysis right and left eye data were combined after inverting left eye data so that corresponding points in the right and left eye were superimposed.

The frequency distributions of field defects in all eyes with AION, LTG, OAG(23–34), and OAG(> 34) are displayed in Fig. 2. In AION the most frequently defective sectors were in the inferior hemifield, especially inferonasally, but also inferotemporally. In LTG and OAG(23–34) the most frequently defective sectors were more often superior than inferior, with a marked predilection for the nasal periphery. In OAG(> 34) the upper and lower fields were more equally involved, with a marked predilection for the nasal field.

Visual field loss in AION was more often severe (involving more than 30 sectors) and less often mild (involving 1 to 15 sectors) than in either LTG or OAG (Table 5). OAG(> 34) tended to have more severe visual field loss than OAG(23–34) (Table 5). To be sure the differences in frequency distribution

119

Table 5. Distribution of visual field defects according to size.

No of sectors	AION (160 eyes) %	LTG (94 eyes) %	OAG(23–34) (143 eyes) %	OAG(> 34) (81 eyes) %
0–15	12.5	31.9	38.5	24.7
16–30	19.4	23.4	21.0	16.0
> 30	68.1	44.7	40.5	59.3

of defects that we found when comparing all eyes in the various diagnostic categories did not reflect these differences in average severity of field loss, we compared only those eyes with mild loss (1 to 15 sectors) or moderate loss (16 to 30 sectors).

The frequency distributions of eyes with mild visual field loss (1 to 15 sectors) are displayed in Fig. 3. The field loss in all four categories tended to be in the nasal periphery. Central loss was common in AION, and defects

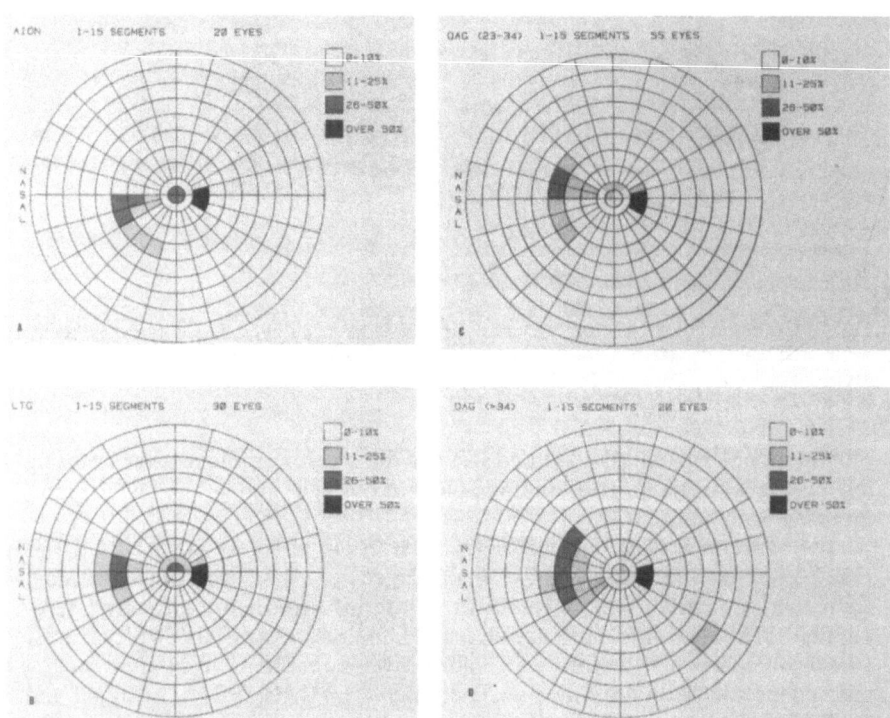

Fig. 3. Frequency distribution of visual field defects in eyes with mild visual field loss (less than 16 sectors); (A) anterior ischemic optic neuropathy; (B) low-tension glaucoma; (C) primary open angle glaucoma (maximum intraocular pressure 22–34 mm Hg); (D) primary open angle glaucoma (maximum intraocular pressure greater than 34 mm Hg).

120

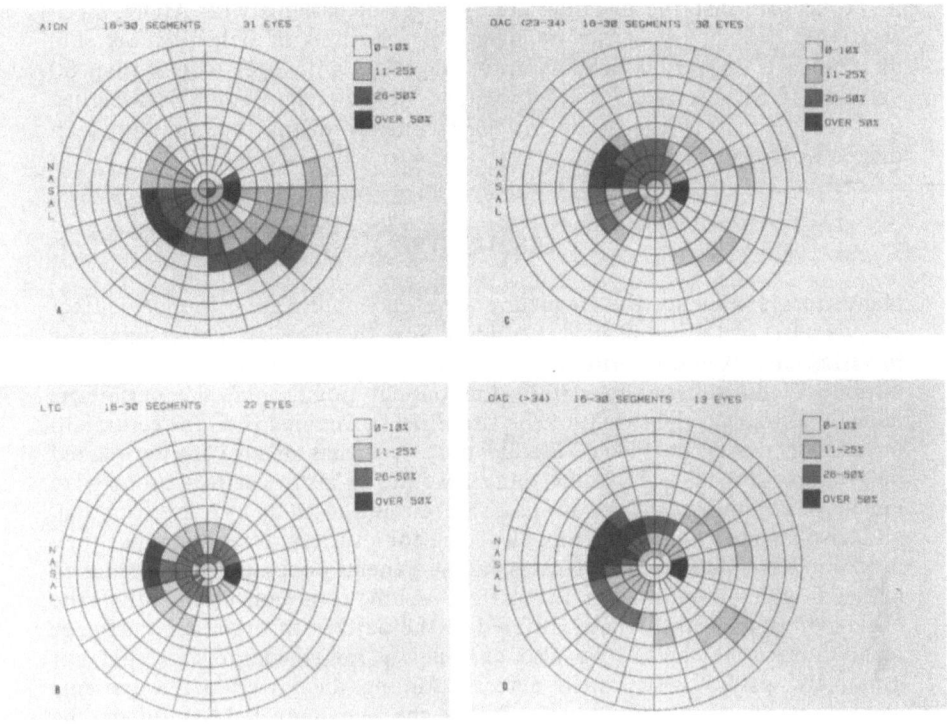

Fig. 4. Frequency distribution of visual field defects in eyes with moderate visual field loss; (A) anterior ischemic optic neuropathy; (B) low-tension glaucoma; (C) primary open angle glaucoma (maximum intraocular pressure 22–34 mm Hg); (D) primary open angle glaucoma (maximum intraocular pressure greater than 34 mm Hg).

close to and just above fixation occurred frequently in LTG and, to a much lesster extent, in OAG.

The frequency distribution for eyes with moderate amounts of visual field loss (16 to 30 sectors) are displayed in Fig. 4. The most frequently involved sectors in AION continue to be in the lower hemifield, while in LTG, OAG (23–34), and OAG(> 34) the upper hemifield is more frequently involved.

When only eyes with extensive field loss (> 30 sectors) were examined (not illustrated here), there was extensive involvement of all parts of the visual field in all diagnostic categories. However, AION continued to preferentially involve the lower hemifield.

A similar computer-assisted analysis was made in which the combined LTG and OAG groups were subdivided into categories separated by different intraocular pressure boundaries (10–19, 20–29, 30–39, 40 mm Hg or higher). In this analysis, also, no significant difference was found between categories in the distribution of defects.

121

To be sure that the differing average ages of patients with AION, LTG, and OAG did not affect the frequency distributions of field loss, we subdivided each diagnostic category into subgroups with ages of less than 60 years, 60 to 69 years, and 70 years or older. No differences could be discerned between the various age groups in the frequency distributions within each diagnostic category.

DISCUSSION

Many factors influence the frequency with which a disease is found to affect various parts of the visual field, including how the cases are ascertained, the inclusion and exclusion criteria, the number of patients studied, the distribution of disease severity within the patient population, the perimetric detection strategy, the extent of the visual field examined (i.e., the central 30 degrees or the entire field), whether only scotomas or also isopter-related defects are studied, and whether only absolute or also relative scotomas are included. For the most part our cases were referred to us by other ophthalmologists and had come under medical care for a variety of reasons; thus they may not be representative of cases in the general population. We excluded patients with other diseases that affect vision; it is conceivable that the excluded patients might have differed in the pattern of optic nerve damage from those we included. We also excluded patients whom we could not accurately test for visual field defects. Among them were a few patients whose loss of vision was so marked that the remaining field could not be reliably plotted. This exclusion biased our study towards less severely affected fields. We had only 59 patients with LTG (including 94 abnormal visual fields); although this constitutes one of the largest series of LTG fields yet reported, the number is too small for definite conclusions.

Our patients with AION differed from those with OAG and LTG in several respects: their average age was less, they more frequently had only one eye involved, and their visual field defects tended to be larger. They had the same kind of visual field loss; no type of defect was found exclusively in AION and not in LTG or OAG. However, there were striking differences in distribution of the defects. We found in AION a strong predilection for the lower and central parts of the visual field, confirming the findings of previous investigators (1, 2). In contrast, LTG and OAG rarely involved the point of fixation, especially early in the course of the disease. The upper hemifield in AION was free of defects in 49% of the eyes.

Patients with LTG differed from patients with OAG in two respects: they were more frequently women, and, on the average, they were older. Otherwise the two conditions were very similar. They were bilateral with equal frequency. They had nearly identical patterns of visual field loss. Both involved the upper hemifield more often than the lower hemifield. Both caused field defects close to fixation with equal frequency. When the defects did encroach on fixation, it was usually from above, confirming an observation made previously by Aulhorn and Karmeyer (7). Both LTG and OAG had a strong predilection for the nasal periphery, a predilection that was perhaps

122

more apparent in this study than in the classic analysis of Aulhorn and Karmeyer because we analyzed the entire field rather than only the central field.

After a comprehensive literature survey and a review of his own patients, Levene concluded that LTG and OAG must have different pathogenic mechanisms (3). Among his evidence for this concusion were the following observations: 1) LTG is more often unilateral than OAG, 2) LTG more frequently causes an early dense field defect within five degrees, and 3) LTG involves fixation early. Our results disagree with the first and third points. A recently completed study by Motolko and Drance also found no evidence that the cental field was involved more frequently in LTG than in OAG (4). As is shown in Fig. 3B, a small number of LTG eyes had early defects very close to fixation. This type of early defect is rare in OAG. Otherwise, there is little, if any, evidence from the patterns of visual field loss that LTG and OAG have different pathogenic mechanisms.

The contrast between AION and the two forms of glaucoma suggests that the pathogenic mechanism in AION differs from that of LTG and OAG. It does not necessarily imply that the mechanism of optic nerve damage in LTG and OAG is non-ischemic. Perhaps, for unknown anatomical reasons, the upper and temporal parts of the optic disc are especially susceptible to acute ischemia while the lower part is more susceptibel to chronic ischemia. On the other hand, it is possible that non-ischemic 'mechanical' damage accounts for some cases of OAG, and, for just as poorly understood anatomical reasons, the lower pole of the disc is the part most susceptible to mechanical damage.

There are limitations on the use of data from a study such as this to derive optimum glaucoma screening protocols, as has been attempted by other investigators (9, 10), because the data depend on the detection strategy we employed in the study. Nevertheless, our results re-emphasize the importance in glaucoma screening of testing the central portion of the visual field with static targets in order to detect isolated scotomas and of testing peripheral nasal isopters with kinetic targets in order to detect isolated peripheral nasal steps. Without both of these manouvers, and especially the latter which is omitted in many of the automated machines now on the market, a number of visual field defects would have been missed.

ACKNOWLEDGEMENTS

This study was supported by Research Grant EY-03330 from the National Institutes of Health.

We are grateful for the skilled assistance of Benita Carney, Ginny Colston, and Miriam Leinen, who tested the visual fields.

REFERENCES

1. Hayreh, S. S. and Podhajsky, P. Visual field defects in anterior ischemic optic neuropathy. Doc. Ophthalmol. Proc. Series 19:53–70 (1979).

2. Aulhorn, E. and Tanzil, M. Comparison of visual field defects in glaucoma and in acute anterior ischemic optic neuropathy. Doc. Ophthalmol. Proc. Series 19:73–79 (1979).
3. Levene, R. A. Low-tension glaucoma: a critical review and new material. Surv. Ophthalmol. 24:621–664 (1980).
4. Motolko, M., Drance, S. M. and Douglas, G. R. Visual field defects in low-tension glaucoma: comparison of defects in low-tension glaucoma and chronic open angle glaucoma. Arch. Ophthalmol. 100:1074–1077 (1982).
5. Armaly, M. F. Selective perimetry for glaucomatous defects in ocular hypertension. Arch. Ophthalmol. 87:518–524 (1972).
6. Drance, S. M., Brais, P., Fairclough, M. and Bryett, J. A screening method for temporal visual defects in chronic simple glaucoma. Can. J. Ophthalmol. 7:478–479 (1972).
7. Aulhorn, E. and Karmeyer, H. Frequency distribution in early glaucomatous visual field defects. Doc. Ophthalmol. Proc. Series 14:75–83 (1977).
8. Zehnder-Albrecht, S. Zur Standardisierung der Perimetrie. Ophthalmologica 120:225–270 (1950).
9. Rabin, S. and Kolesar, P. Mathematical optimization of glaucoma visual field screening protocols. Doc. Ophthalmol. 45:361–380, (1978).
10. Johnson, C. A. and Keltner, J. L. Computer analysis of visual field loss and optimization of automated perimetric test strategies. Ophthalmology 88:1058–1064 (1981).

Author's address:
Dr Charles D. Phelps
Dept. of Ophthalmology
University of Iowa Hospitals
Iowa City, IA 52242
U.S.A.

124

DISCUSSIONS

E. L. Greve: The four studies discussed in this part are the following:
1. 'A comparative study of visual fields of patients with low-tension glaucoma and those with chronic simple glaucoma', by S. Anderton and R. A. Hitchings.
2. 'Comparison of glaucomatous visual field defects in patients with high and with low interaocular pressures', by E. L. Greve and H. C. Geijssen.
3. 'The visual field defects of low-tension glaucoma (A comparison of the visual field defects in low-tension glaucoma with chronic open angle glaucoma)', by M. Motolko, S. M. Drance and G. R. Douglas.
4. 'Visual fields in low-tension glaucoma, primary open angle glaucoma, and anterior ischemic optic neuropathy', by C. D. Phelps, S. S. Hayreh and P. R. Montague.

The set-up of the four studies differs in some respects (Table 1). There seems to be a difference in referral pattern. The numbers in study 1 and 2 are small. The selection criteria for IOP are comparable in studies 2 and 4 to a certain extent. Studies 1 and 3 separate at one IOP level. Study 2 selected patients partly on the basis of disc features. Study 3 matched the primary open angle glaucoma (POAG) and low-tension glaucoma (LTG) group for cup—disc ratio (CDR), so as to compare LTG and HTG at the similar states of involvement.

Visual field: The detection phase of the visual field examination used the Armaly-Drance method in studies 1, 3 and 4 and a modified Visual Field Analyser (150 positions) with additional kinetic perimetry in study 2. All four studies used meridional static perimetry. The method of examination therefore was comparable in all studies.

Type of comparison: Study 1 examined steepness of the defect and distance to the center in matched visual field defects. Study 2 compared homogeneity of defects; distance to the center and size of the defect in upper and lower visual field half. Study 2 excluded high myopic refractions; study 3 depth and width of scotoma, position of scotoma in the field distance from center. Study 4 compared type of defect, distance to the center and frequency of affected visual field units.

From Table 1 it is clear that considerabe differences in selection and comparison exist in the four studies. These could account for the differences in the results. The authors of studies 3 and 4 concluded that there is no

Table 1. Discussion Greve.

	Anderton et al.	Greve et al.	Motolko et al.	Phelps et al.
Referral	?	– (general practice)	+ (glaucoma clinic)	+ (glaucoma clinic)
Numbers	small	small	large	large
Age	?	HTG: 52 LTG: 82, 72 resp.	OAG and LTG; 72 (mean)	OAG: 65, LTG: 69
Examination:				
IOP	diurnal	diurnal	diurnal	diurnal
IOP Separation	< 21; > 22	< 26; > 40 highest IOP	< 21 highest IOP	< 22; > 23 < 22; 23–24; > 35 30–39; > 40 highest IOP
Disc	?	stereophoto selection based on disc appearance	stereophoto matched for similar CDR	stereophoto
Visual field	Armaly-Drance detection meridional static perimetry matching of visual fields	Visual Field Analyser (Amsterdam frontplate) + peripheral kinetic meridional static perimetry no central islands	Armaly-Drance detection meridional static perimetry	Armaly-Drance detection meridional static perimetry only I/4/e-defects
Comparison	distance to center slope of defects	distance to center size of defect in upper and lower half myopes excluded	density of defect width of scotoma distance from center	distance to center; type frequency per visual field unit

difference in distribution of glaucomatous visual field defects in primary open angle glaucoma and low-tension glaucoma and that more defects are located in the upper visual field half of both groups. Study 2 (small numbers) found an approximately equal distribution over the upper and lower half in high-tension glaucoma and a predominance of defects in the upper half of the visual field in low-tension glaucoma. It is interesting that in study 4 in high-tension glaucoma (HTG 34 mm Hg) 77% of visual field defects were found in the upper half and 67% in the lower half of the visual field. This result is comparable to that of study 2. The authors of study 4, however, stated that the difference they found between open angle glaucoma (23–34) and open angle glaucoma (HTG > 34) was due to a more extensive amount of visual field loss in HTG. In study 4 (Fig. 3D) it was shown that the distribution of visual field defects over the lower and upper half in mild visual field defects is about equal in HTG (> 34). However in cases with moderate visual field loss this was not so. The authors of study 1 stated that visual field defects in LTG had steeper slopes and occurred closer to fixation than visual field defects in primary open angle glaucoma. The first finding has not been investigated in the other studies; the second finding is in contrast to the findings of the three other studies.

G. L. Spaeth: It seems to me that the differences between papers may be to some extent explained by different methods of selecting the patients. There was the greatest similarity of selection of patients between the two American studies and their results were most similar. The patients that were from The Netherlands clearly had a higher upper level of intraocular pressure and I think that the distinction between these three groups was made at least partly on the appearance of the optic nerve head itself rather than on the nature of IOP.

In the British group the results are a bit hard to understand because that seemed to be selected mostly in IOP itself. It may be that the difference reported by the groups represents a real difference depending on how the patients were selected. We have examples in our own group of low-tension glaucoma that were more similar to the ones that Erik has described. We certainly do not find anywhere near 1/3 of the patients with hemodynamic crisis. That is a very different population than, I think, most people would include in low-tension glaucoma, at least for us. The thing that I can recognize behind these different conditions, still is not quite answered.

S. M. Drance: All these studies were carefully done and obviously different results mean that they did not use identical techniques and different selections in polulation. Dr Motolko and I selected patients for equal amount of cupping. It is obvious that the low-tension glaucoma patients are normally only discovered because somehow the cupping and the field loss are sufficiently severe that those characteristics alone bring these patients to the attention of the clinician whereas IOP often brings the high-tension patients to the attention of the clinician at a time when they can still have had much less cupping or field loss. This may be one explanation of the different findings in these studies.

127

It is interesting to note that the cases with previous hemodynamic crisis, though admittedly far more than one would normally see in unselected low-tension glaucoma, did not have different fields from those without crisis, which speaks against selection being the important factor accounting for differences.

B. Schwartz: I believe that the paper by Anderton and Hitchings would benefit from a more detailed statistical analysis. This analysis should especially confirm that the differences in slope of the visual field defects, as well as the closeness of the visual field loss due to fixation, are significantly different in patients with chronic simple glaucoma than in ones with low-tension glaucoma.

In the paper by Motolko, Drance and Douglas, apparently the subjects with low-tension glaucoma and chronic open angle glaucoma were matched, having a similar degree of optic nerve change, but this change was in cupping or contour of the optic disc. Our previous studies have shown that pallor is probably a better indicator of visual field loss than cupping (1). Furthermore, open angle glaucomatous patients with visual field loss have advanced degrees of cupping (2). Therefore, it may be pertinent to have matched these patients by pallor or color changes, rather than cupping, especially since we have shown that the area of pallor, but not cupping, is significantly larger in ocular hypertensive eyes than normal eyes (3).

It would also be of value to compare the frequency distribution of visual acuities in these studies since changes of visual acuity may point to visual field loss approaching fixation.

As a final point, it is not surprising to me that the visual fields of open angle glaucoma patients may not be significantly different from those of low-tension glaucoma patients. If we recall that in all the studies done on the frequency distribution of ocular pressures in populations, about 50% of the populations have ocular pressures less than 15 to 16 mm Hg. Therefore, one would expect many persons whose normative pressures may be 12 to 15 mm Hg or less to show visual field loss with significant increases of pressure. Yet, when they are diagnosed initially, their pressures, associated with visual field loss, would be less than 21 mm Hg. This concept, therefore, implies that chronic open angle glaucoma and low-tension glaucoma are really the same disease in many individuals.

REFERENCES

1. Schwartz, B. Correlation of pallor of optic disc with asymmetrical visual field loss in glaucoma. Acta XXII Concilium Ophthalmologicum, Paris, 1974, 2:633–638. Masson Publishers (1974).
2. Schwartz, B. Differences between cupping and pallor of the optic disc in glaucomatous and neurological optic nerve disease. Transactions of the XXII International Congress of Ophthalmology, Kyoto, Japan, 1978. Amsterdam, Excerpta Medica, pp. 1108–1111 (1979).
3. Schwartz, B. Optic disc changes in ocular hypertension. Surv. Ophthalmol. 25: 148–154 (1980).

DETERIORATION OF THRESHOLD IN GLAUCOMA
PATIENTS DURING PERIMETRY

ANDERS HEIJL and STEPHEN M. DRANCE

(Malmö, Sweden/Vancouver, British Columbia, Canada)

Key words. Increment threshold, time changes, glaucoma.

ABSTRACT

Chronic open angle glaucoma patients and glaucoma suspects were subjected to continuous contrast threshold measurement using automatic and manual perimetric techniques. The results show, that an increment of contrast threshold over time is a frequent finding in glaucoma patients and that this increment can be large especially close to existing field defects. It is reproducible and independent of background illumination and can be demonstrated in the same test points both with automatic and manual testing.

The results, which may have some important implications for visual field testing in glaucoma, are discussed.

INTRODUCTION

In patients with disease of the optic pathways, posterior to the lamina cribrosa, a marked increment in the differential threshold has been reported during 'flashing repeat static testing'. The reduction in sensitivity which accompanies the increment of the threshold was termed 'visual saturation or visual fatigue-like effect' (8, 2). The phenomenon was described with high background luminosities of 31 cd/m^2 (100 asb) and was lessened or eliminated by diminished background luminosity. The changes were reported to be consistent in patients with optic nerve disease behind the lamina cribrosa and were not present in patients suffering from glaucoma (1, 3). Using automatic perimetry others have reported that normal subjects maintained a stable level of differential threshold during a continuous 30 min examination while many glaucoma patients showed a fairly marked increment of contrast threshold during such a test. Larger changes of threshold often occurred in areas in the vicinity of field defects or relative disturbance (5, 7). A reduction of the stimulus exposure time from 0.5 sec, which was the standard in these investigations, to 0.25 sec augmented these changes (7).

The apparent discrepancies of these findings sparked us to study the time dependence of the differential threshold during automatic and manual perimetry of glaucoma patients, to see whether a deterioration could also be observed with manual perimetry, whether there was an association between changes in the threshold and location of the stimulated area in or out of a visual field defect, and whether it was reproducible and dependent on the background illumination. We were also interested to see whether there was a correlation between the automatic and manual modes of testing.

METHODS

All automatic perimetry was performed with the Competer computerized automatic perimeter (6). Six points were tested in each patient. A short pre-test of approximately 1 minute was used to establish the initial thresholds of the points to be tested. The patients were then allowed to rest with their eyes closed for five minutes and following that, a continuous recording of differential thresholds was carried out continuously for approximately 30 minutes. The computer used as its starting point, the threshold measurements obtained at the pre-test. The differential threshold was determined through a repetitive up-and-down stair case method, which has been described elsewhere (5). The 30 minute test was continued without interruption, but was subsequently divided into 12 equal periods for calculation of results. During each period the stimulus was presented 10 times at each of the 6 test points and in the blind spot of the tested eye. The order in which the stimuli were presented was randomized. Any stimulus seen was always followed by one 0.3 log units fainter, and any stimulus not seen was increased by 0.3 log units. The reliability of fixation was ascertained by exposing the stimuli into the blind spot. The computer also calculated the mean of the intensity levels used at each point during each of the 12 periods and printed out a fixation quotient. The duration of the stimulus was 0.25 seconds. A stimulus diameter 14', and background illumination $1.0 \, cd/m^2$ (3.14 asb) were used. In order to study the effects of the background illumination, tests were also done with 0.1 and $10 \, cd/m^2$ backgrounds.

All manual perimetry was performed on a Tübingen perimeter, and the testing procedure described by Enoch (8) was followed as closely as possible. Prior to the test, the patients kept their eyes closed for a few minutes. The stimulus was then presented every $\frac{1}{2}$ to 1 second with an exposure time of 100 msec. It was first presented with subliminal intensity, and the intensity was rapidly increased in steps of 0.1 log units, being exposed several times at each level until the patient indicated that the stimulus was seen. The intensity was then decreased by 0.3 to 0.5 log units and the procedure repeated. The tests were continued manually for approximately 12 minutes at each test location. The perimetrist presented the stimuli and checked fixation while the threshold values and time were recorded by an assistant. The background intensity was usually $20 \, cd/m^2$, but in some patients a background of $10 \, cd/m^2$ was tested as well.

The points tested were chosen so as to be in an area of relative visual field defect or a suspect area close to an existing visual field defect as plotted on the Tübingen perimeter. In many instances each point was matched by testing the corresponding mirror point in the area of the normal visual field. The patients were corrected for their refractive errors and given a full correction for near, both for the automatic and manual perimetry. On manual perimetry, the changes of differential threshold were calculated as the differences between the mean threshold during the first minute and the last minute of the test while in automatic perimetry the changes were calculated as the difference between the average threshold during the 1st period and the 12th period.

MATERIAL

21 patients with glaucomatous visual field defects were tested. One showed unreliable fixation during the test and the results were not included. 11 patients were tested both manually and automatically, and 10 were tested only on the automatic perimeter. Two patients with suspect glaucoma but no visual field defects were also tested but only on the automatic perimeter.

RESULTS

18 of the 20 patients had the visual field defects in the central part of the field which was the area of the continuous automatic or manual differential threshold recording. Of the 11 patients who were tested manually only, a total of 20 points was tested. 11 of these points showed stable thresholds, i.e. -0.2 to $+0.1$ log units over a 12 minute period, while 9 points showed the increment in the differential threshold ($+0.3$ to $+1.0$ log units) with a mean change of $+0.54$ log units. In the automatic mode, 108 points (6 in each patient) in the 18 patients tested showed much greater changes in differential threshold with time. 14 of the 108 points tested, showed very few responses by the patient during the entire 12 minute period, as they happened to be situated in an unexpectedly dense part of the visual field defect. 17 other points showed a marked change in the threshold, so that after some time of testing the maximum luminosity of the automatic perimeter was reached and the resulting curve relating threshold against time therefore became truncated (compare Fig. 1). The mean increment in threshold of those 17 points was $+0.91$ log units (S.D. ±0.39), with the maximal change being $+1.7$ log units. In the remaining 77 points, the mean increment of the threshold was $+0.27$ log units (S.D. ±0.36). 50 points showed an increase in differential threshold greater than 0.3 units, while only 5 points showed a decrease in threshold greater than 0.3 log units and in only one of those was the decrease greater than 0.4 log units.

In 4 patients who had either no field defects at all, or whose visual field disturbance was not in the central field, the mean threshold change was only $+0.01$ log units.

In the 3 patients whose tests were performed at three levels of background luminance, the results were very similar at all three background illuminations (Fig. 1). At the lowest background illumination, fewer of the curves were

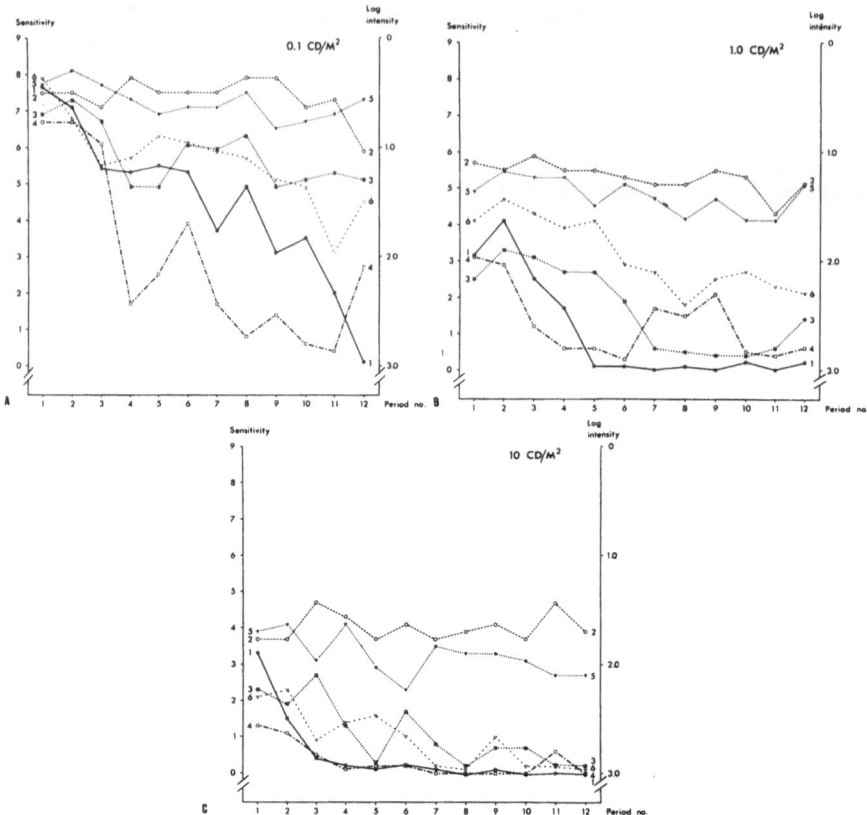

Fig. 1. Continuous automatic threshold recording of six test points during 30 minutes which have been divided into 12 equal periods. The y-axis shows the sensitivity levels of the Competer on the left side and the relative stimulus intensities in arbitrary units on the right side. Some points show pronounced deterioration of sensitivity with increasing test time and this occurs at all three background levels (0.1, 1.0 and 10 cd/m²). The location of points 1–6 tested are shown in Fig. 2. The most stable points 2 and 5 are situated closest to fixation in the least disturbed inferior half of the field. Reproduced with permission from the British Journal of Ophthalmology.

truncated because of the greater margin between the initial threshold and the maximum stimulus luminosity of the computerized perimeter. Two of these patients were tested manually at 2 background luminosities and the results were very similar.

The 6 points tested in each patient on the automatic perimeter were classified into three groups according to their relationship to defective areas. The classification was done without access to the results of the continuous threshold recordings.

Group 1 included points from defective parts of the visual field. Group 2 consisted of those points outside an existing field defect so situated that if any progression in the visual field defect were to occur it might involve the point tested. Group 3, consisted of points in the normal parts of the visual

132

Table 1. Mean increment of differential threshold over 30 minutes of automatic testing in relationship to proximity to existing field defects.

Patient group	Mean increment in threshold in log units	
1	+ 0.57	S.D. ± 0.47
2	+ 0.44	S.D. ± 0.47
3	+ 0.10	S.D. ± 0.27

Group 1: test points from defective parts of the visual field.
Group 2: test points close to existing field defects.
Group 3: test points in normal parts of the visual field.
1 > 2; $p < 0.05$ ⎫
2 > 3; $p < 0.05$ ⎬ one-sided sign test.
1 > 3; $p < 0.01$ ⎭

field well removed from existing visual field defects as judged from previous manual kinetic and static and automatic fields.

In 14 points which happened to be in more grossly defective areas than suspected from manual perimetry very few responses were elicited and they could therefore not be used in the analysis. The mean increase in differential threshold of the points in each of the above three groups are presented in Table 1. The results show that during a 30 minute automatic perimetric testing session, points tested in a relative visual field defect or in areas of the visual field adjacent to a visual field defect, showed more increment in threshold than points situated in normal areas of the visual field away from existing defects ($p < 0.01$ and $p < 0.05$, respectively – one-sided sign test). The means given for groups 1 and 2 are probably an underestimate of the actual change as some of the threshold changes reach the maximum stimulus

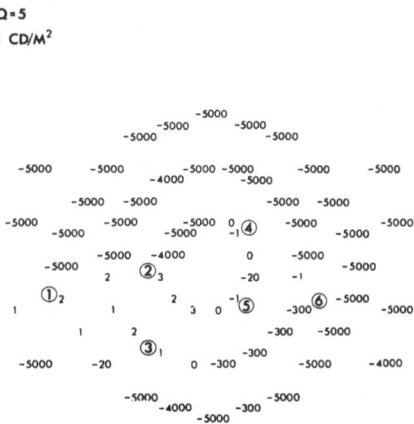

Fig. 2. Competer visual field of the eye tested in Fig. 1. The points tested are situated 5–20° from fixation with the three circles at 5, 10 and 15° respectively, negative numbers indicate areas with depressed sensitivity and the field thus shows a complete Bjerrum scotoma upwards and an arcuate scotoma connecting with the blind spot inferiorly. The location of the points illustrated in Fig. 1 are shown by circles. Reproduced with permission from the British Journal of Ophthalmology.

133

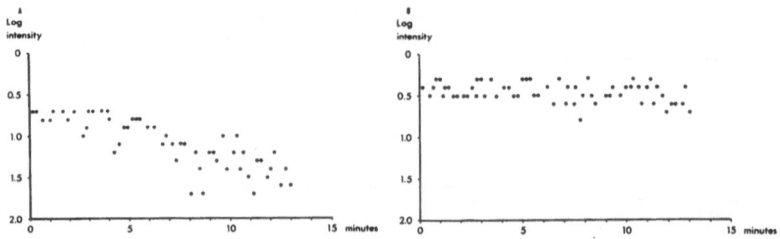

Fig. 3. Result of continuous manual threshold recording. Log stimulus intensity on the y-axis. Two points have been tested, one in a slightly disturbed part of the field (Fig. 3a) and one in the corresponding mirror point in a normal part of the field (Fig. 3b). The test point in the pathological part of the field shows decreased sensitivity with time, while the point in the normal part of the field remains more stable. Reproduced with permission from the British Journal of Ophthalmology.

intensity of the automatic perimeter and the curves relating threshold increment and time were therefore truncated.

There was a statistically significant correlation between the results obtained on manual and automatic testing (Spearman's rank coefficient = 0.49; $p <$ 0.05 — one-sided test).

The changes in threshold on manual testing were usually a good deal smaller. In those points tested with both methods the mean increment of the threshold on automatic testing was +0.67 log units, whereas on manual testing it was +0.19 log units. The greater change shown on automatic perimetry was present even when the increment was calculated at the end of 12 minutes of the 30 minute automatic testing in order to correspond to the average duration of the manual tests. As one might have expected the correlation between the 12 minute automatic results and the manual results was better than between the 30 minute automatic and the manual results (Spearman's rank correlation coefficient = 0.77; $p < 0.01$ — one-sided test).

No difference was found between the results obtained from patients with chronic open angle glaucoma and low-tension glaucoma. There was also no difference between those patients who had recently shown progression of their visual field defects and those whose visual fields were stable.

CONCLUSIONS

The study suggests that:
1. An increment of the differential threshold during prolonged continuous threshold recording is a common phenomenon in patients with glaucoma.
2. This increment in threshold was demonstrated both in automatic and manual perimetry.
3. The increment is larger in the automatic than manual mode of perimetry.
4. Areas in a relative scotomata or immediately adjacent to it show a more pronounced deterioration of threshold than normal points well away from field defects.
5. The increments of threshold occurs at different background luminosities, both in automatic and manual perimetry.

134

6. Those points showing an increment of threshold manifested them both at automatic and manual testing, whereas those points being stable were usually stable in both modes of testing.

DISCUSSION

Our study shows a definite deterioration of the differential threshold with time during continuous threshold determinations. In accordance with two previous studies (5, 7) we found this phenomenon common in patients with glaucoma. The present study further shows that it can be elicited on manual perimetry and is independent of background luminosity. These results are different from those of Enoch (1, 3) but we would point out that he showed increments of threshold of 1 or 2 log units over a 5 minute period in patients with pathology behind the optic disc (2, 8), while in our studies the increments were often smaller and appeared later during the test. Since the changes are independent of the background luminosity it must be questioned whether these are really the same saturation-like phenomena, which Enoch described. We used the optimum eccentric lens correction giving the minimum threshold (4) in only a few cases, but since these showed the same type of response as the rest of the patients we have no reason to believe that this could play any major role in our results.

Since the threshold changes in glaucoma patients still can be quite large especially near to existing field defects, they may have important implications. First, one cannot assume an increase in the accuracy of measuring the differential threshold if procedures like averaging of many responses are used and a continuous mode of testing is utilized. Secondly, the length of a test in a glaucoma patient should preferably be standardized if one wants to use the information to determine whether a glaucomatous field defect has progressed or not. Thirdly, the present results indicate that a moderate decrease in sensitivity at repeated static testing cannot be taken as a sign pointing only to a non-glaucomatous lesion. Further, the increment of differential threshold during prolonged testing might be a sign of impending damage because it is much more common in areas where one might expect progression of a field defect to occur as compared to those areas well away from a scotoma. It might therefore provide information about early disturbance and be a possible perimetric provocative test indicating the possiblity of subsequent visual field damage. This will, however, require prospective studies.

ACKNOWLEDGEMENTS

This study was supported by the E. A. Baker Foundation, Medical Research Foundation of Canada, MT 1578, Swedish Medical Research Council grant # B81-17F-5900-01 and Alcon Pharmaceuticals Ltd.

REFERENCES

1. Enoch, J. M. Quantitative layer-by-layer perimetry. Invest. Ophthalmol. 17:199–257 (1978).
2. Enoch, J. M., Berger, R. and Birns, R. A static perimetric technique believed to test receptive field properties: extension and verification of the analysis. Doc. Ophthalmol. 29:127–53 (1970).
3. Enoch, J. M. and Campos, E. C. Analysis of patients with open angle glaucoma using perimetric techniques reflecting receptive field-like properties. Doc. Ophthalmol. Proc. Series 19:137–49 (1979).
4. Fankhauser, F. and Enoch, J. M. The effects of blur upon perimetric thresholds. Arch. Ophthalmol. 68:240–51 (1962).
5. Heijl, A. Time changes of contrast thresholds during automatic perimetry. Acta Ophthalmol. 55:696–708 (1977).
6. Heijl, A. and Krakau, C. E. T. An automatic perimeter for glaucoma visual field screening and control. Albrecht von Graefes Arch. Klin. Exp. Ophthalmol. 197:13–23 (1975).
7. Holmin, C. and Krakau, C. E. T. Variability of glaucomatous visual field defects in computerized perimetry. Albrecht von Graefes Arch. Klin. Exp. Ophthalmol. 210:235–50 (1979).
8. Sunga, R. N. and Enoch, J. M. Further perimetric analysis of patients with lesions of the visual pathways. Am. J. Ophthalmol. 70:403–22 (1970).

Authors' addresses:
Dr S. M. Drance
Dept. of Ophthalmology
University of British Columbia
2577 Willow Street
Vancouver, B.C.
Canada V5Z 3N9

Dr A. Heijl
Dept. of Ophthalmology
University of Lund
Malmö General Hospital
S-214 01 Malmö
Sweden

136

CONSTANCY OF SENSITIVITY IN TIME IN PATIENTS WITH OPEN ANGLE GLAUCOMA: FURTHER RESULTS

EMILIO C. CAMPOS and SILVIA BELLEI

(Modena, Italy)

Key words. Visual field, glaucoma, static perimetry, sensitivity, time-dependent functions.

ABSTRACT

Years ago Enoch et al. showed a decay in sensitivity in time in the visual field of patients with active optic nerve disease, with the Flashing Repeat Static Test (FRST). Recently, Drance and Heijl found, with a different technique, similar changes in open angle glaucoma patients. In this paper results are presented taken from an additional group of 10 open angle glaucoma patients, examined with the FRST. No significant decrease in sensitivity in time was found. Tentative explanations for the discrepancy in results are provided. It is concluded that functional responses of patients with open angle glaucoma are different from those of patients with optic nerve disease.

INTRODUCTION

Various psychophsical paradigms have been described for studying the visual field layer-by-layer along the visual pathway (3, 5, 8). Two functions, reflecting receptive field-like properties have been localized in the inner retina. A third paradigm, called the Flashing Repeat Static Test (FRST) provides information about lesions in the retro-laminar portion of the optic nerve. The two functions, which reflect receptive field-like properties have been showed to be altered, among other diseases, in open angle glaucoma (3—5, 8). The FRST elicits a decay in sensitivity in time (in a 5 minute period) in patients with active optic nerve diseases (3, 5, 8). Further, measurement of contrast sensitivity, i.e. visual acuity, at high luminance levels with an interferometric acuity device, reveals a loss of such property in time in patients with optic nerve disease (1, 3—8). These effects are not manifest in many patients when adapted to low levels of luminance (1, 3—8).

The FRST appeared normal in patients with open angle glaucoma (8). This was shown even over a one-year testing period. Conversely, other visual functions (V.A., visual field, receptive field-like properties) fluctuated and eventually deteriorated in many patients. Recently Drance and Heijl (2) showed a decay in sensitivity in time in patients with open angle glaucoma and they were kind enough to let us know their results.

We examined an added further group of patients with open angle glaucoma in order to verify whether previous data obtained in Enoch's laboratory were repeatable. The FRST was administered and in some of these same patients interferometric acuity in time was measured.

MATERIAL AND METHODS

Ten patients with open angle glaucoma were considered. Intraocular pressure (IOP) with medical therapy ranged from 17 to 32 mm Hg. The eyes which were tested did not show significant corneal or lens changes, which could lead to erroneous results, because of optical reasons. Each patient showed significant visual field deficits attributable to glaucoma. An example is shown in Fig. 1A. The FRST was performed if possible at two symmetrical points in the two eyes. If visual function was altered in the second eye, two points in the same eye were chosen, equidistant from the point of fixation. The point which was actually tested was in or closely adjacent to an area of visual field deficit. The control point was in a normal response area.

The FRST was examined on a Goldmann perimeter and was conducted as follows: the patients, wearing their optimal optical correction were kept for ten minutes in a darkened examining room, with the only light source provided by the cupola of the Goldmann perimeter, set at $31.5 \, asb = 10 \, cd/m^2$. Then a first increment threshold was taken in the point to be tested, to provide a rough control of the level of sensitivity. After this, the patients were asked to close their eyes for a 5 minute period. Then as many as possible increment thresholds were taken sequentially for a testing period of 5 minutes. Each determination was an ascending threshold, i.e., the target was brought from not seen to just seen.

The size of the target used for the test was based on kinetic perimetric findings in the area to be tested.

In seven of the ten patients the Interferometric Acuity in Time (IAIT) was measured as well.

The IAIT was tested with a Takata Interferometric Acuity Device.* The procedure was the same as for the FRST. The patients were adapted for 10 minutes and a first determination was performed. Then they were kept for 5 minutes with both eyes closed. Then, repeated determinations of visual resolution were performed over a 5 minute period of time. All tests were performed by the second author (SB) as the senior author (ECC) had been involved in previous studies on this subject and did not want to introduce a bias in the results.

RESULTS

None of the ten patients examined by us exhibited a significant decay in sensitivity in time when measuring the FRST. Indeed, fluctuations were

*Courtesy: Amplimedical S.p.A., Milano.

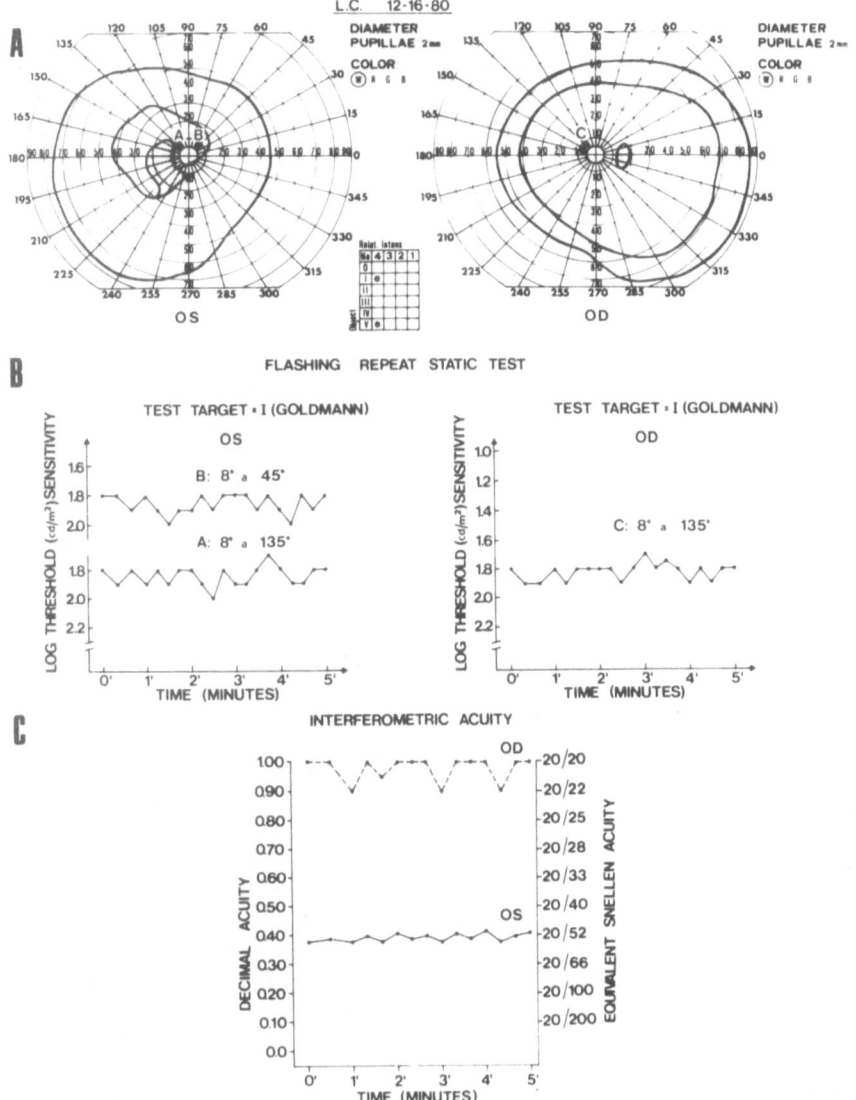

Fig. 1. (A) Kinetic perimetry in one of the patients with open angle glaucoma considered in this study; (B) Flashing Repeat Static Test (FRST) in the same patient, indicates no decay of sensitivity in time; (C) Interferometric acuity measured in time in the same patient of A and B. No decrease of visual acuity in time is detected.

noticed, as can be seen in Fig. 1B. However, the end result, after five minutes of testing did not depart from the initial result. This was constantly evident in all patients. In many patients reduced sensitivity was found in areas of their visual field. However, such reduction in sensitivity was constant and stable in time.

139

The IAIT, performed on 7 patients showed results which were stable in time as well. Again, contrast sensitivity was often anomalous, i.e., lower than 6/6, but no decay in sensitivity in time was observed (Fig. 1C).

DISCUSSION AND CONCLUSIONS

Our results indicate that in the group of patients considered for this study there was no evidence of decay in sensitivity in time. Clearly, the level of sensitivity was altered, i.e., it was reduced on several observers at the points tested. This has to be expected, because a loss of sensitivity is present when a visual field deficit is detected. It has to be stressed, however, that sensitivity was not altered and did not progress during the 5 minute test sessions. Fluctuations were found, but never of significant importance. In fact, in previous experiments conducted in Enoch's laboratory by the senior author a FRST was considered pathological only if a decay in sensitivity was found greater than 1/2 log unit. This was never the case in the population examined for this study.

Purposely, we did not test patients for a period of time longer than five minutes. Five minutes is the time span during which clear alterations in the increment threshold are found in patients with optic neuritis. Indeed, in the latter group of patients, changes are observable as early as the first or second minute of testing. The test was prolonged to five minutes for safety. We do not exclude that a fatigue phenomenon could be observed, testing glaucoma patients in longer sessions. Nevertheless, if changes should be present using prolonged testing times, they could not be superimposed to the results obtained in patients with optic neuritis. In any event a difference should exist between these two types of pathologies. In optic neuritis a fatigue phenomenon is observed very early and the two other psychophysical paradigms, which reflect retinal receptive field-like properties are normal. On the other hand in glaucoma, the receptive field-like properties are both pathological; the FRST is normal and, possibly, a decay in sensitivity in time may be found beyond 5 minutes of testing as stated by Drance and Heijl. We have no reason to doubt Drance and Heijl's results. However, we like to stress that functional differences do exist between patients with glaucoma and patients with optic neuritis.

We interpreted such differences as due to the fact that myelin sheets do not exist in the prelaminar portion of the optic nerve. Myelin is involved in conducting the visual information. If a pathology involves myelin, then a decay in sensitivity in time is observed. This could explain the different functional behaviour found in patients with open angle glaucoma and patients with optic neuritis. In both cases the pathology involves the same cells, i.e., the ganglion cells. The type of involvement, however, should be different because evidently the cells and their fibers react differently when they are or they are not surrounded by myelin.

Clearly further studies on this subject are necessary to clarify these points. More pathologies should be analyzed and the experiments should be repeated in various laboratories with the same techniques.

ACKNOWLEDGEMENTS

This research has been supported in part by National Eye Institute Grant No. EY-03674 to J. M. Enoch, National Institutes of Health, Bethesda, Maryland.

REFERENCES

1. Campos, E. C., Enoch, J. M., Fitzgerald, C. R. and Benedetto, M. D. A simple psychophysical technique provides early diagnosis in optic neuritis. Doc. Ophthalmol. 49:325 (1980).
2. Drance, S. and Heijl, A. Personal communication (1980).
3. Enoch, J. M. Quantitative layer-by-layer perimetry. Invest. Ophthalmol. and Visual Sci. 17: 208 (1978).
4. Enoch, J. M. and Campos, E. C. Analysis of patients with open angle glaucoma using perimetric techniques reflecting receptive field-like properties. Doc. Ophthalmol. Proc. Series 19:137 (1979).
5. Enoch, J. M. and Campos, E. C. New quantitative perimetric tests designed to evaluate receptive field-like properties in diseases of the retina and the optic nerve. In: Electrophysiology and Phychophysic: Their Use in Ophthalmic Diagnosis. Int. Ophthalmol. Clinics 20: 83 (1980).
6. Enoch, J. M., Campos, E. C. and Bedell, H. E. Visual resolution in a patient exhibiting a visual fatigue or saturation like effect. Arch. Ophthalmol. 97:76 (1979).
7. Enoch, J. M., Campos, E. C., Greer, m. and Trobe, J. Measurement of visual resolution at high luminance levels in patients with possible demyelinating disease. Int. Ophthalmol. 1:99 (1979).
8. Enoch, J. M., Fitzberald, C. R. and Campos, E. C. Quantitative layer-by-layer perimetry. An extended analysis. Grune and Stratton, New York (1980).

Author's address:
Dr E. C. Campos
Clinica Oculistica dell' Università
Via del Pozzo 71
Modena
Italy

DISCUSSION

Discussion on 'Constancy of sensitivity in time in patients with open angle glaucoma: Further results', by E. C. Campos and S. Bellei.

J. M. Enoch: Two issues need to be considered here: 1) in essence Heijl and Drance question whether Flashing Repeat Static Testing (FRST), as defined in my laboratory, has validity as a discriminator between post- and pre-laminar functional anomalies. Anomalies of the post-lamina are characterized by a visual saturation or fatigue-like effect which is adaptation-level-dependent and is clearly observed in cases of optic neuritis and has not been observed in open angle glaucoma patients; 2) have Heijl and Drance defined a separate time-dependent response with a different time course based on use of a different test which may show alteration in glaucoma? They claim that their finding is independent of the light-adaptation level.

The answer to the first question is that they never performed our test, although they claim to have duplicated it as closely as possible. We ordinarily use a Goldmann perimeter at the usual $10 \, cd/m^2$ level. We use as small a stimulus as possible (Goldmann 0, I or II, i.e. ca $3'$, $6'$ or $12'$ diameter); we provide a 5 min eyes closed pre-exam period and record the static threshold over a 4—5 min test period. We always come from not seeing to just seeing and immediately drop the luminance of the test target (to a subliminal value) the instant we get a positive response. We use the smallest target possible and non-seeing to first seeing because we find that the presence of a visible target influences threshold and causes increased fluctuant behaviour and apparent loss in sensitivity. We discontinue after 5 min because we find that subjects (particularly the elderly) become impatient and variance tends to increase. Further, if the visual fatigue or saturation-like response that we describe is present, it usually manifests itself in an unambiguous fashion within about 3 min. That is, sensitivity falls rapidly and profoundly, usually by 1 log unit or more. Heijl and Drance compare the first and the twelfth minutes in their test data, claiming to test the FRST. We have never measured beyond 5 or 6 min. I do not want to say that we ignore the first min, because in many optic neuritis cases, on many occasions, if you do not record the first min, sensitivity falls so that you obtain virtually nothing. In normals and in open angle glaucomas that we have studied, we tend not to base our judgments on the first several readings because after 5 min with eyes closed the patient has partially dark-adapted. Upon opening the eyes, the patient light-adapts and visual sensitivity will normally fall 0.1 to 0.3 log units, generally during the first minute of the test. This is a strictly physiological change in sensitivity. To be sure that I had not somehow erred, when Professor Drance told me of his study, I asked Professor Campos to conduct further tests. He is familiar with our techniques and has reported confirmatory results today. I can only conclude that Heijl and Drance did not conduct the FRST test as we have reported it.

Have Heijl and Drance revealed a different phenomenon? First, whatever they report is not luminance-dependent. Our test is highly luminance-dependent. Visual saturation or fatigue-like effect is increased at higher luminances and reduced at lower light levels (or eliminated). They get mixed results with their two instruments/methods. In their automated procedure, they use 0.3 log unit steps and bracket the threshold and use larger targets than we do. If a patient uses a slightly conservative criterion and has reasonably good fixation, this test technique could easily result in apparent sensitivity loss over time. That is, such a technique can cause adaptation to a higher light level. Are the patients fresh, do they provide reliable data over so extended a test period? I feel that Heijl and Drance have more work to do to establish their position firmly. If a separate time-based alteration in sensitivity is present in glaucoma, this could be a valuable contribution.

S. M. Drance: Dr Enoch has alluded to the differences between our results in the automatic and manual mode of continuously testing the differential threshold in patients with glaucoma. That such a difference exists is indeed interesting and requires further study as it may lead to an understanding of the underlying light threshold disturbances in glaucoma. There remains, however, the discrepancy between his and Dr Campos' findings and our findings done on the Tübingen perimeter. Our tests reproduced Enoch's technique almost exactly so that the background illumination was in the same low photopic range, the stimulus size was usually small (10'), we always approached threshold from seeing to non-seeing in a staircase method, we corrected optically at the outset for the areas tested but found this not to be of major consequence, we adapted the patient in an identical preadaption followed by closing the eye for 5 min. In spite of this similar approach we had some patients who in defective areas or areas adjacent to defects showed a fairly marked impairment of the differential threshold of 0.6 log units with 5 min. Dr Enoch considers 1 log unit significant in his post-laminar cases but even if there were only 2 or 3 of our patients who showed similar change to his this would throw serious doubt on the FRST being fundamentally different in optic neuritis and glaucoma. It is important to study the reasons for our differences as we may learn about the glaucomatous process as opposed to differences between glaucoma and post-laminar optic nerve disease. The differences between our results should stimulate further study and a re-examination of the concept that they indicate, a difference in behaviour according to site of optic nerve involvement. It may be that glaucomatous eyes even with early field defects may behave differently during or shortly after progression of a field defect even if it is so subtle as to escape detection as opposed to other stages of the disease.

THE EFFECT OF A NUMBER OF GLAUCOMA MEDICATIONS ON THE DIFFERENTIAL LIGHT THRESHOLD

JOSEF FLAMMER* and STEPHEN M. DRANCE**

(Vancouver, British Columbia, Canada)

Key words. Glaucoma medication, differential threshold.

ABSTRACT

The influence of acute pressure reduction on the differential light threshold was studied in 113 eyes of 75 patients with elevated intraocular pressure or very early stages of chronic open angle glaucoma. Systemic acetazolamide showed a tendency to improve the visual function, whereas topical epinephrine and timolol showed a tendency to decrease visual function while placebo and pindolol appeared to have no influence on the differential threshold.

INTRODUCTION

A number of investigators have studied the effects of acute reduction of intraocular pressure, produced by medications on the differential light threshold (4—6). The published data are sometimes contradictory. Clear-cut improvements in visual function and also a tendency to deterioration in visual function have both been reported. In addition to the obvious clinical significance such findings are of interest in the understanding of the effects of pressure on visual function. An improvement in visual function following the reduction in intraocular pressure suggests that intraocular pressure is a damaging factor in the disease and also suggests that at least in some glaucomatous patients, the first stage of the disease is a functional disturbance which is reversible and not yet accompanied by irreversible morphological changes. Depending on their findings, some authors have supported the pressure damaging theory (4), whereas others have denied its importance (5). In various studies the changes in intraocular pressure were produced by various medications such as acetazolamide and timolol. The purpose of our study was to examine whether the differences reported in the literature might be produced through the use of various medications used to reduce intraocular pressure. The

*In receipt of a Fellowship from the Swiss National Fund and the Verry Foundation.
**To whom requests for offprints should be addressed.

present pilot study summarizes the action of epinephrine, pindolol, timolol, acetazolamide and placebo.

PATIENTS AND METHODS

One hundred and thirteen eyes of 75 patients were examined. The intraocular pressure was reduced in 18 eyes (10 patients) with 1% epinephrine, 14 eyes (8 patients) with 1% pindolol, 28 eyes (16 patients) with 0.5% timolol and 25 eyes (25 patients) with 750 mg of oral diamox, while 28 eyes of 16 patients were treated with a placebo (eye stream). All eyes were suspect glaucomas without localized visual field defects or very questionable early field abnormalities. Only in the diamox group were there two patients with definite nerve fiber bundle defects. The mean age was 60 years, with a range of 22 to 82. The age was the same in the various groups treated with the drug. None of the patients were on any glaucoma medication.

All eyes were examined both with and without topical medication or tablets a week apart. The untreated or treated examination were randomly alternated in a block design. The drops or placebo were topically instilled one hour prior to the examination of thresholds whereas the diamox tables were given in three equal doses 12 hours prior to the examination with the last dose being given two hours before the examination. The differential thresholds were measured with Program JO on the Octopus perimeter (2).

RESULTS

The influence of the various drugs on intraocular pressure and differential threshold are summarized in Table 1. The placebo showed no reduction in intraocular pressure while epinephrine showed only a slight pressure reduction at the end of an hour, it is known to reduce pressure later than that. Pindolol and timolol showed a definite reduction in intraocular pressure. Acetazolamide lowered the intraocular pressure even more, which appears to be due to the pressure measurements being done 12 hours after the beginning of therapy.

The effects on the differential threshold was varied. The placebo showed none, while pindolol had virtually no effect on differential threshold. Epinephrine, and even more so, timolol showed a tendency for the visual function to deteriorate, whereas acetazolamide showed a very clear tendency to

Table 1.

	Number of eyes	Change in differential sensitivity after treatment	Change in IOP after treatment
Placebo	28	+0.01 ± 0.7 dB	+0.1 ± 2.5 mm Hg
Epinephrine	18	−0.32 ± 0.6 dB	−1.6 ± 5.0 mm Hg
Pindolol	14	−0.07 ± 0.6 dB	−5.1 ± 3.2 mm Hg
Timolol	28	−0.59 ± 1.0 dB	−5.2 ± 3.3 mm Hg
Diamox	25	+0.79 ± 2.3 dB	−8.5 ± 7.0 mm Hg

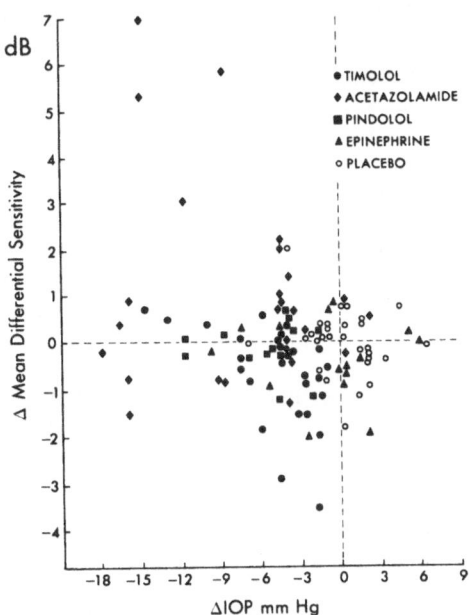

Fig. 1. Correlation between intraocular pressure changes and changes in the differential light threshold. The various symbols show the results obtained by the various glaucoma medications used.

improve visual function. An examination of the relationship of the intraocular pressure reduction with the changes of differential threshold showed that most of the eyes in all groups remained within the area of scatter which was also observed after placebo. Such a scatter is a resultant of the learning effect, experimental error and long-term fluctuation (3). The block design, however, makes the expected effect of such fluctuations on the mean to be zero. By looking at the outlyers, one can see that the outlyers following diamox therapy are all displaced toward improvement in visual function, whereas those following timolol are all displaced towards a deterioration in visual function (Fig. 1).

DISCUSSION

The pressure reduction produced by acetazolamide is associated with a tendency to improve the differential light threshold while in those eyes treated with timolol a tendency to deterioration in visual threshold is shown. These results confirm the results described in the literature (4–6). Placebo and pindolol showed no effect on the differential threshold, whereas epinephrine showed a small tendency towards deterioration. The influence of epinephrine on differential threshold has not been reported, to the best of our knowledge, in the literature.

The divergence of the effects of various medications, suggests that the effects produced by the drugs on differential threshold cannot be explained

147

by the medically obtained intraocular pressure reduction. This suggests that the published support or lack of support for the hypothesis that acute intraocualr pressure lowering changes visual function may not be valid. Intraocular pressure reduction either has no effect on the differential threshold or the effect is over-shadowed by other actions of the medications.

The differences cannot be explained through a change in pupil size or changes in blood pressure, as neither the beta-blockers nor acetazolamide produced a change in the size of the pupil. the blood pressure was reduced only in the acetazolamide-treated group.

The cause of the different effects of the medications on the differential threshold remains unclear. Hypothetically, one could assume that this might be effected through changes in the blood supply of the posterior segment of the eye. In monkeys following acetazolamide a clear improvement in blood supply on choroid and brain have been demonstrated (7), whereas propranolol shows a clear reduction in the cerebral blood flow (1). The lack of change in visual function following pindolol could be explained by its intrinsic sympathomimetic activity.

ACKNOWLEDGEMENT

This study was supported in part by the E. A. Baker Foundation for the Prevention of Blindness and Medical Research Council of Canada, Grant No. MT 1578.

REFERENCES

1. Aqyagi, M., Deshumukh, V. D., Meyer, J. S. et al. Effect of beta-adrenergic blockade with propranolol on cerebral blood flow, autoregulation and CO_2 responsiveness. Stroke 7:291 (1976).
2. Flammer, J., Drance, S. M., Jenni, A. et al. JO and STATJO: Programs for investigating the visual field with the Octopus automatic perimeter. Can. J. Ophthalmol. (in press).
3. Flammer, J. and Drance, S. M. The long-term fluctuation of the differential light threshold. Doc. Ophthalmol. Proc. Series (to be published).
4. Heilmann, K. Augendruck, Blutdruck und Glaukomschaden. Vergleichende perimetrische Studien des Zusammenhanges von Augendrucksteigerung, Blutdrucksenkung und Glaukomschaedigung bei primaeren Glaukomen. Buecherei des Augenarztes, Vol. 61, 72 Stuttgart, Ferdinand Enke (1972).
5. Holmin, C. and Krakau, C. E. T. Short-term effect of timolol in chronic glaucoma. Acta Ophthalmol. 60:00–00 (1982).
6. Paterson, G. Effect of intravenous acetazolamide on relative arcuate scotomas and visual field in glaucoma simplex. Proc. Roy. Soc. Med. 63:865 (1970).
7. Wilson, T. M., Strang, R. and MacKenzie, E. T. The response of the choroidal and cerebral circulations to changing arterial P_{Co_2} and acetazolamide in baboon. Invest. Ophthalmol. Visual Sci. 16:576 (1977).

Authors' address:
Dept. of Ophthalmology
University of British Columbia
2577 Willow Street
Vancouver, B.C.
Canada V5Z 3N9

TIME RESOLUTION IN GLAUCOMATOUS VISUAL FIELD DEFECTS

P. ROSSI*, G. CIURLO, C. BURTOLO and G. CALABRIA

(Genoa, Italy)

Key words. Flicker fusion, temporal resolution, glaucoma.

ABSTRACT

Flicker fusion frequency determination using threshold stimuli in each point shows that glaucoma specifically affects the time resolution properties of the visual system.

INTRODUCTION

Flicker fusion frequencies (FFF) have been reported among the earliest functional alterations in glaucoma (1, 2). In a previous study (4) we stressed the need that FFF should be assessed using threshold-related stimuli in each tested point. This study reports and discusses the results of flicker perimetry using liminal stimuli in glaucomatous patients.

MATERIAL AND METHOD

Seven patients affected by open angle glaucoma and visual field (VF) defects within the central 10° were studied. Flicker fusion frequencies were assessed by means of a rotating sector device mounted on a Goldmann perimeter, as previously described (3). FFF were assessed within the central 10° of the VF with a descending method using targets with diameters of 1/4 and 4 mm² and the corresponding threshold luminance. The mean value and the standard deviation of 8 measurements were calculated. For each patient the differences in FFF between the central point and a scotomatous area of the VF were evaluated by means of Fisher's test.

RESULTS

Table 1 reports the FFF of the central and the scotomatous area on reported values, together with the corresponding *t* value.

*To whom requests for offprints should be addressed.

Greve, E. L., Heijl, A. (eds.) Fifth International Visual Field Symposium.
©1983 Dr W. Junk Publishers, The Hague/Boston/Lancaster.

Table 1. Results: mean values and standard deviation of FFF in normal and scotomatous areas.

Patient No.	Area			Area		
	Normal	Scotomatous	Fisher's t	Normal	Scotomatous	Fisher's t
1	12.50 ± 0.9	4.25 ± 0.5	18.39	14.2 ± 0.70	6.1 ± 0.5	17.44
2	15.75 ± 0.5	10.2 ± 0.81	12.9	15.6 ± 0.40	9.3 ± 0.36	25.2
3	12.75 ± 0.95	2.75 ± 0.57	17.3	13.25 ± 0.85	4.2 ± 0.20	21.241
4	12.25 ± 1.0	7.75 ± 0.5	8.05	12.50 ± 0.89	7.12 ± 0.40	11.04
5	12.00 ± 1.15	5.6 ± 0.89	6.27	14.1 ± 1.1	5.8 ± 0.81	12.17
6	12.1 ± 0.2	4.5 ± 0.57	25.76	13.45 ± 0.75	6.1 ± 0.25	18.52
7	11.75 ± 0.5	7.25 ± 0.9	8.75	12.75 ± 0.90	8.5 ± 0.75	7.03
Target diameter	1/4			4		mm^2

DISCUSSION

Previous results allow the following considerations: 1) flicker fusion frequency evaluation using threshold stimuli in combination with a descending method is a quite reliable examination, as indicated by the low scattering of the measurements; 2) flicker fusion frequencies decreased significantly within scotomatous areas.

In a previous study (4) we reported that, when threshold stimuli are used in each point, FFF's do not significantly change in the central visual field of normal people; the time resolution properties of the visual system therefore will look constant throughout the central VF. The present study shows that, within scotomata, FFF's are lowered and, therefore, that glaucoma affects the time resolution properties of the visual system, besides light threshold. These results correspond with those of previous authors who showed FFF's to be altered in glaucoma at an early stage. It should however, be stressed that such authors tested FFF using the same stimulus in VF areas having different light thresholds. In this way FFF alterations are related not only to the actual time resolution properties of the retinal area tested, but also to the degree of supraliminality of the testing stimulus in that point.

The higher the light sensibility, the higher will be the FFF, and vice versa. FFF within scotomata will therefore appear lower than in normal areas mainly because the stimulus will be only slightly supraliminal within the former and highly supraliminal within the latter: changes in FFF will therefore especially reflect changes in light threshold.

CONCLUSION

FFF's tested with liminal stimulus show that glaucoma specifically affects the time resolution properties of the visual system. FFF alterations assessed using a constant stimulus throughout the area examined are more related to light threshold differences than to the time resolution properties.

REFERENCES

1. Hylkema, B. S. Fusion frequency with intermittent light under various circumstances. Acta Ophthalmol. 20:159 (1942).
2. Miles, P. W. Flicker fusion fields. III. Findings in early glaucoma. Arch. Ophthalmol. 43:661 (1950).
3. Rossi, P., Ciurlo, G. and Suetta, G. Nuovo apparecchio per Flicker-perimetria. Min. Oftal. 20:61−68 (1978).
4. Zingirian, M., Ciurlo, G., Rossi, P. and Burtolo, C. Flicker fusion and spatial summation. Doc. Ophthalmol. Proc. Series 26:127−130 (1981).

Author's address:

Dr P. Rossi
University Eye Clinic
Viale Benedetto XV, 5
16132 Genoa
Italy

THE LOCATION OF EARLIEST GLAUCOMATOUS VISUAL FIELD DEFECTS DOCUMENTED BY AUTOMATIC PERIMETRY

ANDERS HEIJL and LEIF LUNDQVIST

(Malmö, Sweden)

Key words. Glaucoma, visual field, glaucoma screening, automatic perimetry.

ABSTRACT

A large material of eyes (2,500–3,000) with ocular hypertension, with or without established glaucoma in the fellow eye, were followed with automatic perimetry on the Competer perimeter for several years. Forty-five eyes showed a documented change from repeated normal fields to reproducible glaucomatous visual field loss. The location of the defective points in the first pathological field of each eye was registered, and a composite figure drawn. The resulting frequency distribution is similar to but not identical with that previously reported by Aulhorn and Karmeyer for their stage II defects found with manual perimetry. Thus, we were able to confirm their observation that in the very central field early glaucomatous visual field loss is more common in the superior than in the inferior half of the field, but we also found that early glaucomatous field loss in general is more common in the superior half of the field.

INTRODUCTION

Knowledge of the nature of glaucomatous visual field defects is of importance not only for the recognition of glaucomatous visual defects as such, but also for understanding the pathophysiology of glaucoma and in designing instruments or test protocols for the early detection of glaucomatous visual field damage. Largely through the work of Aulhorn and Harms the earlier opinions of enlargement and baring of the blind spot as early glaucomatous field defects have been replaced by the modern concept of small paracentral defects with or without nasal steps as being typical signs of early damage (1). These findings have later been confirmed by others (e.g. 2).

In 1977 Aulhorn and Karmeyer published a report on the frequency distribution of so-called stage II glaucomatous defects (i.e. defects with an asbolute nucleus but no connection to the blind spot) using manual static and kinetic techniques on the Tübingen perimeter (3). This report has later been followed by others using manual or semi-automatic perimetric techniques (4, 5).

Greve, E. L., Heijl, A. (eds.) Fifth International Visual Field Symposium.
©*1983 Dr W. Junk Publishers, The Hague/Boston/Lancaster.*

The aim of the present study was to investigate the frequency distribution of the locations of the *earliest* glaucomatous visual field loss using automatic perimetry in order to see whether this would give similar results to those previously published.

MATERIAL AND METHODS

Since we wanted to know the distribution of early glucomatous field loss we studied only eyes which had been shown to change from normal to pathologic when followed with automatic perimetry. The Competer computerized perimeter (6) was used and only eyes which had shown repeated (at least two) normal fields later followed by repeated (at least two) pathological fields were included in the study. Ophthalmoscopy was used to sort out field defects due to other reasons than glaucoma.

The eyes studied came from two sources:

1. Twenty-two eyes of 21 patients from a material of 907 eyes with increased intraocular pressure (≥ 22 mm Hg) followed with computerized perimetry in a prospective way for a period of at least three years.
2. Twenty-three eyes of 18 patients retrospectivley found in a larger material of approximately 2000 eyes with ocular hypertension.

The material consisted of both treated and untreated eyes. Some of the eyes were second eyes in patients with manifest glaucoma in one eye.

The patients had been followed with the supraliminal screening technique of the Competer or with the threshold technique of the same instrument in which actual threshold measurements were performed in each of the 64 points tested.

The interpretation of the fields followed criteria, which have been previously described (7, 8). In the 45 eyes studied the positions of all points with a sensitivity below the stipulated limit in the first pathologic field were plotted in two composite figures, one showing all points with pathologically decreased sensitivity (Fig. 1) and one (Fig. 2) with only absolute defects (maximum luminosity defects on the Competer). All fields from left eyes were converted to the corresponding right eye fields.

RESULTS

The results are shown in Figs. 1 and 2. Quite naturally the largest number of missed points is in the physiologic blind spot area at 15° eccentricity on and around the horizontal meridian. The pathologic points are most numerous in the nasal field and superiorly. In the central field 5° from fixation there is a striking preponderance of defective points superiorly particularly nasally. Disturbances are more common in the superior half of the field.

DISCUSSION

The results show that also with automatic techniques and very early field defects one arrives at a frequency distriution similar to that of Aulhorn and Karmeyer.

154

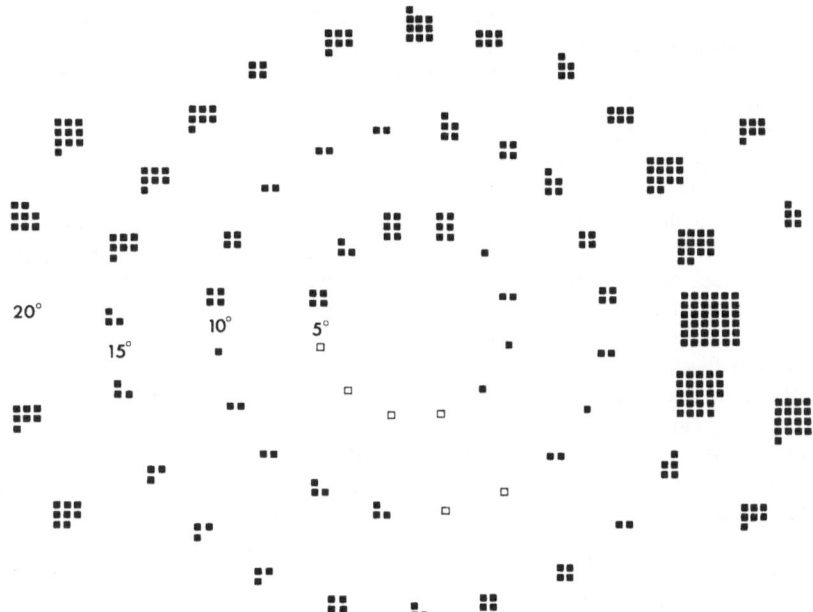

Fig. 1. All points with pathologically decreased sensitivity. Each black square represents one pathological point in one patient.

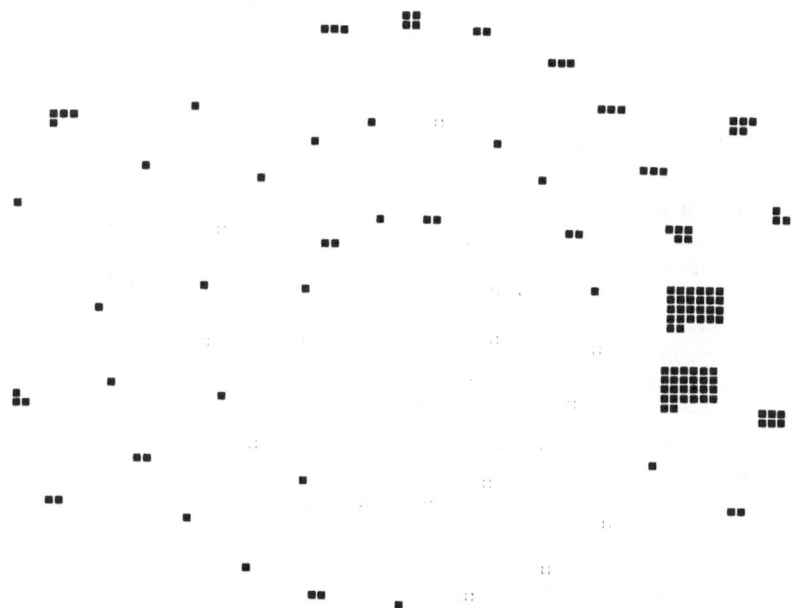

Fig. 2. Points with maximum luminosity defects on the Competer.

In manual perimetry one only finds the defects that one looks for. This is true to some degree also for automatic perimetry of course, since also the automatic instruments have been programmed to test for defects in certain areas and with certain techniques. However, automatic perimetry is free from perimetrist-bias, employs sensitive static testing and tends to test a larger number of positions in the central field than is usually done in manual perimetry. It was therefore a possibility that the results of this study would differ a great deal from those of earlier studies. It might be reassuring to see that also in this study the results are rather similar to those previously published. Thus, defects are more common nasally and occur more centrally in the superior than in the inferior field. The large number of missed points around the blind spot should not be taken as a sign indicating that glaucomatous field loss is particularly common there, since small defects due to angioscotoma are common in this region even in normal subjects (9).

Pathological field loss was more common in the superior than in the inferior half of the field in the present study. This is contrary to the results of Aulhorn and Karmeyer (3) but agrees with other studies (4, 5, 10). This might perhaps be explained by the recent observation that optic disc haemorrhages are more common in the inferotemporal than in the superotemporal part of the disc (11).

An interesting observation is that as many as 21 of the 45 visual fields demonstrated at least one test point (outside the blind spot) with a maximum luminosity defect on the Competer. This might be taken as a confirmation of previous opinions that early glaucomatous field defects, though mostly shallow, often contain some deep nucleus. Other factors may also play a role. Thus, early models of the Competer used fairly low-output light emitting diodes (the only ones available at that time) giving a quite limited practical stimulus range. Another contributing factor might be the fact that field defects often appear deeper on automatic than on manual perimetry (12). Furthermore, the interpretation criteria for abnormality referred to above are somewhat conservative in order to limit the frequency of false positives. Commonly a computerized comparison of consecutive fields can show suspicious areas with increased scatter and inconstant relative disturbances before the criteria used here become positive (13).

The tested area in this study includes only the central field. Defects situated only outside this area must have been missed. We believe that only a few percent of the total number of defective fields have been missed in this study, since in one study, in which the ability of the Competer to detect glaucomatous field loss was compared to that of very careful combined static and kinetic manual perimetry, only a few percent of the field defects were missed by the automatic instrument (18). Even if one recent study using automatic perimetry (10) indicates that glaucomatous field defects up to stage II increase in frequency nasally from the point of fixation up to 30° eccentricity this does not mean that the whole defect must be situated outside the area covered by our stimulus pattern. At the same time it cannot be denied that the present data cannot be used to confirm or reject the results of Gramer et al. (10).

The results of this study can, and probably should, be used as a help in designing test protocols for the detection of early glaucomatous field loss. It is tempting to use the results to device some sort of very limited but still efficient test point pattern, particularly since 82% of the pathological fields of this study could be identified just by looking at the test result in eight test points. We refrain from giving such a very reduced test point pattern, however, for two reasons: first, the present results are based on only 45 eyes which have been observed to convert from normal fields to showing glaucomatous field defects; secondly, one cannot be sure that the 82% of the defective fields in this material would have been detected by using the eight points referred to above. The reason for this is that the increment thresholds in glaucomatous eyes cannot be regarded as static even during one and the same test session, but instead areas of relative disturbance or areas in the vicinity of field defects frequently show progressively deteriorating sensitivity during a test session (14) (pp. 00–00, this volume). This means that defects are easier to detect when the perimetric testing has been going on for a while than at the very beginning of a test. A very quick test using only few test points might therefore not show pathology which is clearly identified in the very same test points on a longer test.

ACKNOWLEDGEMENT

This study was supported by the Järnhardt foundation.

REFERENCES

1. Aulhorn, E. and Harms, H. Early visual field defects in glaucoma. In: Glaucoma Symposium Tutzing Castle 1966, Karger, Basel-New York, pp. 151–86 (1967).
2. Drance, S. M., Fairclough, M., Thomas, B., Douglas, G. R. and Susannna, R. The early visual field defects in glaucoma and the significance of nasal steps. Doc. Ophthalmol. Proc. Series 19:119–126 (1979).
3. Aulhorn, E. and Karmeyer, H. Frequency distribution in early glaucomatous field defects. Doc. Ophthalmol. Proc. Series 14:75–83 (1977).
4. Furuno, F. and Matsuo, H. Early stage progression in glaucomatous visual field changes. Doc. Ophthalmol. proc. Series 19:247–53 (1979).
5. Coughlan, M. and Friedmann, A. I. The frequency distribution of early glaucomatous field defects in glaucoma. Doc. Ophthalmol. Proc. Series 26:345–9 (1981).
6. Heijl, A. and Krakau, C. E. T. An automatic perimeter for glaucoma visual field screening and control. Construction and clinical cases. Albrecht von Graefes Arch. Klin. Exp. Ophthalmol. 197:13–23 (1975).
7. Heijl., A. Automatic perimetry in glaucoma visual field screening. A clinical study. Albrecht von Graefes Arch. Klin. Exp. Ophthalmol. 200:21–37 (1976).
8. Heijl, A., Drance, S. M. and Douglas, G. R. Automatic perimetry (Competer) Ability to detect early glaucomatous field loss. Arch. Ophthalmol. 98:1560-(1981).
9. Heijl, A. Unpublished results.
10. Gramer, E., Gerlach, R., Krieglstein, G. K. and Leydhecker, W. Zur Topographie früher glaukomatöser Gesichtsfeldausfälle bei der Computerperimetrie. Klin. Mbl. Augenheilk. 180:515–523 (1982).
11. Airaksinen, P. J., Mustonen, E. and Alanko, H. I. Optic disk hemorrhages. Analysis of stereophotographs and clinical data of 112 patients. Arch. Ophthalmol. 98: 1795–1801 (1981).

12. Heijl, A. Time changes of contrast thresholds during automatic perimetry. Acta Ophthalmol. 55:696–708 (1977).
13. Heijl, A. Unpublished results.
14. Heijl, A. and Drance, S. M. Deterioration of threshold in glaucoma patients during perimetry. Doc. Ophthalmol. Proc. Series 35:129–136 (1983).

Authors' address:
Dept. of Ophthalmology
University of Lund
Malmö General Hospital
S-214 01 Malmö
Sweden

THE COURSE OF EARLY VISUAL FIELD CHANGE IN GLAUCOMA AS EXAMINED BY PUPILLOGRAPHIC PERIMETRY

TATSUYA AOYAMA* and KIMITOSHI MATSUNO

(Osaka/Hyugo, Japan)

Key words. Pupil, pupillographic perimetry, glaucoma, visual field defect.

ABSTRACT

Objective visual field changes in 5 cases of early open angle glaucoma were followed by pupillographic perimetry. Our experiments suggested that pupillographic perimetry was a useful method to detect the effect of treatment in those cases. Reversibility of glaucomatous visual field change was detected in 3 of the 5 cases by pupillographic perimetry after appropriate control of intraocular pressure.

INTRODUCTION

Previously, the authors reported that pupillographic perimetry (PP) was an effective method for glaucoma diagnosis since it could detect early visual field changes in the Bjerrum area in glaucoma cases where routine subjective perimetry was normal (1, 2).

In the present study, the authors selected several follow-up cases and examined the course of subjective and objective visual field change at the same time.

SUBJECTS AND METHODS

The subjects included one normal control and 5 patients with early glaucoma who showed normal visual field with kinetic and static perimetry, but reduction of pupillary sensitivity in the Bjerrum area at the first examination. All patients were controlled with intraocular pressure (IOP) within normal levels by the use of miotics, epinephrine hydrochloride and β-blockers. The apparatus and the experimental procedures were the same as described in the preceding papers (1, 2).

*To whom requests for offprints should be addressed.

Greve, E. L., Heijl, A. (eds.) Fifth International Visual Field Symposium.
©*1983 Dr W. Junk Publishers, The Hague/Boston/Lancaster.*

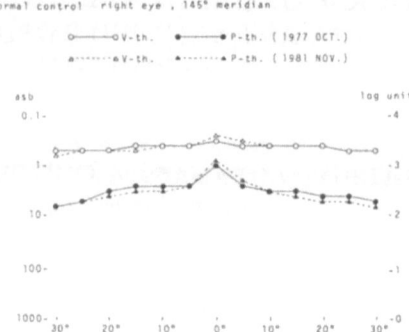

Fig. 1. Pupillographic perimetry in a normal control.

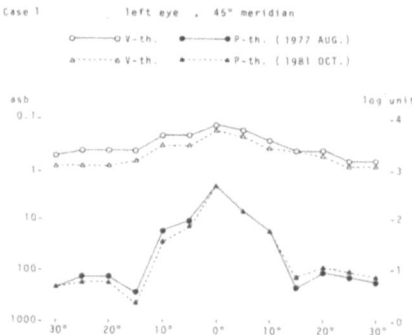

Fig. 2. Pupillographic perimetry in case 1.

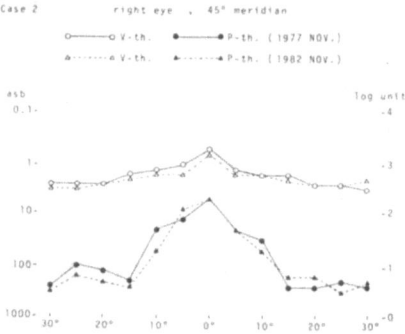

Fig. 3. Pupillographic perimetry in case 2.

RESULTS

In normal controls, no visual change could be found between the first and second exmaination by static perimetry and PP (Fig. 1). In our follow-up examinations, no cases showed significant visual field change by static perimetry. On the other hand, by PP, reversibility of glaucomatous visual field

160

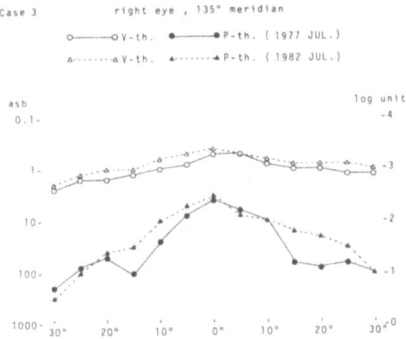

Fig. 4. Pupillographic perimetry in case 3.

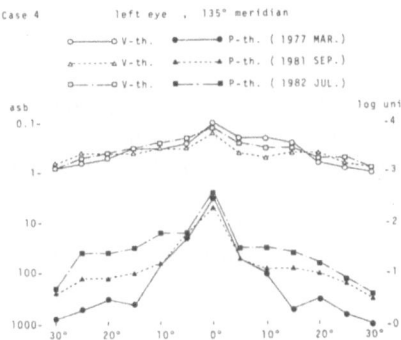

Fig. 5. Pupillographic perimetry in case 4.

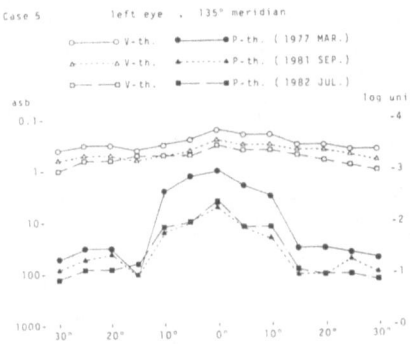

Fig. 6. Pupillographic perimetry in case 5.

changes could be found in 3 cases (cases 3, 4, 5), while in 2 other cases no change could be detected during follow-up (cases 1, 2).

Case 1: a 22-year old woman. The left eye had an IOP of 25 mm Hg and showed depression of the pupillary sensitivity at 15° in August, 1977. Following the control of IOP by use of miotics, the depression remained unchanged using PP on October, 1981 (Fig. 2).

161

Case 2: a 66-year old woman. Her right eye had an IOP of 20 mm Hg and showed depression of the pupillary sensitivity at 15° on November 1977. In this case, no treatment was given between the first and second examination. No change could be found in PP (Fig. 3).

Case 3: a 13-year old woman. Her right IOP was 28 mm Hg and this eye showed depression of the pupillary sensitivity at 15° in July, 1977. Following the control of IOP by use of miotics and epinephrine hydrochloride, the depression of pupillary sensitivity at 15° disappeared and PP showed a normal pattern in July, 1982 (Fig. 4).

Case 4: a 35-year old man. His left IOP was 25 mm Hg and this eye showed depression of the pupillary sensitivity at 15° in March, 1977. Following the control of IOP by use of miotics and β-blockers, the depression of the pupillary sensitivity at 15° recovered and reached normal values of PP in July, 1982 (Fig. 5).

Case 5: a 44-year old woman. Her left IOP was 30 mm Hg and this eye showed depression of the pupillary sensitivity at 15° in March, 1977. In spite of the control of IOP by use of miotics, PP remained pathological in September, 1981. After that, the IOP was controlled by a β-blocker. In July, 1982, the pattern of PP became almost normal, although the pupillary sensitivity still showed depression at the central retinal area (0°–10°) (Fig. 6).

DISCUSSION

PP is not easily applied in the routine examination since the pupillary reflex is easily affected by patient's mental state. Furthermore, it is difficult to measure precisely in glaucoma patients who are controlled by the autonomic nervous system. When observing the course of glaucomatous visual field changes by PP, it is important to give attention not to the change of the actual value of the pupillary sensitivity but more to the change of the pattern of PP.

Several studies have been reported concerning reversibility of galucomatous visual field change and it has been mentioned that this is not a frequent phenomenon (3, 4, 5). In this investigation by PP, reversibility of glaucomatous visual field change could be found in 3 of 5 cases following appropriate control of IOP. This suggests that the reversibility appears more frequently in the earliest stage of glaucoma, in which glaucomatous visual field change can be detected only by PP.

REFERENCES

1. Aoyama, T. Pupillographic perimetry — The application to clinical cases. Acta Soc. Ophthalmol. Jap. 81:1527–1538 (1977).
2. Aoyama, T. Visual field change examined by pupillographic perimetry in glaucoma. Doc. Ophthalmol. Proc. Series 19:265–271 (1978).

3. Armaly, M. F. Reversibility of glaucomatous defects of the visual field. Doc. Ophthalmol. Proc. Series 19:177–185 (1978).
4. Greve, E. L. et al. The clinical significance of reversibility of glaucomatous visual field change. Doc. Ophthalmol. Proc. Series 19:197–204 (1978).
5. Phelps, C. C. Visual field defects in open angle glaucoma: Progression and regression. Doc. Ophthalmol. Proc. Series 19:187–196 (1978).

authors' addresses:
Dr T. Aoyama
Osaka Central Hospital
2-8-2 Sonezaki, Kita-ku
Osaka 530
Japan

Dr K. Matsuno
Dept. of Ophthalmology
Hyogo College of Medicine
1-1 Mukogawa-cho, Nishinomiya
Hyogo 663
Japan

THE OCCUPATIONAL VISUAL FIELD

I. Theoretical aspects: the normal functional visual field

GUY VERRIEST (editor), LUIGI BARCA, ANDRÉ DUBOIS-POULSEN,
M. J. M. HOUTMANS, BORIS INDITSKY, CHRIS JOHNSON,
IAN OVERINGTON, LUCIA RONCHI and SERGIO VILLANI
(Ghent, Belgium)

Key words. Visual field, behavior, binocular vision, visual lobe, conspicuity, attention, eye and head movement.

ABSTRACT

This official report from the IPS Group on Functional Visual Field describes the concept of functional visual field and defines the differences between it and the diagnostic visual field. In comparison to clinical perimetric findings, the behavioral visual field is generally binocular, the target acquisition level often must be higher than for simple detection, targets are generally suprathreshold, and both the target and background can be complex. Attention, pre-existing knowledge and training can considerably affect performance, and the target as well as the observer's eyes, head and body are often moving. The major theoretical components of the functional visual field consist of models of visual physiology and visual performance, and distinctions among different types of functional visual fields.

The *functional visual field* is defined as the spatial area that can be monitored by a subject while performing a given visual task (Sanders, 1962) or, alternatively, as the visual field extent that is useful for a specific visual task. The terms 'ergonomic', 'behavioral' or 'occupational' visual field would be less confusing for ophthalmologists. However, the use of 'functional' visual field is already well established in other disciplines.

Although it is well known that individuals with tunnel vision exhibit severe visual impairment, research pertaining to the functional visual field has only been conducted in recent times. The first concerted research efforts were performed in the Netherlands by Sanders and by Engel in the 1960's, followed by the work of Ikeda in Japan during the 1970's. A historical overview of this discipline is available in the review papers by Villani (1979) and Barca and Fornaro (1980). Currently, the concept of the functional visual field is incorporated in mathematical models of visual performance developed in the

United Kingdom and the United States for lighting engineering, military applications and aeronautics.

The complexity of the functional visual field can best be demonstrated by *comparing it to the clinical visual field evaluated by ophthalmologists.* Perimetry, or clinical visual field testing, is designed to generate a topographical representation of sensitivity to light for a stationary eye. This is typically accomplished by placing the eye to be examined at the center of curvature of a uniform hemisphere, with the fellow eye occluded. The eye under examination maintains fixation on a small target at the center of the bowl, while the examiner determines the light sensitivity at various locations in the visual field by projecting a small, round stimulus to various parts of the hemispherical bowl. Stimulus visibility is increased by incrementing its luminance or size, or by moving it closer to the fixation point, while the subject reports (either verbally or by pressing a button) the first instance that the stimulus is detected. These clinical perimetric tests are only relevant to the rare ergonomic situations that involve detection tasks without visual scanning. Specialized forms of clinical perimetry such as color fields, flicker fusion fields, delay fields, double flash fields, motion fields, and stereoscopic depth fields (Regan, 1980) may be relevant to a small number of specialized work conditions. Similarly visual fields for low spatial frequencies (2−4 c/deg) are relevant to low-contrast (e.g. foggy) conditions, as when driving or flying. These fields cannot necessarily be predicted from the acuity field (Regan, 1982).

In most instances, the functional visual field of importance to the ergonomics specialist is considerably different from clinical visual fields measured by ophthalmologists. First of all, workers use both eyes rather than just one for most occupational situations. Often, it is necessary to recognize or identify a target as well as detect its presence. The targets employed for clinical perimetric testing are usually near threshold, whereas the worker is generally presented with suprathreshold stimuli that are more visible. In work environments, it is seldom that small round white targets are observed on a homogeneous background: workers are normally confronted with complex stimuli that are superimposed on textured or structured backgrounds. Vision is normally tested at a constant background luminance level while in practice the level might vary between very high (e.g. sea, snow) to very low (e.g. night traffic). Clinical perimetry attempts to minimize the influences of attention, learning, expectation, prediction and fatigue, whereas these factors need to be carefully evaluated in functional visual field studies. For many work environments, especially in traffic situations, the objects of regard are moving with reference to the observer. Perhaps the most significant difference between functional and clinical visual fields concerns the fixation patterns of the eyes. Clinical perimetry is performed with stable fixation of the eye, in contrast to work situations in which gaze is unrestricted and complex eye, head and body movements frequently occur.

The remainder of this report will review each of the factors mentioned above, and will provide a brief overview of the mathematical models that have been proposed to account for them.

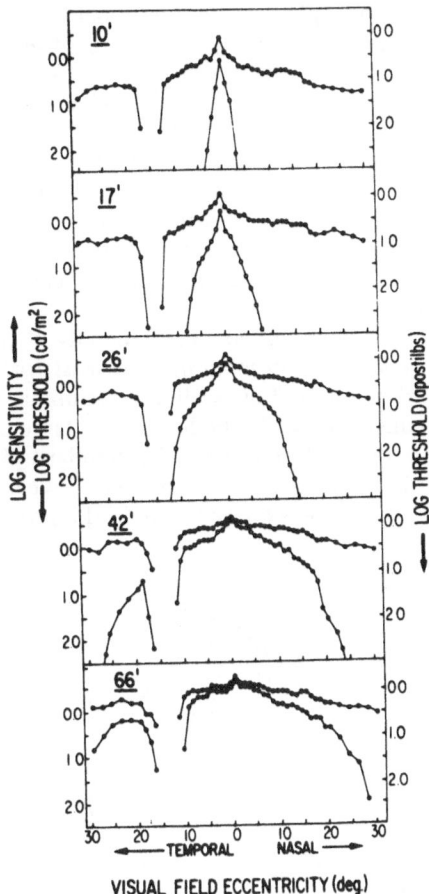

Fig. 1. Detection (●, top curves) and resolution (○, bottom curves) threshold sensitivities plotted as a function of stimulus eccentricity for 5 target sizes in the horizontal meridian. from Johnson, Keltner and Balestrery (1978).

As mentioned previously, one of the differences between clinical and functional visual fields is that *both eyes* are normally used for daily activities, while monocular testing is usually performed for clinical perimetry. The binocular visual field of a normal subject is not only larger than the monocular field, but it is also often more sensitive in the region of overlap between the two eyes. This is true for depth perception as well as absolute thresholds, differential thresholds and visual acuity. Recent studies have shown that when a target stimulates precisely corresponding retinal points in the two eyes, the gain sensitivity can be greater than that predicted on the basis of probability summation (Thorn and Boynton, 1974; Westendorf and Fox, 1977).

167

Overington's (1976) concept that the functional visual field depends upon the target acquisition level (detection, class recognition, detail recognition, full identification) is also of importance for our purposes. In work situations, detection of a target is often followed by its identification through resolution of critical details. The Tübingen perimeter, an ophthalmologic instrument, permits direct comparison of detection and resolution thresholds by using round and square luminous targets of the same approximate area. Johnson, Keltner and Balestrery (1978) utilized this technique to demonstrate that resolution gradients exhibit steeper slopes than detection sensitivity profiles (see Fig. 1). Thus target detection can be carried out over a larger area than target identification.

Objects in actual work environments are generally of sufficient luminance and size to be readily seen, or *supraliminal*, at least for central vision. The term 'visibility' is used to define how well a supraliminal target can be seen. Blackwell (1981) defines the visibility level of a target as the ratio of its actual contrast to the threshold contrast of a standard disc target, although this formulation has been questioned by others (Boyce, 1981). For low to moderate target visibility, there is a rapid drop in the probability of detection

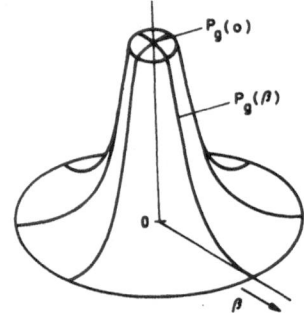

Fig. 2. Schematic illustration of detection probability per fixation. From Inditsky and Bodmann (1980).

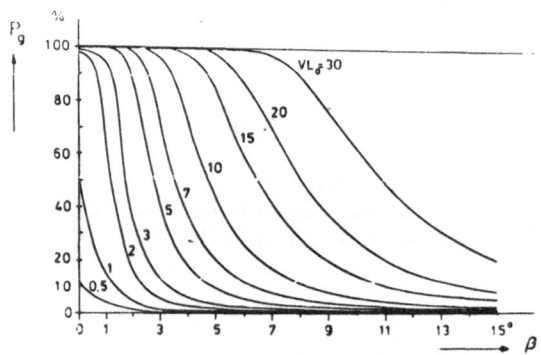

Fig. 3. Detection probability profiles per fixation (parameter VL_0 = 'on-axis' visibility level). From Inditsky and Bodmann (1980).

168

from the fovea out to the periphery. The most recent models of visual performance for a single glimpse (Inditsky and Bodmann, 1980; Overington, 1980) are based on both the perimetric sensivity gradient and the frequency of seeing curve. This combination of parameters generates a graph referred to as a 'visual lobe', which defines the probability of perception as a function of eccentricity (see Fig. 2). If the contrast of a target is increased, the central portion of the visual lobe will be flat, since each point will correspond to 100% probability of perception (see Fig. 3). The central portion of the visual lobe will also be flat when the target size is increased or the acquisition level is reduced. However, there are occasions, particularly for large targets or low image quality, where visual lobes can be much shallower and not reach a plateau of 100% probability of perception (Overington, 1982). Inditsky and Bodmann (1980) consider the on-axis visibility level as the most suitable parameter for the visual lobe. Inter-observer variability in the sensitivity gradient and long-term changes in perception probability (Ronchi and Salvi, 1973) are accounted for by Overington's model.

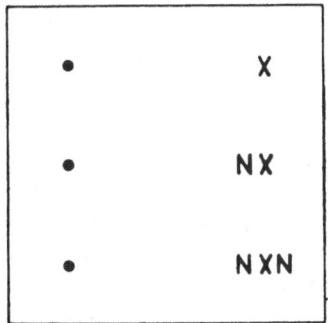

Fig. 4. Demonstration of the lateral inhibition effect. When the dot on the left is fixated the letter on the right, seen in peripheral vision, is less well recognized the more it is surrounded by other items. From Sanders (1970).

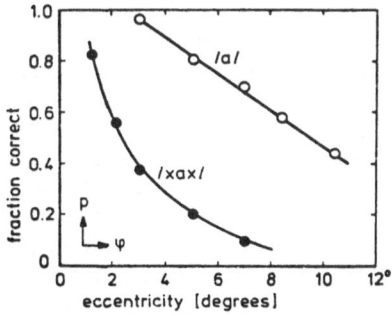

Fig. 5. Embedding randomly chosen target letters between two letters x̄ (indicated as |xax|) makes recognition scores in eccentric vision drop sharply as compared with the non-embedded situation (indicated as |a|). The diameter of the corresponding useful visual field shrinks to about 30% of its non-embedded value. From Bouma (1980).

169

Let us now consider the topic of *complex targets* and *complex back-grounds*. This concept is difficult for the ophthalmologist to address, because quantitative perimetry (as defined by Goldmann and Harms) consists of the assessment of luminance contrast thresholds. For simple targets on complex backgrounds, and particularly for complex targets on complex backgrounds, it becomes difficult to define contrast thresholds because the target and background luminances are non-uniform. It is also not clear what stimulus cues are being used to perform visual tasks when there is a complex display (Boyce, 1981). In fact, luminance contrast thresholds cannot account for all of our perception of real visual scenes. Color contrast and especially contour perception and lateral inhibition have also significance for observation of complex targets and complex visual environments. Overington (1982) discussed the importance of effective perimeter data to visual performance at the input to the perceptual levels of the visual system. For simple objects with little internal structure the effective perimeter is the geometrical perimeter. However, for objects having fine protuberances (such as an aircraft viewed head-on) or having strong internal structure it may be that the effective perimeter is very different from the geometrical perimeter. Lateral inhibition was demonstrated by Mackworth (1965) when he found that the addition of extra letters to a stimulus display seriously impaired the ability to accurately compare three letters; he concluded that 'visual noise causes tunnel vision'. Lateral inhibition becomes more important for more peripheral vision, when target acquisition levels are higher and when the target is more closely surrounded by confounding structures. This is illustrated in Fig. 4. By fixating the black dot and viewing the letters with peripheral vision, it can readily be observed that the isolated X is more legible than the X that is preceded by an N, which in turn is more legible than the X flanked by an N on both sides. Figure 5 presents a quantitative description of this effect. Onset of interference for smaller separations is progressive and relatively slow; it depends greatly on the relative contrasts of the target and the parasitic structure, so that for considerably closer separations the interference is not generally catastrophic. As a general approximation, 'visual isolation' (absence of interference effects) requires a homogeneous background region surrounding the target over a distance equal to one half of the target's eccentricity (Mackworth, 1965; Wolford and Hollingsworth, 1974; Bouma, 1970, 1980). Moreover, we must distinguish between such local interactions by lateral inhibition from stimuli within the vicinity of the target, and global interactions as by objects similar to the target which may produce false alarms and lengthen visual search time (Mutschler, 1981). In the presence of a highly structured global context, the detection of forms and details becomes necessary in order to differentiate the target from confounding stimuli (Scanlon, 1977). On the other hand, movement of a target is detected better on a structured background than on a homogeneous background.

Engel (1971) showed that peripheral target acquisition on a structured background can be specified by the *conspicuity field*, which consists of the perimetric area in which a briefly-presented target (e.g., 75 msec) can be acquired at a given level (when the subject has no pre-existing knowledge of its location). Of course, this area will be larger on an unstructured background

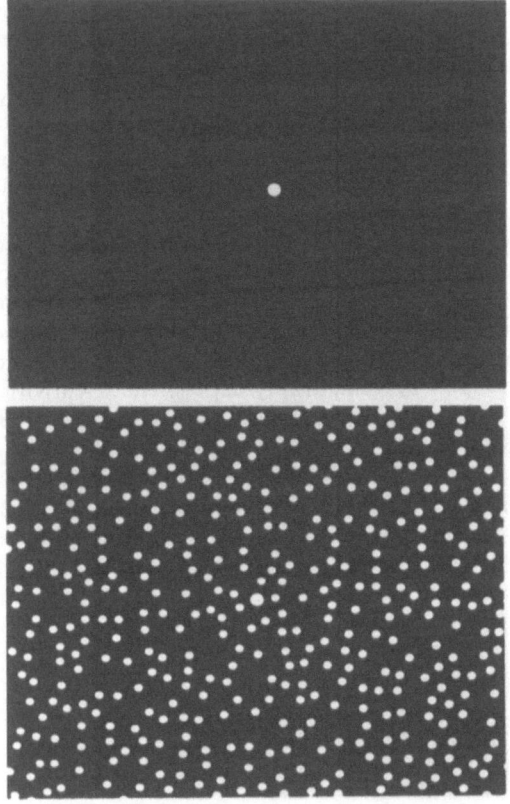

Fig. 6. As can be judged by eccentric fixation, the perceptibility of the test disc is decreased through the addition of background discs. From Engel and Bos (1973).

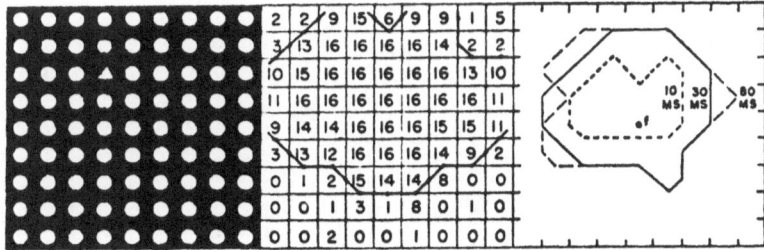

Fig. 7. (Left) a sample stimulus matrix containing one triangle. (Middle) a sample frequency table of positive responses (triangle seen), with liminal points and a liminal contour connecting them; the fixation point lies in the central cell. (Right) three liminal fields for one subject, obtained with exposures of 10, 30 and 80 msec, respectively; f = fixation point. The angular width of the 10 msec field is 2.23', approximately the size of the fovea. Three other subjects had much larger fields at these short exposure times. From Chaikin, Corbin & Volkmann (1962).

171

than on one saturated with figures resembling the target (see Fig. 6). Chaikin, Corbin and Volkmann (1962) reported that the conspicuity field becomes larger as exposure time is increased, and that it can have an irregular shape (Fig. 7). Indeed for reading, recognition is better in the right visual field than in the left (Terrace, 1959; Bouma and Van Rens, 1970).

Most ophthalmologists are aware of the alterations of perimetric sensitivity profiles produced by the state of *adaptation*. In photopic conditions there is a central sensitivity peak; in scotopic conditions there is a central sensitivity dip, the so-called central scotoma in darkness, while in mesopic conditions the sensitivity profile is flat. However these ophthalmological concepts concern artificial steady adaptation states. In driving and in other human activities adaptation is generally rapidly changing, e.g. when gaze moves through differently lit scenes. Boynton and Miller (1963) showed that such transient adaptations always temporarily depress the sensitivities. Accordingly, Blackwell (1981) introduced a transient adaptation factor in his model of visual performance.

Webster and Haselrud (1964) have demonstrated that a central task can increase the luminance thresholds for peripheral stimuli. The effect is small for pure detection and greater for higher order tasks. However for higher order tasks the effect is largely a matter of training and expectancy (the information is available at the perceptual level but sharing of attention requires training and briefing). Ikeda and Takeuchi (1975) applied these findings by defining the *working conspicuity field* as the alteration in the conspicuity field produced by a foveal load, resulting from concentration of

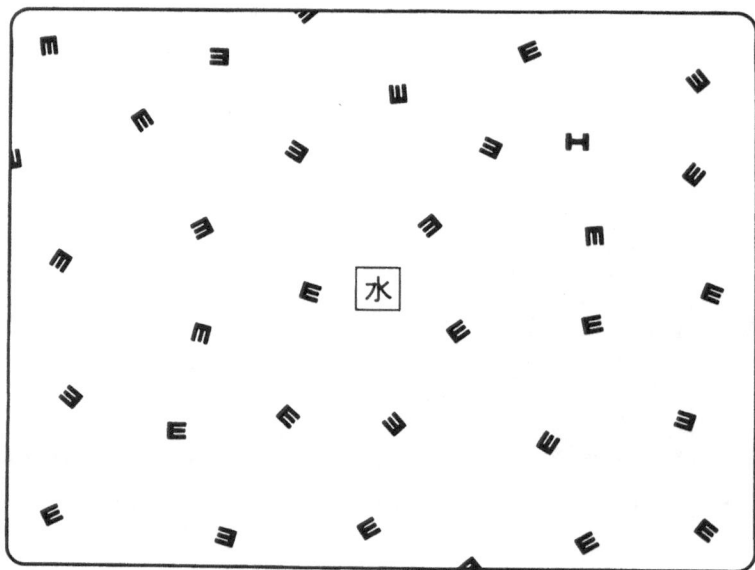

Fig. 8. An example of display to determine the working conspicuity visual field. The subject is asked to read the central letter 'water' and to detect the peripheral target 'H'. From Ikeda (1978).

172

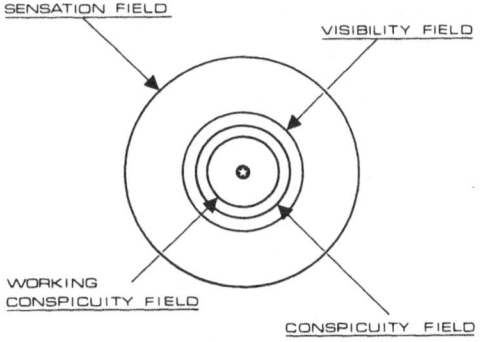

SENSATION FIELD

VISIBILITY FIELD

WORKING
CONSPICUITY FIELD

CONSPICUITY FIELD

Fig. 9. Four kinds of static functional visual field. From Ikeda, Uchikawa and Saida (1979).

attention on the fixation area. For example, in Ikeda's experimental procedure illustrated in Fig. 8, the subject's task was to recognize the H-shaped target embedded among the E-shaped targets while identifying foveally presented characters.

These different concepts are summarized in Fig. 9, taken from a paper by Ikeda (1979). What Ikeda unfortunately refers to as the 'sensation field' extends to the absolute limits of the visual field, while the smaller 'visibility field' is the area in which a given target can be seen against a homogeneous background. Within this region is a smaller 'conspicuity field' in which the target can be perceived within a structured background. Finally, the 'working conspicuity field' is the area for the same target on the same structured background in the presence of a foveal load, where attention is concentrated on the center of the visual field. Alternately it can also be said that the visual lobe is smaller not only for less visible targets, but also for more complex backgrounds, greater target—nontarget similarity, higher spatial or temporal uncertainty of the target's appearance and higher perceptual load.

Attention can also be directed to a peripheral portion of the visual field, thereby producing an enlargement in the conspicuity area in that direction (Engel, 1971) as shown in Fig. 10. This concentrated attention that is directed to the fixation region or to a specific visual field area must be distinguished

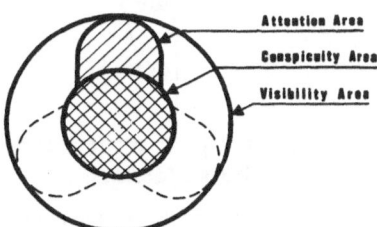

Attention Area

Conspicuity Area

Visibility Area

Fig. 10. Schematic diagram of the relation between the corresponding conspicuity, visibility and three attention areas. From Engel (1970).

173

from generalized attention to the entire visual field. According to Grindley and Townsend (1970), attention acts selectively in peripheral vision, where the pattern of stimulation is complex.

Sanders (1967) has pointed out that attention also pays a significant role in *temporary memorization* of details in a briefly presented scene. In this regard, Mackworth (1965) introduced another concept of the functional visual field referred to as the 'useful field of view'. It consists of 'the area around the fixation point from which information is being temporarily stored and then processed during a visual task'. Sperling (1960) has previously reported that when many visual targets are presented for a brief exposure, the material remains available to be 'read out' for a period of time following the presentation. This is usually referred to as 'short-term visual memory'.

The above-mentioned effects of attention must be distinguished from the influences of *prior knowledge* and *training*. In real life situations man, due to previous experiences, always expects and predicts what might happen. These central higher order functions are very important for our functional visual field. Prior knowledge of peripheral target location increases the proportion

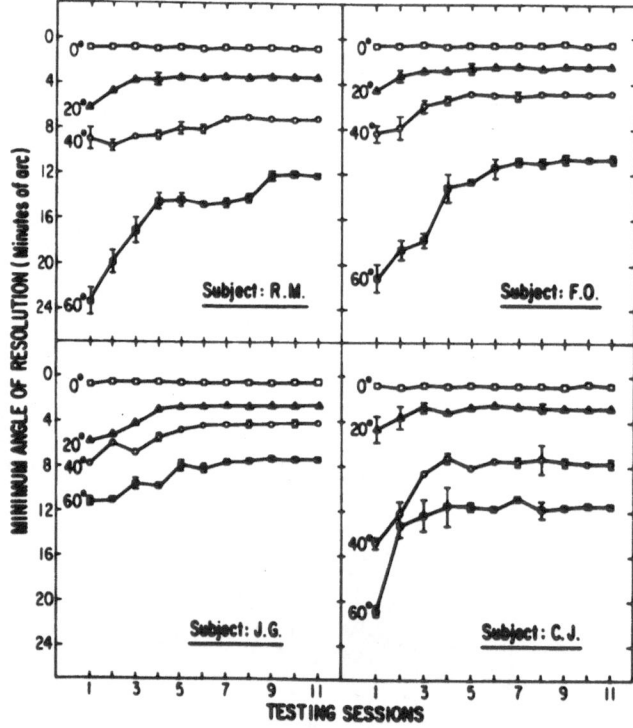

Fig. 11. Visual resolution thresholds as a function of the number of testing sessions at 0° (open squares), 20° (filled triangles), 40° (open circles) and 60° (filled squares) of visual eccentricity. The vertical bars present ± 1 standard deviation. From Johnson & Leibowitz (1979).

174

of correct responses (Grindley and Townsend, 1968; Keely, 1969) and enhances threshold sensitivity (Lie, 1969). Training can greatly improve visual performance, especially in the periphery (see Fig. 11) and if feedback is provided to the subject (Engel, 1971; Johnson and Leibowitz, 1974, 1979). Moreover, the contraction of the functional visual field produced by a foveal load is less pronounced in trained subjects (Ikeda and Takeuchi, 1975).

Although there is no development of the real visibility field from the age of 5 years on the functional visual field of children is narrower than that of adults because of such conceptual and attentional factors as foveal load and prior knowledge. In infants a single stimulus can capture the entire span of attention; the functional visual field is even contracted by non-visual competing activities as sucking, while the ability to respond to more distant objects develops only gradually (for the references see Verriest, 1982).

So far, we have only considered static observation conditions, whereas in real life, visual targets and the observer's eyes and head are nearly always *moving*.

Let us now consider the case of a *target moving* relative to a stationary direction of gaze. When a near-threshold target is moved in the visual field, it is detected earlier than expected from the static sensitivity profile, presumably because of the recruitment of receptor cells as a consequence of the movement (Dubois-Poulsen, 1981). However, movement sensitivity decreases progressively from the fovea to the peripheral visual field, with peripheral movement sensitivity being more greatly influenced by the area and luminance of the target than foveal movement thresholds (Johnson and Scobey, 1980). This is shown in the upper and middle panels of Fig. 12. The well-known statement that the periphery is exquisitely designed for detection of movement is based on the fact that movement displacement sensitivity decreases less rapidly than resolution sensitivity as visual field eccentricity becomes greater (lower panel of Fig. 12). It has been difficult to integrate target movement characteristics into visual performance models. Overington and Brown (1979) attempted to base their model for simple movements on a two-channel spatiotemporal response, with one channel representing the midget bipolars and sustained ganglion cells, and the other channel representing the diffuse bipolars and transient ganglion cells.

We will now consider *eye and head movements*, which can greatly augment the amount of space that can be visually inspected by combining the stationary binocular visual field with the binocular field of gaze and the head field. When the 'display angle' is progressively increased, eye movements appear, followed by the introduction of head movements, and subsequent increases in the magnitude of both eye and head movements, as shown in Fig. 13. (The display field is defined as the angular extent over which the target to be acquired can appear.) In one of the first papers specifically designed to examine the functional visual field, Sanders (1962) showed that the curves depicting a gradual decrease in performance with increasing eccentricity had two abrupt transition points corresponding to rapid performance decrements. The first abrupt transition occurs at an eccentricity of about 20—30 degrees, and corresponds to the first eye movements. The second transition point appears at approximately 80—90 degrees, and coincides with the first head

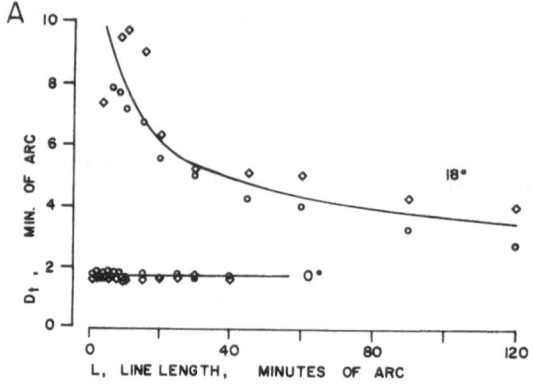

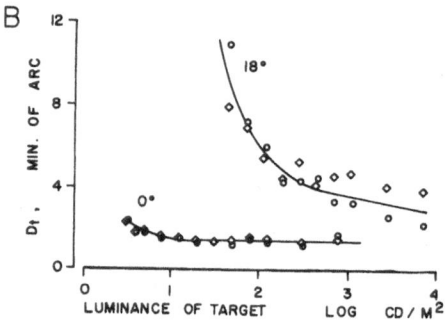

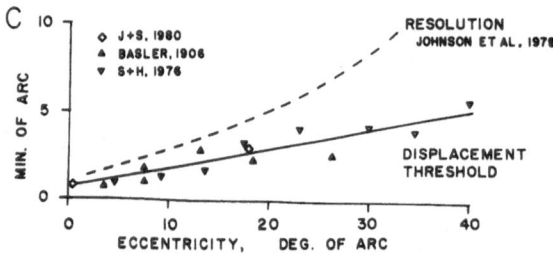

Fig. 12. (A) The displacement threshold as a function of line length in foveal vision (0°) and in peripheral vision (18°); (B) the displacement threshold as a function of target luminance; (C) the displacement threshold as a function of eccentricity. For comparison, the normal resolution properties determined with stationery flashing spots is shown as the dotted line. From Scobey (1981).

movements (see Fig. 14). Sanders showed that these rapid drops in performance are due to an increase in the complexity of the perceptual process created by these movements. Using a very different type of task requiring visual scanning, Enoch (1959) had previously reported a performance decrement for visual displays larger than 9 degrees, probably as a result of non-uniformities in the distribution of eye movements. For smaller display sizes,

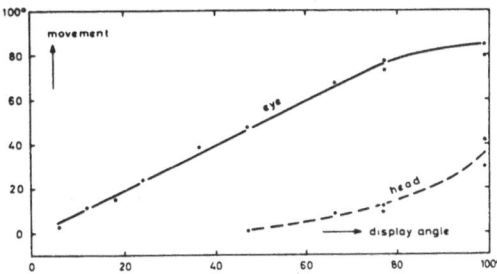

Fig. 13. Eye and head movements as a function of display angle. Results from two groups of 6 subjects. From Sanders (1970).

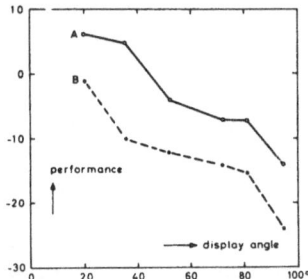

Fig. 14. Performance as a function of display angle and discriminability (A: 2, 3 dots; B; 4, 5 dots). From Sanders (1970).

duration of fixation increased, interfixation distances decreased, concentration of attention in the central area increased, and efficiency (defined as the percentage of eye fixations within the display area) decreased.

There are two types of *eye movements* that are of particular importance in ergonomic contexts: smooth pursuit and saccades. An important finding with regard to smooth pursuit eye movements is that visual acuity for moving targets (dynamic visual acuity) decreases as the angular velocity of the target increases. According to Burg (1967), the dynamic visual acuity of drivers correlates better with traffic accident rates than does standard static visual acuity measurements.

Saccadic eye movements consist of an abrupt displacement of the direction of gaze from one point in the visual scene to another, with an accuracy of approximately one tenth of the total excursion distance (Wolf, 1978). The residual error is then corrected by one or two additional saccades with shorter latencies. In daily life the eyes spend about 90% of the time engaged in stationary fixation, although the duration of each fixation is only about 0.3 sec (Overington, 1981: duration of fixation is likely to be 0.5 sec or larger for very demanding tasks). These fixational pauses are separated by one or more ocular saccades. Vision is attenuated during saccadic eye movements for a period of 40 msec prior to and 60 msec following the saccade (Wolf, 1978). This phenomenon is often referred to as 'saccadic suppression'. Saccadic eye

177

movements are the means by which targets that are detected in the periphery are fixated by the foveal region for detailed inspection and identification. However extrafoveal visual guidance is used only when it is needed, i.e. when it contributes significantly to the speed of visual search as with tasks of low visibility and small density of the background objects. The latency of such saccadic eye movements depends upon the target contrast, target eccentricity and retinal adaptation state. Moreover, the right hemifield may exhibit a shorter latency than the left hemifield (Santucci and Chevaleraud, 1974).

Saccades are also used for scanning a visual scene. It is by means of a series of appropriate saccades that we are able to read textual material, perceive the essential features of a scene, or examine a work of art such as Hiroshige's 'Sudden Shower' (Fig. 15). Analysis of eye movement records demonstrates that scans overlap considerably to assure good perception of the pattern (Saida and Ikeda, 1979). The type of scanning pattern employed depends upon the content of the scene. The simplistic approach assuming a random-control (or involuntary) eye guidance disregards the continuous cognitive analysis of the perceived information and fails to explain the pecularities of the highly organized and adaptive visual scanning behaviour of man. Figure 16 shows the variation of relative fixation frequency among the different segments of a 30 degree circular area of expected random search, in which the observer was required to detect a stimulus that could appear at any location in the circular region (Ford, White and Lichtenstein, 1959). It is apparent that the distribution of fixations is not random, but is instead concentrated in the mid-periphery region of the display area where the visual lobe is most effective. These kinds of experiments indicate that random search models are reliable only under some real conditions with intelligent assumptions about effective search area. Still more caution is recommended for models based on 'quasi-random scanning' in which the observer is expected to detect the fine details of many highly visible objects by directly fixating each object successively. Indeed, the probability of direct fixations decreases as the visibility level increases, because the scanning strategy changes to minimize the visual work load (Inditsky and Bodmann, 1980).

The analysis of the body of existing experimental evidence using the stochastic search models (Inditsky, 1978) reveals that the scanning strategy in every particular case approaches an optimal one, whether it is quasi-random or quasi-systematic scanning. Thus the 'intelligence' is a most common feature of human visual scanning. Once a given scanning pattern is assumed the corresponding model equations incorporating the physiological data on single glimpse detection probabilities can be developed to predict such performance parameters as a mean search time, its cumulative distribution function, etc. The modelling also proved to be very useful for the deeper understanding of visual acquisition processes and development of optical viewing systems. Surprisingly enough most search experiments so far analyzed in terms of cumulative probability distributions are nearly consistent with the random search model, in particular if extra-foveal guidance of saccades (Inditsky, 1978) is incorporated. This led Bodmann to qualify the random search model as a first order approximation of much more sophisticated strategies of scanning. By assuming a random distribution of fixation

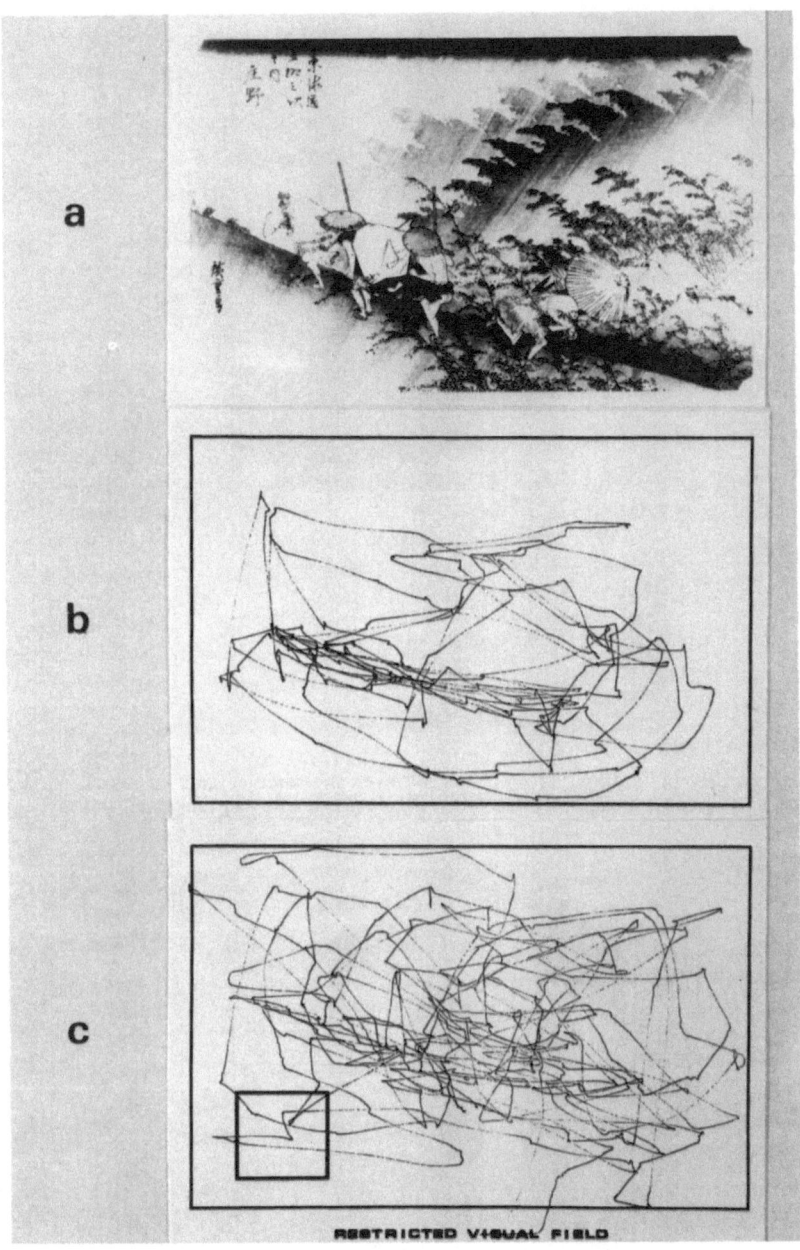

Fig. 15. (a) The woodcut print *A sudden Shower* by Hiroshige; (b) eye movement traces from viewing the print for 1 min without any restriction in the visual field; (c) eye movement traces from viewing the print for 1 min with a visual field restricted to the size shown by the square. From Ikeda, Uchikawa and Saida (1979).

179

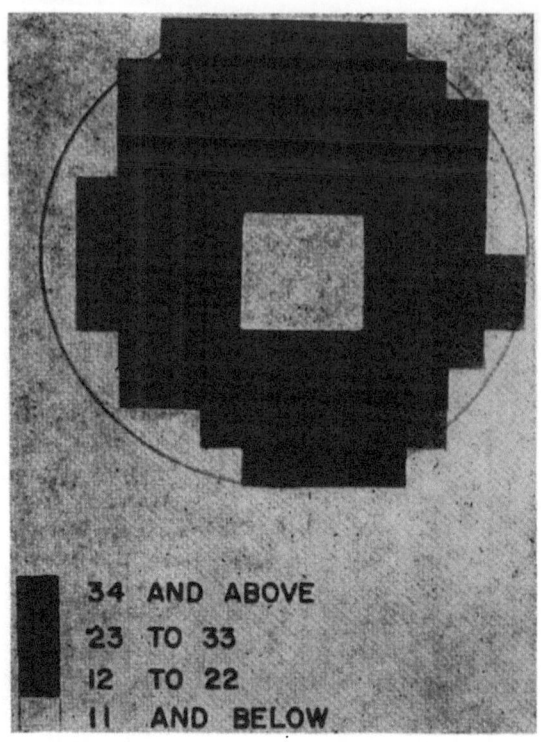

34 AND ABOVE
23 TO 33
12 TO 22
11 AND BELOW

Fig. 16. Density of fixations plotted in cells over the circular area of search to show regions of concentration and neglect. From Ford, White and Lichtenstein (1959).

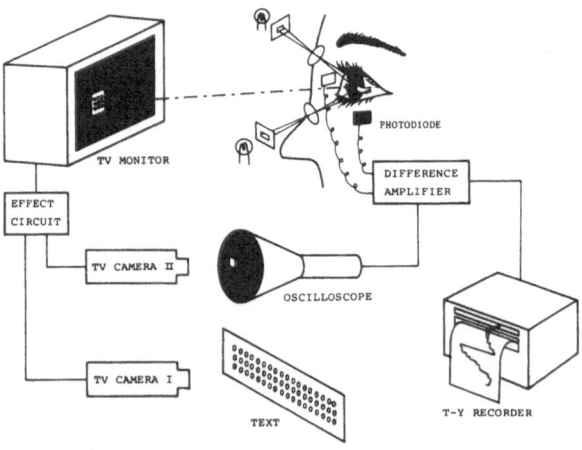

Fig. 17. Experimental arrangement for determining the dynamic functional visual field. From Ikeda and Saida (1979).

180

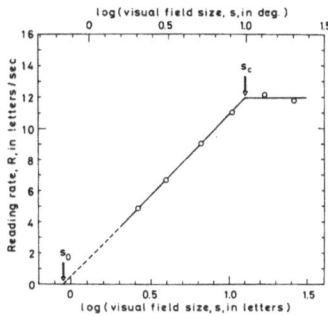

Fig. 18. The reading speed as a function of the visual field size. From Ikeda and Saida (1979).

positions over the display area during search, Engel (1977) was able to relate experimentally the cumulative probability of target discovery against search time with the size of the target conspicuity area.

Let us now consider Ikeda's concept of the *dynamic functional visual field.* In contrast to the static functional visual field, this concept pertains to the actual functional visual field that is present between ocular saccades. Utilizing Watanabe's (1971) technique Ikeda has investigated the dynamic functional visual field by means of an electronic system limiting always the field of view to the chosen area around the fixation point in spite of any eye movements that may occur (see Fig. 17). By plotting visual performance as a function of visual field size, the dynamic functional visual field corresponds to the field size from which there is no further improvement in performance (Fig. 18). This technique indicates that for reading, approximately 10 to 17 letters can be acquired simultaneously. When this finding is compared to the number of fixation shifts, we must conclude that reading includes more verifications than expected (Ikeda and Saida, 1978). Fast readers have a wider dynamic functional visual field (Marcel, 1974). With regard to the acquisition of complex scenes, the lower panel of Fig. 15 shows that the scanning strategy of the 'Sudden Shower' print is highly disorganized when the field of view is limited to the area depicted by the lower left-hand square. Saida and Ikeda (1979) reported that for such tasks, the useful visual field corresponds to about 50% of the entire scene. Korn (1981), using a technique similar to that of Watanabe, found that detection of a 1 degree vehicle in a complex scene became dramatically reduced as the visual field size was changed from 6 degrees to 3 degrees. Ikeda (1978) evaluated the dynamic functional visual field by dividing the scene into individual segments and showing them separately to the subject. Osaka (1980) used in children and in adults peep-holes mounted in underwater goggles and showed that recognition latency for pictures changed as a cube-root function of aperture area. The dynamic functional visual field increases by sequential redundancy in non-linguistic visual tasks (Sanders, 1970) and by more effective use of context in reading (Marcel, 1974). Just as with the static functional visual field, dynamic

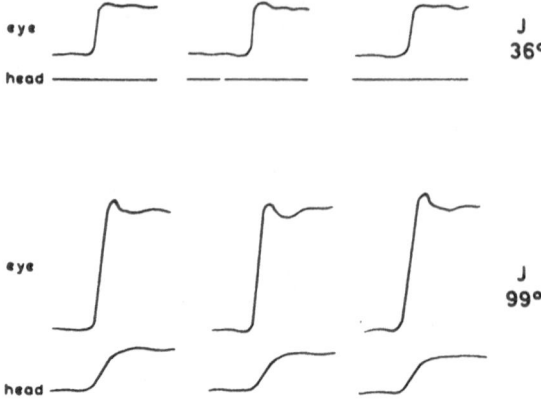

Fig. 19. Records of eye and head movements. From Sanders (1970).

functional visual field size can be reduced by a foveal load ('dynamic working conspicuity field': Ikeda).

As was derived from the search time data, the effective sizes of the conspicuity areas during search were found to be about 30% smaller than the conspicuity areas determined by means of single tachistoscopic presentations (Engel, 1977).

With regard to *head movements* used to increase the size of the functional visual field, Sanders (1970) has shown that at larger target eccentricities the eyes and head begin moving at about the same time, but that the head movements are slower, producing a compensatory eye movement in the reverse direction (Fig. 19). Head movements in drivers are larger in town, especially for round-abouts, than on highways (Åberg and Rumar, 1975). On highways there are nearly no eye and head movements, and the functional visual field becomes more constricted as we go faster and look progressively farther in front of the car, because of the optical flow pattern or 'speed smear' of objects in the periphery (Danielson, 1957).

CONCLUSIONS

A first conclusion of this report will concern the striking evidence of the importance of off-axis vision in human behavior. In a simple search task with vacant background it would take 10 to 100 times more time to discover a target when the glimpse visual field is reduced to the foveal region. The role of peripheral vision is still more important in tasks with complex backgrounds, requiring effective saccadic guidance. Extrafoveal information governs saccadic guidance and changes scanning behavior to optimize performance.

A second conclusion is that the recent and growing topic of the functional visual field has a great importance for ophthalmologists. This is so not only for our general understanding of human vision mechanisms, but also for judging the effects of visual impairment on behavior and for determining how better visual field job standards could be established.

BIBLIOGRAPHY

Åberg, L. and Rumar, K. Head movements of drivers, equipment and exploratory study. Report 182, Department of Psychology, University of Uppsala, Sweden (1975).

Barca, L. and Fornaro, G. The functional visual field, A preliminary annotated bibliography. Atti Fond. G. Ronchi 35:491–510 (1980).

Blackwell, H. R. (ed.). An analytic model for describing the influence of lighting parameters upon visual performance. CIE publication 19/2 (1981).

Bouma, H. Interaction effects in parafoveal letter recognition. Nature 226:177–178 (1970).

Bouma, H. Visual search and reading, eye movements and functional visual field: A tutorial review. In: R. S. Nickerson (ed.), Attention and Performance. Lawrence Erlbaum Ass., Hillsdale, New Jersey (1980).

Bouma, H. and Van Rends, A. L. M. Reading processes: On the recognition of single words in eccentric vision. IPO Ann. Progr. Rep. 5:99–106 (1970).

Boyce, P. R. Contrast as a metric of visibility. Contribution for the CIE TC 3.1 meeting in Gouvieux (1981).

Boynton, R. M. and Miller, N. R. Visual performance under conditions of transient adaptation. Illum. Engrng. 58:541–550 (1963).

Burg, A. The relationship between vision test scores and driving record: general findings. UCLA Department of Engineering, Report No. 67–24 (1967).

Chaikin, J. D., Corbin, H. H. and Volkmann, J. Mapping a field of short-time visual search. Science 138:132–1328 (1962).

Danielson, R. W. The relationship of fields of vision to safety in driving, with a report of 680 drivers examined by various screening methods. Am. J. Ophthalmol. 44:657–680 (1957).

Dubois Poulsen, A. Contribution to this paper (1981).

Engel, F. L. Visual conspicuity and directed attention. IPO Ann. Progr. Rep. 5:123–128 (1970).

Engel, F. L. Visual conspicuity, directed attention and retinal locus. Vision Res. 11:563–576 (1971).

Engel, F. L. Visual conspicuity, visual search and fixation tendencies of the eye. Vision Res. 17:95–108 (1977).

Engel, F. L. and Bos, T. M. Visual conspicuity related to generalisation of background irregularities. IPO Ann. Progr. Rep. 8:35–41 (1973).

Enoch, J. M. Effect of the size of a complex display upon visual search. J. Opt. Soc. Am. 49:280–286 (1959).

Ford, A., White, C. T. and Lichtenstein, M. Analysis of eye movements during free search. J. Opt. Soc. Am. 49:287–292 (1959).

Grindley, G. C. and Townsend, V. Voluntary attention in peripheral vision and its effects on acuity and differential thresholds. Quart. J. Exper. Psychol. 20:11 (1968).

Ikeda, M. A new look at the functional visual field. Proc. ICO-11 Conf., Madrid, Spain, pp. 3–10 (1978).

Ikeda, M. and Saida, S. Span of recognition in reading. Vision Res. 18:83–88 (1978).

Ikeda, M. and Takeuchi, R. Influence of foveal load on the functional visual field. Perception and Psychophysics 18:225–260 (1975).

Ikeda, M., Uchikawa, K. and Saida, S. Static and dynamic functional visual fields. Optica Acta 8:1103–1113 (1979).

Inditsky, B. Analysis of visual performance. Theoretical and experimental investigation of visual search. Thesis, Karlsruhe (1978).

Inditsky, B. and Bodmann, H. W. Quantitative model of visual search. Proc. 19th Sess. CIE, Kyoto, 1979, Paper P-79-33. Publ. CIE N° 50, pp. 197–201 (1980).

Johnson, C. A., Keltner, J. L. and Balestrery, F. Effects of target size and eccentricity on visual detection and resolution. Vision Res. 18:1217–1222 (1978).

Johnson, C. A. and Leibowitz, H. W. Practice, refractive error, and feedback as factors influencing peripheral motion thresholds. Perception and Psychophysics 15:276–280 (1974).

Johnson, C. A. and Leibowitz, H. W. Practice effects for visual resolution in the periphery. Perception and Psychophysics 25:439–442 (1979).

Johnson, C. A. and Scobey, R. P. Foveal and peripheral displacement as a function of stimulus luminance, line length and duration of movement. Vision Res. 20:709–715 (1980).

Keely, S. M. Visual detection as a function of attentional demands and perceptual system error. Perception and Psychophysics 6:73 (1969).

Korn, A. Visual search: Relation between detection performance and visual field size. Proc. of the First European Annual Conference on Human Decision and Manual Control, Delft, May 25–27, 1981.

Leibowitz, H. W. and Appelle, S. The effect of a central task on luminance thresholds for peripherally presented stimuli. Human Factors 11:387–392 (1969).

Lie, E. The momentary sensitivity contour of the retina: an approach to the study of attention. Stud. Psychol. 11:157 (1969).

Mackworth, N. H. Visual noise causes tunnel vision. Psychon. Sci. 3:67–68 (1965).

Marcel, T. The effective visual field and the use of context in fast and slow readers of two ages. Br. J. Psychol. 65:479–492 (1974).

Mutschler, H. Zusammenfassende Darstellung der Beobachterleistung bei ferngelenkten Flugkörpern (RPVS). Forschungsbericht aus der Wehrtechnik, BMVg-FBWT 81–3 (1981).

Osaka, N. Effect of peripheral visual field size upon visual search in children and adults. Perception 9:451–455 (1980).

Overington, I. Vision and Acquisition. Pentech Press, London (1976).

Overington, I. A review of visual acquisition modelling. Br. Aerospace Dynamics Group, Bristol Division, Rep. N° BT 10635 (1980).

Overington, I. Observations to CIE publication 19/2. Contribution for the CIE TC 3.1 meeting in Gouvieux, 1981.

Overington, I. Towards a complete model of photopic visual threshold performance. Optical Engineering 21:2–13 (1982).

Overington, I. and Brown, M. B. Modelling of visual threshold performance in the presence of image motion. Br. Aerospace Dynamics Group, Bristol Division, Rep. N° ST 23217 (1979).

Regan, D. New visual tests in multiple sclerosis. In: H. S. Thompson (ed.), Topics in Neuro-Ophthalmology. Williams and Wilkins, Baltimore (1980).

Regan, D. and Beverley, K. I. Visual fields described by contrast sensitivity, by acuity and by relative sensitivity to different orientations. Invest. Ophthalmol. Vis. Sci. (in press).

Ronchi, L. and Salvi, G. Performance decrement, under prolonged testing, across the visual field. Ophthalmic Res. 5:113–120 (1973).

Saida, S. and Ikeda, M. Useful visual field size for pattern perception. Perception and Psychophysics 25:119–125 (1979).

Sanders, A. F. Studies into the functional visual field. I. Performance as a function of display angle. Inst. for Perc. RVO-TNO, Rep. N° IZF 22 (1962).

Sanders, A. F. Informatie verwerking in het funktioneel gezichtsveld. Ned. T. Psychol. 22:137–149 (1967).

Sanders, A. F. Some aspects of the selective process in the functional visual field. Ergonomics 13:101–117 (1970).

Santucci, G. F. and Chevaleraud, J. Influence de l'excentricité et de la couleur du stimulus lumineux sur le délai de réponse oculomotrice. C. R. 1er Congr. int. Vision Sécurité Routière, Paris, 1975.

Scanlan, L. A. Target acquisition in realistic terrain. Proc. of the Human Factors Society, 21st Annual Meeting, 249–253, 1977.

Scobey, R. P. Psychophysical and electrophysiological determinants of motion detection. Doc. Ophthalmol. Proc. Series 26:63–70 (1981).

Sperling, G. The information available in brief visual presentations. Psychol. Mon. 74/11 (1960)

Terrace, H. S. The effects of retinal locus and attention on the perception of word. J. Exper. Psychol. 58:382 (1959).

184

Thorn, F. and Boynton, R. M. Human binocular summation at absolute threshold. Vision Res. 14:415−455 (1974).

Verriest, G. Visual field in childhood. Bull. Soc. Belge Ophthalmol. 202:41−58 (1982).

Villani, S. Some ergonomical terms. Visual vs. functional visual field. Atti Fond. G. Ronchi 34:706−717 (1979).

Watanabe, A. Fixation points and eye movements. Oyo Buturi 40:330−334 (1971).

Webster, R. G. and Haslerud, G. M. Influence on extreme peripheral vision of attention to a visual or auditory task. J. Exper. Psychol. 68:269 (1964).

Westendorf, D. H. and Fox, R. Binocular detection of disparate light flashes. Vision Res. 17:697−702 (1977).

Wolf, W. Visuelle Detektion bei sakkadischen Augenbewegungen. Thesis, Techn. Universität München (1978).

Wolford, G. and Hollingsworth, S. Lateral masking in visual information processing. Perception and Psychophysics 16:315−320 (1974).

Editor's address:
Dr G. Verriest
Oogheelkunde
Akademisch Ziekenhuis
De Pintelaan 185
B-9000 Ghent
Belgium

185

FUNCTIONAL SCORING OF THE BINOCULAR VISUAL FIELD

BEN ESTERMAN

(New York City, New York, U.S.A.)

Key words. Binocular field, functional field, grid, relative values, enhancement.

ABSTRACT

The pressing need for a way to evaluate total 'binocular' peripheral acuity has been pointed out by the International Council of Ophthalmology. It has set 1982 as a target date for its tentative adoption as an international standard. The present offering is an attempt to fill this need until a better method is devised.

The new method is based on 'function' instead of on anatomy alone. It starts by imitating nature in plotting the total field *binocularly*, eliminating the error created by combining the two conventional monocular fields (which overlap and duplicate each other extensively). The resulting binocular isopter is then scored (according to the author's theory of relative values) by means of a new binocular scale in the form of a weighted grid which assigns higher scores to the 'functionally' more important parts of the human field – the center, the lower hemisphere and the horizon. The new method also led to the rediscovery of 'binocular enhancement', which produces scores more realistic than was formerly possible. Especially useful to ophthalmic consultants for evaluating visual capability or disability in industry, law and government (social security, motor vehicle, workers compensation, aviation, military) the new system works accurately and rapidly with most existing perimeters, manual or automated.

THE PROBLEM

Until now there has been no correct way to assess the efficiency of the total (binocular) peripheral field on the basis of function. Yet there is need for such a scale, analogous to the Snellen scale for central acuity. The answer to the question: 'How useful to him is the patient's field?' is important not so much diagnostically as medico-socially and medico-economically. It helps tell us how he functions: in industry – how well he can do a job; in government

Greve, E. L., Heijl, A. (eds.) Fifth International Visual Field Symposium.
©1983 Dr W. Junk Publishers, The Hague/Boston/Lancaster.

— how safely he can drive a car or fly a plane or engage in combat; in social security, workers compensation, medico-legal, or low-vision determinations — to what percent his vision is impaired.

To be realistic, such a scale should have two qualities: it must be based not on area alone, but also on function and it must measure the entire (*binocular*) field. Functional scoring became available in 1968 (1,2) with the theory of relative values: 'For human activity, certain parts of the field are more important than others — the center, the lower hemisphere and the horizon'. These parts are assigned higher percentages when scored on a relative-value scale in the form of a weighted grid. This scale has been in use since its approval in 1969 by the American Committee on Optics and Visual Physiology.

However, this scale scores only the *monocular* field whereas most patients are *binocular*. It was at first assumed that the binocular score could easily be derived by simply combining both monocular percentages — and this was the method until now. But the results were obviously wrong because in real life, both fields extensively overlap (dotted line, Fig. 1G); blind areas in one are cancelled by seeing areas in the other. Attempts to correct this by complicated mathematical formulas brought no solution. In 1978 the International Council of Ophthalmology targeted 1982 as the year for the adoption of some workable binocular scale.

MATERIAL AND METHODS

The present binocular scale became possible only after breaking away from the long-standing tradition that all fields must plotted monocularly. Perimetry had always been monocular; properly so because for diagnosis that is the only way. But binocular scoring is not concerned with diagnosis, so the new method completely by-passes monocular perimetry. It plots and scores the field *binocularly*, exactly as the patient sees it, without occluding either eye. By thus imitating nature, we obtain a more accurate score because we eliminate the error caused by the overlapped fields and incidentally save much time and work.

The new scale is not really new. It is merely the monocular one expanded to binocular simply by fusing right and left along the mid-line (Figs. 1F and 1G) just as occurs in the act of seeing.

More important, in expanding the grid from a 100-unit monocular to a 120-unit binocular, there is *no change in the size and distribution of the units*, so the relative values remain unchanged. *This gives the new binocular scale the same validity as the approved and accepted monocular one.*

Because the standard test object must remain uniform for all patients, the old standard 1/2 degree white is retained. This has long been accepted as workable, being neither too demanding nor too easy for the average patient. Its approximate equivalent on Goldmann-type perimeters or on computerized perimeters is $4\,mm^2$ white at 1000 asb with a background of 31.5 asb.

188

PROCEDURE

1. Plot the binocular field on to the binocular chart using any standard perimeter or suitably programmed computerized perimeter. The chin-rest is positioned in the mid-line, neither eye is occluded and *both* eyes (or the dominant eye) look at the fixation target.
2. Transfer the isopter to the scale on the back of the chart — simply by retracing it over carbon paper with carbon side up.
3. Count the units whose dots lie wholly within the field. Omit those dots touched by the boundary or by scotoma.

The total, multiplied by 5/6 is the score in percent. Steps 2 and 3 (after perimetry) take about one minute — or a fraction of a second when the computerized perimeter has been used. (Why 5/6? Because the original full, 100% monocular field contained *100* units; on the same scale, *expanded to binocular*, the full, 100%, binocular field contains *120* units; 100/120 = 5/6.)

ENHANCEMENT

The binocular method yielded another unexpected dividend. Although it had been assumed that the binocular field (Fig. 1E,F) would be larger than either monocular field (Fig. 1A–D), careful scoring disclosed that often the total was *still larger* than anticipated (Fig. 1G,H). For lack of a better term I call this 'enhancement' and it is probably due to the availability of *two* sets of retinal receptors, where the fields extensively overlap. A similar phenomenon, of course, occurs in *central* vision; we are all familiar with Snellen readings of OD = 20/70, OS = 20/50 but with *both maculae*, OU = 20/30.

None of this is new. What is new is that, with the availability of scoring which is *both functional* and *binocular*, it is now possible to demonstrate it *quantitatively*. Its practical significance is that a total field, so measured, may yield a score up to 20% higher. It supports my thesis that the *only* realistic and accurate way to assess total peripheral function is to plot and score it *binocularly*.

WHAT BINOCULAR SCORING DOES NOT DO

It has no value in diagnosis. It merely measures the functional field. It is not a substitute for diagnostic perimetry that must still be done conventionally with each eye separately. It ignores central acuity, already scored by the Snellen scale. It ignores the normal blind spots; there are none in the binocular field.

ATTRIBUTES OF THE NEW METHOD

The new method outlines the total field binocularly, without occlusion, just the way it is used in nature. It scores functionally, giving greater weight to the

189

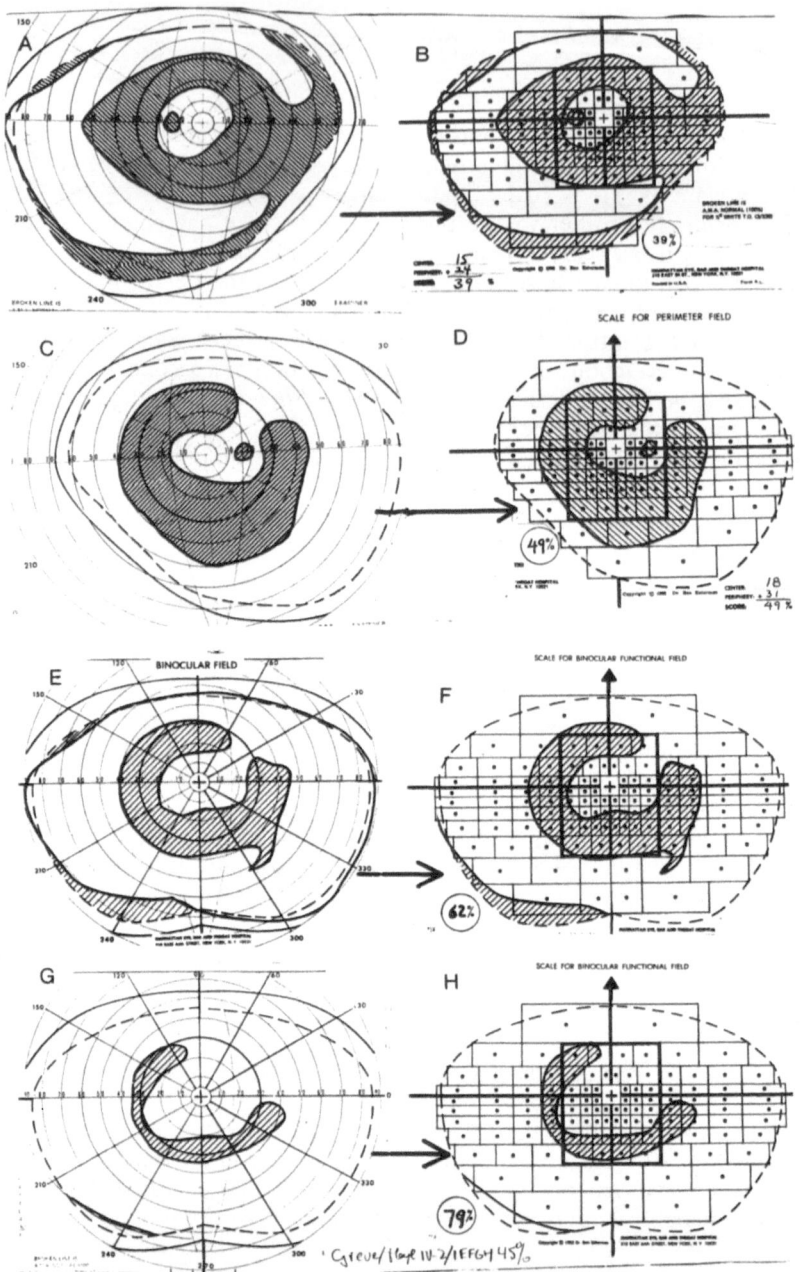

Fig. 1. (A–H) Pigmentary degeneration of the retina; (A and C) left and right monocular fields; (B and D) scores: L 39%, R 49%; (E) 'theoretical' binocular field, created by merging (A) and (B); (F) 'theoretical' binocular score = 62%; (G) 'enhanced' binocular field: the true field, true because it is plotted *binocularly*, as seen by the patient; (H) true score: 79%. The 17% difference between the *theoretical* and the *actual* is the 'enhancement'.

190

more important areas. It scores defects within the field (scotomata) with the same facility as defects in the periphery (contraction). It includes the effect of binocular peripheral 'enhancement' in the final functional score. It is based on reasonable, workable, and long-accepted standards. It is fully and easily reproducible. It is adaptable to most existing perimeters without new apparatus, requiring only specially printed paper charts. It is adaptable to most automated and computerized perimeters, making these marvelously time-saving and labor-saving machines even more attractive to industry and to government agencies for individual or mass screening. It is easily susceptible to quality control and future modification by an international ophthalmologic body.

COMMENT

Some experts have suggested lowering the standards for specific groups, such as the elderly, aphakes, certain occupations, etc. However, thoughtful consideration would probably lead to retention of the single standard, while reducing the percentage accepted as normal for certain disabilities: thus, 85% for the elderly, 50% to 80% for aphakes, etc. depending on type of spectacles or other kinds of refractive correction, etc.

In any case, national bodies such as health ministries, ophthalmologic societies, and certain industries or agencies will probably reserve to themselves the right to set their own minimum standards.

Other authorities have suggested grouping into classes of visual disability: A = excellent, B = good, C = fair, D = poor, and E = blind. With greater precision now available in the form of percentages, this would seem a step backward.

Nor is there any real advantage to combining the scores of several functions such as central acuity, peripheral acuity, and muscle balance all into one unified score. Expressing them as separate entities is more descriptive and medically more useful.

SUMMARY

A new scale evaluates the total (binocular) field on the basis of function. It does for peripheral vision what the Snellen scale has done for central acuity. The functional nature of the score is achieved by a binocular relative-value grid that assigns proportionally higher values to the more important parts of the field. Because the calculations are already built into the grid, scoring in percent is quick and easy without need of new equipment, special training, or complex formulae.

The new scale, combined with a new method of perimetry — binocular, instead of the conventional monocular — lead to the re-discovery of another dimension called 'enhancement', which yields a truer and more realistic appraisal of how well the patient sees than has heretofore been possible. It is a socioeconomic, rather than a diagnostic, tool.

191

The method is applicable universally as a standard for all patients, on almost all existing perimeters, manual or computerized, for individual or mass screening.

REFERENCES

1. Esterman, B. 'Grids for scoring visual fields'. I. Tangent screen. Am. Arch. Ophthalmol. 77:780–786 (1967).
2. Esterman, B. 'Grids for scoring visual fields'. II. Perimeter. Am. Arch. Ophthalmol. 79:400–406 (1960).
3. Esterman, B. 'Functional scoring of the binocular field'. AAO Ophthalmology 89/11 (1982).

Author's address:
Dr Ben Esterman
Glaucoma Clinic
Manhattan Eye, Ear and Throat Hospital
210 East 64th Street
New York, NY 10021
U.S.A.

THE REPRESENTATION OF THE VISUAL FIELD

RONALD P. CRICK, JONATHAN C. P. CRICK and LIONEL RIPLEY
(London, England)

Key words. Visual field, parabolic projection, numerical field cross, octopus perimeter, practical visual field, functional visual field.

ABSTRACT

Any projection of the visual field is a manipulation. It is therefore essential to select a projection which gives the most useful representation of the field and its clinical defects. It should also provide a uniform numerical assessment of the sensitivity of vision throughout the field and incorporate a percentage functional field estimate along the lines proposed by Dr Esterman.

To study these requirements a mathematical system of representation of the visual field which progressively augments it parabolically towards the centre is proposed. It is applicable to all types of perimetry but the Octopus perimeter has been used as a test-bed employing the Sargon programme with both the traditional and the sine-bell stimulus. This work and the case for the adoption of the system are briefly presented.

PROPOSITIONS

The basis of this paper can be expressed as a few simple propositions.
1. Any projection of the visual field is a manipulation. Geographers have had the same problem.
2. The manipulation should be convenient in use and have as much physiological and pathological justification as possible so that it inclines towards the representation of what seems reality in so far as our limited understanding allows.
3. The isometric or linear projection on which degrees subtended at the eye are represented in terms of equal distances on the chart has been traditional. It has little to recommend it except a general plausibility.
4. The projection must be mathematically expressed for transposition to any other mathematical projection when this is required.
5. The objects of visual field examinations are (a) diagnostic; (b) the determination of the progress of a field defect; (c) the assessment of functional

193

handicap resulting from the degree and distribution of defects in the visual field.

6. For diagnosis, the test and its representation need to be as detailed as practicable using a programme appropriate to any particular condition suggested by other parts of the clinical examination. It should provide a uniform numerical threshold assessment throughout the field.

7. For clinical follow-up, especially at intervals over a long period, the field of vision must be capable of being represented numerically in a simple, easily visualised and readily calculated manner. For those who prefer isopters, symbols or profiles these are also readily available but it is considered that numerical methods of representation and interpretation will be gradually adopted in the future.

8. Functional assessment is an extremely complicated matter involving varying occupational threshold requirements but Dr Esterman has made a great initial advance in devising his grid by providing a practical measure to take account of differential functional field loss in general (1). Both automation of output and ergophthalmology will also be able to make great contributions to this important facet of perimetry.

9. Perimetry in the past has been almost as flexible and individual as the consulting room door on which Bjerrum first plotted his patients' fields but now with the advent of automated perimetry it behoves us to pay attention to the problem so that we avoid to some extent the difficulties of language which have bedevilled the computer scene. If we accept that the linear projection is inadequate and needs replacing we could well agree to adopt one which in the simplest manner tries to satisfy the theoretical and practical requirements of perimetry. One such projection is here described for your consideration.

THE PROJECTION

When adopting an isometric scale what we are doing is shown on Fig. 1. The points where perpendiculars are dropped, when joined up describe a curve which represents the projection. A chart which gives adequate central representation would be enormous if extended to the periphery on the same scale and the frequent use of separate charts for central and peripheral fields is evidence that an isometric projection is unsatisfactory because it gives a cramped recording of the central 30—40° of field and yet is prodigal of space in the usually less informative periphery. Goldmann charts and the usual type of Octopus charts share this disadvantage. Practical dissatisfaction with isometric projection in the past had led to some other arbitrary modifications. But, not only convenience is concerned. The magnified central field recording can reasonably be related to: (1) the clinical finding that, apart from local retinal peripheral disturbances and lesions affecting the unpaired visual field, the change in the central field of 40° is a reliable indicator of the visual field state as a whole; (2) the increased concentration of retinal receptors in the central area as emphasised by Dannheim (personal communication); (3) the increased representation of the central retina in the visual cortex.

194

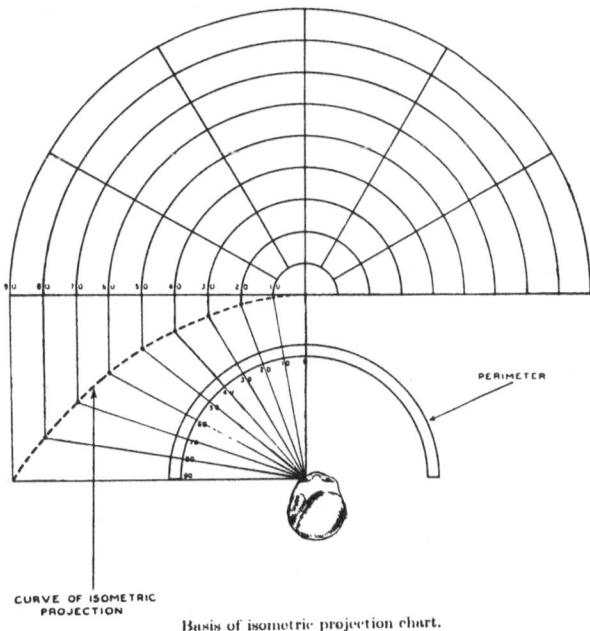

Basis of isometric projection chart.

Fig. 1. Curve of isometric projection.

At the same time the peripheral representation must not be so miniscule as to prevent changes in the periphery being recognised. With these criteria in mind one of us proposed many years ago the use of a convenient non-linear mathematical projection which was based on a parabolic curve having the formula $5y = x^2$. This gave a satisfactory magnification in the central $40°$, reasonable size from $40-70°$ and still tolerable representation from $70-90°$. The projection of the parabola is shown in Fig. 2 and the formation of the field chart in Fig. 3.

This system was presented by one of us at the Oxford Congress in 1957(2) and has been on trial at King's College Hospital during the last 25 years. It was found to be of practical value, at first in conjunction with the use of a modified Lister perimeter and later with the Friedmann Analyser. More recently with the kind cooperation of Professor Fankhauser, Mr Zülkhe and Miss Rhyner of Interzeag parabolic displays have been devised for the Octopus using the Sargon programme and their use will be described. In addition to the benefits of larger central representation itself the positioning of stimuli for static perimetry on regular co-ordinates superimposed on the parabolic projection places them much more usefully in the field and lends itself to functional field assessment. In the grid coordinates of the stimuli as used in the standard Octopus programmes which at present employ an isometric projection the ratio of central ($0-30°$) to peripheral ($30-60°$) representation is less than 1/5 of that in the Octopus parabolic programmes. In addition within the $30°$ zone in e.g. Octopus programme 32, of a total of 76 stimuli

195

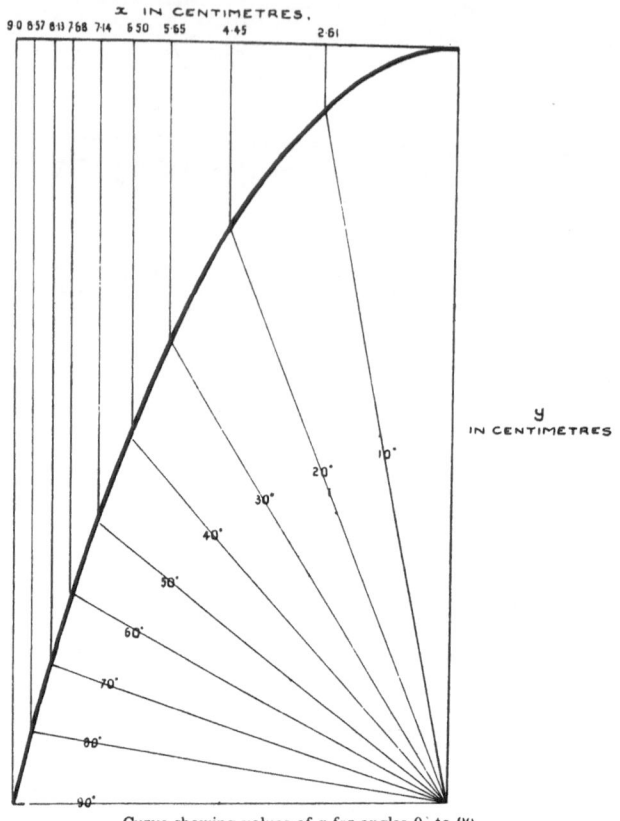

Curve showing values of x for angles 0° to 90°

Fig. 2. Projection of parabola $5y = x^2$.

there are (Fig. 4A): 12 stimuli for the central 10° (16%); 20 stimuli for the area 10–20° (26%); and 44 stimuli for the area 20–30° (58%).

The corresponding 30° representation employing a 1 cm square grid superimposed on a parabolic projection of the field where 90° = 9 cm is much more useful because, of a total of 96 stimuli, there are (Fig. 4B): 24 stimuli for the central 10° (25%); 36 stimuli for the area 10–20° (37.5%); and 36 stimuli for the area 20–30° (37.5%).

Having plotted a 1 cm grid on the parabolic projection it is necessary to consider what it is best to measure in order to assess the field numerically. There are many aspects to this including:

1. What is the shortest test which will give a satisfactory assessment of the important parts of the field.
2. How can extraneous factors such as brow, nose and lid configuration be eliminated so as not to affect a numerical score indicating as reliably as possible the total average state of the field.
3. How can the outer parts of the field be included in the assessment when

196

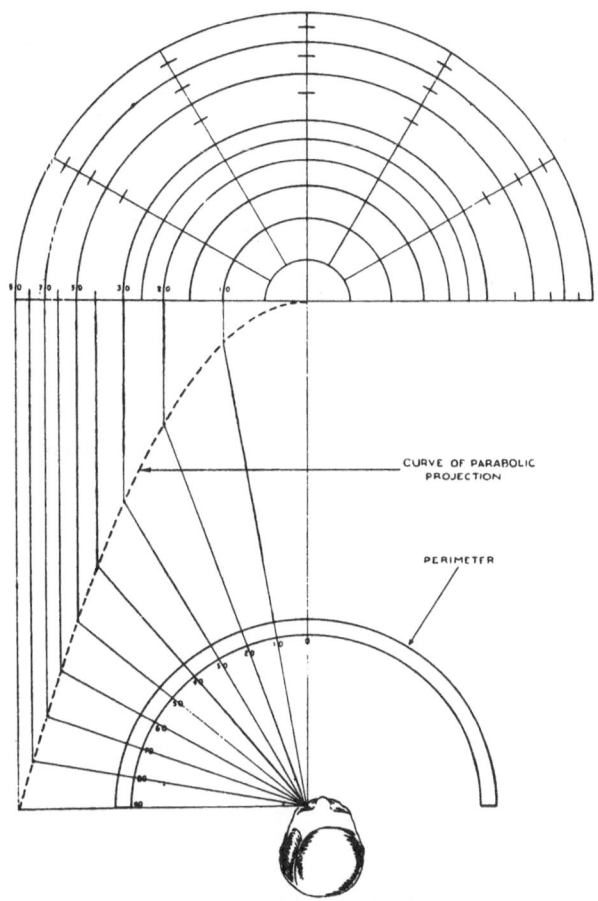

CURVE OF PARABOLIC
PROJECTION

PERIMETER

Basis of parabolic projection chart.

Fig. 3. Formation of parabolic visual field chart.

desired and added to that of the central field to make a uniform parabolic projection of the whole field.

To satisfy these requirements (Fig. 5) it is clear that the useful field would extend horizontally to 40° on each side. This would show a nasal step if present and be well clear of the blind spot so as to reveal wedge defects on the temporal side which Drance has shown to be important in glaucoma. It would not extend upwards more than 20—25° to avoid the eyelids and brow affecting the score but downwards about 30° would be appropriate. There would be advantages in basing the display on 100 stimuli so that a percentage score could readily be calculated (2 stimuli placed in the blind spot are ignored and can act as a test for false positives so that in all 102 stimuli are shown). The central field thus delineated is symmetrical horizontally, but vertically it extends further downwards than upwards. This has the advantage

197

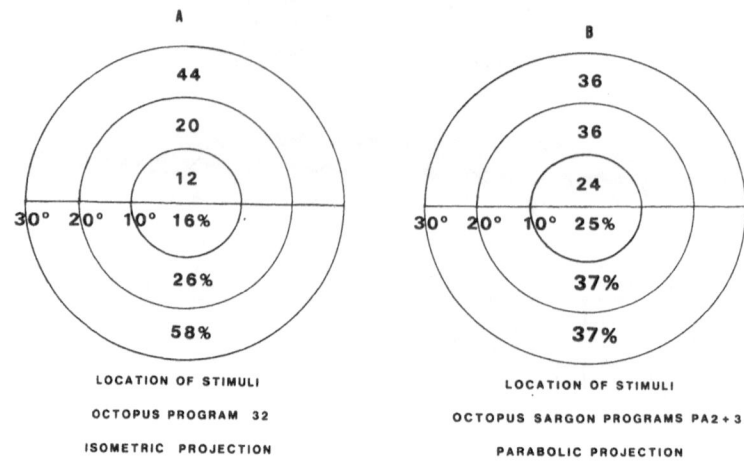

Fig. 4. (A) Distribution of stimuli in isometric projection; (B) distribution of stimuli in parabolic projection.

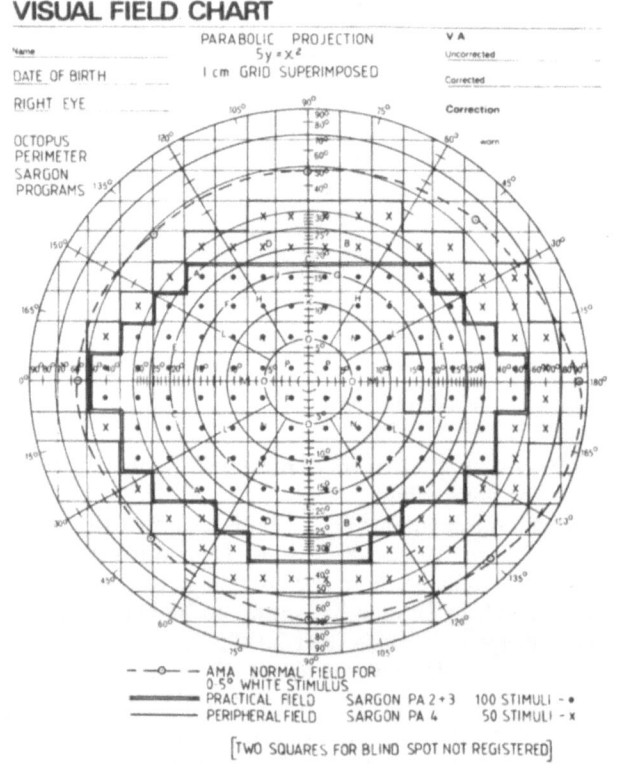

Fig. 5. Parabolic visual field chart showing centimetre grid, 'practical field' and 'peripheral field'.

198

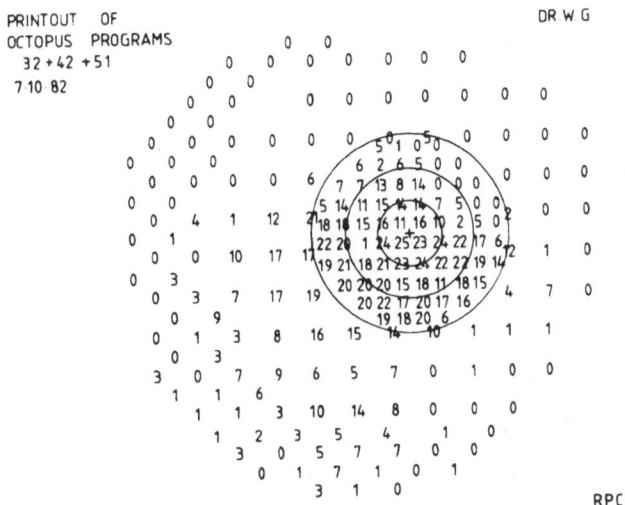

PRINTOUT OF
OCTOPUS PROGRAMS
32 + 42 + 51
7 10 82

DR W G

RPC

Fig. 6. Plot of Octopus programmes 32, 42 and 51.

that it would include the risk areas for primary open angle glaucoma as determined by Professor Aulhorn (3). These were displayed on a non-isometric projection but the units are not specified, Dannheim and Greve have also shown work based on non-linear projection charts. The visual field delineated above could be described as the 'practical visual field' to avoid confusion with the usual conception of the central field. An investigation is in progress to determine the extent, if any, to which a very short 50 stimuli test with stimuli placed exclusively in the high risk area is inferior in glaucoma detection and follow-up to the longer examination with a wider display. The peripheral field which adds another 50 stimuli would not ordinarily have to be used but it is desirable to have it available when its use seems applicable. It extends in all directions to be suitably within the peripheral isopter of the 0.5° white test object 3/330 (AMA standard). Figure 6 shows the plot of Octopus programmes 32 and 42 and 51 indicating the result of 45 minutes actual testing, even so the central area requires Programme 31 to be added to give adequate central representation.

NUMERICAL REPRESENTATION

When using the Octopus perimeter the 0.1 log unit (decibel) of filter with a standard stimulus brightness of 1000 apostilb (1 asb = 0.318 candela/metre^2) and a standard background luminance of 4 asb expressed the threshold sensitivity of the retina at the stimulated point. In this way a visual field score can be obtained in a manner used for 14 years at King's College Hospital for computerised numerical glaucoma field assessment employing a 'field cross' in which the field is divided into four quadrants each with three zones. The average score for each zone is simply calculated by mental arithmetic using a unit of 4 decibels (quadecibel). The average for the field is

199

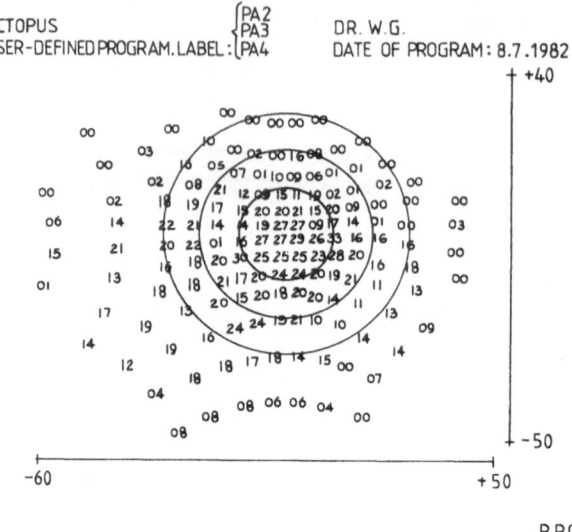

Fig. 7. Parabolic projection.

expressed as an Average Threshold Score (4). A similar scoring procedure can be applied to the parabolic Octopus programmes (PA 2/3/4) and the result delivered immediately by its microprocessor printout. This removes unnecessary drudgery and presents the clinician, once he has made the very slight effort to visualise what the figures mean, with a labour saving, 'at a glance', method of assessing visual fields and their progress. We are using it at present, adapting the 'field cross' to Octopus Programmes 32 and 42 in a long-term visual field and treatment study and find it invaluable.

Figure 7 demonstrates the more advantageous distribution of stimuli provided by a parabolic projection which compared favourably with Fig. 6.

Figure 8 shows the 'practical visual field' with 100 stimuli and contrasts the ease of interpretation using single figure units of 4 dB instead of higher numbers of 1 dB units.

Figure 9 portrays the left parabolic chart in quadecibel units using a colour code. 'Field crosses' and 'average thresholds' for both unspecialised functional fields and conventional threshold fields are included in the printout.

FUNCTIONAL FIELD SCORE

We are all familiar with Dr Esterman's valuable concept of functional field scoring. It is clear that in the parabolic system each unit of field in the centimetre grid represented by the stimulus at its centre can be allotted a Functional Factor which when multiplied by the threshold in quadecibels gives a Functional Value for that unit of field area. From this it is easy to calculate an unspecialised Average Functional Value for the whole of the field under test. This would be routinely provided at the touch of a key by the

200

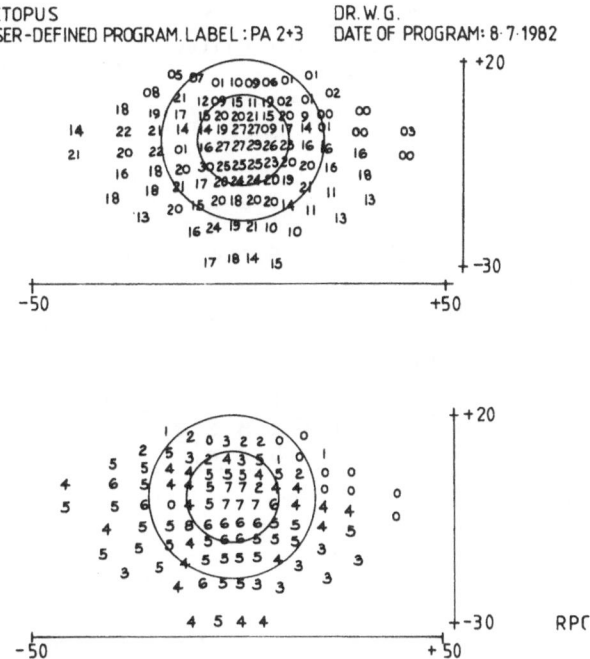

OCTOPUS
USER-DEFINED PROGRAM. LABEL : PA 2+3   DATE OF PROGRAM: 8·7·1982   DR. W. G.

Fig. 8. 'Practical' visual field.

microprocessor of an automatic perimeter in the same manner as the Average Threshold Scores and because the use of such instruments will soon become general, the time is already overdue for us to cease thinking in isopters and while working in 1 dB units to embrace the simplicity and informativeness of output in single digit quadecibel numerical grids without interpolation.

As Professor Krakau has emphasised the literal meaning of interpolation is to 'polish' or even 'falsify' (5) and though infilling is a temptation it is one we must strongly resist in the interests of reality and the hope of progress. Use of a large sine-bell stimulus may give true information about the field between the centres of stimuli (6) (7).

The Octopus has been fitted with a 'sine bell' aperture and work on this and other aspects of stimuli lacking high spatial frequency components is continuing. The traditional 'island of vision' has been shown to be a 'composite' (Fig. 10) and the degree of independence from the effect of refractive error is being evaluated. Much of the Esterman Central Rectangle has a Functional Factor close to unity. Thus it was a matter of some satisfaction to find that the Esterman analysis of the functional value of different parts of the field corresponded well with the value given by the type of parabolic projection chosen, so that function, physiology, and mathematical precision as well as practical convenience all combine to support this projection or one closely resembling it.

201

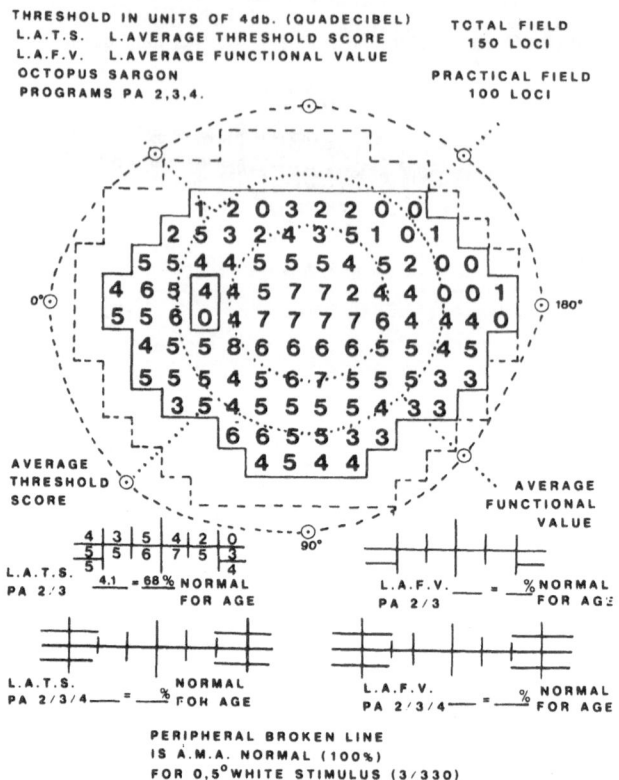

THRESHOLD IN UNITS OF 4db. (QUADECIBEL)
L.A.T.S.   L.AVERAGE THRESHOLD SCORE
L.A.F.V.   L.AVERAGE FUNCTIONAL VALUE
OCTOPUS SARGON
PROGRAMS PA 2,3,4.

TOTAL FIELD
150 LOCI

PRACTICAL FIELD
100 LOCI

Fig. 9. Parabolic chart for left eye with colour coded quadecibel units, field crosses and average threshold scores for direct and functional field assessment.

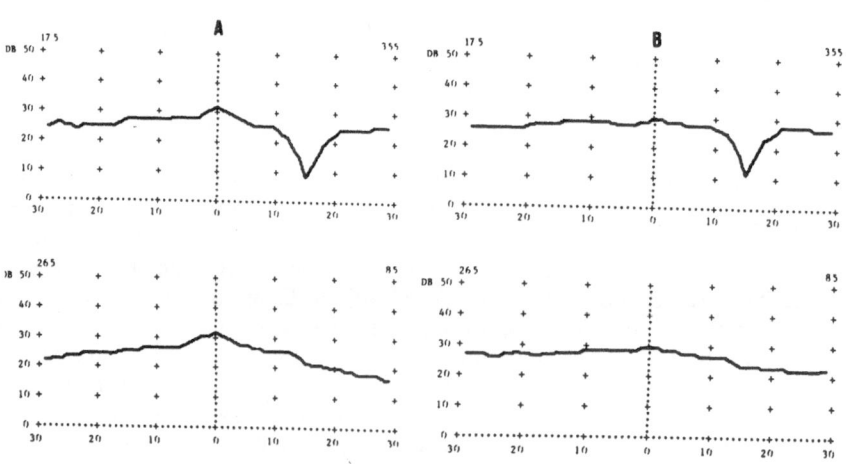

Fig. 10. Profile (A) normal stimulus; (B) sine bell stimulus.

202

ACKNOWLEDGEMENTS

Our thanks are due to all our ophthalmic colleagues at King's College Hospital especially Dr Patricia Reynolds, Glaucoma Research Fellow, to our Glaucoma Technicians Miss Louise Lee, Mrs Elaine Hammond, Mrs Eileen Cobb and Miss Judith Alexander, to Mrs Ann Warwick, Senior Ophthalmic Medical Secretary, Miss Eileen Creaby, Glaucoma Secretary, Mrs Jean Curtis, Glaucoma Research Secretary and Mr Colin Clements, Ophthalmic Medical Photographer.

The Octopus perimeter was generously provided by the Stanley Thomas Johnson Trust of Berne, by Merck Sharp and Dohme Ltd., and by the B.U.P.A. and we are indebted for construction and fitting of the sine-bell aperture and the Sargon programmes to Miss Helen Rhyner, Mr Spälte and Mr Zülkhe of Interzeag, Switzerland.

REFERENCES

1. Esterman, B. Grids for functional scoring of visual fields. Doc. Ophthalmol. Proc. Series 26 : 373–380 (1981).
2. Crick, R. P. A system of visual field testing and recording using a parabolic projection. Trans. Ophthalmol. Soc. U.K. 77 : 593–606 (1957).
3. Aulhorn, E. Comparative visual field study in patients with primary open angle glaucoma and anterior ischaemic optic neuropathy. Doc. Ophthalmol. Proc. Series 22 : 3–13 (1980).
4. Crick, R. P. Prevention of blindness from glaucoma using the KCH computerised problem orientated medical record. Br. J. Ophthalmol. 59 : 236–248 (1975).
5. Krakau, C. E. T. Aspects on the design of an automatic perimeter. Acta Ophthalmologica 56 : 389–405 (1978).
6. Crick, J. C. P. and Crick, R. P. The application of signal processing theory to perimetry. Res. and Clin. Forum 2/1: 109–115 (1980).
7. Crick, J. C. P. and Crick, R. P. The sine bell stimulus in perimetry. Doc. Ophthalmol. Proc. Series 26 : 239–246 (1981).

Author's address:
Dr R. P. Crick
Dept. of Ophthalmology
King's College Hospital
Denmark Hill
London SE5 9RS
England

INVESTIGATIONS ON SPACE BEHAVIOUR OF GLAUCOMATOUS PEOPLE WITH EXTENSIVE VISUAL FIELD LOSS*

G. CALABRIA, P. CAPRIS and C. BURTOLO

(Genoa, Italy)

Key words. Glaucoma, binocular visual field, behaviour difficulties.

ABSTRACT

Glaucomatous patients with extensive visual field defects often show more important difficulties in behaviour than patients with visual field defects of a similar extent but of different origin. In order to investigate this problem, the binocular visual field for these groups of patients was tested. Glaucomatous patients in binocular vision often show a sensitivity summation less efficient than other subjects. Further examinations were therefore carried out. It appears that different also non-perimetric factors play a role in the disability seen in glaucomatous patients.

INTRODUCTION

Glaucoma is often an extremely incapacitating disease: glaucomatous patients affected by severe visual field defects exhibit severe behaviour problems. Visual function often appears more seriously compromised than what would be expected by traditional functional examinations (visual acuity, kinetic perimetry).

Moreover it is commonly observed that patients having severe perimetric defects of a non-glaucomatous nature (e.g. diabetic retinopathy, photo-coagulative retinal ablation, post-surgical retinal detachment, hemianopsias due to neurological lesions, etc.) appear more capable of using their residual vision in overcoming their perimetric defects.

In order to try to explain this clinical phenomenon we studied the binocular visual field in binocular vision of patients with glaucomatous and non-glaucomatous perimetric defects.

In fact, because unclarified phenomena have been noted in the monocular

---

*Requests for offprints should be addressed to: Miss Vanna Re, Librarian of the University Eye Clinic, Viale Benedetto XV, 16132 Genoa, Italy.

Greve, E. L., Heijl, A. (eds.) Fifth International Visual Field Symposium.
©1983 Dr W. Junk Publishers, The Hague/Boston/Lancaster.

visual field in binocular vision conditions (e.g. blind spot enlargement) we verified how, in binocular conditions, superimposition and/or eventual integration of two abnormal monocular visual fields occur (4,5).

Moreover we studied how visual field defects of a different nature and morphology superimpose and integrate.

Finally, because from a practical point of view, two monolateral visual field defects seemed to superimpose and integrate in the same manner in normal, glaucomatous and non-glaucomatous patients we hypothesized that the visual problems of glaucomatous patients also derive from non-perimetric causes.

Therefore in some patients we carried out various preliminary functional examinations (adaptometry, flicker fusion perimetry, colour tests, reaction times) searching for different results in glaucomatous and non-glaucomatous patients.

MATERIALS AND METHOD

Patients (110) with binocular perimetric defects greater than 40% were examined. These patients presented with: chronic glaucoma (57); diabetic retinopathy (15); optical pathways lesions (13); pigmentary retinopathy (8); moreover 12 patients previously underwent retinal detachment surgery and 5 patients submitted to photocoagulative retinal ablation.

The patients ranged from 22 to 60 years of age. After a standard ophthalmological examination each patient was submitted to the following tests: monocular kinetic and static photopic perimetry (using a standard Goldmann perimeter); binocular kinetic and static perimetry (using a standard Goldmann perimeter. The same conditions and objects of monocular perimetry were utilized. The test was carried out after correction of existing presbyopia and refractive errors, studying the central and paracentral visual field; monocular and binocular static photopic campimetry (using the Grignolo-Tagliasco-Zingirian projection campimeter).

These tests were carried out only in patients having a residual visual field less than 30° wide.

Moreover, in 15 patients presenting glaucomatous visual field defects and in 10 patients affected by visual field defects of a non-glaucomatous origin, the following examinations were performed:
— light sensitivity evaluated by the Goldmann-Weeckers adaptometer;
— colour vision evaluated by the Farnsworth-Munsell 100 Hue test;
— flicker fusion frequencies evaluated in monocular and binocular vision by a Goldmann perimeter equipped with an electrically driven rotating semi-circular sector. The examination has been carried out according to a new method using supraliminal stimulation and a photometric equivalent target (9);
— measurement of reaction times. For this examination of a luminous spot (100 nits intensity 704 mm^2 surface area) was presented 36 times to each subject testing the macular region and the four quadrants at 30° eccentricity. The reaction times were measured by a millisecond chronometer connected to a microcomputer (10).

RESULTS

Normal binocular visual field

In the normal subject the binocular visual field is the result of superimposition of the two monocular visual fields. The resulting visual field is almost 180° wide. The central part (about 130°) depends on both eyes. The two exterior portions depend on one eye only. In these areas integration or summation phenomena are not possible. The lateral portions are crescent-shaped and their width changes with convergence. The greater sensitivity of the temporal hemifields creates an enlargement of the internal isopters.

Also the binocular static curve is the result of the interaction between the two monocular curves.

Beyond 30° the threshold corresponds to that of the more sensible eye, while inside 30° a certain summation is noted for which the binocular sensitivity curve appears slightly elevated. In the horizontal meridian such sensibility increase is obviously not seen in the coecal area.

Binocular visual field in glaucoma

In all the glaucomatous subjects with binocular perimetric damage the peripheral limits integrate without presenting unexpected phenomena: when one eye shows an absolute sectorial defect and normal sensitivity in the corresponding area of the opposite eye is present, integration of the peripheral limits occurs.

An isopter enlargement, when two normal visual field portions superimpose, was seen in 22 glaucomatous patients, as in normal behavior.

Besides, in 35 patients, no sensitivity summation happened when a deep perimetric defect corresponded to a normal area. Static perimetry clearly shows this phenomenon.

The binocular curve is exactly that of the better eye. These patients were affected by very severe defects in one of two eyes (e.g. fascicular defect, more than one quadrant wide).

Binocular visual field in non-glaucomatous pathology

In 12 patients with optical pathways diseases and perimetric defects the integration of the monocular visual fields is comparable to that of normal subjects. The binocular visual field of a patient affected by meningioma has shown an area of sensitivity that the monocular examination did not reveal.

In 42 subjects (80%) with retinal diseases (diabetic retinopathy, pigmentary retinopathy, photocoagulative retinal ablation, post-surgical retinal detachment), binocular kinetic and static perimetry showed normal integration in both eyes with binocular sensitivity increase.

In three patients affected by pigmentary retinopathy an island of sensitivity not detected in monocular examination has been shown with binocular perimetry.

The low visual acuity and fixation difficulties have invalidated the examination results of 5 patients.

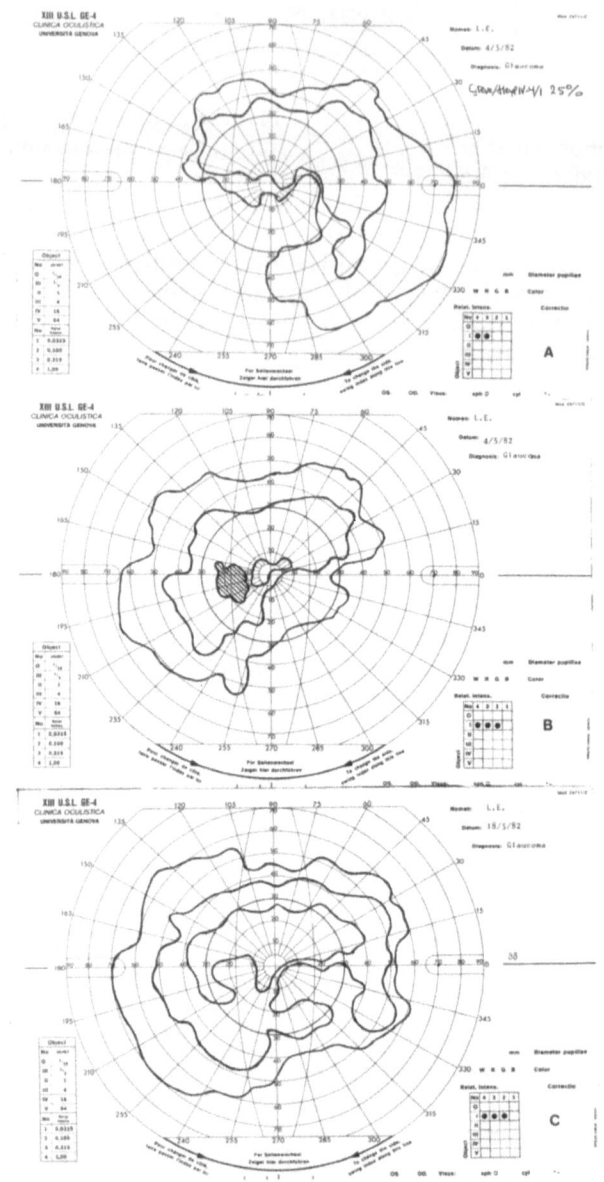

Fig. 1. Glaucomatous visual field (mild): severe perimetric damage. Binocular examination (C) shows a summation of two monocular visual fields (A, B).

208

Light sensitivity test

All patients with perimetric defects depending on glaucoma, pigmentary retinopathy, photocoagulative retinal ablation revealed a pathological light sensitivity curve of dark adaptation (e.g. prolonged times in scotopic and photopic adaptation). The patients who underwent retinal detachment have shown fewer alterations in adaptation times. Only three patients with optical pathway diseases have demonstrated severe alterations.

Colour vision

Alterations in colour vision (e.g. dichromatopsies without a preferential axis) are connected to visual acuity loss. There is little correlation between visual field defects and colour alterations in all subjects. No significant differences were revealed in various diseases.

Flicker perimetry

Flicker fusion frequency confirmed low sensitivity in the affected area of the visual field and variable results were noted in the other areas. No significant differences were revealed in the various diseases.

Reaction times

In all the subjects, using our method, no significant differences were noted between the four quadrants of the visual field.

Comparing various groups of patients a slight increase in reaction times was noted for glaucomatous patients.

CONCLUSIONS

We have not obtained any particular datum that would satisfy our objective to explain why glaucomatous and non-glaucomatous patients with visual field defects show different behaviour difficulties.

However, the vast majority of phenomena obtained in this study is generally negative in the patients affected by perimetric defects of a glaucomatous nature.

In particular the binocular visual field in glaucomatous patients often shows a sensitivity summation less efficient than that encountered in normal and pathological non-glaucomatous patients. In glaucoma a loss of sensitivity summation is more evident when one of the two visual fields is seriously compromised. A minor enlargement of the binocular isopters and a smaller increase in the central binocular static curve was noted. In contrast in cases of serious perimetric defect of a non-glaucomatous nature (particularly in pigmentary retinopathy, diabetic retinopathy and in neurological defects) efficient integration and summation phenomena are present.

We think that actual techniques of perimetric investigation may not be

209

able to define and clarify binocular phenomena, because these techniques are developed exclusively for monocular investigation. Beside other non-perimetric functional examinations have not shown substantial differences among the various groups. Consequently, a deeper and more widespread utilization of these diagnostic means is not encouraged. Only reaction times appear slightly longer in glaucomatous patients, but this fact can be indicative of a general decay of neuronal functions not necessarily of ophthalmological origin.

In conclusion it is possible to hypothesize the coexistence of various negative factors in order to explain the behaviour difficulties of glaucomatous patients. These factors can be of a various nature but are linked together to affect visual function. In particular we refer to ocular factors (myosis; incipient cataract, drug-induced conjunctivitis etc.) and general factors (advanced age, psychological constitution, psychotic problems induced by the disease, etc.) (1,7,8). On the basis of the perimetric data gathered it is possible to hypothesize that in glaucomatous patients inhibition phenomena (2,3) from the damaged visual field disturb residual visual function. Our techniques are only sufficient to suggest but not to explain these phenomena.

REFERENCES

1. Cazzullo, C. L. L'indirizzo psiconeurotico nello studio del glaucoma primario. Riv. Pat. Nerv. Ment. 75:581 (1954).
2. Critchley, M. The problem of awreness or non-awreness of hemianopic field defects. Trans. Ophthalmol. Soc. U.K. 69:95−109 (1949).
3. Dannheim, F. and Drance, S. M. Psychovisual disturbance in glaucoma. A study of temporal and spatial summation. Arch. Ophthalmol. 91:463 (1974).
4. Dubois-Poulsen, A. and Le champ, visuel. Parigi, Masson and Cie ed. (1952).
5. Dubois-Poulsen, A. The enlargement of the blind spot in binocular vision. Doc. Ophthalmol. Proc. Series 19:423−426 (1979).
6. Grignolo, A., Zingirian, M. and Rivara, A. Campimetry with two variables and a new projection compimeter. Am. J. Ophthalmol. 58:839−849 (1964).
7. Levi-Minzi, S. and Segato, T. La componente psichica nella patogenesi del glaucoma. Boll. Ocul. 59:457 (1971).
8. Marcenaro, M., Rasore, E., Savelli, P., Rolando, M. and Calabria, G. Glaucoma cronico e problemi psicoreattivi. Min. Oftalmologica (1981).
9. Rossi, P. L., Ciurlo, G. and Burtolo, C. La frequenza critica di fusione nell'area maculare. Boll. Ocul. 3:243−246 (1981).
10. Tartaglione, A., Cocito, L. and Favale, E. Ulteriori indagini sulle variazioni del tempo di reazione in funzione della frequenza spaziale e del contrasto dello stimolo. Atti Fond. G. Ronchi 33:571−578 (1978).

Author's address:
Dr G. Calabria
University Eye Clinic
Viale Benedetto XV, 5
16132 Genoa
Italy

CORRELATIONS BETWEEN PERIPHERAL VISUAL FUNCTION AND DRIVING PERFORMANCE

JOHN L. KELTNER* and CHRIS A. JOHNSON

(Davis, California, U.S.A.)

Key words. Peripheral vision, driving performance.

ABSTRACT

An automated visual field screening test was administered to 10,000 volunteers (20,000 eyes) at two California Department of Motor Vehicles driver's license offices. The incidence of visual field loss was 3.0 to 3.5% for individuals between the ages of 16 and 60, but rose to approximately 13% for the population over 65 years of age. Over half of the individuals with abnormal visual fields (57.6%) were previously unaware of any problem with peripheral vision. The relationship between peripheral vision and driving performance was determined by examining accident and conviction rates for three years prior to our testing. Drivers with binocular visual field loss had accident and conviction rates that were twice as high ($p < 0.005$) as those of an age and sex-matched control group with normal visual fields, whereas drivers with monocular visual field loss had accident and conviction rates that were equivalent to those of their age and sex-matched control group.

INTRODUCTION

It is a common clinical observation that patients with severe visual field loss have difficulty with locomotion and other forms of visually guided behavior. Therefore, it might be expected that peripheral vision is an important determinant of visuomotor tasks such as driving an automobile. However, studies by Burg (2–4, 7) and others (6, 14, 15) have reported little or no relationship between visual field size and driving performance. It is difficult to evaluate the significance of these findings because of several methodologic problems in their investigations. First, the perimetric technique used to obtain measurements was a non-standard procedure that had not been validated. The extent to which their tests could distinguish between normal and abnormal visual

---

* To whom requests for offprints should be addressed.

Greve, E. L., Heijl, A. (eds.) Fifth International Visual Field Symposium.
©*1983 Dr W. Junk Publishers, The Hague/Boston/Lancaster.*

fields is therefore not known. A second difficulty is that the tests were performed with no method of controlling or monitoring fixation, and were administered by personnel with no previous perimetric training. Also, the tests did not perform a full visual field evaluation, but rather measured only two locations along the horizontal meridian to determine lateral visual field extent.

Recently, Fishman et al. (6), using standard clinical perimetric techniques, found that retinitis pigmentosa patients with marked visual field loss had significantly worse driving records than an age-matched control group with normal visual fields. Since their results are contrary to previous studies, this again raises the question of relationships between peripheral visual function and driving performance.

The present study was designed to re-examine this issue by testing a large driving population of 10,000 individuals. In particular, we were interested in two basic questions: 1) what is the incidence of visual field loss in a driving population for various age groups, and 2) is there a relationship between peripheral visual field abnormalities and driving performance?

METHODS

A modified Fieldmaster Model 101-PR was used to conduct visual field screening exams, since previous clinical validation studies have shown that it can accurately distinguish between normal and abnormal visual fields (8,10, 12,13). Based on results from a pilot study of 1,017 eyes (11), a background luminance of 31.5 asb and a target luminance of 1,270 asb (Goldmann I/4c equivalent) were employed. A reduced target pattern consisting of 78 visual field locations (see Figs. 1 and 2) were used to provide adequate coverage of the visual field and minimize examination time. The average testing time was one minute and 54 seconds per eye (including instructions, alignment, etc.), with an additional one minute and 57 seconds required to record answers to the questions in Table 1.

The subject population consisted of 10,000 volunteers (20,000 eyes) from driver's license applicants at two California Department of Motor Vehicles offices. Perimetric test results and answers to questions were recorded on magnetic storage media and analyzed with an LSI 11/23 computer system. Abnormal and questionably abnormal visual field results were also evaluated manually according to previously developed criteria (8,10–13). Answers to questions and visual field results were then correlated with Department of Motor Vehicles driving conviction and accident records for three years prior to the test date.

RESULTS

Due to incomplete information or data transmission errors, results from 2,466 of the 20,000 eyes could not be included for analysis. The incidence of visual field abnormalities for the remaining 17,534 eyes was between 3.0 and 3.5%

212

Table 1. Questions asked of each study participant.

1. Name
2. Address
3. City and State
4. Telephone number
5. Driver's license number
6. Yearly mileage driven
7. Age
8. Sex
9. Years since last eye exam
10. Are glasses worn?
11. Are contact lenses worn?
12. Is refractive error large ($> 3D$)?
13. Do you have glaucoma?
14. Any family history of glaucoma?
15. Other serious eye problems?
16. Visual acuity
17. If results indicate a possible problem, do you wish to be notified?

for individuals under 60 years of age. This value doubled (6%) for individuals between 61 and 65, with the age group over 65 showing a 13% incidence of abnormal visual fields. Approximately one third of the total number of individuals with visual field abnormalities had binocular involvement. Follow-up reports indicated that the most common ocular disorders contributing to visual field defects were glaucoma, cataracts and retinal disorders. Our estimate of the incidence of false alarms is less than 1%, based on our follow-up reports and the results of similar mass screening studies using automated perimetry (1). In the present investigation, most of our documented false alarms were attributable to high refractive errors. More detailed information pertaining to other aspects of visual field characteristics in this population is presented in another paper (9). Figures 1 and 2 present examples of homonymous hemianopsias and severe binocular visual field loss that were found in this study.

To examine the relationship between driving performance and visual field loss, we examined each participant's driving accident and conviction record for a period of three years prior to the visual field test. Individuals with visual field loss were classified according to whether they demonstrated monocular or binocular visual field loss. For comparison, each of these groups were paired with an age and sex-matched control group with normal visual fields in both eyes. The average number of accidents and convictions per 100,000 miles are presented in Table 2 for each of the groups.

For individuals with monocular visual field loss, there was no statistically significant difference in accident and conviction records, as compared to their control group ($\chi^2 = 1.195$, df $= 1$, $p > 0.20$ for accidents; $\chi^2 = 1.244$, df $= 1$, $p > 0.20$ for convictions). However, the results for individuals with visual field loss in both eyes were quite different. Accident and conviction rates for this group were more than twice as high as for their control group. The differences were statistically significant ($\chi^2 = 8.25$, df $= 1$, $p < 0.005$ for accidents; $\chi^2 = 15.25$, df $= 1$, $p < 0.001$ for convictions). These findings clearly indicate a relationship between binocular visual field loss and driving

213

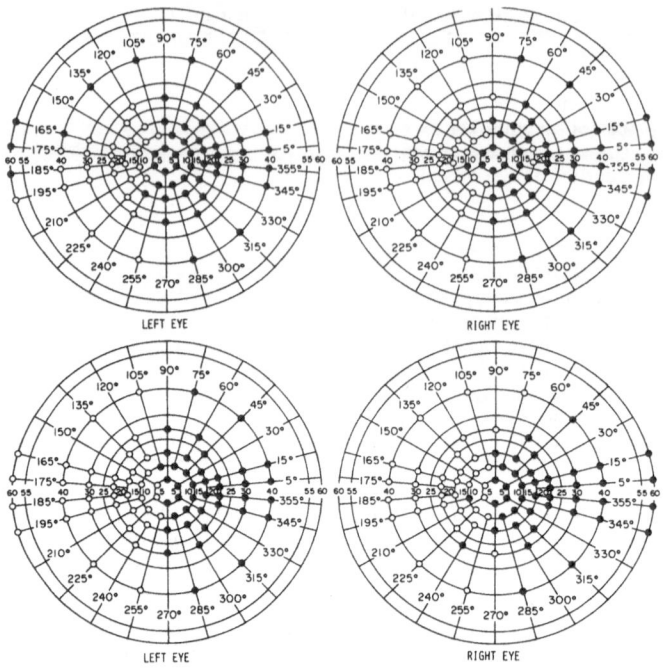

Fig. 1. Examples of homonymous hemianopic visual field loss found in our mass visual field screening study.

performance. Differences between the two control groups for accident and conviction rates are probably related to the age differences of the two populations.

DISCUSSION

Our results indicate that the overall incidence of visual field loss in a driving population is approximately 3.3%, a value that compares favorably with previous mass visual field screening studies utilizing automated perimetry (1,11). More than half (57.6%) of the individuals with visual field loss were previously unaware of any visual field abnormalities. Bengtsson and Krakau (1) have previously reported that 48% of their population with visual field loss were not previously aware of any abnormality. These findings indicate that mass visual field screening with automated perimetry is an effective method of finding previously undetected visual field abnormalities.

Our findings for relationships between binocular visual field loss and driving performance are contrary to those reported by Burg (2–4,7) and others (6,14,15) but are consistent with those reported by Fishman et al. (6) for retinitis pigmentosa patients. We feel that the studies by Burg (2–4, 7) and others (6,14,15) have several methodologic problems associated with their peripheral visual field measurement technique, as noted previously.

214

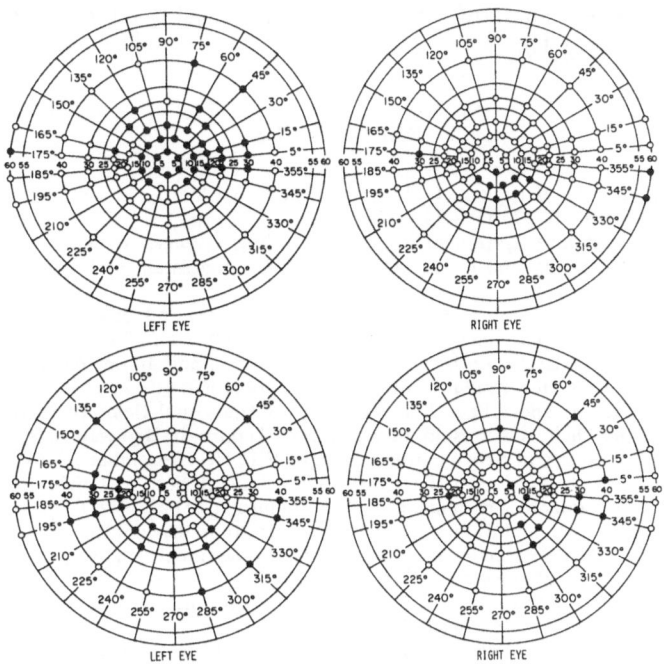

Fig. 2. Examples of severe binocular visual field loss found in our mass visual field screening study.

Table 2. Average number of accidents and convictions per 100,000 miles.

	Accidents	Convictions
Monocular loss	0.80	2.40
Age and sex-matched control group	0.68	2.20
Binocular loss	1.34	2.90
Age and sex-matched control group	0.64	1.50

In the present study and that of Fishman et al. (6), validated clinical perimetric procedures were employed, and a significant relationship was found between peripheral visual function and driving performance. These data suggest that a re-evaluation of visual screening procedures for driving would be useful.

ACKNOWLEDGEMENTS

We are grateful to Synemed, Inc. for their assistance and technical support, to the California Department of Motor Vehicles for their cooperation and help, to Jan Horton for the development of data analysis software used in this study and Shirley Bingham for typing the manuscript and handling the correspondence for our follow-up letters to participants.

215

This study was supported in part by the National Eye Institute Grant No. EY-03424 (to C.A.J.).

REFERENCES

1. Bengtsson, B. and Krakau, C. E. T. Automatic perimetry in a population survey. Acta Ophthalmol. 57:929–937 (1979).
2. Burg, A. An investigation of some relationships between dynamic visual acuity, static visual acuity and driving record. UCLA Department of Engineering Report No. 64–18 (1964).
3. Burg, A. The relationship between vision test scores and driving record: General findings. UCLA Department of Engineering Report No. 67–24 (1967).
4. Burg, A. The relationship between vision test scores and driving record: Additional findings. UCLA Department of Engineering Report No. 68–27 (1968).
5. Council, F. M. and Allen, J. A. A study of the visual fields of North Carolina drivers and their relationship to accidents. Report of Highway Safety Research Center, University of North Carolina, Chapel Hill, NC (December 1974).
6. Fishman, G. A., Anderson, R. J. Stinson, L. and Haque, A. Driving performance of retinitis pigmentosa patients. Br. J. Ophthalmol. 65:122–126 (1981).
7. Henderson, R. L. and Burg, A. Vision and audition in driving. Report No. DOT-HS-801-265, US Department of Transportation, National Highway Traffic Safety Administration, Washington, DC (November 1974).
8. Johnson, C. A. and Keltner, J. L. Automated suprathreshold static perimetry. Am. J. Ophthalmol. 89:731–741 (1980).
9. Johnson, C. A. and Keltner, J. L. The incidence of visual field loss in 20,000 eyes and its relationship to driving performance. Arch. Ophthalmol. 101:371–375 (1983).
10. Johnson, C. A., Keltner, J. L. and Balestrery, F. G. Suprathreshold static perimetry in glaucoma and other optic nerve disease. Ophthalmology 86:1278–1286 (1979).
11. Keltner, J. L. and Johnson, C. A. Mass visual field screening in a driving population. Ophthalmology 87:785–790 (1980).
12. Keltner, J. L. and Johnson, C. A. Effectiveness of automated perimetry in following glaucomatous visual field progression. Ophthalmology 89:237–254 (1982).
13. Keltner, J. L., Johnson, C. A. and Balestrery, F. G. Suprathreshold static perimetry: Initial clinical trials with the Fieldmaster automated perimeter. Arch. Ophthalmol. 97:260–272 (1979).
14. Shinar, D. Driver visual limitations: Diagnosis and treatment. Report No. DOT-HS-5-01275, US Department of Transportation, National Highway Traffic Safety Administration, Washington, DC (September 1977).
15. Shinar, D., Mayer, R. M. and Treat, J. R. Reliability and validity assessments of a newly developed battery of driving related vision tests. Proceedings of the 19th Annual Meeting of the American Association for Automotive Medicine, San Diego, 209–225 (November 1975).

Author's address:
Dr J. L. Keltner
Depts. of Ophthalmology, Neurology and Neurological Surgery
University of California
Davis, CA 95616
U.S.A.

NON-LINEAR PROJECTION IN VISUAL FIELD CHARTING

FRITZ DANNHEIM

(Hamburg, FRG)

Key word. Perimetry.

ABSTRACT

Visual field charts with a non-linear projection for eccentricity enlarging the central field correspond with psychophysical data and practical demands. An application to clinical perimetry proved their usefulness.

INTRODUCTION

Any flat representation of the function of the spherically arranged retina will necessarily introduce distortion (8). The isometric projection of the conventional visual field charts with equidistant representation of the eccentricity from 10 to 10 degrees (Fig. 1E) may appeal as a logical solution. It results in a considerable distortion, however, enlarging the peripheral field disproportionately. The spatial dimensions of the retina call for a more refined representation of the central field (6) (Fig. 1D). The finer network of receptive fields in the retina (9) or the cortical representation of the field (10) are in favour of an even larger representation of the central portion. An additional demand is the functional importance of the central field (7) and the practical requirement to record small paracentral defects.

A larger scale for the central field within $30°$, as used for campimetry and in perimeters with different transmission, may satisfy some of these needs. Two or more different graphs are then necessary, however. A non-linear scale for the eccentricity which represents the whole field of an eye in one graph, may at the same time allow enough resolution in the central portion.

PROGRESSION OF NON-LINEAR SCALES

The Hamblin projection perimeter already applied a non-linear scale for eccentricity (11). The enlarging effect in the center was relatively mild, less

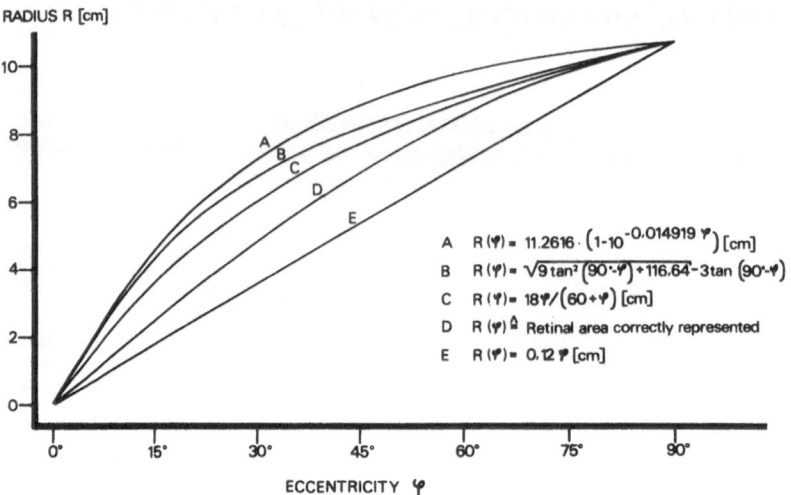

Fig. 1. Different projections of angle of eccentricity φ in visual field charting, related to a standard Goldmann chart with a radius of 10.8 cm and an equidistant linear projection E; (A) receptive fields invariantly represented; (B) 'parabolic' projection (2); (C) projection of the Peritest; (D) retinal area correctly represented (6).

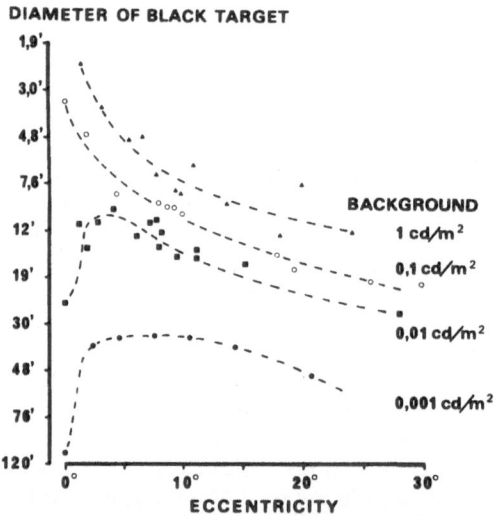

Fig. 2. Size of smallest just visible circular black target in relation to eccentricity, plotted for 4 background luminances. Curves resemble those of light difference sensitivity (1) and represent a functional meshwork of the retina.

pronounced than the one of a projection representing retinal area correctly (6) (Fig. 1D).

A projection which reflects receptive fields throughout the visual field might be an even more functional approach. Resolution of black targets

218

reveals a functional meshwork of receptive elements (1). We therefore measured the diameters of the smallest just visible black targets within the central visual field for different background luminances (Fig. 2).

This series of curves correspond to different non-linear nets. Some representative values for a slightly brighter background luminance of 3.2 cd/m² in a group of normal subjects are about 4′ at 5°, 10′ at 30°, 20′ at 60° and 120′ at 90° eccentricity. These data do correlate fairly well with the size of receptive fields in spider monkeys (9). A projection which invariantly represents this functional grid throughout the visual field is given in Fig. 1A.

The enlargement of the center was felt to be too pronounced for practical purposes, since the periphery, which is responsible for the orientation in space, is compressed inappropriately. A projection with a slightly lesser enlargement of the center (Fig. 1B) was successfully applied to kinetic (2) and computerized static perimetry (3).

We found another arbitrary projection lying just between the 'functional' (Fig. 1A) and the 'anatomical' meshwork (Fig. 1D) to be a suitable compromise (Fig. 1C). This projection has demonstrated its usefulness in grid perimetry (5) (Fig. 3) as well as in static and kinetic manual perimetry (4).

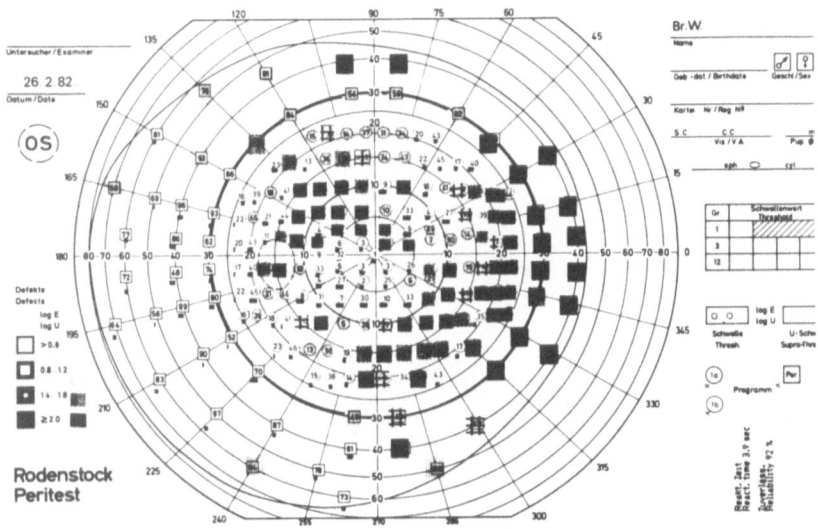

Fig. 3. Glaucomatous paracentral and peripheral defects plotted with a non-linear projection (Fig. 1C) in automated grid perimetry (Peritest). 30°-parallel accentuated, showing the enlargement of the central field. Absolute and relative depression of sensitivity marked with grey scale symbols.

219

REFERENCES

1. Aulhorn, E. Über die Beziehung zwischen Lichtsinn und Sehschärfe. Albrecht von Graefes Arch. Klin. Exp. Ophthalmol. 167:4–74 (1964).
2. Crick, R. P. A system of visual field testing and recording using a parabolic projection. Trans. Ophthalmol. Soc. U.K. 77:593–607 (1957).
3. Crick, R. P., Crick, J. C. P. and Ripley, L. The representation of the visual field. Doc. Opthalmol. Proc. Series 35:193–203 (1983).
4. Dannheim, F. Perimetry in Glaucoma I: Methods. Doc. Ophthalmol. Proc. Series 22.29–38 (1980).
5. Dannheim, F. Clinical experiences with a new automated perimeter 'Peritest'. Doc. Ophthalmol. Proc. Series 35:309–312 (1983).
6. Drasdo, N. and Fowler, C. W. Non-linear projection of the retinal image in a wide-angle schematic eye. Br. J. Ophthalmol. 58:709–714 (1974).
7. Esterman, B. Grid for scoring visual fields. II. Perimeter. Arch. Ophthalmol. 79:400–406 (1968).
8. Frisén, L. The cartographic deformations of the visual field. Ophthalmologica 161:38–54 (1970).
9. Hubel, D. H. and Wiesel, T. N. Receptive fields of optic nerve fibres in the spider monkey. J. Physiol. 154:572–580 (1960).
10. Miller, N. R. Walsh and Hoyt's Clinical Neuro-Ophthalmology, 4. ed. Williams and Wilkins, Baltimore, pp. 93–95 (1982).
11. Walker, C. B. Cited after Crick, R. P. (see Ref. 3).

Author's address:
Dr F. Dannheim
Dept. of Ophthalmology
Eye Clinic of the University of Hamburg
Martinistr. 52
D-2000 Hamburg 20, FRG

DISCUSSION

G. Verriest: All these considerations are very important. The first conclusion we have to make is that in a conventional perimetric chart we must not test every point at the same angular distance, as for example the Octopus device does. The physiological reality is that a defect of the same extent is less important in a peripheral region of the visual field as in the central region.

I would like to ask a question to Dr Esterman. I examine also binocular visual fields, with the Goldmann perimeter, but I wonder if because of the convergence of the eyes the binocular visual field is not restricted laterally when compound to a greater distance tracing. You can measure the effect by making a drawing.

B. Esterman: I'll answer the last question first. We measured that and it actually comes to less than 5% and since most human errors are more, at least 10%, we know that we are not in much trouble. The answer to the first question is very interesting. If you have been an ophthalmologist in length of time, you all will have had the experience that if you take a patient's central acuity with the Snellen chart and you take the right eye and let's say you get 20–70 and you take the acuity of the left eye and you get 20–50 and if you take both eyes you get 20–30. A similar phenomenon may be happening here, I think.

When you take the field binocularly with the two eyes simultaneously you get the effect of two sets of retinal receptors, so that you get sharpened acuity in the central area, therefore any scotoma that you would get by artificially combining the two fields would be larger than the scotoma that actually exists because you have two sets of retinal receptors zeroing on the central field and therefore your scotoma will be smaller.

G. Verriest: It is already known that for many visual functions there is improvement in binocular vision when compared to monocular vision. Recently I published data for the 100-Hue Colour Vision Test: when you do it in binocular vision you have better mean scores than if you do it in monocular vision. That is for similar visual acuity and many other functions. But there seem to be other factors in ocular pathology and therefore your contribution is very interesting.

Greve, E. L., Heijl, A. (eds.) Fifth International Visual Field Symposium.
©*1983 Dr W. Junk Publishers, The Hague/Boston/Lancaster.*

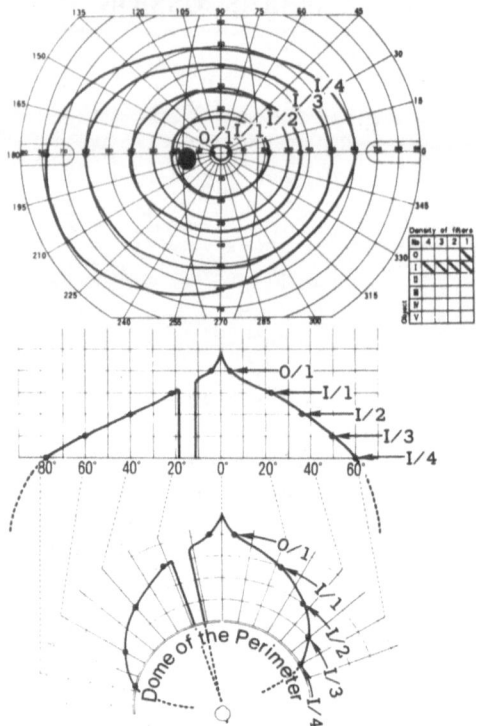

Fig. 1.

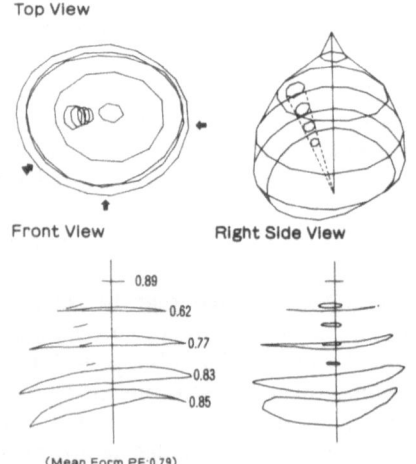

Top View

Front View   Right Side View

(Mean Form PE:0.79)

Fig. 2.

222

G. Calabria: I think that in retinopathia pigmentosa it was an expected phenomenon to see that the binocular visual field is better, because sometimes people affected by this disease have a very bad visual behavior. Anyway, I think that the monocular visual field, the absolute peripheral visual field is maybe not realistic. Maybe the making between a summation to a complete absolute visual field is possible to have some new visual field islands is useful for the behavior of the patient.

G. Verriest: I am personally happy of what you said because I have always proclaimed that the contradictory results of a prior investigation of Burg were not significant because of the lack of an adequate method of examination. Thus now an important problem is solved. But which methods of examination could be recommended?

The Fieldmaster is a rather expensive apparatus for such purposes. I personally believe in simple methods. Santucci also stated an higher accident rate in people with visual field defects and his study was made simply by means of an attachment to a multiphasic visual screener (the Campitest attached to the Vislotest). Once we know that visual field has importance for driving and for job fitness we have to find methods for examination of visual field that could be applied for drivers, in industry and so on.

F. Furuno: I wish to briefly show you our ideas concerning functional scoring of visual field. This is a profile of the visual field sensitivity in which the degrees from fixation are marked in angular degrees, rather than linearly along the x-axis in the conventional method, as you are used to seeing. By this technique, an onion-shaped 3-dimensional representation of the visual field was calculated by integration of the kinetic result using a micro-computer.

As you know, from a clinical point of view the central field is more important than the periphery, therefore if only the volume of the conventional visual field island were measured, it might not indicate the visual function and it is therefore necessary to give some greater weight to the central field rather than the periphery for accurate evaluation. Giving weight to the central field volume was reasonably achieved in our onion-shaped representation of the visual field.

We also measured the coefficient of the form of each isopter and the volume of the onion-shaped visual field was multiplied by their mean value. The resulting value was called the modified volume. The evaluation of the quantitative perimetry was considered satisfactory by this method.

METHODOLOGICAL ASPECTS OF CONTRAST SENSITIVITY MEASUREMENTS IN THE DIAGNOSIS OF OPTIC NEUROPATHY AND MACULOPATHY

IVAN BODIS-WOLLNER

(New York, New York, U.S.A.)

Key words. Contrast sensitivity, optic neuropathy, macular disease.

ABSTRACT

Spatial contrast sensitivity and visual evoked potential studies reveal defects not tapped by visual acuity measurements in patients suffering from maculopathy and optic neuropathy. Differential diagnosis can be aided, since in maculopathy the loss is of the high frequency type, in glaucomatous optic neuropathy it shows up best as a loss of dynamic, low spatial frequency detection, and in demyelinating optic neuropathy it may occur only for selected orientations and/or spatial frequency of the pattern.

INTRODUCTION

Undoubtedly, ophthalmoscopy is one of the most useful clinical tools for differentiating maculopathy from optic neuropathy. Unfortunately, this is not always sufficient. For instance, problems arise when a patient who has already had macular changes begins to complain of more recent visual loss. In doubtful cases one may resort to widely validated objective clinical tests, which may include fluorescein angiography or occasionally an electrophysiological test such as the ERG and EOG. Some psychophysical tests, such as color vision testing, static perimetry, and the use of the Amsler grid, may all give help. However in recent years several new techniques have emerged which appear to open new avenues in the exploration of the pathophysiology of visual disorders in general, and carry the promise of being useful in the differential diagnosis of macular and optic nerve diseases. One of these techniques, called 'layer perimetry', was pioneered and explored by Enoch and his co-workers (16). Another widely used new technique is called contrast sensitivity measurements (5), a procedure utilizing sinusoidal grating pattern stimuli. The methodology, general sensitivity, and specificity of psychophysical and electrophysiological measurements using sinusoidal gratings have been described earlier. Here those aspects of the methodology of contrast sensitivity measurements will be emphasized which are immediately relevant to the question of maculopathy versus optic neuropathy. In addition, a brief review of recent data using contrast sensitivity measurements and electrophysiological studies which pertain to the diagnosis of optic neuropathy and maculopathy will be provided.

RELEVANT METHODOLOGY

Definitions

The stimuli employed in the studies to be reviewed here consist of sinusoidal grating patterns (Fig. 1a) and occasionally checkerboard patterns. Such patterns have several variables, all of which must be taken into account when comparing different studies. Spatial frequency is the number of bars subtended in one degree of visual angle. Conversely, the size of a band of a grating can be defined by its width, calculated by the formula $W = 60/2f$, where W is in minutes of arc and f is spatial frequency in cycles/degree. Conversely, the fundamental spatial frequency of a check pattern (12) can be expressed as $f = 60/1.4W$, where f is in cycles/degree and W is the width of the check in minutes of arc. Contrast is the luminance difference of adjacent dark and bright bands given a constant level of luminance. The mean luminance of the pattern is the average luminance of the screen. It is kept constant if spatial frequency is the variable being explored. In most studies

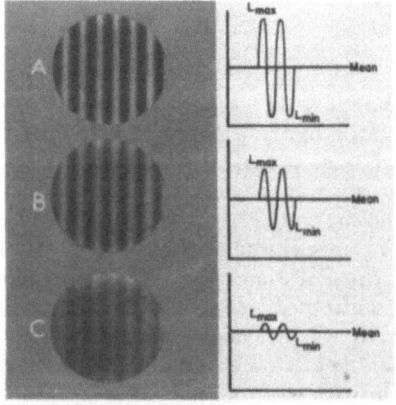

Fig. 1a. Photographs (left) and luminance profiles (right) of sinusoidal grating patterns, electronically generated at three levels of contrast. The contrasts of the gratings were 85% (A), 50% (B), and 10% (C). Contrast is defined as the maximum and minimum luminance divided by their sum, i.e., $(L_{max} - L_{min})/(L_{max} - L_{min})$. Maximum luminance is labeled 'L_{max}' and minimum luminance 'L_{min}' on the profiles at right. The mean luminance of the pattern remains constant as contrast is changed. (Illustration from Wolkstein et al. Ophthalmology 87:1140–1149, 1980. Reproduced with permission).

226

the mean luminance is fixed around $10 \, cd/m^2$, although some studies indicate that the effect of exploring contrast sensitivity at several mean luminance levels may provide information. Pattern field size is usually circular, and in many studies it is surrounded by a larger field of the same mean luminance as the prestimulus field. Spatial contrast sensitivity is the inverse of the minimum contrast which is needed for an observer to detect a given spatial frequency. The general shapes of these curves vary as a function of mean luminance (36). Both the cut-off frequency (which is roughly equivalent to a visual acuity measurement using grating patterns), the spatial frequency at which peak sensitivity occurs, and the peak contrast sensitivity value, shift as a function of luminance. However in a wide photopic range $(6–600 \, cd/m^2)$, there is little change.

Other relevant variables concern the size of the field. In normals, spatial contrast sensitivity at a given spatial frequency does not appreciably change once the stimulus contains at least 7–8 cycles of the pattern. The pattern also has to be long enough. A circular field with a diameter of 480/f will express in minutes of arc the minimum stimulus area which is needed for optimal sensitivity, where f is the spatial frequency in cycles/degree of the pattern. For instance, for optimal detection of fine patterns, a relatively small field with a diameter of 16 min of arc is sufficient. Conversely, if one cannot provide a field larger than 1 degree in diameter, it is important to know the lowest spatial frequency which can be explored without distorting the results. This can be easily calculated as $f = 480/d$, if f is in cycles/degree and d is the diameter of the field in minutes of arc. In the specific example ($1°$ field), a 6 cycles/degree pattern is the lowest spatial frequency which can be explored without distorting the absolute contrast sensitivity value.

The two-fold effect of cycloplegia needs to be considered. Spatial contrast sensitivity will be degraded if the pupil is either too large or too small. In the case of a large pupil the intrusion of the effects of the degraded optics of the eye will distort the data, and in the case of a too small pupil the reduced mean luminance will have the same effect. Thus in the exploration of a patient's contrast sensitivity, one must take pupil size into account. Practically speaking, a patient's pupil between 2.8 and 5 mm will not seriously influence contrast sensitivity in the photopic range (14), and given the spread of normal contrast sensitivity values (8), the exact pupil size in this range can be neglected.

Refractive errors

Refractive errors will not uniformly degrade contrast sensitivity. The highest spatial frequencies are affected first, but with an increase in the number of diopters of error, eventually sensitivity to low spatial frequencies becomes degraded. The peak of the contrast sensitivity curve, however, is remarkably immune to refractive error. Myopic defects are greater: at least in young people a refractive error which causes hypermetropia can be compensated for by accommodation (13).

Age

Age has an appreciable effect on the contrast sensitivity curve, and

227

abnormalities have been reported both in the high and low spatial frequency range. For clinical work it is most important to establish normative values in age-matched controls for the particular methodology in use, rather than attempting to rely upon data already published, as normative data are still being worked out (29).

Color displays

There have been relatively few studies dealing with contrast sensitivity using isoluminance color contrast. However colored filters over the whole display have established that green and red patterns yield similar contrast sensitivities, whereas the contrast sensitivity curve to blue patterns will be lower (15). Contrast sensitivity studies employing alternating isoluminance colored bars would require technology which is not easily available. This is unfortunate since displays which would allow one to change hue without changing the luminance, and vice versa, could be of great value in studies of maculopathy versus optic neuropathy (1).

Visual evoked potential studies

While not a psychophysical technique, some pertinent VEP data will be considered. Although most clinical VEP studies employ checkerboard patterns as stimuli, some have used sinusoidal gratings (Figs. 1a, 1b), and some studies have even established contrast sensitivity using VEP measurements. However some relevant data concerning the use of checkerboard stimuli will also be mentioned in conjunction with psychophysical data. The routine methodology of VEP recordings concerning techniques of averaging and electrode placement over the inion have been described previously.

Pattern electroretinogram (ERG)

These measurements have come into vogue during the last two years, following the demonstration by Maffei and colleagues (22) that cats with transsection of the optic nerve showed deterioration of pattern ERG responses, while the flicker ERG remained intact. Histological studies of the retina of optic-nerve-transsected cats showed that the ganglion cell layer had degenerated, while the preganglionic layers were intact. These studies suggested that the ganglion cell layer contributes heavily to pattern ERG responses. Such data have been somewhat conflicting, however most authors agree at the moment that ganglion cell pathology can degrade the pattern ERG signal.

CLINICAL STUDIES

1. Retinitis pigmentosa

Although the hallmark of retinitis pigmentosa (RP) is a 'typical' annular scotoma, foveal defects occur in many patients late in the disease and in

228

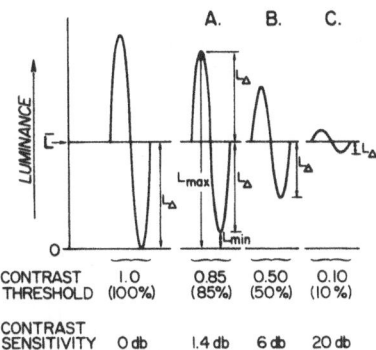

CONTRAST THRESHOLD	1.0 (100%)	0.85 (85%)	0.50 (50%)	0.10 (10%)
CONTRAST SENSITIVITY	0 db	1.4 db	6 db	20 db

Fig. 1b. Contrast thresholds and contrast sensitivity. Curves A, B, and C are the luminance profiles of the three gratings shown in Fig. 1a. $\bar{L}$ is the mean luminance level of each grating. This is held constant. L_{max} indicates the luminance values at the centers of the light bars, and L_{min} is the luminance at the centers of the dark bars. Contrast is defined as $(L_{max} - L_{min})/(L_{max} + L_{min})$. This is equivalent to the absolute difference between peak luminance and mean luminance (L_{Δ}) divided by the mean luminance $(\bar{L})$. That is,

$$\text{Contrast} = L_{\Delta}/\bar{L}, \text{ where } L_{\Delta} = [L_{max} - \bar{L}] = [L_{min} - \bar{L}].$$

Contrast can theoretically vary from a maximum of one to a minimum approaching zero. The theoretical maximum contrast possible is one because the minimum luminance physically cannot be less than zero. In this situation, $L_{\Delta} = \bar{L}$ and contrast = $L_{\Delta}/\bar{L} = 1$. Four luminance profiles with contrasts ranging from 1.0 to 0.10 are diagrammed here. Each grating shown represents the contrast threshold for a different subject. The threshold is the contrast of that grating which is detected 50% of the time. The contrast sensitivity is then defined as the inverse value of the contrast threshold.

some concurrently with or even prior to peripheral defects. Indeed, foveal contrast sensitivity may be impaired even when visual acuity is intact. Wolkstein and his colleagues studied two sisters with tapetoretinal degeneration (37). Both sisters had visual acuities of 20/20, and although the older sister complained of visual problems, and had difficulty in reading the eye chart, she could do so. Her contrast sensitivity was markedly attenuated compared to the normal, and compared to that of her own sister, who was normal. Subsequent studies of more patients (38) suggested that indeed contrast sensitivity defects in RP may indicate that there are at least two different forms of the disease, or two stages of the disease process (Fig. 2). Recently a detailed study was published by Hyvarinen et al. (17) of eleven patients in three different stages of RP. The visual field sizes used were 5.5 to 40 degrees, both monocular and binocular viewing were explored. The mean luminance was 10 cd/m^2 for all patients, but in addition luminance levels of 1 and 0.1 cd/m^2 were explored. In very severe RP, both contrast sensitivity and grating acuity were essentially impaired. However in the 'severe' group with peripheral scotoma (but not necessarily a complete ring scotoma), contrast sensitivity differed from patient to patient. The severity of reduction in contrast sensitivity was poorly correlated with visual acuity, field size, and age. Visual acuity therefore predicts neither the maximum contrast sensitivity nor the spatial frequency of maximum sensitivity in RP.

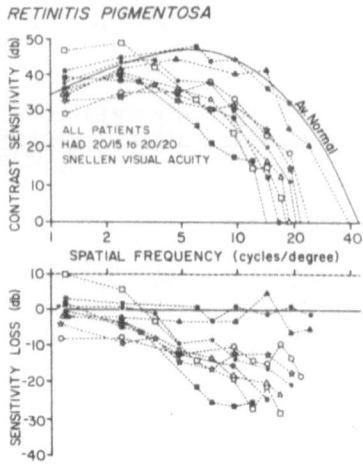

Fig. 2. Grating detection of patients with retinitis pigmentosa. In retinitis pigmentosa patients with 20/20 or better acuity, seven of nine curves showed losses at high spatial frequencies. Their cut-off frequencies were markedly less than 42 cycles/degree, the average cut-off of normal subjects with 20/20 vision. (Illustration from Wolkstein et al. Ophthalmology 87:1140–1149, 1980. Reproduced with permission.)

2. *Macular involvement in diabetes*

Contrast sensitivity studies (20) have been performed in patients prior to and following laser therapy, after which the sensitivity of patients' treated and untreated eyes were compared. This study demonstrated that foveal contrast sensitivity (5° field) can be uniformly decreased in patients who had had only peripheral laser treatment. Contrast thresholds of diabetic patients were determined with psychophysical and visual evoked potential methods using checkerboard patterns (40). The pattern elements were 15 min of arc and were presented in a 2.5° field, below fixation, with a pattern reversal rate of 12 Hz. Mean luminance was 10 cd/m². Both the visual evoked potential and contrast sensitivity were reduced even in the absence of clear-cut retinopathy. Wolkstein and colleagues (39) found that diabetic patients without clear-cut diabetic retinopathy may have abnormal contrast sensitivity.

At the moment it is not clear whether contrast sensitivity deficits are due to subclinical diabetic retinopathy, or represent optic nerve pathology rather than retinal maculopathy. One of the important questions which always arises with regard to a diabetic patient is whether all visual changes can be attributed to retinal disease, or whether a concomitant small vessel disease of the optic nerve or brain structures accounts for the visual sensitivity deficits.

Thus there are a few promising studies which suggest that contrast sensitivity measurements and concomitant visual evoked potential measurements may be useful in following the progression of diabetes, and in assessing the effects of therapy. However the distinction of whether or not foveal visual

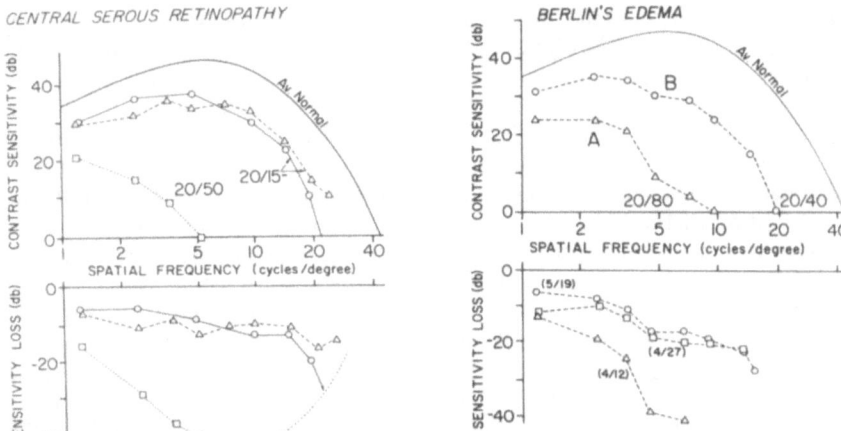

Fig. 3a. Grating detection of patients with central serous retinopathy. Contrast sensitivity losses were noted throughout the spatial frequency spectrum in spite of only moderately reduced Snellen acuities. The cut-off frequencies were less than would have been expected from the patients' Snellen acuities. (Illustration from Wolkstein et al. Ophthalmology 87:1140–1149, 1980. Reproduced with permission.)

Fig. 3b. Grating detection by a patient with Berlin's edema. Contrast sensitivity curves are given in upper plot, visuograms below. Contrast sensitivity curves successively improved, and losses decreased as edema resolved. (Illustration from Wolkstein et al. Ophthalmology 87:1140–1149, 1980. Reproduced with permission.)

changes found in the diabetic patient do represent maculopathy, or an abnormality at some other site in the visual system, has not been established by the present data.

3. *Acute maculopathy*

Apparently one may find a surprisingly small contrast sensitivity (CS) deficit in central serous retinopathy, but occasionally CS is more profoundly affected than the visual acuity (38) (Figs. 3a, b). It is apparent that contrast sensitivity measurements reveal deficits which are not quantified by visual acuity testing (2). Kayazawa and colleagues (18) found that in the recovery stage of central serous retinopathy and retinal branch occlusion, the contrast sensitivity function shows delayed recovery compared to visual acuity improvement. There may be a simpler relationship between CS and visual acuity following surgical reattachment of the macula: the recovery can be assessed equally well by either measurement (2).

The latency of the visual evoked potential, which is thought to be a measure of optic neuropathy (ON), has also been shown to be affected in patients with clear-cut maculopathy without evidence of ON. Lennerstrand (19) reported a study of 16 patients with different forms of maculopathy (most of them categorized as having had Stargardt's), who demonstrated abnormal evoked potential latency even with fairly good visual acuity.

Lennerstrand's experience is certainly not unique. Both Nath, Sherman and Bass (23) and Bodis-Wollner and Feldman (9) reported abnormal VEP latencies in patients with clear-cut maculopathy and relatively good visual acuity (better than 20/50). In the study by Bodis-Wollner and Feldman, patients who were suffering from toxoplasmosis and central serous maculopathy were compared. Abnormal VEPs occurred in both groups, though in one patient involved in the study latency returned to normal following reabsorption of the clinically visible changes. The same effect, in one patient with central serous retinopathy, was reported in the study of Nath et al. (23). It is important to note that in both studies the pattern element size was near the peak of the contrast sensitivity curve (13' grating band and 14' and 7' checks, respectively). Selecting the proper element size is important in studying foveal responses. Unfortunately, visual field size was not parametrically varied in either of these studies. Rover et al. (27) found that checkerboard patterns with an individual check size of 25 min of arc elicit high amplitude visual evoked potentials from an annular region outside the central 2.5 degrees. Thus it is apparent that 25' checks are nonoptimal for detecting foveal abnormalities.

4. Senile macular degeneration

Most patients with senile macular degeneration have high frequency losses (18,31,32,38). Generally, however, these studies do not differentiate among patients with different degrees of maculopathy. Although there is agreement among authors that high frequency losses almost always occur in maculopathy, there is some misunderstanding about a general loss, as this term has been used differently by different investigators. Bodis-Wollner and Diamond (8) defined a level loss as a visuogram without a particular slope. This is not the case in any of the published data regarding maculopathy patients. Rather, the loss may involve all spatial frequencies, but the high frequency region is always affected to a greater degree. Recently 14 patients with senile maculopathy were studied by Schmidt et al. (27). Visual fields were normal. The correlations between visual acuity, cut-off frequency, and the peak contrast sensitivity value were poor. Sjostrand (31) compared contrast sensitivity using very small (1.4°) and large (6–24°) fields, and found remarkable differences, i.e., with a small field CS was frequently abnormal, while with a large field it could be normal in the same patient. A comparison of the large and small field data show that at those high spatial frequencies where even the small field was of sufficient size for a normal observer to obtain optimal CS, the patient required a larger area of stimulation. This result suggests either that these patients benefited from sampling with multiple fixations, or that in patients the boundaries of traditional grating summation area is pathologically altered to include a *wider* area of sensitivity summation. Varying the area of the field was suggested to be useful to differential or early diagnosis of multiple sclerosis by Rossini et al. (26). These authors found a normal, straightforward relationship of the visual evoked potential using central, foveal, or a larger field stimulus. Exploring VEP latency to different levels of luminance, pattern element size, and field size can reveal

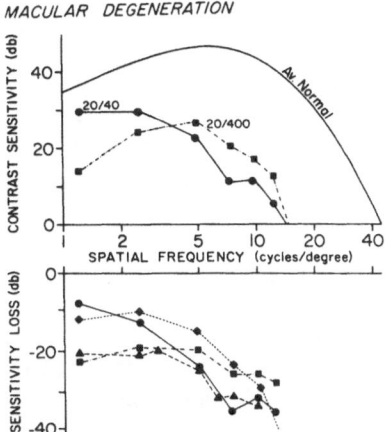

Fig. 4. Grating detection of patients with macular degeneration. All curves show both low frequency and high frequency losses. All cut-off frequencies were reduced. In three of the four patients tested, however, the cut-off frequency was better than would have been predicted from the patient's Snellen acuity. (Illustration from Wolkstein et al. Ophthalmology 87:1140–1149, 1980. Reproduced with permission.)

abnormalities in a greater number of MS patients than measurement of VEP latency to macular stimulation alone.

5. Glaucoma

Several studies (3,4,7,35) have revealed that contrast sensitivity deficits and visual evoked potential loss (6) are dominant at low spatial frequencies at fast reversal rates in glaucoma. This is not to say that high frequency losses do not occur, but rather that the distinguishing mark of glaucoma is this type of low spatial frequency loss, which does not occur in maculopathy. In addition to a demonstration of VEP attenuation and delay, pattern ERG recordings have recently revealed abnormalities in patients with glaucoma and retrobulbar neuritis (21). Pattern ERG losses can be demonstrated in a high proportion of glaucoma patients, whereas VEP changes are less common in demyelinating types of optic neuropathy, where the opposite seems to occur. In maculopathy, pattern ERG data are not yet available.

6. General considerations concerning the differential diagnosis of ON and maculopathy

There have been few direct attempts (33) to address the issue of macular versus optic nerve pathology of recent onset. In general, it would appear that VEP studies which attempt to evaluate the possibility of maculopathy should vary pattern element and field size (23). Another stimulus manipulation which may be considered in attempting to use the VEP to study retinopathy versus multiple sclerosis is based on a study by Camisa and colleagues (12).

233

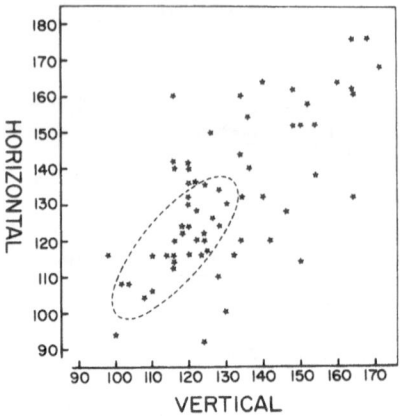

Fig. 5. The 95% probability ellipse based on the normal bivariate distribution for vertical and horizontal gratings found in 56 normal eyes. Each of the start plotted in this figure represents the latency (msec) for vertical (abscissa) and horizontal (ordinate) gratings in 1 of the 74 patient eyes tested. Stars falling inside the ellipse therefore represent normal VEP latencies for both orientations, and those outside, abnormal latencies. Forty-seven of the 74 patient eyes fell outside the ellipse. Nine of the patient eyes produced latencies greater than 190 msec and are not represented in the figure. The 47 stars outside the ellipse represent abnormal monocular VEP latencies. Of these, 16 eyes had abnormal latencies in only one orientation; thus the proportion of monocular meridional abnormality in 16 of 47 (34%). This means that if only one orientation had been used, 17% of the patients would have been misclassified as normal. (Illustration from Camisa et al. Annals of Neurology 10:532–539, 1981. Reproduced with permission.)

They showed that in many multiple sclerosis patients the VEP latency depends on the orientation of the pattern (Fig. 5). Given that Bodis-Wollner and Feldman (9) were able to show that in maculopathy the orientation of the grating pattern does not influence VEP latency, orientation of the pattern may be a useful stimulus parameter to manipulate. Contrast sensitivity studies by Regan and colleagues (25) yielded similar data: that is, patients with demyelinating disease were shown to have an orientationally dependent loss in contrast sensitivity. Furthermore, MS patients may have a notch loss of contrast sensitivity even with preserved visual acuity (24).

DISCUSSION

One is accustomed to thinking that good foveal vision is synonymous with good visual acuity, yet the anatomical and functional fovea is larger than the peephole occupied by the tiny optotypes which are detected by an observer with good visual acuity. Contrast sensitivity measurements offer a new technique to bridge the gap between the endpoint 'acuity' measure of central gaze, and visual field testing with small, discrete light patches. As we have seen, contrast sensitivity measurements reveal abnormalities which are not encompassed either by acuity measurements or visual field testing.

When we compare the maculopathy data with those of optic neuropathy, there are a few useful facts to consider. First of all, the size of the stimulus area and of the pattern element are of crucial importance. In cases of maculopathy a small field is very likely to elicit abnormalities, and small pattern elements are useful for the VEP. The relevance of field size and pattern element size has not been studied in optic neuropathy, but available data indicate that both of these stimulus variables are less crucial for the diagnosis of this disease. The effect of mean luminance of the field has not been employed systematically in the two conditions. Visual evoked potential data suggest that low mean luminance is especially degrading to evoked potential responses in optic neuropathy (10). Spatial frequency losses in maculopathy are almost always of the high frequency type, perhaps with superimposed low frequency loss, whereas in optic neuropathy due to demyelinating diseases, the loss may involve only a band of spatial frequencies, and both the CS loss and the VEP abnormality may be orientationally dependent. In the glaucomatous type of optic neuropathy, contrast sensitivity and VEP changes are prevalent at low spatial frequencies.

In sum, then, contrast sensitivity measurements and evoked potential and ERG tests utilizing patterned stimuli demonstrate abnormalities which are not revealed by either visual acuity or visual field studies. By stimulus manipulation one can increase the specificity of these tests, and differentiate maculopathy from optic neuropathy. The new tests carry the promise of becoming useful in exploring different types of pathologies affecting different parts of the visual pathways.

ACKNOWLEDGEMENTS

This research was supported in part by grant No. EY 01708 of the National Eye Institute, N.I.H.; grant No. NS 11631 of the Clinical Center for Research in Parkinson's and Allied Diseases; N.I.H. grant No. RR-00071 of the Division of Research Resources, General Clinical Research Center Branch; and Core Center grant No. EY01867 of the National Eye Institute.

We thank Ms Caroline Leake, who transcribed and edited the manuscript.

REFERENCES

1. Adams, A. J. Selective loss of blue cone mechanism in central serous choroidopathy. Invest. Ophthalmol. Visual Sci. Suppl. 22(3):62 (1982).
2. Anderson, C. and Sjostrand, J. Contrast sensitivity and central vision in reattached macula. Acta Ophthalmol. 59:161–169 (1981).
3. Atkin, A., Bodis-Wollner, I., Anders, M., Kels, B. and Podos, S. Interocular comparison of contrast sensitivities in glaucoma patients and suspects. Br. J. Ophthalmol. 11:858–862 (1980).
4. Atkin, A., Bodis-Wollner, I., Wolkstein, M., Moss, A. and Podos, S. Central vision in glaucoma: abnormalities of spatiotemporal contrast sensitivity. Am. J. Ophthalmol. 88:205–211 (1979).
5. Bodis-Wollner, I. Detection of visual defects using the contrast sensitivity function. In: *International Ophthalmology Clinics*, S. Sokol (ed.), Electrophysiology and

Psychophysics: Their Use in Ophthalmic Diagnosis, Vol. 20, Boston, Mass., Little, Brown and Company, pp. 135–153 (1980).

6. Bodis-Wollner, I. Differences in low and high spatial frequency vulnerabilities in ocular and cerebral lesions. In: *Pathophysiology of the Visual System*, L. Maffei (ed.), The Hague, Dr W. Junk Publishers, pp. 195–204 (1981).

7. Bodis-Wollner, I., Atkin, A., Podos, S., Wolkstein, M., Mylin, L. and Nitzberg, S. VEP latency in ocular hypertension and glaucoma. Invest. Ophthalmol. Visual Sci. Suppl. 22(3):95 (1982).

8. Bodis-Wollner, I. and Diamond, S. The measurement of spatial contrast sensitivity in cases of blurred vision associated with cerebral lesions. Brain 99:695–710 (1976).

9. Bodis-Wollner, I. and Feldman, R. Old perimacular pathology causes VEP delays in man. American EEG Society, Chicago, Ill., p. 85 (1981).

10. Cant, B. R., Hume, A. L. and Shaw, N. A. Effects of luminance of the pattern visual evoked potential in multiple sclerosis. Electroencephalog. Clin. Neurophysiol. 45:496–504 (1978).

11. Camisa, J. and Bodis-Wollner, I. Stimulus parameters and visual evoked potential diagnosis. In: *Annals of the New York Academy of Sciences*, Vol. 388, *Evoked Potentials*, I. Bodis-Wollner (ed.). New York Academy of Sciences, pp. 645–647 (1982).

12. Camisa, J., Mylin, L. and Bodis-Wollner, I. The effect of stimulus orientation on the visual evoked potential in multiple sclerosis. Ann. Neurol. 10:532–539 (1981).

13. Campbell, F. W. and Green, D. C. Optical and retinal factors affecting visual resolution. J. Physiol. 181:576–593 (1965).

14. Campbell, F. W. and Gubisch, R. W. Optical quality of the human eye. J. Physiol. 186:558–578 (1966).

15. Daitch, J. and Green, D. Contrast sensitivity of the human peripheral retina. Vision Res. 9:947–952 (1969).

16. Enoch, J. M., Fitzgerald, C. and Campos, E. *Quantitative Layer by Layer Perimetry: An Extended Analysis*. New York, Grune and Stratton (1980).

17. Hyvärinen, L., Rovamo, J., Laurinen, P. and Peltomaa, A. Contrast sensitivity function in evaluation of visual impairment due to retinitis pigmentosa. Acta Ophthalmol. 59:763–773 (1981).

18. Kayazawa, F., Yamamoto, T. and Itoi, M. Contrast sensitivity measurements in retinal disease by laser generated sinusoidal gratings. Arch. Ophthalmol. 60:511–524 (1982).

19. Lennerstrand, G. Delayed visual evoked cortical potentials in retinal diseases. Arch. Ophthalmol. 60:497–504 (1982).

20. Long, J., McCormick, A. J. A., Yeo, W. C., Keesey, U. T. and Davis, M. D. Diabetic retinopathy, photocoagulation and contrast sensitivity (unpublished observations).

21. Maffei, L., Bodis-Wollner, I., Harnois, C., Bobak, P. and Podos, S. A preliminary study of pattern VEP and ERG in glaucoma and RBN. Invest. Ophthalmol. Visual Sci. Suppl. 22(3):258 (1982).

22. Maffei, L. and Fiorentini, L. Electroretinographic responses to alternating gratings before and after section of the optic nerve. Science 211:953–955 (1981).

23. Nath, S., Sherman, J. and Bass, S. J. VEP delays in macular disease. Invest. Ophthalmol. Visual Sci. Suppl. 22(3):60 (1982).

24. Regan, D., Murray, T. J. and Silver, R. Effect of body temperature and visual perception in multiple sclerosis. J. Neurol. Neurosurg. Psychiat. 40:1083–1901 (1977).

25. Regan, D., Whitlock, J. A., Murray, T. J. and Beverley, K. I. Orientation-specific losses of contrast sensitivity in multiple sclerosis. Invest. Ophthalmol. Visual Sci. 19:324–328 (1980).

26. Rossini, P. M., Pirchio, M., Sollazzo, D. and Caltagirona, C. Foveal versus peripheral retinal responses. A new analysis for early diagnosis of multiple sclerosis. Electroencephalog. Clin. Neurophysiol. 47:515–523 (1979).

27. Rover, J., Schaubele, G. and Berndt, K. Macula and periphery: their contribution to

236

the visual evoked potential (VEP) in humans. Albrecht von Graefes Arch. Klin. Exp. fur Ophthalmol. 214:47–51 (1980).

28. Schmidt, M. J., Camisa, J. and Faye, E. Is contrast sensitivity useful with low vision patients? American Academy of Ophthalmology Program 89:195 (1982).

29. Sekuler, R., Hutman, L. P. and Owsley, C. Human aging and spatial vision. Science 209:1255–1256 (1980).

30. Sekuler, R., Hutman, L. P. and Owsley, C. Assessing spatial vision in older patients. Am. J. Optometry Physiol. Optics (in press).

31. Sjostrand, J. Contrast sensitivity in macular disease using a small-field and a large-field TV-system. Acta Ophthalmol. 57:832–845 (1979).

32. Sjostrand, J. and Frisen, L. Contrast sensitivity in macular disease. Acta Ophthalmol. 55:507–514 (1977).

33. Skalka, H. W. Comparison of Snellen acuity, VER acuity, and Arden grating scores in macular and optic nerve diseases. Br. J. Ophthalmol. 64:24–29 (1980).

34. Sokol, S., Domar, A., Moskowitz, A. and Schwartz, B. Pattern evoked potential latency and contrast sensitivity in glaucoma and ocular hypertension. Doc. Ophthalmol. Proc. Series 27:79 (1981).

35. Towle, V., Sokol, S., Moskowitz, A. and Schwartz, B. The visually evoked potential in glaucoma: effects of check size, field size, and alternation rate. Invest. Ophthalmol. Visual Sci. Suppl. 20(3):22 (1981).

36. Van Ness, F. L. and Bouman, M. A. Spatial modulation transfer in the human eye. J. Opt. Soc. Am. 57:401–406 (1967).

37. Wolkstein, M., Atkin, A. and Bodis-Wollner, I. Grating acuity in two sisters with tapetoretinal degeneration. Doc. Ophthalmol. 12:41–46 (1977).

38. Wolkstein, M., Atkin, A. and Bodis-Wollner, I. Contrast sensitivity in retinal disease. Ophthalmology 87:1140–1149 (1980).

39. Wolkstein, M., Atkin, A. and Bodis-Wollner, I. Contrast sensitivity and diabetic retinopathy (unpublished observations).

40. Yamasaki, H., Adachi-Usami, A. and Chiba, J. Contrast thresholds of diabetic patients determined by VECP and psychophysical measurements. Acta Ophthalmol. 60:368–392 (1982).

Author's address:
Dr I. Bodis-Wollner
Depts. of Neurology and Ophthalmology
The Mount Sinai School of Medicine
Fifth Avenue at 100th Street
New York, NY 10029
U.S.A.

VISUAL FIELDS VERSUS VISUAL EVOKED POTENTIALS IN OPTIC NERVE DISORDERS

TAKAHIRO OHNUMA*, YUSAKU TAGAMI and YOSHIMASA ISAYAMA

(Kobe, Japan)

Key words. Visual fields, visual evoked potentials.

ABSTRACT

Visual evoked potentials (VEPs) and static central visual fields were examined in 55 patients with optic neuropathies. There were no significant correlations between the VEP peak latencies and Tübinger static central fields. In 7 clinically definite multiple sclerosis (MS) patients who had a documented episode of optic neuritis, the VEPs showed remarkable prolongation of the latency in spite of good results in psychophysical tests such as visual acuity and static fields. Normal VEPs were obtained from 2 patients with MS, who had no involvements of visual pathways. Therefore MS should be suspected when patients with recovered optic neuropathies have delayed VEPs despite of normal psychophysical tests. Both VEPs and visual fields are necessary for assessing functional losses and predicting the prognosis in optic neuropathies.

INTRODUCTION

During the last decade many investigators have demonstrated that the measurement of visual evoked potentials (VEPs) is one of the most reliable methods for assessing functional losses in optic nerve disorders — especially in cases with multiple sclerosis (MS) (2,3,5). But there are few articles about the relationship between VEPs and conventional function tests such as the visual fields in clinical ophthalmology. In the present study, we examined checkerboard pattern reversal VEPs in patients with optic neuropathies and compared the results with visual acuity and static visual fields.

SUBJECTS AND METHODS

Forty-five subjects (90 eyes) without any ophthalmological abnormalities were used as normal controls. The age range was 6–70 years with a mean of

*To whom requests for offprints should be addressed.

Greve, E. L., Heijl, A. (eds.) Fifth International Visual Field Symposium.
©1983 Dr W. Junk Publishers, The Hague/Boston/Lancaster.

33 years. Seventy-two patients (102 eyes) with recovered optic neuropathies (ON) participated in this study. They were in a steady-state period at least 2 months after they regained their best visual acuity. The age range of the patients was 17–65 years and the mean was 38 years.

Anterior ischemic optic neuropathy was diagnosed in 5 cases (8 eyes), rhinogenic optic neuropathy 6 cases (6 eyes), ethambutol-induced toxic optic neuropathy 8 cases (16 eyes), compressive optic neuropathy due to chiasmal tumor 6 cases (12 eyes) and clinically definite multiple sclerosis with a history of at least one attack of optic neuritis (MS with ON) 7 cases (13 eyes). In the other 40 cases (47 eyes), the causes were not determined. Two multiple sclerosis patients (4 eyes) with no involvement of visual pathways (MS without ON) were also included.

The stimulus for VEPs was generated on a TV screen controlled by a microcomputer. The black and white checkerboard pattern was monocularly presented at 2 m distance subtending a visual angle of $4° \times 6°$. The size of each single square (check size) was $0.45°$ with a contrast of 97% and the pattern reversal frequency was 1.7 Hz. The mean luminance of the pattern was $100\,cd/m^2$. The active electrode was placed 2.5 cm above the inion in the midsagittal plane with the reference electrode on the ear lobe. Hundred sweeps of the signals were amplified through a filter (0.1 to 100 Hz, Time Constant 0.3) and averaged by a computer.

The static central fields were examined using a 7' white stimulus with the background illumination of 10 asb on a Tübinger perimeter. The sensitivities of 7 points on the horizontal meridian were averaged and the results were used as the central visual sensitivities (CVS). As controls, 10 normal subjects were used (age 18–55 years) their mean CVS being 23.5 dB.

RESULTS

A typical recording of the checkerboard pattern reversal VEP in a normal subject is shown in Fig. 1. The mean and the standard deviation of the P2 peak latency in 45 normal subjects (90 eyes) was 109.1 ± 10.8 msec. The sex and the age differences of the latency were not found.

In 19 out of 74 patients (22 eyes) with ON, the VEP could not be recorded. In these cases, large central scotomas were detected and the visual acuity was < 0.1.

The relationships of the P2 peak latency to the visual acuity and the static

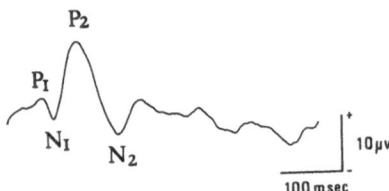

Fig. 1. A typical recording of the checkerboard pattern reversal VEP in a normal subject.

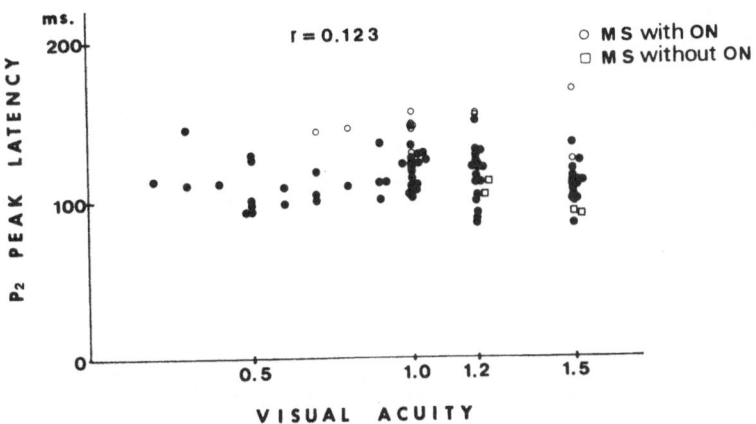

Fig. 2. Correlations between the P2 peak latency of the VEP and the visual acuity in 55 patients (84 eyes) with optic neuropathies. Open circles and squares indicate MS with and without ON, respectively.

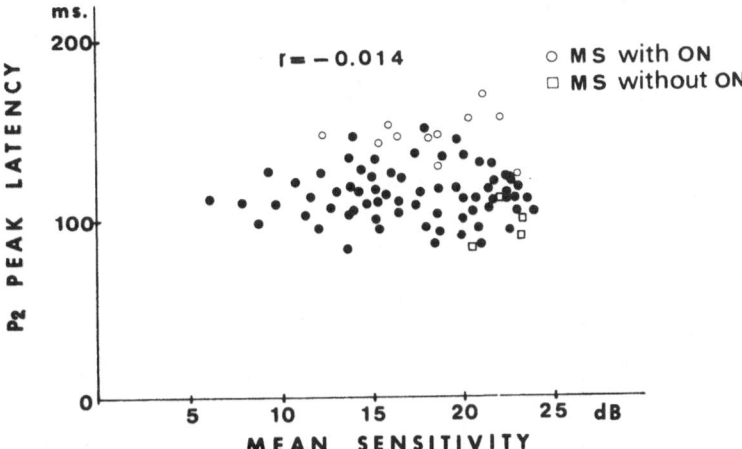

Fig. 3. Correlations between the P2 peak latency of the VEP and the central visual field (central visual sensitivity, CVS) in 55 patients (84 eyes) with optic neuropathies.

central visual fields (CVS) in 55 patients (84 eyes) are shown in Figs. 2 and 3, respectively. There is no significant correlation between the latency and the visual acuity, or the visual fields.

In Fig. 4, the P2 peak latencies in 55 patients (84 eyes) with ON of various causes is illustrated. The dotted line indicates the level of mean latency + 2SD in the normal controls. Only the patients with MS and ON have significant prolongation of the P2 peak latencies as compared with the normal controls ($p < 0.01$). MS without ON have normal P2 peak latencies.

The results in 7 MS patients with ON (13 eyes) are presented in Table 1.

241

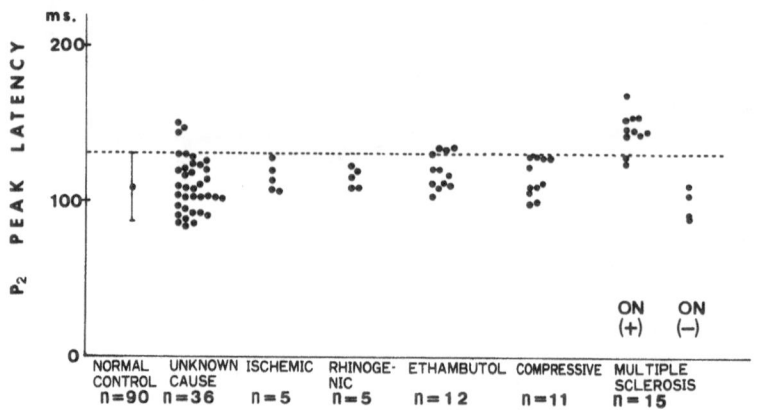

Fig. 4. Distribution of the P2 peak latencies in 55 patients (84 eyes) with optic neuropathies of various causes. The dotted line indicates the level of the mean + 2 SD of the normal controls.

Table 1. The examined results in 7 MS patients with ON.

| case | sex | age | side | visual acuity $\binom{R}{L}$ | Tübinger's perimetry | | VEP |
					profile depression pattern $\binom{R}{L}$	central visual sensitivity $\binom{R}{L}$ (dB)	P₂ peak latency $\binom{R}{L}$ (msec)
1	F	18	Bil	1.0	sieve-like	18.6	147.2
				1.0	sieve-like	18.6	129.4
2	F	28	Bil	1.0	sieve-like	16.4	146.2
				1.0	sieve-like	15.4	142.9
3	F	36	Bil	1.2	minimal	20.9	153.9
				1.2	minimal	22.5	154.4
4	M	31	Bil	20cm/n.d.	—	—	—
				1.5	minimal	21.3	169.3
5	M	41	Bil	1.0	sieve-like	17.0	140.2
				0.7	sieve-like	13.5	145.0
6	F	35	R	1.5	minimal	23.0	125.1
				1.5	minimal	23.2	93.3
7	F	18	Bil	0.02	—	—	—
				0.8	sieve-like	19.0	142.6

M : Male F : Female Bil : Bilateral R : Right L : Left

Ten out of 13 eyes have relatively good central vision by psychophysical methods (CVS 19.7 dB, visual acuity of more than 1.0) in spite of their abnormal VEPs.

For example, a VEP recording in a 36-year old MS with ON patient (case 3 in Table 1) is shown in Fig. 5 with the Tübinger static central fields. She has a visual acuity of 1.2 in each eye and the central profile showed a minimal depression. The CVS are 20.9 and 22.5 dB in the right and left eyes respectively. On the contrary, the P2 peak latency of VEPs are remarkably prolonged.

242

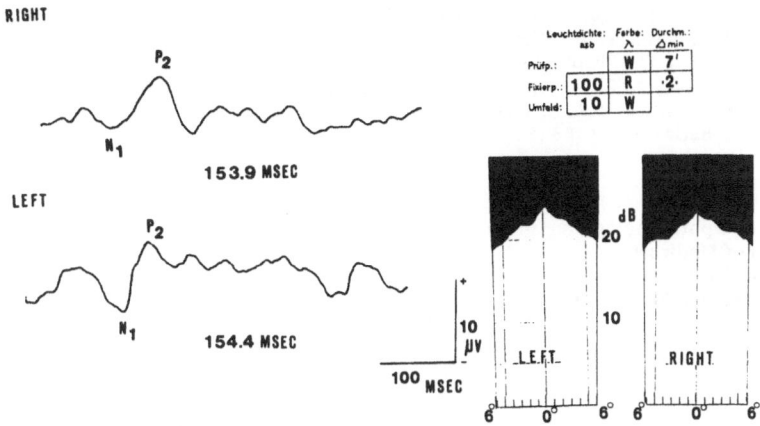

Fig. 5. A VEP recording in a 36-year old MS with ON patient (case 3 in Table 1) with Tübinger's static central fields.

DISCUSSION

In the present study, the P2 peak latency of the checkerboard pattern reversal VEP was not correlated with the visual acuity and the static visual field. Therefore it is suspected that the VEPs reflect some other pathological aspect which cannot be detected by the conventional psychophysical methods used. The conduction delay in the optic nerve axons or the impairment of the synaptic transmission may cause the prolongation of the peak latency (1,4).

The usefulness of VEPs for the diagnosis of MS have been emphasized in some papers (2,3,5). Our results showed significant delay of the latency in patients with definite MS in spite of their relatively good visual acuity and static fields. Our results also demonstrated that MS patients with abnormal VEPs always had a documented episode of optic neuritis. In other words, the VEPs showed no abnormality in MS patients without involvements of the visual pathways. These results indicate that MS should be suspected when patients with recovered optic neuropathies have delayed VEPs despite otherwise normal psychophysical tests.

In conclusion, both VEPs and visual fields are necessary for assessing functional losses and predicting the prognosis in optic neuropathies.

REFERENCES

1. Bornstein, M. B. and Crain, S. M. Functional studies of cultured brain tissues as related to 'demyelinative' disorders. Science 148:1242–1244 (1965).
2. Halliday, A. M., McDonald, W. I. and Mushin, J. Visual evoked responses in the diagnosis of multiple sclerosis. Br. Med. J. 4:661–664 (1973).
3. Khoshbin, S. and Hallett, M. Pattern-reversal visual evoked potentials in patients

with multiple sclerosis. Neuro-Ophthalmology Focus, pp. 229–235. Masson Publishing U.S.A. Inc., New York (1980).

4. McDonald, W. I. Pathophysiology in multiple sclerosis. Brain 97:179–196 (1974).
5. Van Dalen, J. T. W., Spekreyse, H. and Greve, E. L. Visual field (VF) vs visual evoked cortical potential (VECP) in multiple sclerosis patients. Doc. Ophthalmol. Proc. Series 26:79–83 (1980).

Author's address:
Dr T. Ohnuma
Dept. of Ophthalmology
School of Medicine
Kobe University
Kusunoki-cho, 7-chome, Chuo-ku
Kobe 650
Japan

244

HOMONYMOUS QUADRANTANOPIA IN A CASE OF MULTIPLE SCLEROSIS
Pupillographic, perimetric and VEP findings

K. A. HELLNER, K. U. HAMANN, W. JENSEN and A. MÜLLER-JENSEN

(Hamburg, FRG)

Key words. Homonymous quadrantanopia, pupillography, VEP, multiple sclerosis.

ABSTRACT

A case of left lower homonymous quadrantanopia and relative left centrocecal scotoma secondary to multiple sclerosis is presented, and the pupillomotor and VEP findings are discussed.

Pupillography combined with VEP provide a valuable tool for the differential diagnosis. There was a discrepancy between the pupillomotor threshold and the density of the visual field defect. These findings are in agreement with known reports on the development of pupillomotor thresholds in homonymous hemianopia of suprageniculate origin.

CASE HISTORY

The patient we would like to present is a 38-year old male, who realized a sudden onset of a sector-shaped visual field defect in the left lower quadrant. Eight days following this event, he was admitted to our hospital for further evaluation. The past history was unremarkable, besides some vague sensory disturbance involving the back and both legs 2 years before. Although the patient admitted to heavy smoking suggesting a vascular accident, the first clinical examination made us alter our tentative diagnosis in favour of a primary inflammatory process. The unaided visual acuity in the right eye was normal, and in the left eye near normal, uncorrectable with glasses. The examination of both eyes with slit-lymp and the three-mirror Goldmann lens revealed no pathologic findings. Visual fields performed with the Goldmann and the Tübinger perimeter consistently detected a quite dense, incongruent left lower quadrantanopia together with a relative left centrocecal scotoma. However, the pupillomotor threshold was only somewhat elevated in the homonymous blind hemifield (Fig. 1).

In this context we would like to recall our previous findings regarding pupillography:

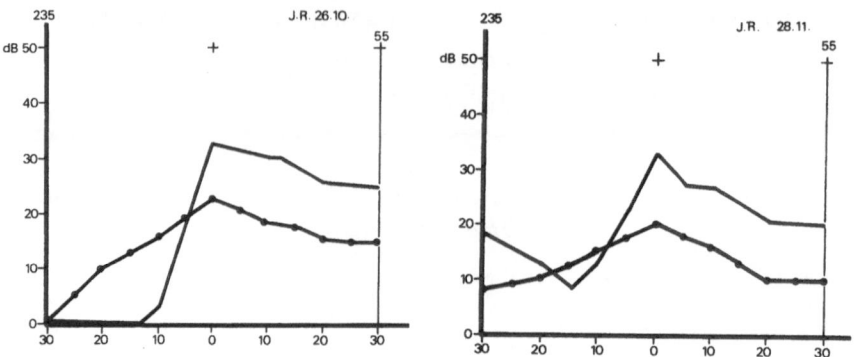

Fig. 1. Sensory and pupillomotor profile; meridian 55°/145° right eye: visual defect; (a) acute stage; (b) 4 weeks later.

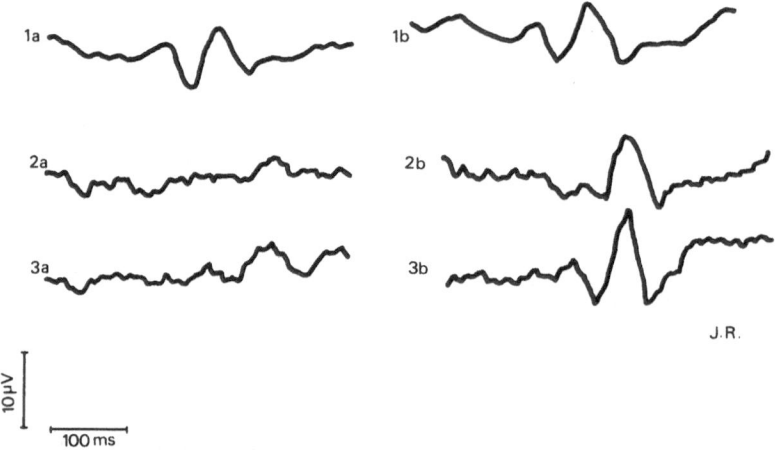

Fig. 2. VEP. (1a/1b) full-field stimulation (r/l eye); (2a/2b) hemifield stimulation; (2a/2b) acute stage; (3a/3b) 2 weeks later.

1. Pupillography represents the essential of objective perimetry. The difference of threshold of the subjective, sensoric perimetry and the objective pupillography amounts to 10 dB. The exact perimetry of the blind spot makes the efficiency of the video-processing pupillography evident (4).
2. Patients suffering from infarctions of the optic radiation, e.g. from occlusion of the posterior cerebral artery are characterized by a fair amount of increase of the pupillomotor threshold within the blind hemifield (3).
3. Extrinsic lesions, e.g. tentorial meningioma with extension to the left, reveal a near normal pupillomotor threshold within the blind hemifield (2).

The VEP in our case showed the following findings: the full-field stimulation of the right eye yielded a near normal latency, whereas the latency of

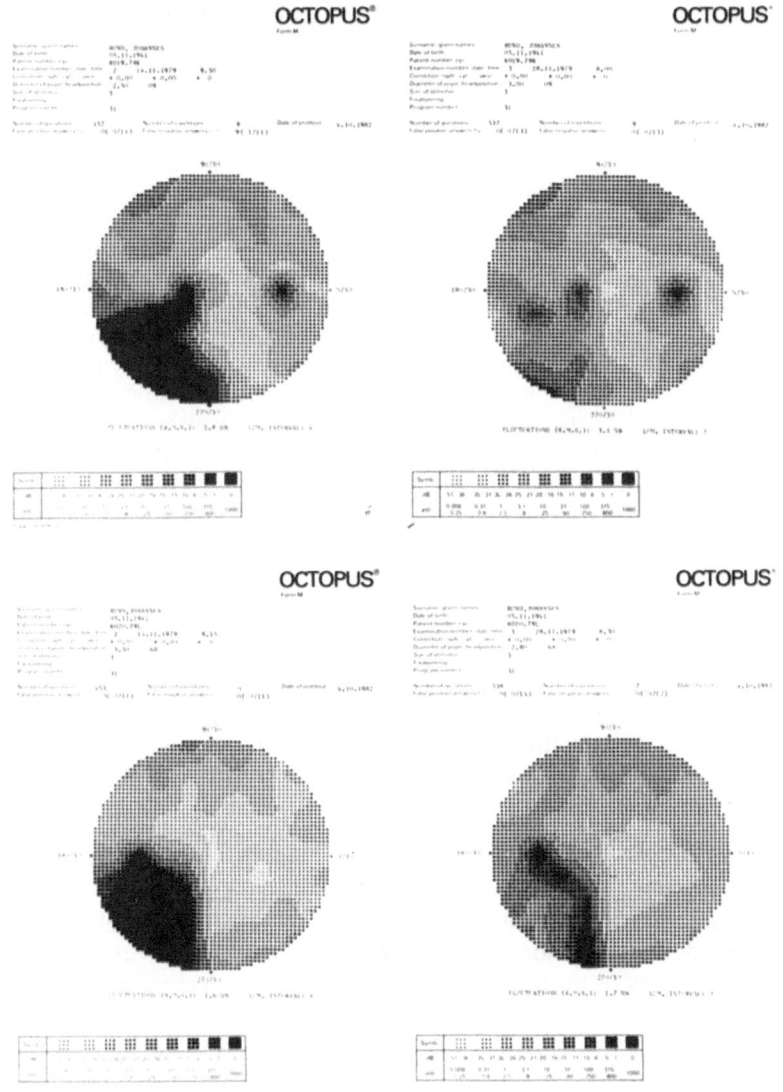

Fig. 3. Visual fields: (Octopus-Perimetry) homonymous, quadrantanopia. Improvement of the defects after 2 weeks.

the left eye appreciably was prolonged. By stimulating the blind hemifields in both eyes no detectable responses were obtained (Fig. 2).

On neurological examination a mild hypermetric finger-to-nose response could be elicited, together with a clumsy steppage-gait. The cerebro-spinal fluid was clear, with an albumin concentration of 395 mg/l, a gamma-globulin content of 38 mg/l and 11/3 cells. The EEG was not contributory, as was the CT scan.

The follow-up examination 6 weeks after admission showed a regression of the visual defect in the left lower quadrant to a relative incongruent homonymous field defect. At this time the pupillomotor threshold in the blind hemifield was back to normal (Figs. 1, 2 and 3).

DISCUSSION

This case history of multiple sclerosis represents an interesting illustration of visual incapability referable to a visual field defect secondary to a lesion of the suprageniculate pathways and not directly to the optic nerve. Visual signs and symptoms in multiple sclerosis are almost always related to optic nerve dysfunction, whereas homonymous field defects are hardly heard of (1) and amounts only to 1.0%. In contradiction, on neuropathological grounds, preferential sites of demyelination of multiple sclerosis were recognized early in the anterior and posterior horns, in the entire corpus collosum, and in the periaqueductal grey matter. This has been confirmed consistently (5).

The VEP of the left hemifield revealed no detectable response, as expected.

The prolonged latency on full field stimulation of the left eye should be interpreted as a subclinical conduction delay of the left optic nerve, compatible with an additional small demyelinating plaque in this area in a case of multiple sclerosis, with a corresponding subclinical centrocecal scotoma. Since we considered only the threshold of the pupillomotor response and not the dynamics, we cannot contribute to the issue of the latency of the pupillomotor response within this subclinical centrocecal scotoma. The course of regression of the homonymous field defect in this case was quite similar to the recovery of function in cases of retrobulbar neuritis.

We are unaware of the amount of demyelinization within the suprageniculate visual pathway necessary to substantially increase the pupillomotor threshold. However, in a visual field defect of this size secondary to tumor invasion or to a vascular infarction, one could anticipate alterations in the CT scan. We conclude, that pupillography combined with VEP could clinch the etiology of the suprageniculate visual field defect in this case.

REFERENCES

1. Boldt, H. A., Haerer, A. F., Tourtelotte, W. W., Henderson, J. W. and Dejong, R. N. Retrochiasmal visual field defects from multiple sclerosis. Arch. Neurol. (Chicago) 8:565–575 (1963).
2. Hamann, K. U., Hellner, K. A., Müller-Jensen, A. and Zschocke, S. Video-pupillography and VEP investigations in patients with congenital and acquired lesions of the optic radiation. Ophthalmologica (Basel) 178:348–356 (1979).
3. Hellner, K. A., Jensen, W. and Müller-Jensen, A. Fernsehbildanalytische pupillographische Perimetrie bei Hemianopsie. Klin. Mbl. Augenheilk. 172:653–657 (1978).
4. Jensen, W. Die Fernsehbildanalyse. Ein Meßverfahren zur objektiven Perimetrie. Albrecht von Graefes Arch. Ophthalmol 201:183–191 (1976).

5. Lumsden, C. E. Clinical manifestations of multiple sclerosis In: Handbook of Clinical Neurology, P. J. Vinken and G. W. Bruyn (eds.), p. 221. North-Holland Publishing Company, Amsterdam (1970).

Authors' addresses:
Dr K. A. Hellner
Dr K. U. Hamann
Dr W. Jensen
University Eye Hospital
University of Hamburg
Martinistr. 52
D-2000 Hamburg 20, FRG

Dr A. Müller-Jensen
University Neurological Hospital
University of Hamburg
D-2000 Hamburg 20, FRG

HIPPOCRATES AND HOMONYMOUS HEMIANOPSIA

H. BYNKE

(Lund, Sweden)

Key words. Hippocrates, homonymous hemianopsia, Hippocratic doctrines, Hippocratic collection.

ABSTRACT

Half-blindness, or homonymous hemianopsia, was known already by the Hippocratians. This symptom was mentioned in the 'Second Book on Disease', written in the 4th century B.C. The present article is a brief presentation of Hippocrates and a review of the Hippocratic collection.

INTRODUCTION

Certain visual field defects were known long before von Graefe (1856) introduced the visual field examination in clinical practice (1). The classic example is the physiological blind spot, which was detected in 1668 by Mariotte (see (3)). According to Hirschberg (2), the great historian of ophthalmology who was recently portrayed by Snyder (8), central scotoma and constriction of the visual field were mentioned by Galen in the 2nd century. Furthermore, Hirschberg stated that as early as the 4th century B.C. the Hippocratians were aware of the existence of homonymous hemianopsia, but according to Polyak, Morgagni described the first case in 1719 (6). These statements are not necessarily inconsistent, though they seem to be.

After consulting a work by Löwegren (5), who was the first professor of Ophthalmology at this university, the author of the present article visited the native island of Hippocrates. He then began to study more closely a few of the Hippocratic writings and read a French translation of the first description of hemianopsia (4).

THE LIFE AND WORK OF HIPPOCRATES

What little we know about the life of Hippocrates, the 'Father of Medicine' (Fig. 1), is based mainly on data provided by his contemporary, the

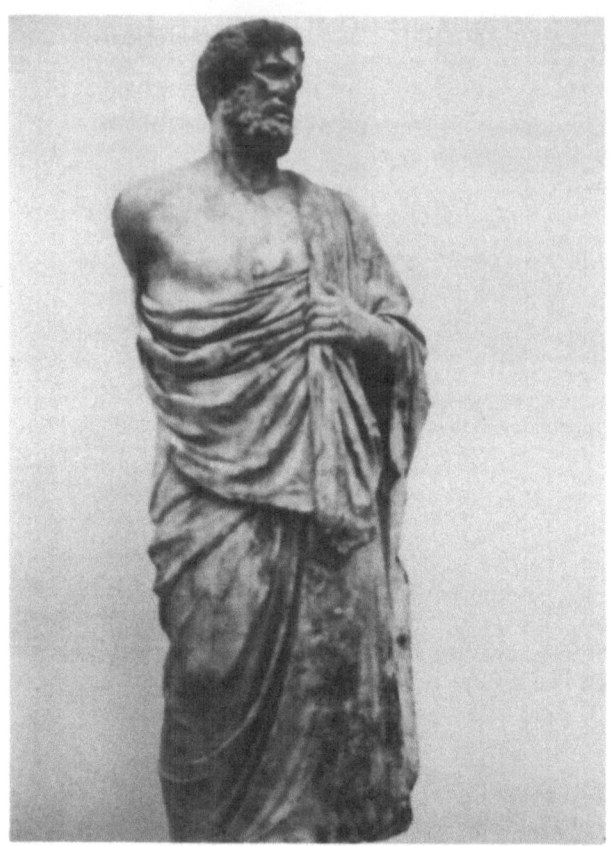

Fig. 1. Statue of Hippocrates from the post-Hellenistic period, excavated in 1929.

philosopher Plato. Hippocrates was born about 460 B.C. in the Greek island of Cos, not far from the coast of Asia Minor, and he died at an advanced age, possibly in Larissa, Thessaly. He was the member of a family of priests and physicians, temple-ministrants at the Coan Asclepion, which was dedicated to Asclepios, the god of medicine. In antiquity numerous Asclepions were erected in Hellas. The Coan Asclepion was discovered in 1902, when excavations began. It consisted of three terraces furnished with ancient temples, other buildings and statues (Fig. 2). Some rooms on the first and third terraces were probably used for patients.

According to tradition, Hippocrates' first teacher of medicine was his father Heracleides. Hippocrates travelled extensively in Hellas and other countries. During the Peloponnesian War he went to Athens. He is said not to have left this city until a plague had been brought under control, an exploit which made him celebrated. After returning to his native island he worked at Asclepion as a physician, medical teacher and author, and made his temple school famous all over the ancient world.

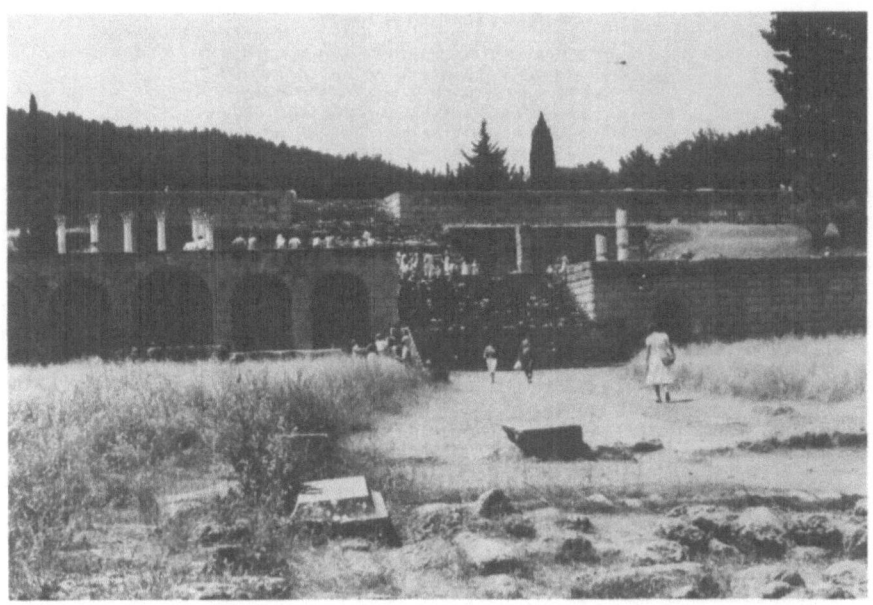

Fig. 2. The Coan Asclepion. The first terrace embanked by the wall with arched cavities. On the second terrace ruins of a Corinthian Apollo temple to the left and two columns of a Ionic Asclepios temple to the right. The third terrace was furnished with a great Doric Asclepios temple.

Hippocrates was in opposition to those philosophic schools which believed that all diseases derived from one or several of the 'elementary qualities' of the body, i.e. heat, cold, drought, and humidity. In fact he rejected all hypotheses; only real observations were of value and experience was the true basis of the art of medicine. However, unable to free himself from all philosophic influence, he adopted a doctrine of the Pythagorean Alcmaeon, which substituted the four 'cardinal humours' mucus, blood, yellow and black bile for the 'elementary qualities'. This was logical, because in Hippocrates' opinion Alcmaeon's doctrine was not hypothetical but based on real observations and facts.

Hippocrates criticized the competing temple school of Cnidos in Asia Minor for giving too much weight to the multiplying of diagnoses, and considered it more important to find out what was common to all disease. He thus became the first to emphasize that external factors such as climate, food and physical work were important to health and disease alike. He also paid much attention to prognosis, which according to the Coan temple school covered not only the future but also the past and present course of an illness. In acute inflammatory disorders the course should be watched carefully, and the physician, being nothing more than a servant of nature, should not interfere until the process had come to maturity ('crisis').

253

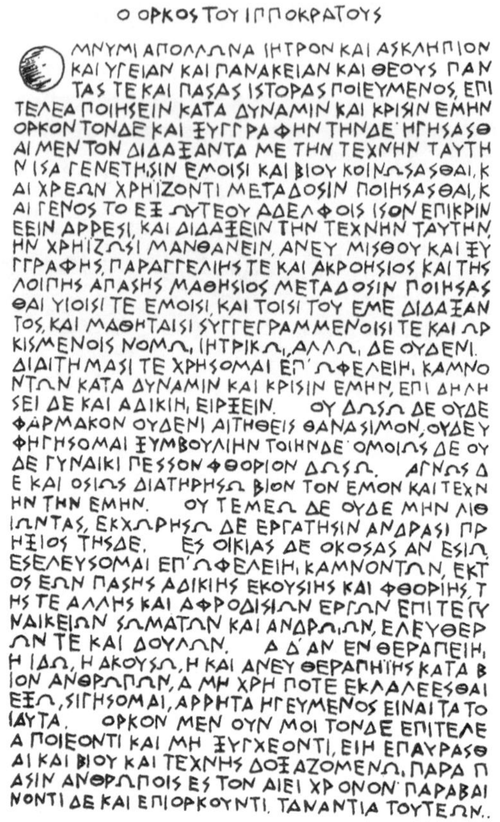

Fig. 3. The Hippocratic oath.

The oath of Hippocrates is a manifestation of his wisdom and noble conception of our profession (Fig. 3). One sentence in this oath, which deals with the obligation of observing secrecy, is still fundamental: 'Whatever I see or hear in the course of my practice as a doctor or outside of my profession, which ought not to be spread abroad, I shall keep secret and shall never reveal'.

THE HIPPOCRATIC COLLECTION

The Hippocratic collection comprises about 70 mutually independent articles of widely different value and constitutes the oldest medical literature preserved. They are probably fragments of a larger collection. A few of the articles are thought to have been written prior to the time of Hippocrates, some by himself and others by his successors. No part of the collection is later than about 300 B.C.

Though he was an ophthalmologist by profession, Löwegren did not

254

mention anything about hemianopsia in his excellent survey of the Hippocratic collection (5). I have therefore consulted a complete translation published in 10 volumes by the French encyclopedist Littré (4). According to Littré five of the authors bore the name of Hippocrates, the great Hippocrates being number II. In the 'Second Book on Disease', dealing with disorders of the head, we find a description of headache connected with bloating of the skin of the head and frequent micturition. These symptoms are said to subside during twenty days and to be followed by impairment of vision: '. . . the light fades and the patient appears to see only half faces. . .'. Complete recovery takes place after forty days, but there is a frequent relapse of the disease after seven or fourteen years (Vol. VII, p. 18–21, 1851). The author of this article, as well as of others, is unknown. Littré first believed that he was Hippocrates III, a grandson of the great Hippocrates, who was active as a writer in about 370 to 350 B.C. Littré later changed his opinion and suggested that the author was from Cnidos and consequently did not belong to the Coan temple school.

COMMENTS

Several of Hippocrates' doctrines are consistent with modern opinion, e.g. his emphasis on the importance of experience and on external factors, his noble conception of the physician as a servant of nature, and particularly his medical ethics as expressed in his oath. Others are based on his primitive humoral pathology and have lost all value.

From a modern medical point of view Hippocrates' negative attitude towards hypotheses seems very strange. Nevertheless it deserves some consideration. It is on hypotheses that improved knowledge is based, e.g. the knowledge about mechanisms underlying physiological and pathological processes. Therefore we must not be averse to hypotheses as such but should still adopt a critical attitude to them: such an attitude is in fact a prerequisite for scientific progress. A prominent feature of the doctrines of the modern philosopher Popper (7) is that hypotheses can never be proved but only disproved, and that we gradually approach the truth by falsifying hypotheses. It is also interesting that Popper — like Hippocrates — stresses the importance of experience.

Hirschberg was right or almost right when stating that already the Hippocratians were aware of the existence of hemianopsia (2). The description in the 'Second Book on Disease' is confusing and seems to deal with a mixture of symptoms of various diseases, but it partly suggests attacks of migraine with hemianopsia, although the course is too protracted and the order of the symptoms is reversed.

It is certainly not surprising that hemianopsia was mentioned as early as the 4th century B.C. This common and disabling symptom must have been noticed even long before that time.

ACKNOWLEDGEMENT

Dr Claude Öhrn, University Eye Clinic, Lund, assisted the author in interpreting the text of Littré.

REFERENCES

1. Graefe, A. von. Ueber die Untersuchung des Gesichtsfeldes bei amblyopischen Affectionen. Arch. Ophthalmol. II (2): 258–298 (1856).
2. Hirschberg, J. Geschichte der Augenheilkunde. In ed. 2 of the Graefe-Saemisch Handbuch der Augenheilkunde. Leipzig, Engelmann, Vol. XII, pp. 97 and 346 (1899).
3. Lebensohn, J. E. An anthology of ophthalmic classics. Baltimore, Williams and Wilkins, 407 pp. (1969).
4. Littré, E. Oeuvres complètes d'Hippocrate. Paris, Baillière, Vol. I–X, 6587 pp. (1839–61).
5. Löwegren, M. K. The Hippocratic writings (in Swedish). Lund, Gleerup, Vol. I–II, 1304 pp. (1909–10).
6. Polyak, S. The vertebrate visual system. Chicago, The University of Chicago Press, 1390 pp. (1957).
7. Popper, K. R. Objective knowledge. An evolutionary approach. Oxford, Oxford University Press, 395 pp. (1979).
8. Snyder, C. Julius Hirschberg, the neglected historian of ophthalmology. Am. J. Ophthalmol. 91: 664–676 (1981).

Author's address:
Dr H. Bynke
University Eye Clinic
S-221 85 Lund
Sweden

CAROTID PERFUSION AND FIELD LOSS

V. J. MARMION and M. ALDOORI
(Bristol, U.K.)

Key words. Visual field loss, intraocular pressure, Doppler ultrasound.

ABSTRACT

Forty patients with known open angle glaucoma were examined by ophthal-modynamometry and Doppler ultrasound to evaluate their carotid flow. The common internal and external carotids were examined at the bifurcation by the A.T.L. 5 MHz real time Duplex Scanner. This provides information on the disturbance and percentage reduction in flow in the affected vessels.

The effect of the reduction in flow is compared with the reduction in field loss as calculated by the Esterman Charts and a computation of the score on the Friedmann Field Analyser. It is noted that there is a better correlation of field loss with lesions at the carotid bifurcation than the presenting level of intraocular pressure.

INTRODUCTION

The optic atrophy of open angle glaucoma is classically ascribed to raised intraocular pressure. Recent papers, Bengtsson (3), Krakau (7), indicate that field loss is not directly related to a specific level of intraocular pressure. Many authors in the past have postulated that there was a vascular element in open angle glaucoma. Goldman (6) proposed several formulae to link the effect of intraocular pressure on circulation. De Laet (7), and Arakawa (1), have used ophthalmodynamometry to explore this possibility further. Changes in retinal artery pressure could be local or related to carotid disease. The development of ultrasonic angiology (Doppler ultrasound) in the past ten years (8) now offers the possibility of determining the relevance of lesions at the carotid bifurcation in open angle glaucoma.

MATERIALS AND METHODS

Forty randomly selected treated patients with open angle glaucoma had an evaluation of the carotid bifurcation using the Advanced Technology

Laboratories 5 MHz range gated duplex scan which combines a B scan capability with a flow meter. Lesions at the carotid bifurcation were classified into: 1) no abnormality demonstrated; 2) flow disturbance/stenosis/calcification; 3) plaques.

Plaques were quantified according to the percentage of the lumen occluded. The intraocular pressures taken for the analysis were those recorded at the first out-patient visit, and before treatment. Goldman fields were scored using the Esterman charts, using the 11/2e isopter. Friedman fields were scored using a whole field computation.

RESULTS

Table 1 shows the age and sex distribution of the group, and the distribution of lesions at the carotid bifurcation. Table 2 shows the distribution of the lesions according to age, the vessel involved, and the degree of involvement. Table 3 shows the compliance of intraocular pressure and carotid lesions to the greater degree of field loss.

A further detailed statistical analysis did not reveal a correlation of significant levels between intraocular pressure and field loss, or the presence of carotid lesions and field loss. The Spearman rank correlation test suggested a weak correlation between field loss and group two lesions. There was no

Table 1. Ultrasound carotid scan in glaucoma.

Lesions shown 54	Absent 26
M/F ratio 19/21	Mean age 69

Table 2. Carotid lesions demonstrated.

Age group		50–59	60–69	70–79	80 +	Total
Common	1	12	24	23	11	70
	2	–	3	2	–	5
	3	–	1	3	1	5
Internal	1	5	11	10	3	29
	2	4	7	13	4	28
	3	3	10	5	5	23
External	1	12	27	25	10	74
	2	–	–	2	–	2
	3	–	1	1	2	4

Table 3. Correlation of field loss.

	Consistent	Not compliant
Intraocular pressure	31	9
Carotid scan	35	5

258

correlation between intraocular pressure and lesions at the carotid bifurcation. The numbers involved did not permit a three-way analysis.

DISCUSSION

The age distribution and field loss characteristics of the group of patients was typical of open angle glaucoma. The absence of a firm statistical correlation between intraocular pressure and the field loss concurs with comments of Kraukau (7), and casts some doubt on the precise role of intraocular pressure. The existence of significantly raised pressure can not be ignored and in conjunction with the deterioration of the vision inspite of reasonable control, observed by Drance (5), raises the question of contributory factors.

The lack of a statistical relationship between intraocular pressure, and carotid lesions would suggest that the raised pressure was not a result of the carotid lesions. A level of 10% of pathological lesions at the carotid bifurcation was expected. The relatively high level of 68% requires an explanation. The distribution of lesions in relation to age did not exhibit any surprising characteristics. The two positive findings in relation to field loss were the lower incidence of false positives in carotid disease, than with intraocular pressure, and a trend developing between field loss and the presence of stenotic lesions in the carotids.

Stenosis in the carotid system would be consistent with the natural history of the disease, and offers a possible explanation for some of the deterioration observed in patients who are well controlled. The natural history of plaques would account for micro infarcts noted in glaucomatous patients, Begg and Drance (2), and sudden change in the visual field of an isolated and non-progressive character.

ACKNOWLEDGEMENTS

We wish to thank members of the Vascular Laboratory of the Bristol Royal Infirmary who have co-operated in this study, John Woodcock, and Jane Snedden. Also Mr A. J. Hughes of Bristol University Medical Statistics.

REFERENCES

1. Arakawa, Y. Ophthalmodynamography of open-angle glaucoma. Jap. J. Ophthalmol. 31:687–693 (1977).
2. Begg, I. S., Drance, S. M. and Sweeney, V. P. Haemorrhage on the disc – a sign of acute ischaemic optic neuropathy in chromic simple glaucoma. Can. J. Ophthalmol. 5:321–330 (1970).
3. Bengtsson, B. Findings associated with glaucomatous visual field defects. Acta Ophthalmol. 58:20–32 (1980).
4. De Laet, H. La Pratique de L'Ophthalmodynamometrie. Soc. Belge D'Ophthal. 127:123 (1961).
5. Drance, S. M., Bryett, J. and Schulzer, M. The effects of surgical pressure reduction on the glaucomatous field. Doc. Ophthalmol. Proc. Series 14:67 (1976).

6. Goldman, H. Open-angle glaucoma. Br. J. Ophthalmol. 56:242 (1972).
7. Krakau, C. E. T. Intraocular pressure elevation — cause or effect in chronic glaucoma? Ophthalmologica 182:141 (1981).
8. Woodcock, J. P. and Skidmore, R. Principles and applications of Doppler ultrasound. New techniques and instrumentation in ultrasound, pp. 166–185 (1981).

Authors' address:

Bristol Eye Hospital
Vascular Laboratory
Bristol Royal Infirmary
Bristol, U.K.

ANTERIOR ISCHEMIC OPTIC NEUROPATHY AND ASSOCIATED VISUAL FIELD CHANGES

LAO YUAN-XIU (KATHERINE LAO)

(Beijing, China)

Key words. Ischemic optic neuropathy, disc edema, papilledema, visual fields.

ABSTRACT

Sixty-seven eyes of 47 patients with anterior ischemic optic neuropathy were studied. These Chinese patients were younger and their visual prognosis was better than those reported in the western literature. Their associated systemic diseases were somewhat different. A particular pattern of visual field loss which aided in the diagnosis was found in almost all cases. This defect consisted of a short arcuate scotoma bridging the blind spot with a 'large patch' of associated visual field loss. If progression occurred, a new 'large patch' of visual field loss suddenly appeared. The study suggests several facts: 1) a sectorial blood supply of the optic disc; 2) the site of the ischemia was in the deeper part of the nerve fiber layer with resulting disc edema; 3) there was frequently an associated 'large patch' of visual field loss; and 4) cupping of the disc was rarely seen. The differential diagnosis between anterior ischemic optic neuropathy and glaucoma was made by comparing the clinical pictures and associated visual field changes.

INTRODUCTION

Extensive studies have been reported on anterior ischemic optic neuropathy (AION) (3,4,5,12,15,19). In 1975 we reported 12 cases for the first time in Chinese literature (15). Since then, the importance of visual field changes for diagnostic purposes has been emphasized. From studying the clinical data of 47 cases, several concepts about the associated visual field changes in AION have been recognized.

CLINICAL STUDY AND RESULTS

Clinical data

The clinical features of AION have been well described in the literature (3,4,5,12,15,19). Only the important features will be summarized below:

Greve, E. L., Heijl, A. (eds.) Fifth International Visual Field Symposium.
©1983 Dr W. Junk Publishers, The Hague/Boston/Lancaster.

1. *Funduscopic changes.* There is usually pale swelling of the optic disc with occasional superficial splinter hemorrhages. There may be a sectorial pattern to the disc power. After a short time, the edema subsides and optic atrophy ensues. The two eyes may be involved simultaneously, but more often one eye is involved with the second eye becoming involved after a subsequent time interval. As a result, the appearance of the fundus between the two eyes may be quite different (Table 1).

Table 1. Disc changes of both eyes (47 cases).

Discs	Male	Female	Total
Edema and atrophy	7	4	11
Edema and edema	2	4	6
Edema and normal	5	10	15
Atrophy and normal	4	5	9
Atrophy and atrophy	1	1	2
Normal and normal	2	2	4

2. *Visual field investigation.* In 44 cases, the correct diagnosis of ischemic optic neuropathy was not made until visual field examination disclosed the typical field defects (Table 2).

Table 2. Diagnosis prior to visual field investigation.

Foster-Kennedy Syndrome	6	Pituitary tumor	2
Papilledema	8	Brain tumor	2
Papillitis	10	Neuro-retinitis	1
Optic atrophy	6	AION	3
Visual acuity reduced (unknown cause)	6	Retrobulbar neuritis	1

3. *Visual acuity.* Patients usually can recall the date of the abrupt onset of the blurred vision. The visual loss is usually not severe and is non-progressive (Table 3).

Table 3. Visual acuity at first visit.

Age	< 20	21 —	31 —	41 —	51 —	61 —
> 1.0	1	1	11	8	5	2
0.9–0.6		1	7	5	2	1
0.5–0.4		1	1	4	2	1
0.3–0.1		3	3	2	1	
< 0.1	1	1		2		

— 32/38 eyes with disc edema, visual acuity above 0.4 — (84.21%).
— 17/24 eyes with optic atrophy, visual acuity above 0.4 — (70.08%).

4. *Associated conditions.* Most commonly associated condition with anterior ischemic optic neuropathy would appear to be vascular disorders (Table 4). In our present study, no patients were diagnosed as having giant cell arteritis (10,14).

Table 4. Associated conditions.

Systemic diseases	No. of cases
Hypertension	11
Diabetes	3
Pituitary tumor	2
Brain tumor with papilledema	2
Pulseless disease	2
Hypotension	1
Chronic nephritis	1
Profuse bleeding	1
Coronary artery disease	1
Migraine syndrome	1
Head injury	1
Oral contraceptives	1
Abnormal laboratory tests:	
Rheumatism; 'o' high	5
Anemia (Hgb 7.6 g)	1
Ocular conditions:	
Acute glaucoma	4
Drusen of disc	1
Perforating corneal wound	1

5. Summary. In China, anterior ischemic optic neuropathy appears to develop in younger people and has a better visual prognosis than reported in the western literature. The clinical appearance and association of systemic diseases would appear to be similar to the previously reported studies (4,7,8,13,14).

Diagnosis of AION

1. *Clinical picture.* Patients with ANION frequently show a similar clinical presentation consisting of the sudden onset of blurred vision with mild or moderate sectorial pale disc edema with small flame-shaped hemorrhages. AION may be quite difficult to differentiate from early cases of papilledema due to intracranial hypertension or papillitis.

2. *Fluorescein angiography.* Fluorescein angiography may be helpful in the diagnosis of AION. Sectorial disc hypoperfusion corresponding to the visual field defect and delayed filling of the choroid in the peripapillary region have been demonstrated. However, the filling defects depend on the age of the lesion since the circulation appears to improve steadily and in some cases, even returns to normal (7,12).

3. *Visual field examination.* It appears that AION produces a characteristic pattern of visual field loss which may aid in the diagnosis. The appropriate clinical history and characteristic fundus appearance, when combined with a typical pattern of visual field loss, should easily facilitate the diagnosis of AION. Because this clinical picture was not appreciated, many patients in our study received repeated neurologic investigations at several hospitals including carotid angiography, pneumoencephalography, ventriculography, and CAT scanning. The neurologic investigation failed to reveal the appropriate

diagnosis. All of the patients had typical visual field defects which should have correctly identified AION as the etiologic condition. For example, in our study, 6 patients were misdiagnosed as having a Foster-Kennedy syndrome from brain tumors (Table 2).

4. *Disc edema.* Disc edema in AION was moderate in degree and subsided within a short time period. Among our 21 cases where disc edema was recorded, there was resolution of the disc edema within two weeks for 5 patients, 3–4 weeks for 6 patients, 1–2 months for 7 patients, and in 5 months for 3 patients.

Site for the lesion in AION

From analysis of our data, several concepts have been developed regarding the site of the ischemic lesion.

1. A characteristic pattern of visual field loss could almost always be demonstrated in cases of AION as shown in Figs. 1, 2 and 3. There is frequently a short arcuate scotoma bridging the blind spot and a 'large patch' of visual field loss. The visual field defects are usually permanent.

The following patterns of visual field loss characterize the visual field defects in our patients.

a. The basic pattern of visual field defect is usually a 'large patch' of visual field loss occupying one quarter of the visual field or a so-called 'quadrantic' defect. This quadrantic defect is not limited by the vertical or horizontal meridians. The quadrantic defect does not resemble any nerve fiber arrangement in the retina and is not similar to a Bjerrum scotoma in appearance. Generally, central fixation is spared, accounting for the good central vision in many cases (Table 3). The quadrantic defect often breaks into the periphery (Table 5) (4).

b. Quadrantic defects may simultaneously or successively attack the same eye in different quadrants. If two quadrants are involved, a hemianopic defect may result. If four quadrants are involved, an irregular central area of 10–20 degrees of visual field remains, which might be misinterpreted as a 'concentric

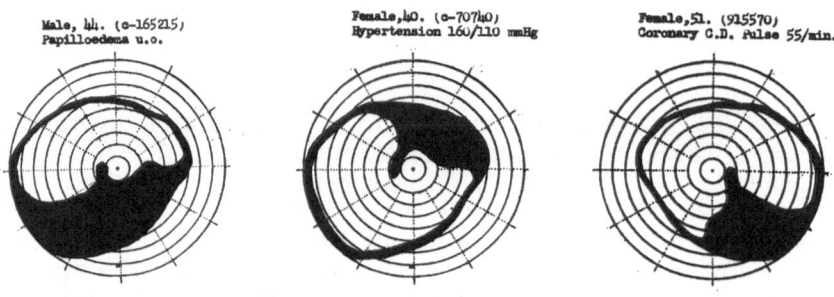

Male, 44. (o-165215)
Papilloedema u.o.

Female,40. (o-70740)
Hypertension 160/110 mmHg

Female,51. (915570)
Coronary C.D. Pulse 55/min.

Typical Pattern of V.F. loss in AION

Fig. 1. Typical pattern of VF loss in AION.

264

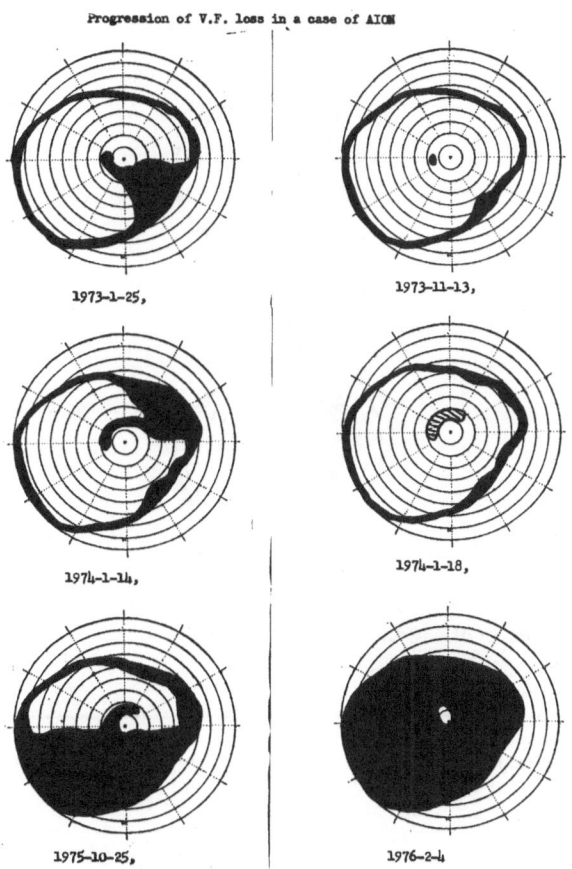

1973-1-25,

1973-11-13,

1974-1-14,

1974-1-18,

1975-10-25,

1976-2-4

Fig. 2. Progression of VF loss in a case of AION.

contraction'. In many cases, the hemianopic defect can be separated into two quadrants when the visual field is tested with targets of different sizes (Fig. 3).

c. If progression should occur, the field defect usually suddenly enlarges with the addition of a new quadrant of loss. The patient is usually aware of the new visual field loss (Fig. 2).

d. If there should be regression of the visual field defect, a residual field loss in the most peripheral part of the field is often found (Fig. 2).

e. The nasal and lower parts of the visual fields are most commonly involved (Table 5).

2. What does the 'large patch' quadrantic defect indicate? According to what we have seen by fluorescein angiography and visual field analysis, basic quadrantic loss suggests a sectorial distribution of the blood supply to the optic disc. As previously described in the literature, the peripapillary vessels

265

Fig. 3

Visual field defect of AION

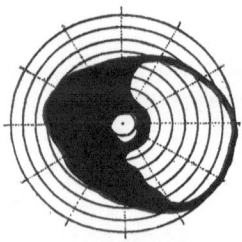

tested with 5/330,white.

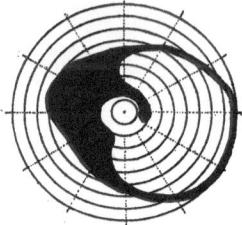

tested with 20/330, white.

Fig. 3. Visual field defect of AION.

Table 5. Visual field defects.

'Quadrantic'			
Nasal lower	20	Temporal lower	2
Nasal upper	2	Temporal upper	0
'Hemianopic'			
Lower	25	Vertical	5
Upper	3		
'Peripheral contraction'	2		
Bjerrum scotoma	1		

of the pre-laminar region may provide subdivisions to the surface nerve fiber layer (1,12). These subdivisions are often seen in the temporal sector of the disc. It is generally believed that nerve fibers entering from the periphery of the retina lie deepest in the nerve fiber layer and enter the periphery of the optic nerve head. Nerve fibers entering from the central area of the retina lie in the inner layer of the nerve fiber layer and enter the central portion of the optic nerve (2,11,17,18). These anatomic relationships in the nerve fiber layer may account for many of the patterns of visual field loss.

Thus, in AION it may be speculated that an occlusion of one of the vessels which supplies the deeper layer of the nerve fibers at the optic disc might produce the sudden onset of a 'large patch' quadrantic visual field defect. This defect usually breaks through the periphery and does not follow a nerve fiber bundle or Bjerrum distribution. In addition, the residual defect at the far periphery may also be explained in a similar fashion. Because these vessels are far from the lamina, its resulting ischemia following the occlusion appears not to result in cupping corresponding to the extent of the field loss. Since the width of the segmental blood supply in the optic nerve head varies, an ischemic infarct in one of these collaterals would produce a corresponding loss of visual field. However, it is unclear why the lower half of the visual field appears to be most commonly involved. The observation is reported by previous investigators (4,7,8,12).

The major factor in ischemic optic neuropathy may not be a pathologic condition of the disc itself. Described in the literature, infarction of the retrolaminar optic nerve, occlusion of the common carotid artery, systemic hypotension, and other conditions have been seen in AION. Thus, the vessels to the particular nerve fiber region may be more susceptible to a fall of perfusion pressure or a rise of intraocular pressure resulting in AION (4,7,8,12).

AION differentiated from low-tension glaucoma (LTG)

In certain cases of primary open angle glaucoma, the pressure is recorded as normal despite progressive field loss, the so-called low-tension glaucoma syndrome. In these cases, perhaps perfusion pressure at the optic nerve head is so marginal that a slight fall in blood pressure or an increase in intraocular pressure may result in ischemic damage to the nerve fiber layer with resulting visual field loss. In both open angle glaucoma and low-tension glaucoma, splinter hemorrhages seen around the disc surface are often associated with nerve fiber bundle visual field defects. These hemorrhages with the ensuing visual field loss are thought to represent small episodes of ischemia in the optic nerve. In our series, patients have developed AION in addition to primary open angle glaucoma. When this occurs, usually some factors other than elevated intraocular pressure were present such as a drop of systemic blood pressure. In addition, an acute rise of intraocular pressure may be associated with AION. In our series, 4 out of 47 cases showed a typical pattern of AION visual field loss but without glaucomatous cupping after an acute attack of glaucoma. From the clinical picture, especially from our visual field data, we are under the impression that there are several apparent differences between AION and low-tension glaucoma (Table 6 and Table 7).

Table 6. Differentiating clinical features of AION and LTG.

AION	LTG
Onset sudden	Chronic
Aware of visual field loss	Unaware visual field loss until late
IOP normal	Normal (diurnal may be abnormal)
C-value normal	C-value low
Often disc edema with pallor	Disc pallor and cupping

Table 7. Differentiating visual field changes between AION and LTG.

AION	LTG
Sudden onset of visual field loss	Chronic visual field loss
Short arcuate defects plus a 'large patch' quadrantic defects	
Visual deficit, permanent and stationary, occasionally progression seen with sudden quadrantic defect appearing	Gradual progression with widening of scotoma
Marked visual field loss but with no glaucoma cupping	Visual field loss usually with associated cupping
If improvement occurs, a residual peripheral visual field defect is left	Usually a segment of the arcuate scotoma remains

REFERENCES

1. Anderson, D. R. Vascular supply to the optic nerve of primates. Am. J. Ophthalmol. 70:341−351 (1970).
2. Anderson, D. R. and Hoyt, W. F. Ultrastructure of intraorbital portion of human and monkey optic nerve. Arch. Ophthalmol. 82:506−530 (1969).
3. Begg, I. S., Drance, S. M. and Sweeney, V. P. Ischemic optic neuropathy in chronic simple glaucoma. Br. J. Ophthalmol. 55:73−96 (1971).
4. Boghen, D. R. and Glaser, J. S. Ischemic Neuropathy. Brain 98:689−708 (1975).
5. Cullen, J. F. Ischemic optic neuropathy. Trans. Ophthalmol. Soc. U.K. 87:759−774 (1967).
6. Drance, S. M. The visual field of low-tension glaucoma and shock induced optic neuropathy. Arch. Ophthalmol. 95:1359−1361 (1977).
7. Eagling, E. M., Sanders, M. D. and Miller, S. J. H. Ischemic papillopathy, clinical and fluorescein angiographic review of 40 cases. Br. J. Ophthalmol. 58:990−1008 (1974).
8. Ellenberger, C., Keltner, J. L. and Burde, R. M. Acute optic neuropathy in older patients. Arch. Neurol. 28:182−185 (1973).
9. Fishbein, S. L. and Schwartz, B. Optic disc in glaucoma. Arch. Ophthalmol. 95:1975−1979 (1977).
10. Foulds, W. S. Visual disturbance in systemic disorders. Trans. Ophthalmol. Soc. U.K. 89:125−146 (1969).
11. Harrington, D. O. The pathogenesis of the glaucoma field. Am. J. Ophthalmol. 47(2):177−185 (1959).
12. Hayreh, S. S. Anterior Ischemic Optic Neuropathy. Springer-Verlag, New York (1975).
13. Henkind, P. et al. Histophthalogy of ischemic optic neuropathy. Am. J. Ophthalmol. 69:78 (1970).
14. Knox, D. L. Optic nerve manifestations of systemic diseases. Trans. Am. Acad. Ophthal. Otol. 83:743−750 (1977).
15. Lao, Yuan-Xiu. Ischemic papilloneuropathy. Chinese Med. J. 1:14−19 (1975).
16. Lichter, P. R. and Henderson, J. W. Optic nerve infarction. Trans. Am. Ophthalmol. Soc. 75:103−121 (1977).
17. Ogden, T. E. The nerve fiber layer of the primate retina. Invest. Ophthalmol. 13:95 (1974).
18. Roth, A. M. and Foos, R. Y. Surface structure of optic nerve head. Am. J. Ophthalmol. 74:977−985 (1972).

19. Sanders, M. D. Ischemic papillopathy. Trans. Ophthalmol. Soc. U.K. 91:360–386 (1971).

Author's address:
Dr K. Lao
Dept. of Ophthalmology
Capital Hospital
Chinese Academy of Medical Sciences
Beijing
China

COMPUTER-ASSISTED PERIMETRY RESULTS IN NEURO-OPHTHALMOLOGY PROBLEM CASES

BRIAN R. YOUNGE

(Rochester, Minnesota, U.S.A.)

Key words. Computer-assisted perimetry, multiple diagnoses, neuro-ophthalmology, Octopus.

ABSTRACT

Computer-assisted perimetry (Octopus) is useful in discerning field defects in patients who have more than one lesion affecting the visual system, largely because of its objective testing strategy and its ability to detect near-threshold abnormalities not found on standard kinetic perimetry.

INTRODUCTION

Patients often present with multiple disorders, complex medical diseases, and a combination of neurologic and ophthalmologic conditions. These patients may have had many neurologic tests before the true nature of the problem was found. In manual perimetry, the patient's responses often are vague and interpretation is difficult and may produce a bizarre-looking visual field. The objectivity of automated perimetry, at least in the gathering of data and their display, is useful in differentiating one disorder from another or in combining known clinical parameters with fields so that two diagnoses can be made simultaneously.

Several cases will be presented in which two or more disorders affected the vision or fields to the degree that the diagnosis was either incorrect or incomplete and in which computer-assisted perimetry contributed to the differentiation of the diagnoses.

METHOD AND MATERIALS

The charts of several patients who were seen in consultation at the Mayo Clinic were reviewed in detail to find those with multiple diagnostic entries of disorders that simultaneously affected the visual system. Among these

Greve, E. L., Heijl, A. (eds.) Fifth International Visual Field Symposium.
©1983 Dr W. Junk Publishers, The Hague/Boston/Lancaster.

disorders were visual field defects due to chiasmal tumors, strokes, and trauma; ocular disorders that also affect fields, such as glaucoma, optic pits, and other disc anomalies; and retinal diseases. Patients who had had visual fields plotted manually and then by computer-assisted perimetry were studied to determine if one field method was more revealing than the other. Several patients had had Goldmann fields determined by their referring physicians, and these patients were retested manually as well as by computer-assisted perimetry. Results of neuroradiologic and electrophysiologic tests were reviewed, as were the general physical and neurologic findings.

ILLUSTRATIVE CASES

Case 1. A 62-year old man was referred for eye examination as part of a general examination for diabetes. For some time, he had complained of failing vision in his left eye, and an ophthalmologist in his home community had been unable to explain the patient's symptoms despite several refractions. Refraction was $-8.50, -1.50 \times 76$ in the right eye and $-8.50, -1.50 \times 108$ in the left, which corrected the vision to 20/25 and 20/20, respectively. He had anomalous optic discs, with very oblique insertions slanted temporally (Fig. 1). The intraocular pressures by applanation were 22 mm Hg bilaterally,

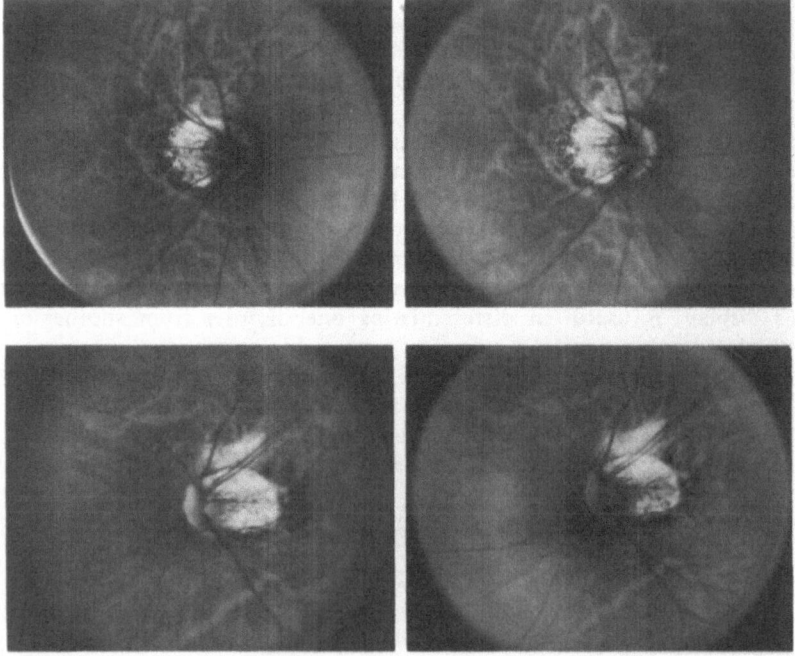

Fig. 1. (case 1). Optic discs view with + 10 lenses. Note tilt toward temporal side, and lack of typical glaucomatous cupping. *Top*, right eye. *Bottom*, left eye.

272

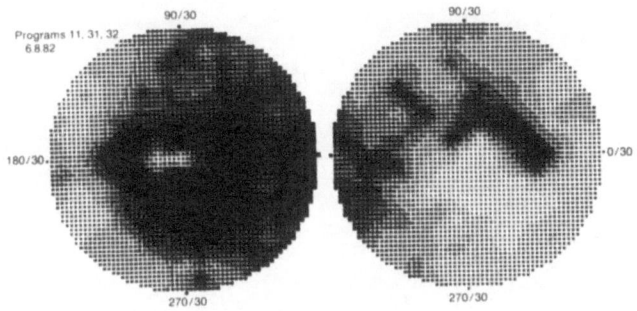

Fig. 2. (case 1). Computer-assisted fields printed as 'gray scales' by the Octopus automated perimeter, programs 11, 31 and 32 combined, size 3 target.

and the confrontation fields were grossly full, with a slight suggestion of a nasal contraction in the left eye. However, the patient complained that he seemed to miss letters when he used his left eye but not when he used his right eye. Because of these symptoms, a computer-assisted field was ordered, and this showed rather striking abnormalities, the right having a superior arcuate defect and the left having double arcs with only a small isle through which the vision was 20/25 (Fig. 2). This was unexpected. Further history obtained at that time revealed that the patient had been involved in six 'fender benders' within the past year, two of which occurred on consecutive days, while he left the same parking space. Stereophotographs of the fundus did not show glaucomatous cupping but did show anomalous tilting to the temporal side. Closer inspection revealed loss of nerve fiber substance in the arcuate areas, as well as choroidal thinning of high myopia. Intraocular pressures were subsequently elevated to 24 mm Hg bilaterally, and the patient was given 0.25% timolol.

Case 2. A 6-year old child who was previously examined in 1979 was referred because of a small-angle esotropia and congenital nystagmus. Previous visual acuity was 20/70 in the right eye and 20/40 in the left, with pictures, consistent with these findings. However, the vision was 20/200 right and 20/40 left, and the optic discs showed 'tract sign' pallor (2) for the first time (Fig. 3). Confrontation fields showed an inconsistent nasal defect in the left eye and a temporal defect in the right. Computer-assisted perimetry showed an incongruous right homonymous defect, more dense in the right eye, suggesting a left-sided chiasmal lesion (Fig. 4). This was confirmed on computed tomographic scanning, and subsequent craniotomy disclosed an optic glioma involving the chiasm and left optic tract. Postoperatively, he was treated with radiation, and his subsequent visual fields showed little change (Fig. 5).

Case 3. A 57-year old woman had cupping and slowly progressive field loss. The intraocular pressure was 17 mm Hg bilaterally while she was on medication. Recently, however, the fields had progressed in an unusual way

273

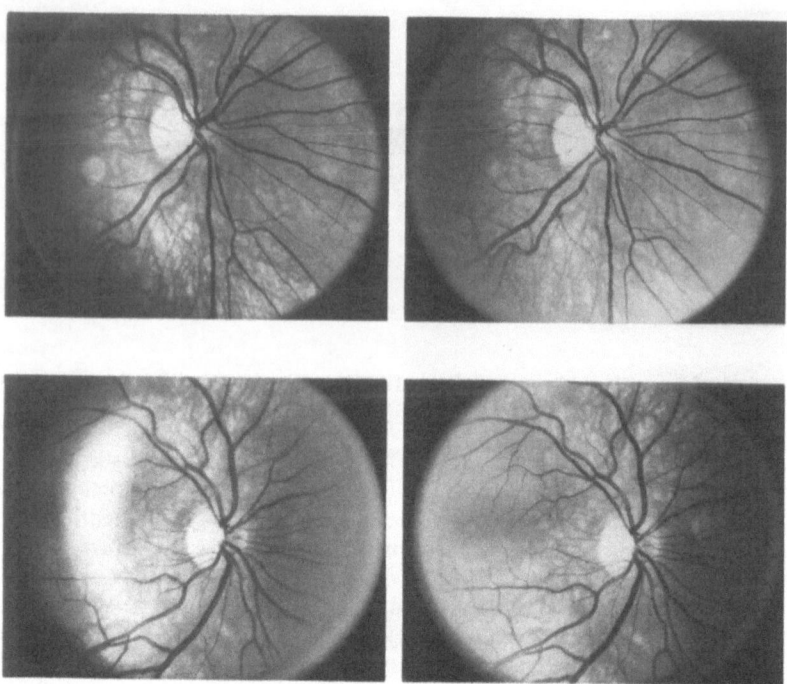

Fig. 3. (case 2). Optic discs showing generalized pallor and 'tract sign' pattern of optic atrophy, that is, preservation of arcuate nerve fiber bundles in the right eye (*Top*), loss of these same fibers in the left eye (*Bottom*), and bow-tie pallor on right (1). View with + 10 lenses.

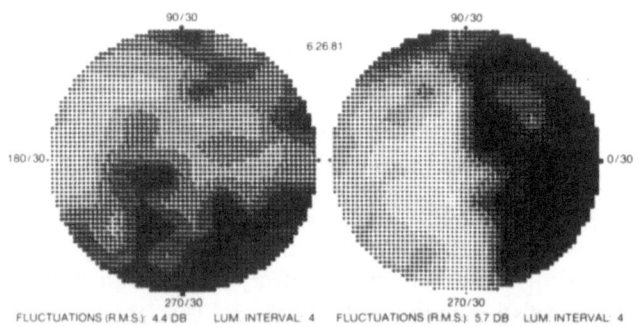

Fig. 4. (case 2). Computer-assisted fields, gray scales, program 32, size 3 target. Pre-operative (June 26, 1981).

that could not be explained on the basis of the glaucoma. There was cupping with notching of the discs inferiorly (Fig. 6). The patient had an afferent pupillary defect in the right eye, and the difference in the appearance of the optic discs was more than could be accounted for by the clear view seen

274

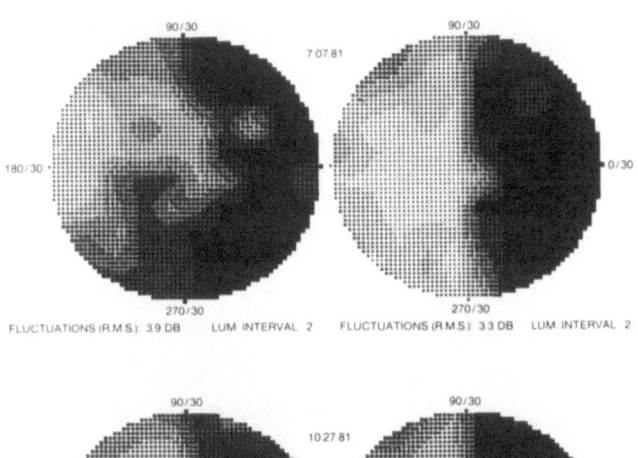

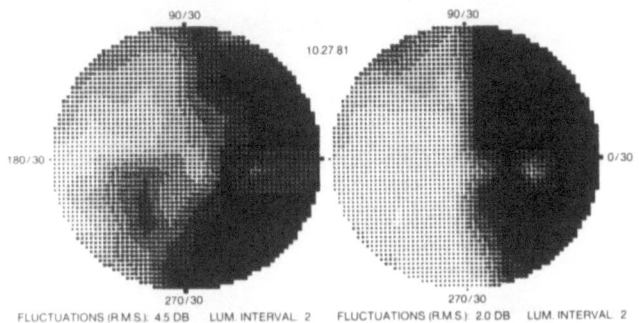

Fig. 5. (case 2). Same examinations postoperatively (July 7, 1981 and October 27, 1981). Note consistency on serial examinations.

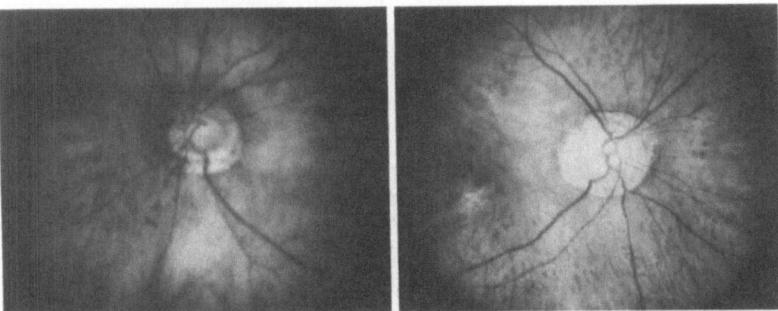

Fig. 6. (case 3). Optic discs as viewed through intraocular right lens and nuclear cataract in left eye. Photograph of left disc is much darker, but optic atrophy was present nonetheless in the right disc, and both discs show cupping due to glaucoma.

through the intraocular lens in the right and the nuclear cataract in the left. Her vision was disappointingly poor after surgery in the previous year, and her vision was 20/400 in the operated eye and 20/70 in the left eye, which had a nuclear cataract. Previous visual fields were confirmed on the Goldmann

275

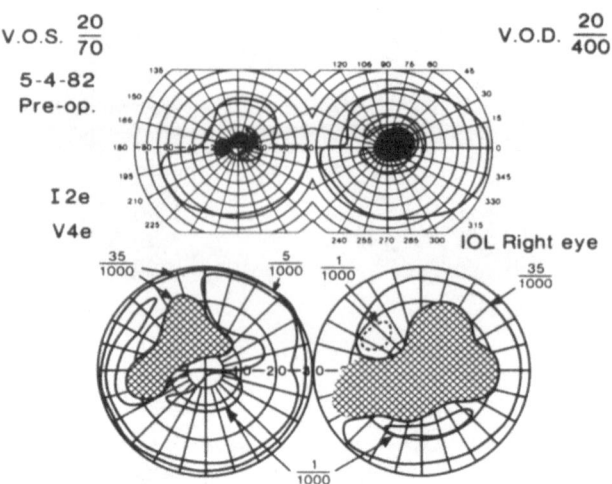

Fig. 7. (case 3). *Top*, Goldmann fields done by the referring physician, and results confirmed by us. *Bottom*, tangent screen examination done by perimetrists and checked by consultant.

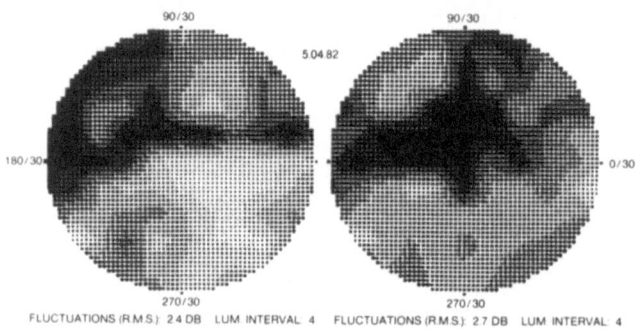

Fig. 8. (case 3). Computer-assisted perimetry, gray scales, program 32, size 3 target. Note arcuate-shaped defects bilaterally, with a superior-temporal depression in each eye, as well as an inferior-temporal depression of the left.

perimeter (Fig. 7 *top*), and tangent screen examinations were done in addition (Fig. 7 *bottom*). Neither of these indicated a localizing lesion, and the patient underwent computer-assisted perimetry (Fig. 8). This showed not only the expected glaucomatous defects but also a central depression in the right eye and relative bitemporal defects superiorly, with fairly distinct midline splitting. There was an inferior temporal depression in the left eye. Roentgenograms showed an enlarged sella, and computed tomography demonstrated a pituitary tumor with suprasellar extension (Fig. 9). Subsequent transsphenoidal surgery was performed without incident. Her postoperative fields showed a significant improvement in the temporal defects (Fig. 10).

276

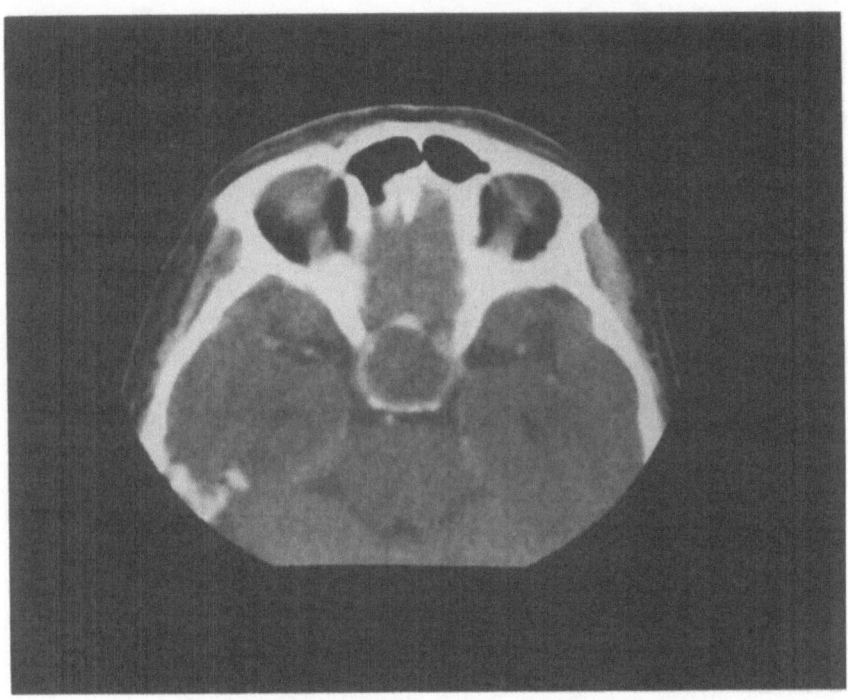

Fig. 9. (case 3). Computed tomography of sellar area, showing sella expanded, with tumor and suprasellar extension.

DISCUSSION

Case 1 illustrates an example of tilted optic discs, a phenomenon that gives rise to relative bitemporal depression crossing the midline (1), particularly when the tilting is inferior. The coexistence of glaucoma was not suspected from the appearance of the optic disc, and intraocular pressures were not inordinately high. However, the density of the field defects indicated more significant disease than could be explained on the basis of the tilted myopic discs.

Case 2 shows the importance of suspecting a problem when the loss of vision seems disproportionate to the findings. The use of automated perimetry was helpful in localizing the pathologic changes to the optic chiasm, despite the presence of nystagmus and the age of the patient. Children often do not complain about loss of vision or visual field, and usually the parents or teachers are the first to become aware of a change in performance or behavior.

Case 3, that of glaucoma coexisting with a pituitary tumor, is a good example of how computer-assisted perimetry is useful in detecting relative defects that are not found on manual perimetry. Although the index of suspicion was high, yet not knowing the actual pathology, the examiners

277

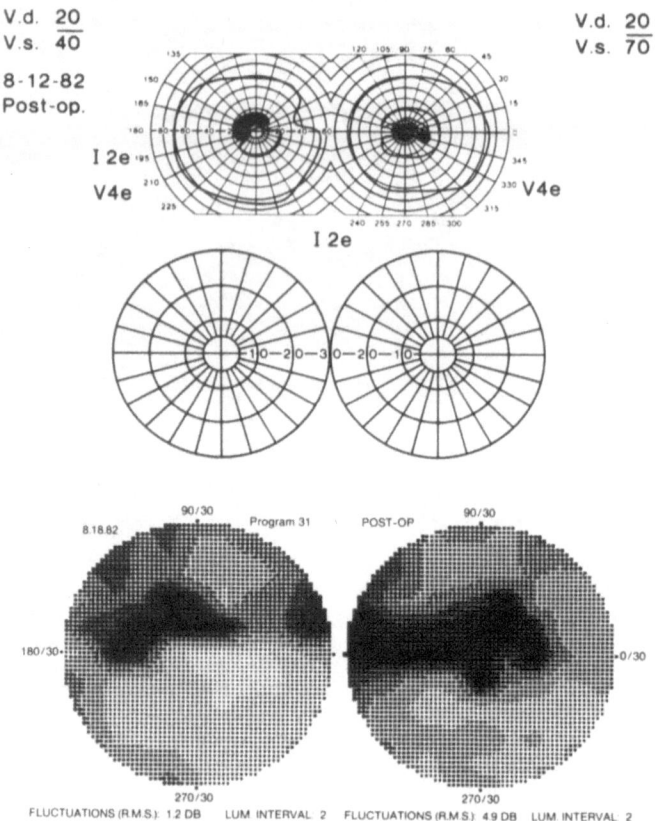

V.d. 20
V.s. 40

V.d. 20
V.s. 70

8-12-82
Post-op.

I 2e
V4e

V4e

I 2e

90/30
8.18.82   Program 31   POST-OP   90/30

180/30

0/30

270/30   270/30
FLUCTUATIONS (R.M.S): 1.2 DB   LUM INTERVAL: 2   FLUCTUATIONS (R.M.S): 4.9 DB   LUM INTERVAL: 2

Fig. 10. (case 3). Postoperative fields, showing considerable resolution of superior-temporal defects, improved visual acuity of the right eye, and even disappearance of the subtle inferior-temporal defect of the left eye. *Top*, Goldmann fields from referring physician. *Bottom*, computer-assisted perimetry, gray scales.

(both the referring physician and the consultant) failed to detect the midline split in the subtle bitemporal depression. One might argue that in retrospect such a diagnosis might have been suspected, but clearly the computer-assisted fields had a major role in diagnosis.

CONCLUSIONS

Combinations of two or more lesions that affect the vision or visual fields are rare, and computer-assisted determination of visual fields is useful in detecting such multiple lesions. Threshold-related automated static perimetry provides some objectivity in determining field defects that are not easily detected by manual perimetry and may even be missed despite knowledge of the condition that produces the field defect (3). The development of such

278

devices adds much to the clinical management of complex diagnostic problems and is of considerable use in follow-up of known field defects.

REFERENCES

1. Rucker, C. W. Bitemporal defects in the visual fields resulting from developmental anomalies of the optic disks. Arch. Ophthalmol. 35:546–554 (1946).
2. Savino, P. J., Paris, M., Schatz, N. J. et al. Optic tract syndrome: a review of 21 patients. Arch. Ophthalmol. 96:656–663 (1978).
3. Younge, B. R. and Trautmann, J. C. Computer-assisted perimetry in neuro-ophthalmic disease. Mayo Clin. Proc. 55:207–222 (1980).

Author's address:
Dr B. R. Younge
Dept. of Ophthalmology
Mayo Clinic and Mayo Foundation
Rochester, MN 55905
U.S.A.

PROPERTIES OF SCOTOMATA IN GLAUCOMA AND OPTIC NERVE DISEASE: COMPUTER ANALYSIS

CHRIS A. JOHNSON* and JOHN L. KELTNER

(Davis, California, U.S.A.)

Key words. Glaucoma, optic nerve disease, computer analysis, scotomata.

ABSTRACT

In a previous study, we determined frequency distributions for the location of visual field loss in glaucoma and other optic nerve disease. A computer algorithm was developed to evaluate these characteristics according to a high resolution grid (approximately 30,000 locations subtending 0.85 by 0.85 degrees). The distributions for glaucoma and optic nerve disease revealed distinct differences, and provided information useful for optimizing target presentation patterns for perimetric testing. This study presents an extension of our earlier work to include frequency distribution characteristics for the size and shape of visual field defects in glaucoma and optic nerve disease. As with the frequency distributions for location of scotomata, the frequency distributions for size and shape of visual field defects are different for glaucoma and optic nerve disease. Scotomata in optic nerve disease have a strong tendency to be round or nearly round in shape, with a relatively equal proportion of small, medium and large sizes. In glaucoma, there is a much greater proportion of small scotomata, and the majority of defects tend to be horizontally oriented, followed by a subgroup of vertically oriented defects, with only a small percentage of round scotomata.

INTRODUCTION

Clinical comparison studies of manual and automated perimetry have established that several forms of automated testing can provide accurate and reliable detection of visual field abnormalities (see e.g., Refs. 2–5,7). The next stage of refining these procedures is to develop optimizing strategies that increase their speed and efficiency. One approach to this problem is to develop a model of visual field testing that is based on *a priori* probabilities. That is,

---

*To whom requests for offprints should be addressed.

Greve, E. L., Heijl, A. (eds.) Fifth International Visual Field Symposium.
©1983 Dr W. Junk Publishers, The Hague/Boston/Lancaster.

if we know which visual field locations are more likely to exhibit visual field loss for specific diseases, then it will be possible to concentrate the major testing efforts in these regions. Similarly, if the frequency distributions for size and shape of visual field defects are known, then it is possible to determine whether a certain region should be examined meticulously with a high density of targets, or whether a lower density target distribution is appropriate. The goal of this approach is to develop a strategy that will obtain the greatest amount of useful information in the smallest amount of time by making use of the known properties of visual field defects associated with specific eye diseases.

In a previous study (6), we determined frequency distributions for the location of scotomata in glaucoma and optic nerve disease. Our results showed that the most frequent areas of visual field loss in optic nerve disease were located in the central and centrocecal regions of the visual field. In comparison, scotomata in glaucoma are most frequently located near the blind spot and at successive locations along the arcuate nerve fiber bundle region out to the nasal horizontal meridian. The present investigation presents an extension of these findings to include frequency distribution characteristics for size and shape of visual field defects in glaucoma and optic nerve disease.

METHOD

A total of 370 scotomata were evaluated, consisting of 260 scotomata from glaucoma patients and 110 scotomata from patients with optic nerve disease. Glaucomatous defects were selected to include a representative sample of early, moderate and advanced visual field loss. For optic nerve disease, scotomata from hereditary optic neuropathies, compressive optic neuropathies, optic neuritis, ischemic optic neuropathy and nutritional amblyopias were included. All visual field defects were entered into an LSI 11/23 computer by means of a digitizing graphics tablet, and were processed by appropriate software algorithms. Details of the selection of cases, the experimental procedure and the strategies employed by the software algorithm have been presented in a previous publication (6). Approximately 30,000 visual field locations (0.85 by 0.85 degrees grid size) were examined.

Frequency distributions for the area (size) of scotomata were determined for both the glaucoma and optic nerve disease populations. For each scotoma, the area enclosed within its boundaries was measured, and was then assigned to one of the size categories consisting of successive 25 square degree increments in area. The frequency of various sizes of scotomata were thereby determined. General shape characteristics were evaluated by determining the maximum horizontal and vertical extent of the scotoma, and computing a horizontal/vertical ratio for each scotoma. Defects which are essentially round would thus have a ratio close to 1.0. Vertically oval scotomata would have a ratio less than 1.0 and horizontally oval scotomata would have a ratio greater than 1.0. For both the glaucoma and optic nerve disease populations, the frequency distributions of horizontal/vertical ratios were determined.

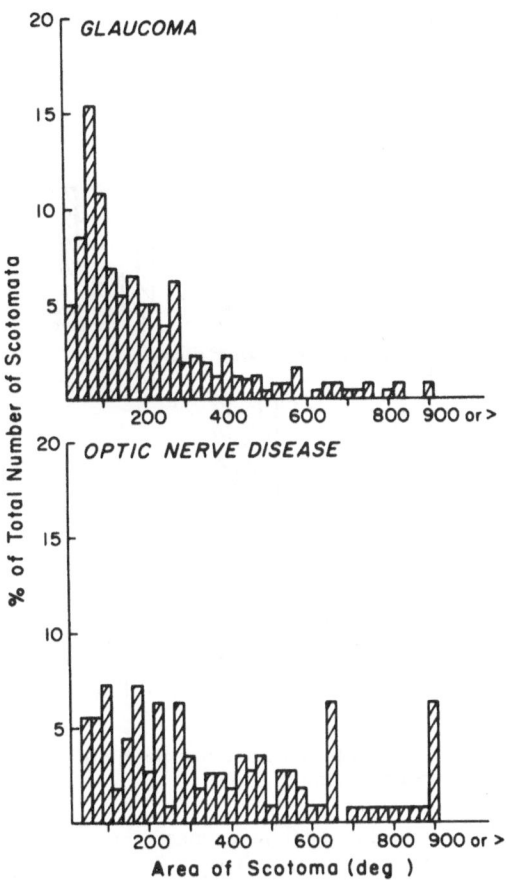

Fig. 1. Frequency distributions of scotoma size for glaucoma (top graph) and optic nerve disease (lower graph).

RESULTS

Figure 1 presents the frequency distributions of scotoma size for glaucoma (top graph) and optic nerve disease (lower graph). The percentage of scotomata falling within successive 25 degree increments of area are plotted. The distribution for glaucoma indicates that the majority of defects tend to be small (less than 150 square degrees). Only a few of the scotomata in glaucoma are large. In comparison, the distribution for optic nerve disease is rather constant throughout the entire range of scotoma sizes. That is, scotomata in optic nerve disease tend to come in all sizes.

In order to obtain a general indication of shape characteristics for scotomata, the maximum horizontal and vertical extents of each defect were determined, and a horizontal/vertical ratio was calculated. Thus, a round

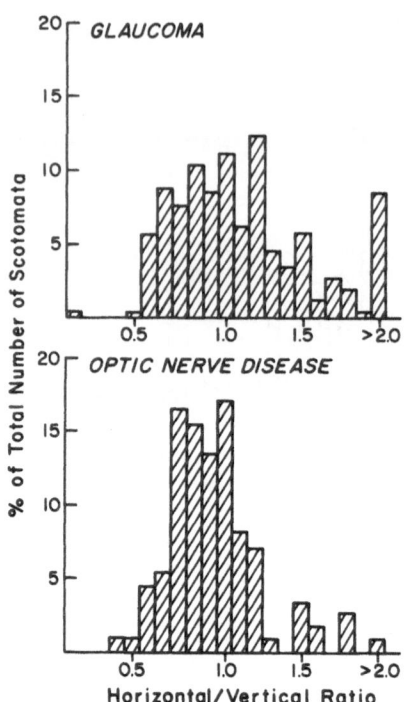

Fig. 2. Frequency distributions for the horizontal/vertical ratio of scotomata in glaucoma (top graph) and optic nerve disease (lower graph).

scotoma will exhibit a ratio equal to or near 1.0, a horizontally oriented scotoma will have a ratio greater than 1.0, and a vertically oriented scotoma will have a ratio less than 1.0. Figure 2 presents frequency distributions for the horizontal/vertical ratio of scotomata in glaucoma (top graph) and optic nerve disease (lower graph).

For glaucoma, most of the defects tend to be horizontally oriented, followed by a smaller group of vertically oriented scotomata. Only about 25% of all of the defects have a horizontal/vertical ratio that is close to 1.0, indicating that most of the scotomata in glaucoma are not round. The distribution for optic nerve disease is quite different, showing a rather high incidence of defects with horizontal/vertical ratios near 1.0, and only a small percentage of scotomata with ratios significantly greater than or less than 1.0. Thus, most of the defects in optic nerve disease tend to be round or nearly round in shape.

DISCUSSION

Previous findings (6) have shown that the frequency distributions for locations of scotomata are quite different for glaucoma and optic nerve disease. The present results indicate that the size and shape characteristics of visual field defects in glaucoma and optic nerve disease are also different. Glaucomatous defects are not usually round, and tend to be rather small in size. Scotomata in optic nerve disease are equally likely to be large or small, and are most often round in shape. These data are important for defining optimal target presentation patterns and test strategies for automated perimetry. Similar analyses for other ocular diseases will also be useful for these purposes.

Our current findings are also relevant to prior determinations of performance characteristics for various perimetric test displays. For example, Fankhauser and his associates (1) have reported the probability of detection values for grid target patterns of predetermined spacing between stimuli. The liklihood of detecting scotomata of various sizes, assuming that all defects were round in shape, was thereby evaluated for a specified grid pattern. According to our present data, the assumption of round scotomata is valid for the majority of defects in optic nerve disease, but is not representative of most glaucomatous scotomata. It would therefore be expected that the calculated probability of detection values would be accurate for optic nerve disease. On the other hand, the calculated probability of detection values for glaucoma would be expected to be an overestimate of actual performance characteristics.

To examine this issue, we conducted a simulation trial in which the 260 glaucomatous defects and the 110 scotomata in optic nerve disease evaluated in this study were processed through grid target patterns of various spacings. Optimal detection rates were thus determined for a variety of grid sizes. In addition, we used the size characteristics (area of scotoma) for each defect to calculate the probability of detection for each grid according to Fankhauser's prior evaluations (1), assuming that all scotomata were round in shape. A comparison of the calculated probabilities of detection, and the detection rates for the simulation trial revealed that there was good agreement between the two sets of values in optic nerve disease. However, the calculated probabilities of detection for glaucoma consistently overestimated the actual detection rates found in the simulation trial. This was true for all grids, except for extremely high densities (greater than 8,000 targets) and extremely low densities (less than 8 targets). These findings confirm our earlier predictions. A more detailed analysis of simulation results will be presented in a subsequent paper.

The population distributions of size, shape and location of visual field defects in various ocular diseases provide an important database for design and evaluation of perimetric testing. Further studies should allow us to derive efficient test strategies for automated perimetry that retain a high degree of accuracy.

ACKNOWLEDGEMENT

This study was supported in part by the National Eye Institute Grant No. EY-03424 (to C.A.J.).

REFERENCES

1. Fankhauser, F. and Bebie, H. Threshold fluctuations, interpolations and spatial resolution in perimetry. Doc. Ophthalmol. Proc. Series 19:295–309 (1980).
2. Fankhauser, F., Spahr, J. and Bebie, H. Three years of experience with the Octopus automatic perimeter. Doc. Ophthalmol. Proc. Series 14:7–15 (1977).
3. Heijl, A., Drance, S. M. and Douglas, G. R. The value of an automatic perimeter (Competer) in detecting early glaucomatous field defects. Arch. Ophthalmol. 95:1560–1563 (1980).
4. Heijl, A. and Krakau, C. E. T. An automatic perimeter for glaucoma visual field screening and control: Construction and clinical cases. Albrecht von Graefes Arch. Klin. Exp. Ophthalmol. 197:12–23 (1975).
5. Johnson, C. A. and Keltner, J. L. Automated suprathreshold static perimetry. Am. J. Ophthalmol. 89:731–741 (1980).
6. Johnson, C. A. and Keltner, J. L. Computer analysis of visual field loss and optimization of automated perimetric test strategies. Ophthalmology 88:1058–1065 (1981).
7. Johnson, C. A., Keltner, J. L. and Balestrery, F. G. Suprathreshold static perimetry in glaucoma and other optic nerve disease. Ophthalmology 86:1278–1286 (1979).

Author's address:
Dr C. A. Johnson
Dept. of Ophthalmology
University of California
Davis, CA 95616
U.S.A.

STATISTICAL ANALYSIS OF NORMAL VISUAL FIELDS AND HEMIANOPSIAS RECORDED BY A COMPUTERIZED PERIMETER

H. BYNKE

(Lund, Sweden)

Key words. Bitemporal hemianopsia, homonymous hemianopsia, normal visual fields, CNS disorders, computerized perimetry, statistical analysis, statistical parameters.

ABSTRACT*

The automatic computerized perimeter 'Competer' was modified in order to become better suited for neuro-ophthalmic examinations. Thus the test point pattern was enlarged and four statistical parameters were elaborated for quantification of the results. Of these, the performance values of the central (Pc) and mid-peripheral field (Pp) express the total ability and the difference values (Dc and Dp) the size of a hemianopsia. The mentioned parameters were evaluated in 75 patients with CNS disorders, who were examined on 1 to 11 occasions. Twenty-two had normal fields, 28 bitemporal and 25 homonymous hemianopsia. In normal fields gradual changes of Pc without any changes of Dc seemed to reflect changes of the general condition. In hemianopsias the changes of P- and D-values were larger, ran more or less parallel, and could be attributed to treatment or to spontaneous progression or regression of the pathological processes. In less alert patients with homonymous hemianopsia false positive defects were recorded in the non-hemianopic hemifields. In alert patients all four statistical parameters were found to be suitable for quantification.

Author's address:
Dr H. Bynke
University Eye Clinic
S-221 85 Lund
Sweden

* The original paper is in press in Neuro-Ophthalmology (Amsterdam).

VISUAL FIELDS IN THE MANAGEMENT OF UNEXPLAINED VISUAL LOSS: A COST-BENEFIT ANALYSIS

JONATHAN D. TROBE, PAULO C. ACOSTA,
JONATHON J. SHUSTER and JEFFREY P. KRISCHER

Key word. Visual field examination.

ABSTRACT

In the investigation of visual loss from anterior visual pathway disease, it is imperative to differentiate the infrequent compressive from the much more common non-compressive lesions. In this task, we compare the cost-effectiveness of two diagnostic strategies, one that uses the results of visual fields as a determinant for ordering neuroradiological studies, and another that disregards the visual field results. The visual field-determined strategy proved more cost-effective only at accuracy levels above those believed to be current in community practice.

Paper published in full in 'Survey of Ophthalmology, 1983.

Greve, E. L., Heijl, A. (eds.) Fifth International Visual Field Symposium.
©1983 Dr W. Junk Publishers, The Hague/Boston/Lancaster.

QUANTITATIVE ISOPTER CONSTRICTION UNDER IMAGE DEGRADATION BY DEFOCUS

A. SERRA

(Cagliari, Italy)

Key words. Refraction scotomata, isopter constriction, defocus.

ABSTRACT

In the present paper a quantitative evaluation of refraction scotomata is attempted. We evalute the narrowing of isopters by degrading the image through a positive lens of variable power placed close to the eye. Average data are produced for a sample of healthy individuals around fifty years of age. An 'increase' in lens power as large as 2.5 diopters beyond the optimal refraction reduces to 50% the extent of the isopter, whatever the meridian considered. In the case of a 'decrease' in lens power, obviously, a partial compensation on the part of residual accommodation occurs.

Deviations from the above behavior on the part of MS patients seems to indicate an impairment in reflex arc subserving accommodative response (supported by a reduction in accommodation amplitude for central vision in the affected eye, compared to the unaffected one).

INTRODUCTION

A sharp retinal imagery is a basic prerequisite in clinical perimetry, to avoid the bias due to 'refraction scotomata' (1,2).

Customarily refraction is corrected when needed, for central vision, by neglecting the possible extra-axial dependencies of best focus conditions.

The question arises how isopter extent is sensitive to the degradation by defocus of the target (of given size), every other thing being kept constant. For this we tested a number of normal and healthy subjects, aging around fifty, representing a control group to which patients could be compared.

MATERIALS AND METHOD

The apparatus used is the Goldmann perimeter. The target used is II/2, the luminance of the background is 45 lux.

Greve, E. L., Heijl, A. (eds.) Fifth International Visual Field Symposium.
©1983 Dr W. Junk Publishers, The Hague/Boston/Lancaster.

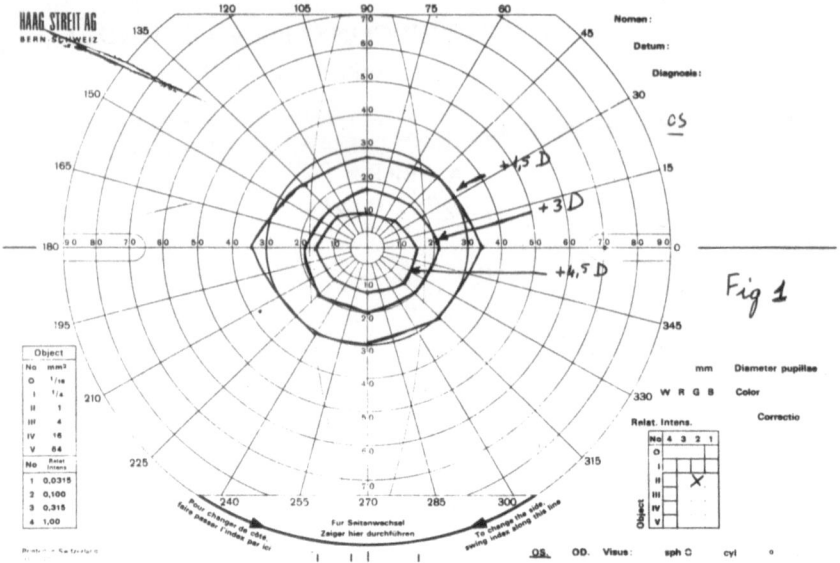

Fig. 1. Isopters recorded from a subject belonging to the control group, by the use of target II/2, for various diopter settings.

We recorded the isopter for different settings of the additional lens placed in front of the eye. We call 'optimal dioptric correction' that condition which corresponds to the largest isopter. As expected, the size of the isopter decreases when the dioptric setting differs from the optimal one (Fig. 1).

To quantify the effect of defocus, we measured the extent of the isopter along every eye meridian. Across-subject averages were calculated, for each meridian. Subjects: the number of the sample of 'normal and healthy' individuals tested by us is ten. Their age ranges from 46 to 55 years. They are highly cooperative and were given a suitable pre-training period. The reliability of their responses was evaluated by comparing the responses after re-testing.

In addition, we tested some young patients with multiple sclerosis (MS), with an history of previous attacks of optical neuritis (ON).

EXPERIMENTAL FINDINGS

The across-subject averages of isopter extent along every meridian are shown in Figs. 2a–2h. Bars denote the standard deviation. The 'zero' point, on the axis of abscissae corresponds to the 'optimal dioptric correction' for each individual.

The lack of symmetry, on either side of the zero point is obviously due to the fact that our subjects exhibit a sort of 'residual accommodation' which allows to compensate for a sub-optimal power of the lens placed in front of their eye. For this we limit ourselves to consider the right branch of the plots shown in Fig. 2. One sees that, in a first approximation, the isopter

290

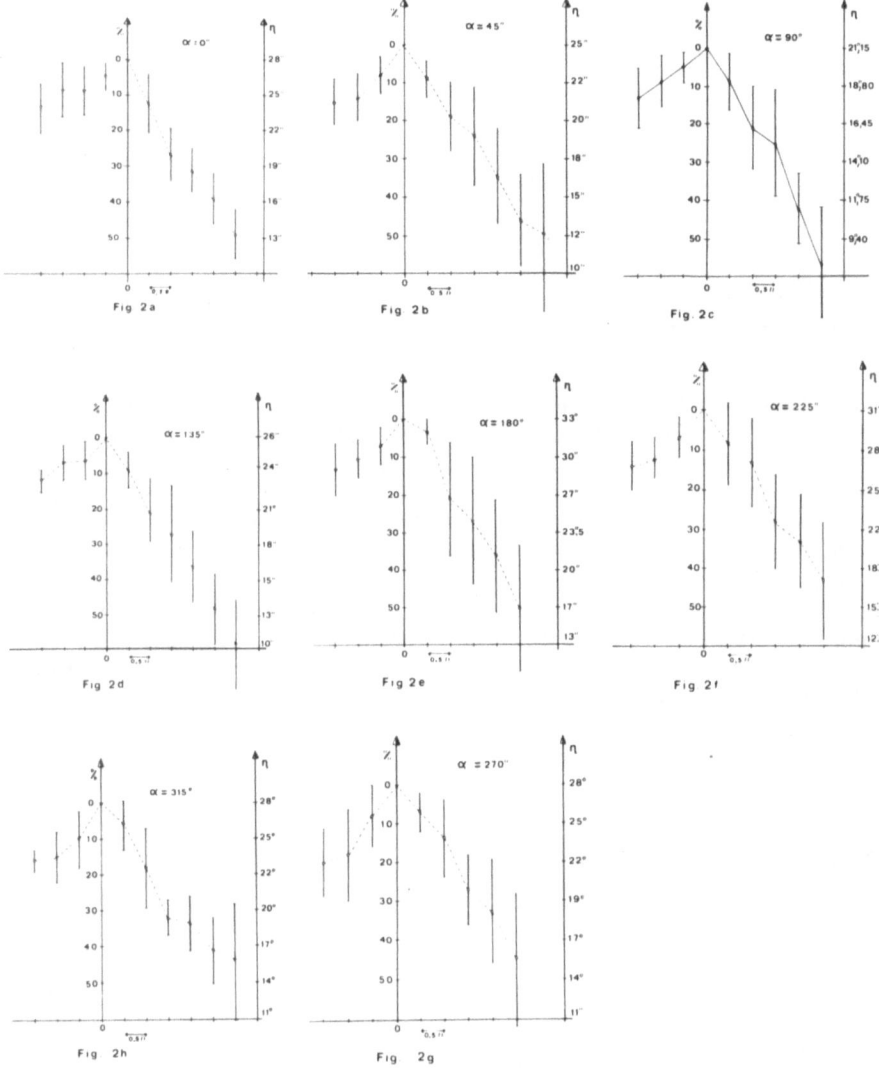

Fig. 2 (a–h) Ordinates: average data for the control group, concerning the meridian defined by its orientation α. Bars denote the across-sample standard deviation. Central axis: percent change in isopter amplitude, referred to the condition where isopter size is maximal. Abscissae: diopter setting.

constriction, on the average, ranges from 22 to 17 degrees per diopter of 'over-correction', according to the meridian considered.

Let us wonder, now, whether, the effect of a given amount of defocus is the same, whatever the eccentricity, or not, in the range attainable by means of target II/2. For this, in Figs. 3a, b, we displayed on the abscissae the

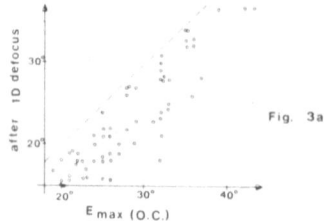 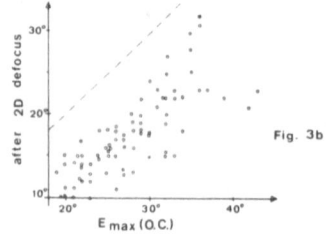

Fig. 3 (a) Abscissae: maximal extent of the isopter, when the dioptric correction is optimal. Ordinates: isopter extent after an overcorrection of 1 diopter. Each point refers to a different observer and/or to a different eye meridian; (b) as for Fig. 3a, but the over-correction is now 2 diopters.

maximal isopter extent (whatever the meridian) and with optimal dioptric correction (say, Emax (O.C.), and on the ordinates the extent after reduction because of a given amount of defocus. The sets of points thus obtained may be fitted by straight lines the slope of which are 1.0 and 0.8 for 1 and 2 diopters of defocus, respectively. The correlation coefficients, $r = 0.95$ for 1 diopter of defocus, $r = 0.94$ for 2 diopters are well above the significance level.

In some pathologies eye lens accommodation capability is indirectly impaired, because of a general deterioration of muscular responsiveness. The question arises whether the rate of isopter constriction because of the addition of positive lenses mirrors the above deterioration.

The answer seems to be affirmative. Let us consider, for instance, Fig. 4, which refers to the horizontal (nasal) eye meridian of an **MS** patient after

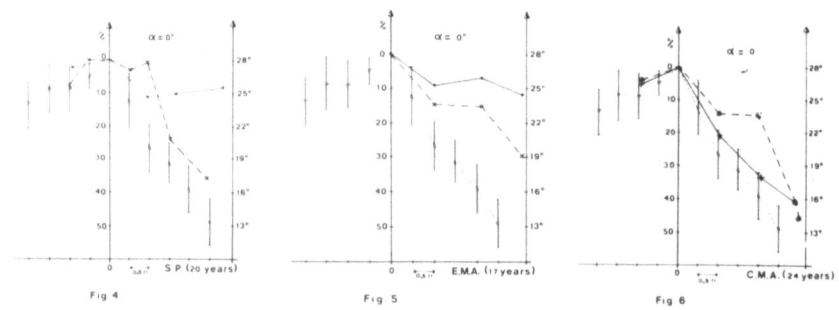

Fig. 4. Abscissae: power to the additional positive lens (the zero corresponding to the diopter setting for which the isopter extent is maximal). Ordinates: extent of the isopter along the nasal side of the horizontal meridian. Open circles: average data for the control group. Crosses: eye after ON attack. Full circles: eye with no ON attack. Age of the MS patient: 20 years.

Fig. 5. As for Fig. 4, the age of the MS patient being now 17 years.

Fig. 6. As for Fig. 4, but the MS patient (with bilateral ON attacks) is 24-years old. Crosses: eye with earlier ON attack. Asterisks: eye with more recent ON attack.

292

unilateral ON attack. Apparently, the affected eye exhibits a greater isopter constriction than the unaffected one, as the power of the additional (positive) lens increases. A differential involvements of right and left eyes is found also for the MS patient after unilateral ON attack shown in Fig. 5.

At last, the MS patient which Fig. 6 refers to, has had ON attacks in both eyes, at different times. Note that the isopter constriction as a function of defocus is the more severe the less recent the attack is.

Note that all the patients above exhibit a 10/10 visual acuity for far vision.

REFERENCES

1. Aulhorn, E. and Garms, H. Visual perimetry. In: Handbook of Sensory Physiol., Vol. VII/4, Visual Psychophysics (D. Jameson, L. M. Hurvich, eds.), Springer Verlag, Berlin, Ch. 5, pp. 113–115 (1972).
2. Fankhauser, F. and Enoch, J. M. The effects of blur upon perimetric threshold. Arch. Ophthalmol. 68:240 (1962).

Author's address:
Dr A. Serra
Dept. of Physiopathological Optics
University of Cagliari
Clinica Oculistica
Via Ospedale
I09100 Cagliari
Italy

VISUAL FIELD DEFECT IN THALAMIC HEMORRHAGE

SYUJI MAEDA, SUMIO USUBA, KEN NAGATA and
SHUICHI MATSUYAMA
(Hirosaki Isezaki, Japan)

Key words. Visual field defect, homonymous field defect, thalamic hemorrhage, cerebro-vascular accident.

ABSTRACT

The visual field was studied using the Goldmann perimeter in 35 cases of thalamic hemorrhage. A homonymous field defect was detected in 12 patients out of these 35 cases. The field defects were classified into four types according to the extent of the defect. Grade I: minimal homonymous defect of the inner isopters in the inferior quadrants, Grade II: homonymous wedge-shaped defect of the inner isopters in the inferior quadrant along the 270° meridian; Grade III: homonymous defect in the inferior quadrant with a wedge-shaped defect of V_4 isopter along the 270° meridian; Grade IV: complete homonymous hemianopia.

A homonymous inferior wedge-shaped defect was thought to be characteristic of a visual field change in thalamic hemorrhage.

INTRODUCTION

Thalamic hemorrhage (TH) is not an uncommon disease, forming about 30% of cerebral hemorrhage. Although there are few reports on the visual field defect in TH and it has been reported that TH can be a cause of contralateral homonymous field defect (2), no reference has been made to the type of the field defect in the cases of TH. In this report, the type of visual field defect in TH were dealt with.

MATERIAL AND METHOD

Out of 430 cases of cerebro-vascular accident who were consulted in Mihara Memorial Hospital and Reimeikyo Rehabilitation Hospital between August 1979 and October 1981, 35 cases of TH were subjected for this study.

Patients in whom precise perimetry was unable to be carried out because of poor general or mental conditions were excluded from this study. There were 23 males and 12 females. Their age distribution was between 45 and 76 years (59 years in average). The period from the onset to this examination was as follows. Nine cases were examined within 6 months after the onset, 10 cases between 6 and 12 months and 12 cases more than 1 year later. In 4 cases the period was unknown. Intracranial complications besides TH were cerebral aneurysm, vertebro-basilar insufficiency, contralateral cerebral infarction and contralateral putaminal hemmorhage.

Prior to the visual field examination, other ophthalmological examinations were made to exclude the field defect due to intraocular causes. Then V_4, I_3, I_2 and I_1 isopters were checked as a standard examination using the Goldmann perimeter. In some cases we could not accomplish the standard perimetry because of poor comprehension and cooperation of the patients. For these patients we applied an expedient technique, by making the patient to look straight ahead in the dome of the Goldmann perimeter and then moving the target centripetally from his anopic field. If the patient recognizes the target, then he turns his eye to the target and this point was taken as an isopter.

RESULTS

On ophthalmological examinations intraocular disorders were found in 4 cases out of 35 of TH; aphakic eyes with or without retinal detachment, corneal leukoma and papilloedema. We could not carry out standard Goldmann perimetry on one third of the patients because of their poor comprehension but employed the above-mentioned expedient technique, judging the patient's eye movement.

As a result, 12 cases (34%) out of 35 cases of TH were proved to have homonymous field defect corresponding to TH. Another two cases, one having concurrent contralateral cerebral infarction and another having concurrent contralateral putaminal hemorrhage, were also proved to have homonymous field defect corresponding to the lesions. Non-homonymous types of field defect were observed in four cases; irregular contraction in the case of retinal detachment, arcuate scotoma due to glaucoma, concentric contraction in two cases of optic atrophy following papilloedema.

These field defects due to TH could be classified into four types according to the extent of the defect (Fig. 1 and Table 1).

Grade I. Minimal homonymous defect of inner isopters in the inferior quadrant. V_4 isopter is intact.

Grade II. Homonymous wedge-shaped defect of the inner isopters along the 270° meridian with minimal depression of V_4 isopter.

Grade III. Marked homonymous wedge-shaped defect of V_4 isopter along the 270° meridian with sharp border in the inferior quadrant but minimal changes in the upper quadrant.

Grade IV. Typical and complete homonymous hemianopia.

There were 3 cases of Grade I, 4 cases of Grade II, 4 cases of Grade III,

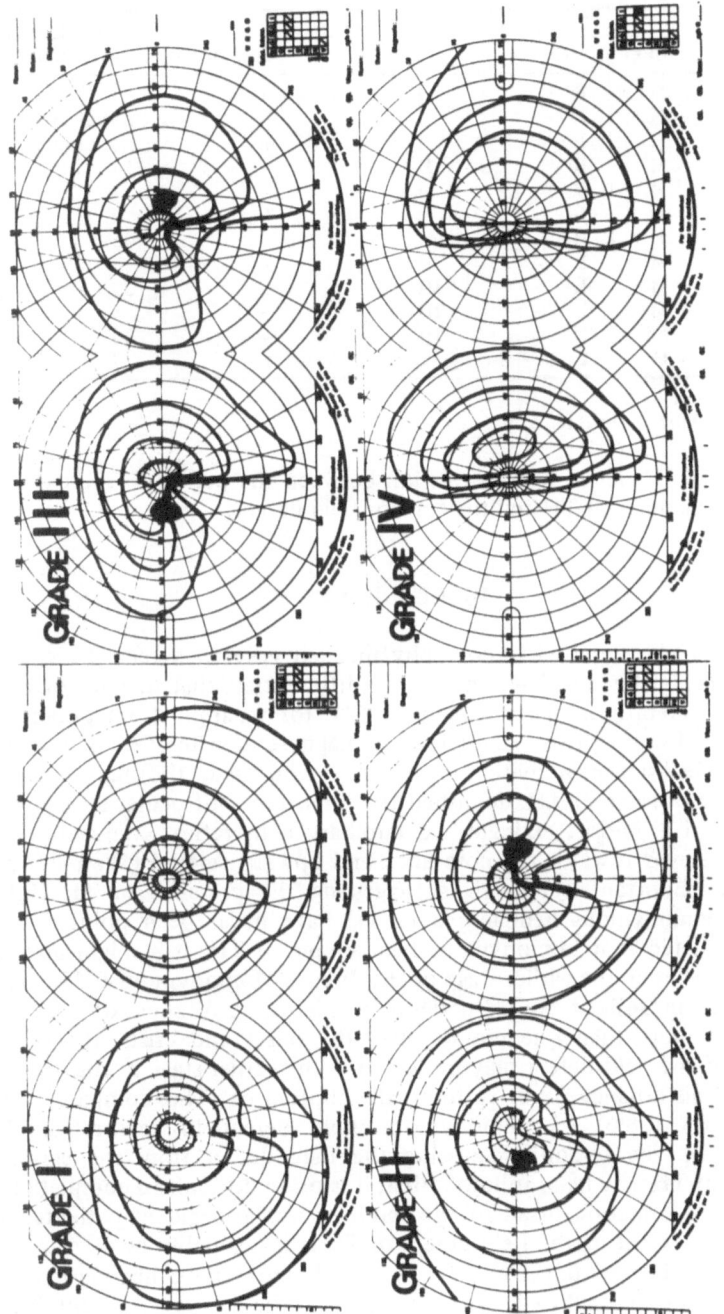

Fig. 1. Typical visual field defect in the cases of thalamic hemorrhage: Grade I (case 1), Grade II (case 4), Grade III (case 8) and Grade IV (case 12).

297

Table 1. Cases of thalamic haemorrhage with homonymous field defect.

Case	Age	Sex	Side of the VFD[a]	Grade of the VFD[a]	Congruity	Period from the onset (month)
1	63	M	R	I	—	3
2	55	F	L	I	—	not clear
3	54	F	L	I	+	not clear
4	45	M	R	II	—	19
5	67	M	R	II	—	2
6	63	F	L	II	?[b]	4
7	58	F	R	II	—	45
8	68	M	L	III	+	8
9	55	M	L	III	+	27
10	73	M	L	III	—	1
11	71	F	R	III	—	30
12	46	F	L	IV	+	7

[a] Visual field defect.
[b] Complicated with corneal leukoma.

and 1 case of IV. There was no relation between the period to the examination from the onset of TH and the type of field defect.

DISCUSSION

Development of computed tomography made it easy to detect the site of minute intracranial hemorrhage and easy to differentiate thalamic hemorrhage from other cerebro-vascular accident (6,10), for example from putaminal hemorrhage. However, it is still difficult to diagnose the site of lesion only by physical or bed-side examination. Fisher (2), who made thorough examinations on many cases of TH, described the importance of ocular signs in the diagnosis of TH. Miosis, extinguished pupillary light reflex, conjugate deviation of the eyes towards the nose apex and upward vertical gaze palsy are said to be important ocular signs suggesting the presence of TH (7,9). However, homonymous hemianopia in TH have never been pointed out. Fisher postulated that homonymous hemianopia in TH, if it might appear, disappear quickly in the earlier stage of the disease. Homonymous field defect was detected in 34% of 35 TH patients in this study. As most of the cases have passed more than one month after the onset and crisis, the actual incidence of the field defect may be higher in the earlier stage of the disease. Visual field disturbance is not an unusual symptom of TH as compared with the incidence (28%) of homonymous field defect in cerebro-vascular accidents (5). The reason of missing the field defect from the cardinal symptoms of TH may be as follows. First, it is often difficult to complete the visual field examination in all of the cerebro-vascular accident patients and secondly, the extent of the field defect in TH is too small to be detected by brief method. Except one case of complete homonymous hemianopia, all other cases showed small wedge-shaped defects in the inferior quadrant. They might be overlooked if we had employed brief visual field testing, i.e. confrontation or cup perimetry.

The thalamus is not a part of the main visual pathway (4). While it is located adjacent to the optic tract, lateral geniculate body and optic radiation, the field defect observed in TH cases is not due to direct effect of thalamic lesion but due to the disorders in visual pathway secondary to TH. With the exception of the area of the lateral geniculate body, upper retinal fibers remain upper, and lower retinal fibers remain lower throughout the visual pathway. In the geniculate body, the upper part of the retinal fibers, which corresponds to the lower part of the visual field, rotates through $90°$ inwards and faces the thalamus (4). This anatomical basis explains the fact that a homonymous visual field defect appeared in the inferior quadrant in these cases.

An incongruous homonymous field defect was found in seven cases. This is thought to be characteristic of the lesion in the lateral geniculate body and optic tract (3). However, it is difficult to explain why only the nasal portion (corresponding to the upper half of the retinal fibers) of the lateral geniculate body is involved, in spite of a very concentrated accumulation of fibers in this small area. Considering this accumulation of the fibers of visual pathways in this very small area and no detection of bilateral optic pallor (optic tract atrophy) which is characterized by ipsilateral temporal pallor and contralateral 'band pallor' (8), it was suggested that the lesion in visual pathway in the cases of TH was located in optic radiation near the lateral geniculate body.

The extent of the field defect which was classified into four grades (Fig. 1), therefore, might reveal the degree of secondary effect of TH on the visual pathway.

In Grades I and II, the defect of inner isopters was more prominent than that of V_4 isopter. This finding corresponds with Blum's opinion (1) that emphasized the importance of changes in the central field on visual field examination.

REFERENCES

1. Blum, F. G. et al. How important are peripheral fields? Arch. Ophthalmol. 61:1−8 (1959).
2. Fisher, C. M. The pathologic and clinical aspects of thalamic hemorrhage. Trans. Am. Neurol. Ass. 84:56−59 (1959).
3. Gunderson, C. H. and Hoyt, W. F. Geniculate hemianopia: incongruous homonymous field defects in two patients with partial lesions of the lateral geniculate nucleus. J. Neurol. Neurosurg. Psychiat. 34:1−6 (1971).
4. Harrington, D. O. The Visual Fields, pp. 66−84. Mosby, St. Louis (1976).
5. Maeda, S. et al. Visual field investigation in cerebrovascular accident. Doc. Ophthalmol. Proc. Series 26:351−357 (1981).
6. Miura, N. et al. A study of hypertensive intracerebral hemorrhage (II)-sequential CT examination and classification. Neurological Surgery 6:635−645 (1978).
7. Mizukami, M. et al. The thalamic hemorrhage − the classification and the clinical pictures. Brain and Nerve 27:195−206 (1975).
8. Savino, P. J. et al. Optic tract syndrome. Arch. Ophthalmol. 96:656−663 (1978).
9. Shizuka, M. et al. Ocular sign in thalamic hemorrhage. Jap. Rev. Clin. Ophthalmol. 74:745−749 (1980).

10. Walshe, T. M. et al. Thalamic hemorrhage: a computed tomographic-clinical correlation. Neurology 27:217–222 (1977).

Author's address:
Dr S. Maeda
Dept. of Ophthalmology
Hirosaki University School of Medicine
5 Zaifu-cho
Hirosaki 036
Japan

300

DISCUSSIONS

Discussion on 'Visual fields versus visual evoked potentials in optic nerve disorders', by T. Ohnuma, Y. Tagami and Y. Isayama.

H. Bynke: Your results are consistent with those of other authors. As a matter of fact the general opinion is that VEPs are more sensitive than perimetry for detecting functional loss in recovered optic neuritis. On the other hand Van Dalen, Spekreyse and Greve have shown that static perimetry is at least as good as pattern VEPs. So there is some disagreement on this point. These divergent results may possibly be ascribed to the methods used. Do you have any comments?

T. Ohnuma: The latency of the checkerboard pattern reversal VEP was not correlated with the static visual field. And our results also showed significant delay of the latency in patients with definite MS in spite of their relatively good static fields. So I think that both VEP and visual fields are necessary for assessing functional losses and predicting the prognosis in optic neuropathies.

H. Bynke: Thank you, and therefore my next question to Dr Bodis-Wollner is, what do you think had happened if we had used your gratings for the VEPs. Would this method have been superior to every visual field examination or what do you think?

I. Bodis-Wollner: Well, I can just echo again the importance of stimulus specification of the human visual system. In the Tübingen perimeter you were using 7' of arc targets. In your study, the VEP check size was 50'. So we are dealing here with apples and pears.

J. L. Keltner: We have found with static automated visual field testing in patients with optic neuritis, that they frequently have 'popcorn fields'. They are multiple missed static spot checks seen more easily on automated perimeters than on kinetic testing because of stato-kinetic dissociation. Certain investigators have felt that the visual fields in patients with optic neuritis have a 'Swiss cheese' type of appearance with multiple holes of a shallow nature. This is confirmed by automated static perimetry.

H. Bynke: Yes, it is an interesting question. Maybe we can be helped out by our educator once again.

I. Bodis-Wollner. Obviously relevant, it is not just an empirical approach we adopted. These patterns looked annoying enough nevertheless single cell physiologists over the last 15 years have been experimenting and trying to find out how neurons along the visual pathway respond best, what kind of stimulus they like. In the early studies of the retina they used spots. Round, spot-like stimuli fit well into the receptive field sampled by retinal ganglion cells, that is also true for the lateral geniculate. So spots or, at crude approximation, checks would fit in nicely. However, in the visual cortex, as a common output for all these observations for the psychophysical and visual evoked potentials, the neurons are not so organized. DeValois and his colleagues directly compared, for instance, the responses of cortical neurons to checkerboard patterns and sinusoidal gratings. Do you remember, I showed you a slide for illustrating that if you were to put together a checkerboard pattern of sinusoidal gratings you would need many, in different orientations. You can logically make the converse step and that is what DeValois did. He compared the checkerboard pattern and the sinusoidal grating response of single cortical neurons and asked: Could I predict, based on the checkerboard response, what kind of a grating this cell would like, and conversely, given the grating response, could I predict how I should rotate my checkerboard pattern and what type of check should I use? And the answer was that he could completely predict each response based on the assumption that what a neuron of the cortex sees from a checkerboard pattern is a single spatial frequency component of that complex pattern. So the reason why sinusoidal gratings are being used is that, after all, the pathway is coming here to the cortex, and by the time we decide seeing something or not, it has to pass through this stage, what some people consider a crucial stage of filtering.

However, clinically we can compare pattern ERGs with pattern VEPs and that I think, is a very good place to start human research. It would be scientifically and clinically very relevant to compare checks and gratings there, too.

Discussion on 'Homonymous quadrantanopia in a case of multiple sclerosis', by K. A. Hellner, K. U. Hamann, W. Jensen and A. Müller-Jensen.

B. R. Younge: Do you state that the field defects represented here are the results of an optic radiation injury?

K. A. Hellner: Certainly, the shape of the visual field defect suggests a lesion in the right parietal lobe. The pupillography proves that the lesion is within the optic radiation.

H. Bynke: I think that the pupillomotor perimetry is a very interesting method. It was detected or worked out by Professor Harms several years ago and in a previous paper you and Dr Jensen demonstrated that in infrageniculate lesions you have very good agreement between the common fields and the results of your method but in suprageniculate lesions there was not such a good correspondence.

K. A. Hellner: First pupillomotor perimetry was done by Harms about 40 years ago, but only under the observation of the naked eye. Alexandridis developed infrared pupillography using large spots. Harms later on used this method. The differences of the methods used are responsible for the discrepancies encountered.

Discussion on 'Carotid perfusion and field loss', by V. J. Marmion and M. Aldoori.

I. Bodis-Wollner: What is the incidence of carotid plaques in an age-matched, non-glaucomatous normal population?

V. J. Marmion: We don't have any control groups for this but what we do have is control of the examination using angiography as a method of determining that this was a satisfactory method of examination. The pathological reports we referred to covered something like 2000 routine autopsies in an age-matched population and in that the level of plugs at the carotid bifurcation was less than 10% and our figures for plugs are considerably higher than that.

S. S. Hayreh: Am I right in saying that you're telling that there were disc changes in these patients we've just seen?

V. J. Marmion: No, you aren't. There weren't disc changes in all patients. What we have not done so far is to analyze the correlation of disc changes and the presence of carotid lesions.

Discussion on 'Anterior ischemic optic neuropathy and associated visual field changes', by K. Lao

H. Bynke: In our experience in Europe the central visual field area is often spared and it appears to me that many of the defects are very similar to what we call glaucoma. But I would like to hear the master of this field, Dr Hayreh.

S. S. Hayreh: There are a certain number of very distinctive differences. I have about 400 patients with AION whom we have studied prospectively and we find that the pattern that we have is very different from that recorded by Dr Lao. Regarding the age profile I have some persons in the early twenties but mostly this is a disease of people sixty years old and over in this country, and in Britain I saw more or less the same distribution. The only thing is that the diabetics are the people who get it at an early age, so that most of the younger group in my collection are patients with diabetes. Regarding the visual acuity, in fact four years ago I presented a paper at the Perimetric Society meeting in Tokyo dealing with visual acuity and field defects in AION. In that analysis we found that the visual acuity in about 40% of the patients was 20/40 or better whereas the rest of the patients had worse vision than that. Some even had a visual acuity of counting fingers. No doubt up to about 40–50% can have pretty good vision. This is a very important fact. Most neurologists and ophthalmologists have a very big misconception that when a person gets AION he has to be stone blind. However, on the whole, the visual acuity in the American patient is much better than what Dr Lao has pointed out. Regarding the visual field I have reported, 4 years ago, that 3 types of visual field defects are common. With a larger target you get inferior nasal quadrantic defects, absolutely classical. With a small target, it is inferior altitudinal hemianopia. Also, central scotoma is a very common defect, which Dr Lao's patients did not have. This is surprising because in numerous studies it has been shown to be one of the most common visual field defects, which distinguishes AION from glaucoma. On the whole, there are quite a number of differences between Dr Lao's series and ours. Whether the Chinese have a different disease or a different response is difficult to say.

J. L. Keltner: I was pleased to hear Dr Katherine Lao's paper from Beijing, China. Dr Lao has recognized that often this condition is misdiagnosed in China and felt to represent a more serious neurologic condition. Certainly in the United States in the last 20 years AION has finally been recognized clinically, where prior to that time it was frequently misdiagnosed as it has been in China.

I do have some questions about the cases on which she reports and whether, indeed, all of these patients would fall under the category of patients we describe in the United States as AION. Unfortunately, Dr Lao did not present fluorescein angiography or fundus photography pictures to confirm if indeed all of her cases, particularly in the younger age groups, truly represent AION. Even in the western literature today, the exact etiology of AION is still somewhat of an enigma even though we call it a 'vascular abnormality'.

Previously in the literature, the incidence of giant cell arteritis has been reported to be low in Chinese and in blacks. Dr Lao did not report any cases of giant cell arteritis in her series, but I did not see any evidence that temporal artery biopsies were performed in any of her patients. There is such a large number of patients in the younger age group with such well-preserved visual acuity, I almost question whether indeed these patients are truly AION or an optic neuropathy from another cause. While the author states that the sed rate was greater than 30 mm/hour in two patients, she does not state whether sedimentation rates were obtained in all the patients nor what laboratory tests were performed.

Dr Lao is to be commended for this study which was performed with a minimum of equipment. We will look forward to future communications from Beijing, China, about AION and hopefully in the future, fluorescein angiography as well as fundus photography will help to document these changes which Dr Lao has described.

I am wondering, Dr Lao, have you found biopsy-proven giant cell arteritis in China?

K. Lao: We never see it.

J. L. Keltner: You don't see it. Do you biopsy the temporal artery at all in China for temporal arteritis?

K. Lao: No we do not, but we also do not see the symptoms of it.

J. L. Keltner: No symptoms of joint pain or headaches, etc., very interesting. Thank you, Dr Lao.

F. Dannheim: The term quadranopic or hemianopic field defect should be reserved for defects due to lesions in the central visual pathways and not be used for definite nerve fiber bundle defects with predominant location in one or two quadrants of the field, as shown by Dr Lao.

H. Bynke: Yes, I agree completely on this point. Well, many things in the world are getting more and more monotonous and uniform, and I think we are happy that there are still differences between China and the U.S. and Europe.

Discussion on 'Properties of scotomata in glaucoma and optic nerve disease: computer analysis', by C. A. Johnson and J. L. Keltner.

C. D. Phelps: This type of study is very important for the derivation of screening strategies, but it has two limitations that must be kept in mind. First, the frequency with which certain parts of the field are found to be abnormal in various diseases depends solely on the screening strategies that were employed by the perimetrists who obtained the visual field data. If, for example, the perimetrists collecting the original data think that the temporal visual field is never involved by glaucoma, they will not look for temporal field defects, they will not find these defects, and the summated field data will show no temporal field defects in glaucoma. A screening strategy based on this summated data would not include a search for temporal field defects, and the failure to find such defects would be perpetuated.

Secondly, the study by Drs Johnson and Keltner looked only at scotomas and not at isopter-related defects. Thus, for example, it does not include peripheral nasal steps among the glaucomatous defects. A screening strategy based solely on the results of their study might therefore fail to search for nasal defects.

B. Schwartz: We may be confronting a philosophical or ethical problem in revising strategies to obtain the maximum efficiency with automated perimetry. If we limit ourselves to testing the central field, we will miss patients with glaucoma and neurological disease who have peripheral field defects. These defects are relatively common in glaucomatous patients and, apparently, relatively rare in neurological patients. However, detection would be important for diagnosis for the one patient, perhaps out of one hundred, with a peripheral defect.

Obviously, we want the greatest cost effectiveness for our visual field techniques. However, we have to provide some means for diagnosing the rare or unusual patient. To obviate this problem, I suggest that, besides detailed central visual field examinations, we incorporate a screening program that encompasses the peripheral fields.

General discussion

H. Bynke: I have a question to Dr Younge. You have used the Octopus now in neuro-ophthalmology cases and I read a paper written by you about two years ago about your first experiences. If I am right it was your suggestion that peripheral programmes were less interesting with the Octopus than central programmes. Do you use only central programmes now or do you always start with the whole examination?

B. R. Younge: We have a lot of experience now with neuro-ophthalmology cases and the Octopus perimeter. It is true that probably 95% of the patients that we do perimetry on, we only do central field examination. The problem is that once you got your screening test of 5–7 minutes done you really want to know what the details are. The most interesting part of the visual field in neuro-ophthalmology is generally speaking the $30°$ central field. I don't like to say that the peripheral field is not important because it certainly is and there are illustrations anybody can bring forward that will show the utility or importance of doing a peripheral visual field, but it is true that most of the visual fields we do, are the $30°$ central programmes. We also use programme 11 which is an extremely sensitive programme for optic nerve diseases. It is as good as anything you can put together in any combination: colour vision. VERs, gratings. That one test alone is probably the best thing the machine has done for us in optic nerve diseases alone.

H. Bynke: Thank you and my next question is to Drs Johnson and Keltner: you demonstrated the extension of the scotomata in optic nerve disease in MS cases and you mentioned that they were often small and round. When we use the Competer we often see scattered scotomata, and although the old idea of central scotomata is true, we know something more now. In cases of slight optic neuropathy due to MS and good vision we often see scattered scotomata over the central field. I think you can agree with that point. Sometimes we also know that homonymous defects exist in MS. I see them 2 or 3 times a year and sometimes I wonder if these defects could be due to suprageniculate lesions. Dr Bodis-Wollner didn't your notches demonstrate that the lesions in MS were often suprageniculate?

I. Bodis-Wollner: Those notches were actually found by Regan. The orientation selective losses are almost compelling to be put in the visual cortex,

306

where as far as we know in primates, is the only place where orientation selection is established. I am afraid this finding is a little bit surprising, it has however been confirmed by totally independent methods, both by Regan and by our laboratories using VEP.

J. D. Trobe: Chris Johnson is very surprised at the low sensitivity for defects. You may say it is not representative and I am happy to agree with you if you were right. But you are not. I shall try to explain to you why. But let me be certain we are all using the same vocabulary. For me a hemianopic defect is one in which there is a difference in threshold across the vertical meridian. Not across the horizontal meridian, and so on. That has nothing to do with nerve fiber bundle defects. We watched the perimetrists while doing their examination and we tried to do the best we could to figure out why they were so insensitive. It is simple. Everybody does glaucoma fields. They don't know about the vertical meridian. They don't see patients with vertical defects. The vast majority of fields that they do are on ocular hypertensives and glaucoma. They are turned to the nerve fiber bundle defects which of course don't stop at the vertical meridians. So that is my explanation. We have not followed these perimetrists to see whether the new information that they learned made them any better. That is another question.

E. L. Greve: I think that the conclusion could be, instead of visual field examination not being important, that you should train your technicians and that is a different conclusion.

J. D. Trobe: I hope you didn't misunderstood me. I would certainly agree with you that there are obviously two answers to this. I am just showing you what exists. The conclusion that you draw from it that if you train people the results will be better, cost a lot of money. I am not sure that training a technician is as cost effective.

S. M. Drance: I want to make a couple of comments. The first one is that I don't think that Dr Trobe needs to apologize for his technicians because they do glaucoma work. It is a question of training technicians. I think that the question you asked: technicians or automatic perimetry is something we have to address ourselves to pretty soon. Actually it may well be that the judgement is already made and we will address ourselves after the fact. But the question that I would like to ask the neuro-ophthalmologists is: when Younge for instance is being pressed by the question of Bynke: you have only shown central fields in neurological cases and what about the peripheral field, is bound to be better in addition to a central field. There is nothing else he could say.

J. D. Trobe: May I make a point to both glaucoma and neurological fields. What we need to do is to get enough stimuli where they are going to be cost effective because time is finite. I would like to suggest something like a non-symmetric or parabolic-type of field representation which was also mentioned by Dr Dannheim. It would be very important to adopt something like that at this stage when automatic perimetry is becoming more popular.

J. L. Keltner: Now in glaucoma work I have chosen for myself that I would never go without the peripheral field. You may miss whatever it is, 10%, 9%, but I think in neuro-ophthalmological work you practically never miss anything if you don't do the peripheral field. I would like the neuro-ophthalmologists to respond to this because it has practical implications. Why should we do a peripheral field in neuro-ophthalmology for diagnostic purposes if in fact this is such a waste of time.

H. Bynke: This is a very important question. Yes, we miss some cases, even in neuro-ophthalmology but there are not so many. About 1% or something like that. You have that problem in glaucoma and we have that problem. Topographical diagnosis. For this I feel that at least I need a periphery in about 20% of all my cases.

E. L. Greve: What about progression? Do you really feel you can do without the periphery for establishing progression?

H. Bynke: I think for detection it is nearly what we want. We don't need the periphery very much for detection nor for follow-up.

CLINICAL EXPERIENCES WITH
A NEW AUTOMATED PERIMETER 'PERITEST'

FRITZ DANNHEIM
(Hamburg FRG)

Key words. Perimetry, automation.

ABSTRACT

The Peritest performs an automated or semi-automated visual field examination in 206 positions by LEDs. The gradient-adapted target luminances are
0.6 log units above the individual threshold, which is first evaluated in representative locations. A further assessment of thresholds in defective areas is
printed out with grey scale symbols. The detection rate of the Peritest turned
out to be superior to that of conventional manual perimetry, and comparable
with the one of the Octopus computer perimeter.

INTRODUCTION

The Peritest had been evaluted in clinical trials with satisfying results (1,2,4).
This further study was carried out to assess the performance in comparison
with conventional kinetic and computerized static perimetry.

MATERIAL AND METHOD

236 eyes of 130 patients from 10 to 77 years of age have been examined with
the *Peritest*, 1/3 with the automated, 2/3 with the manual, semi-automated
mode. Details of the test strategy are given elsewhere (1,4,5). The diagnosis
was chronic glaucoma (65 eyes), lesions of the intracranial visual pathways
(50 eyes), other lesions of the optic nerve (36 eyes), retinal and choroidal
disease (30 eyes), other disorders (12 eyes), and no abnormalities (45 eyes).

The visual fields of 124 eyes could be compared with conventional kinetic
fields, with fields of the Octopus 201 perimeter, or with both.

The *kinetic fields* where retrospectively evaluated from the patients'
files and had been plotted on Goldmann perimeters by residents without
knowledge of any other perimetric findings. A conventional but not standardized technique with 2—5 isopters was used.

Greve, E. L., Heijl, A. (eds.) Fifth International Visual Field Symposium.
©1983 Dr W. Junk Publishers, The Hague/Boston/Lancaster.

For the *Octopus fields* different programs had been applied: the scanning programs 03 and 07, and programs 31–34 and 44.

Manual kinetic and computerized static perimetry cannot directly be correlated. The comparison was thus limited to the statement whether or not the defects were found with roughly adequate position, size and depth. Differing findings between the Peritest and manual kinetic perimetry were reexamined with the Octopus, whenever possible. All defective fields were arbitrarily divided into two groups according to the severity of defects in the Peritest fields.

COMPARISON WITH KINETIC PERIMETRY

A. *Unaffected fields*: 34 eyes had corresponding results, 4 eyes misleading kinetic fields (false defects or refractional defects).

B. *Moderate disturbance*: 14 eyes showed corresponding results, 19 eyes significantly less or no defects in kinetic perimetry (Fig. 1).

C. *Severe disturbance*: 22 eyes had corresponding results, 11 eyes significantly less or no defects in kinetic perimetry.

COMPARISON WITH OCTOPUS COMPUTER PERIMETER

A. *Unaffected fields*: 10 eyes had corresponding results, 2 eyes showed no blind spot in the Octopus field due to an inappropriate distribution of targets.

B. *Moderate disturbance*: 16 eyes had corresponding results (Fig. 1), 1 eye presented an inadequately mild central scotoma due to optic neuritis in the Octopus field.

C. *Severe disturbance*: all 32 eyes showed corresponding results.

CONCLUSIONS

The clinical trial revealed some favorable features:

Programs: small number and easy choice, stepwise increasing spatial resolution and/or accuracy of threshold assessment. Distribution of targets optimal both for nerve fiber defects and lesions of the central visual pathways.

Automated mode: simple operation, relatively quick examination, which can be followed on an LED monitor, interrupted, and manually continued.

Manual, computer-assisted mode: very fast in nearly normal fields. Reasonable performance in patients with limited cooperation, when no automated test is tolerated. Simple re-test in questionable findings.

310

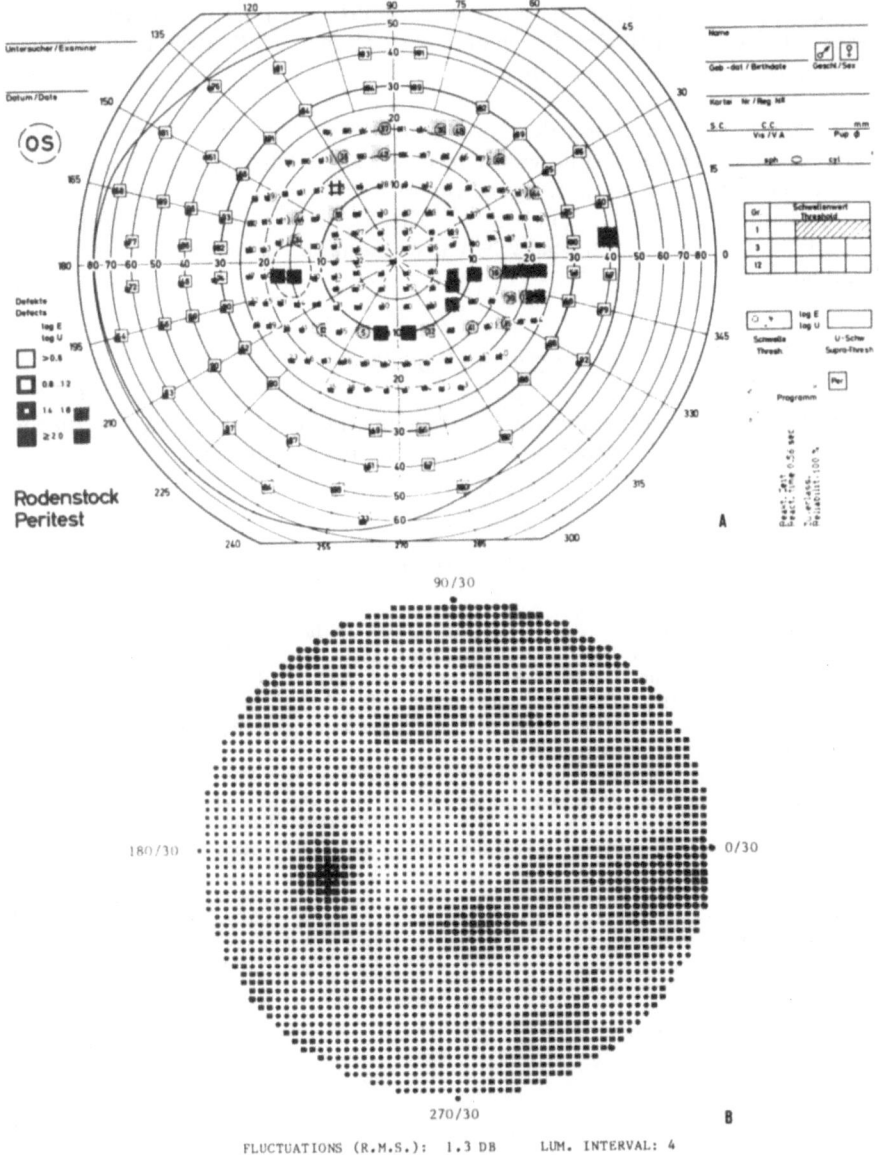

FLUCTUATIONS (R.M.S.): 1.3 DB   LUM. INTERVAL: 4

Fig. 1. Left visual field in chronic glaucoma. Relatively dense and circumscript arcuate defect inferiorly, minimal depression superiorly. Similar findings for Peritest, whole field (a), and Octopus, program 32 (b). Manual kinetic visual field inconspicuous (not presented).

Printout: grey scale symbols only in defects easy to interpret. Non-linear scale for eccentricity with good resolution of the central field, and whole field on one graph (3), see pp. 217–220 of this volume.

311

Comparison with conventional manual perimetry: manual test dependent on the skill of the operator. In general performance of Peritest far superior, especially in eyes with moderate disturbance.

Comparison with Octopus: detection rate of both instruments comparable. The Octopus has more abilities for refined assessment and graphical display of defects, provided ample time for the examination; a permanent storage of data facilitates statistical calculations. The Peritest, however, is superior in visual field screening, especially when examination time or cooperation is limited.

ACKNOWLEDGEMENT

The author, who was involved in the development of the Peritest, is thankful for some technical assistance provided by the manufacturer, Rodenstock Instruments, in preparation of the poster.

REFERENCES

1. Greve, E. L. and Bakker, D. Some possibilities of the Peritest automatic and semi-automatic perimeter. Doc. Ophthalmol. Proc. Series 35:313–321 (1983).
2. Dannheim, F. Zur Anwender-Software für die neuen Rodenstock-Perimeter. B. Klinische Erfahrungen. Der Augenspiegel 28:60–74 (1982).
3. Dannheim, F. Non-linear projection in visual field charting. Doc. Ophthalmol. Proc. Series 35:217–220 (1983)
4. Greve, L. E., Dannheim, F. and Bakker, D. The Peritest, a new automatic and semi-automatic perimeter. Internat. Ophthalmol. 5:201–214 (1982).
5. Guilino, G. Zur Anwender-Software für die neuen Rodenstock-Perimeter. A. Konzept des (Glaukom-) Untersuchungsprogramms. Der Augenspiegel 28:47–58 (1982).

Author's address:
Dr F. Dannheim
Dept. of Ophthalmology
Eye Clinic of the University of Hamburg
Martinistr. 52
D-2000 Hamburg 20, FRG

SOME POSSIBILITIES OF THE PERITEST AUTOMATIC AND SEMI-AUTOMATIC PERIMETER

ERIK L. GREVE and DOUWE BAKKER

(Amsterdam, The Netherlands)

Key words. Automated perimetry, visual field examination, glaucoma.

ABSTRACT

The Peritest is a computer-assisted perimeter which purposely offers the possibility of both automatic and semi-automatic examination modes. A fast multiple-stimulus screening is possible next to extensive automatic assessment. The instrument uses LEDs for the 206 stimuli, of which 151 are located within $25°$ eccentricity. The examination strategy uses the system of threshold-related suprathreshold presentations. The assessment phase may use 0.2 or 0.6 log unit steps. The progress of the examination can be followed on a LED monitor. The experience of over 800 examinations with the Peritest has shown that the instrument is able to do a relatively quick examination with reproducible results. The examination time varies from 4 minutes for a semi-automatic screening to 15 minutes for a completely automatic detection and assessment. The detection rate is better than that of classical kinetic perimetry. This is demonstrated by the fact that 70% of early glaucomatous defects which are usually overlooked by kinetic perimetry are detected. The non-interpolated grey scale printout on a special chart demonstrates the configuration of defects satisfactorily and makes comparison with classical kinetic perimetry possible. The defect volume in separate areas of the visual field or in the whole visual field can be easily expressed in numbers. With some precautions this could be used for describing changes in the visual field.

DESCRIPTION

The Peritest is a new automatic and semi-automatic perimeter which aims at a fast and efficient detection and assessment of visual field defects. First descriptions of the apparatus have been given by Greve et al. (8, 11). The technical data on the Peritest are given in Table 1 and the major points of the Peritest concept are given in Table 2. The Peritest uses light-emitting diodes (LEDs) as light sources and has a total of 206 stimulus positions of which

Table 1. Technical data of the Peritest.

Type	: hemispherical perimeter; radius 30 cm; separate operation desk
Background L	: 1 cd/m²
Stimuli	
L source	: light-emitting diodes; LED
L steps	: 0.2 log units
L range	: 3.0 log units (25° eccentricity)
colour	: peak at 560 mm
size	: 30'
duration	: 0.2 s
presentation automatic	: static, single stimulus
presentation semi-automatic	: static, single and multiple stimulus
positions	: fixed, reproducible
number and distribution	: see Figs. 2–4; total of 206; 151 positions inside 25° eccentricity including central stimulus; 55 positions in peripheral field; different positions for R and L eye.

Table 2. The Peritest concept.

1. Automatic and semi-automatic
2. Large number of stimulus positions → intermediate resolution
3. Large dynamic luminance range
4. INSC; fast detection strategy separating LRS-GRS
5. Intermediate assessment with 0.6 log unit steps or 0.2 log unit steps (threshold)
6. Continuous LED monitoring of performance
7. Special chart for both central and peripheral VF
8. Non-interpolated grey scale printout

151 are inside 25° eccentricity. This includes the measurement of central sensitivity. A choice has been deliberately made for an instrument that offers the possibilities for both automatic and semi-automatic visual field examination. The advantages of an additional semi-automatic, manual mode are presented in Table 3. In practice these possibilities have been proven to be very useful and valuable. A particularly interesting feature is the possibility to do a very fast multiple-stimulus detection. The manual mode can also be used if more extensive instruction is needed in cases of slow comprehension or in cases of simulation of aggravation. Aphakic patients have a peripheral threshold (without correction) that is higher than in phakic patients and comparatively higher than the central threshold (with correction). The points 5 to 9 of Table 3 deal with the possibility to check measurements of the automated examination. After any examination, whatever the instrument, there is a possibility of false and improbable responses. With the Peritest it is possible to check such cases in an easy and quick way.

In point 4 of Table 2 the examination strategy of the Peritest is mentioned. INSC stands for the measurement of the individual normal sensitivity curve. Details on this strategy have been described elsewhere (3,6,7,8,10,11). Briefly it means that first threshold measurements are performed on a few representative positions which are then followed by a fast detection at a 0.6 log unit suprathreshold level. Apart from having the advantage of being a

314

Table 3. Advantages of the possibility of an additional semi-automatic examination mode.

1. Multiple stimulus very fast detection
2. Instruction, slow comprehension
3. Simulation, aggravation
4. Periphery aphakes
5. Check isolated defects
6. Check isolated normal positions
7. Check improbable change
8. Check blind spot
9. Check INSC

rapid detection method, this strategy immediately separates local reduction of sensitivity (LRS) and general reductions of sensitivity (GRS) (6,9). The Peritest offers a possibility for assessment of defect intensity with steps of 0.6 or 0.2 log unit. The 0.2 luminance steps are also used for the threshold measurements of the INSC.

In our experience it is advantageous if the examiner can follow the progress

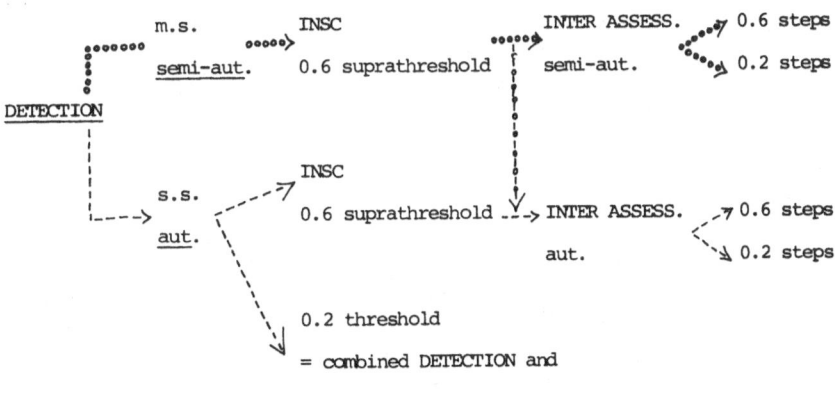

Fig. 1. Possibilities of the Peritest. In the detection phase the fast multiple stimulus semi-automatic mode (dotted line) may be used or the single-stimulus automatic mode (interrupted line). In the semi-automatic mode the INSC (Individual Normal Sensitivity Curve) is first determined, followed by 0.6 suprathreshold testing. After this threshold-related suprathreshold detection an Intermediate Assessment of defects can be done either with steps of 0.2 log unit or of 0.6 log unit. In the automatic mode either a similar threshold-related supradetection can be done or one can start immediately with threshold measurements at all selected positions (combined detection and intermediate assessment). After the suprathreshold detection phase an intermediate assessment can be done using 0.2 log unit or 0.6 log unit steps. The word Intermediate Assessment is used for an assessment phase using an intermediate resolution, arbitrarily 3° to 5°. The word limited assessment is used for an assessment phase with a resolution of 6° or more. In both cases the defect intensity measurements are done at the positions of the detection phase without extension. If a high resolution of 2° or less is used we speak of an extended assessment phase. In this case usually the high resolution is used in selected areas of the visual field at more positions than those of the detection phase. At present the commercially available Peritest does not have all of the above-mentioned possibilities.

315

of the examination continuously. In the case of the Peritest this possibility is given by a LED monitor. The Peritest presents the result on a specially developed chart, purposely using non-interpolated grey scales.

The possibilities of the Peritest are illustrated in Fig. 1. Basically one may choose between an automatic or a semi-automatic mode. Next one can choose between immediate threshold determinations or determination of the INSC followed by suprathreshold detection. Again the intermediate assessment (LA) can be done either automatically or semi-automatically, in steps of

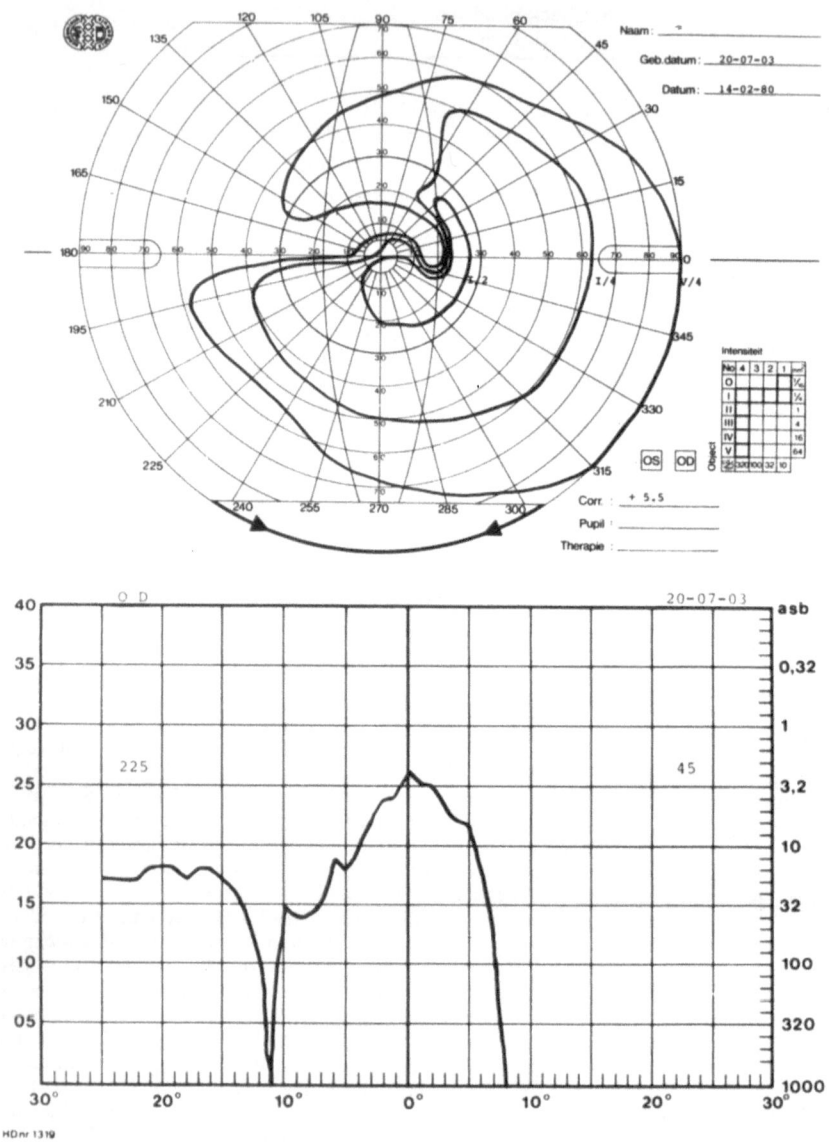

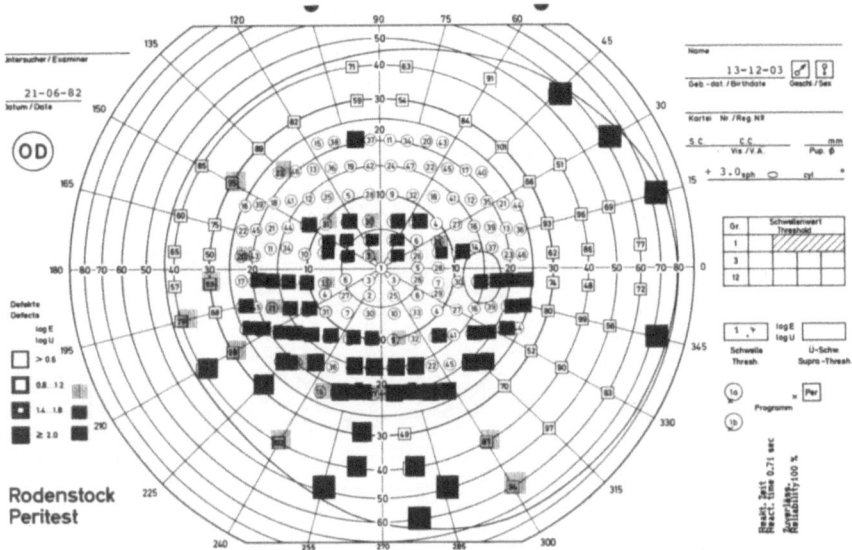

Fig. 2. Example of a male patient with low-tension glaucoma. There is a general reduction of sensitivity of 0.4 log unit, indicated in the rectangle in the middle right-hand side of the chart (Schwelle/Thresh.). The upper half of the visual field shows a large nerve fiber bundle defect for maximum luminance. The configuration of the defect can be easily compared to that of classical manual kinetic perimetry. The lower half of the visual field shows an early inferonasal defect. The Peritest result shows the inferonasal defect better than classical manual kinetic perimetry. Manual meridional static perimetry demonstrates a defect in the 225° meridian.

0.6 log unit or in steps of 0.2 log unit. The Peritest can and has been used for mass screening, routine detection, clinical detection and assessment, and follow-up examinations.

The performance of the Peritest has been tested in over 800 visual field examinations. The performance will be illustrated with two examples (Fig. 2 and Fig. 3). The results of visual field examination with the Peritest have been compared to classical kinetic and static perimetry and with automatic perimeters like the Octopus (4, 5) and Scoperimeter. A number of examinations with the Peritest has been done twice to test its reproducibility.

It is relatively easy to measure the volume of the defect from the Peritest result. The visual field is divided into several parts (Fig. 4): the central 25°' visual field is separated from the peripheral visual field, the upper half is separated from the lower half, finally the central measurement (cent.), the cecocentral measurements (ceco.) and the blind spot (bl. sp.) measurements are separated (Table 4). The INSC/threshold value is also recorded (thr.). The defect volume **(DV)** is calculated by adding the individual defect intensities. The DV is defect intensity x number of defect positions. A class I defect has an intensity of 12 tenth of a log unit (dB), a class II defect of 18 tenth of log unit and a class III defect of 24 tenth of a log unit. In the case of Fig. 3c the individual threshold is 0.4, the central threshold is 0.4; there is no defect

317

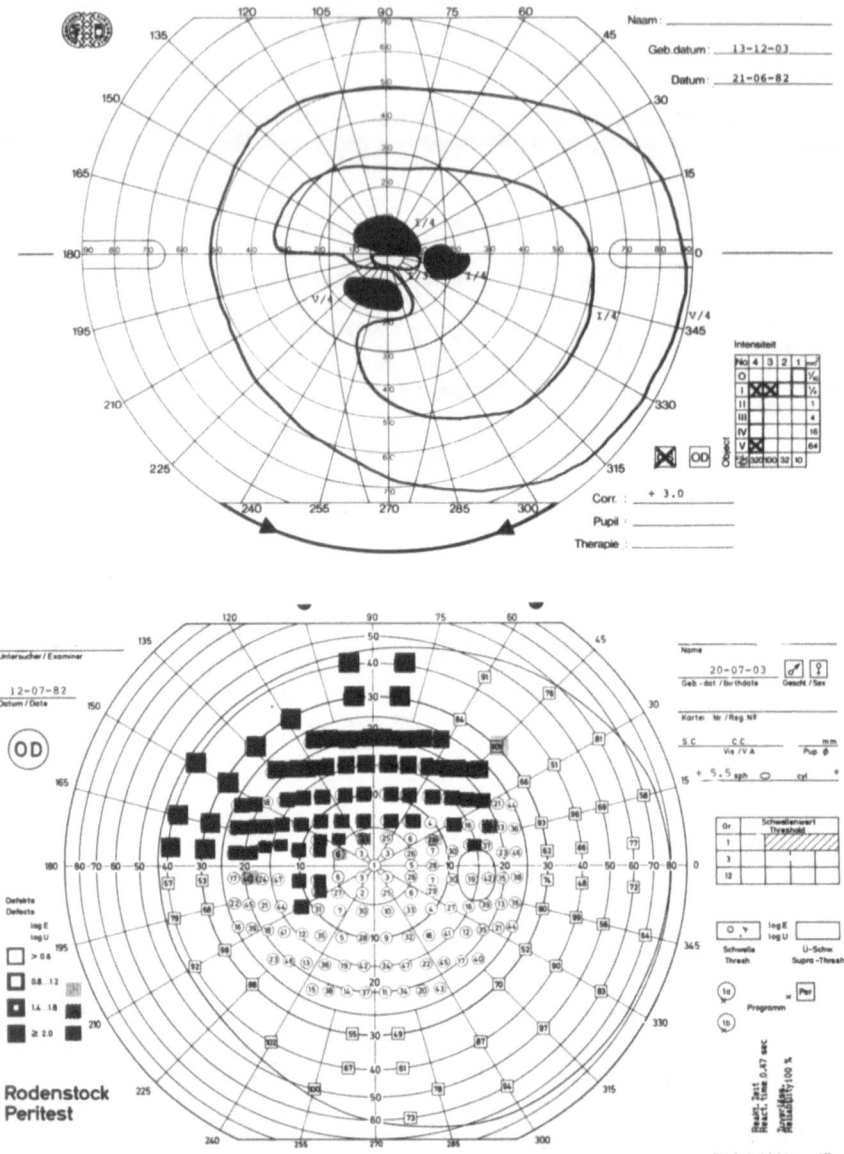

Fig. 3. Example of a male patient with glaucoma and cataract. There is a general reduction of sensitivity of 1.4 log unit. This demonstrates the large dynamic range of the Peritest and the effective functioning of this type of strategy which separates local reduction of sensitivity from general reduction of sensitivity. There is a large nerve fiber bundle defect in the lower half of the visual field with breakthrough into the nasal periphery. The configuration of the defect is well demonstrated as is the extension into the periphery. The upper half demonstrates a paracentral nerve fiber bundle defect. The defect is essentially the same as shown by kinetic perimetry, however the central visual field is shown better because of the enlargement of this part of the chart.

318

in the centrocecal area and the blind spot defect is 24. The defect in the upper half of the 25° visual field has a DV of 1308, etc. The total DV is 1734. If the eye is blind the total DV is 4944.

In the case of Fig. 2 (Table 4) 35% of the maximum possible DV is affected. This DV calculation does not give the number of defect positions. This could easily be added per visual field area including the average defect intensity per area. Finally if a number of measurements have been repeated the statistical variation of measurements and of the respective DV could be given.

DISCUSSION

Our experience has shown that the Peritest is able to do a quick and efficient automatic visual field examination, even in persons of over 90 years of age. The examination time is relatively short as compared to automatic perimeters that perform at the same level (4,5). The usual examination time for a semi-automatic detection phase in normal or almost normal visual field is 4 minutes. The usual examination time for the automatic mode in the presence of substantial visual field defects is 15 minutes.

It is our experience that the INSC-suprathreshold strategy is reproducible and that this strategy also functions in the presence of central defects or central islands in glaucoma. The strategy and the large dynamic range function especially well in cases where a large general reduction of sensitivity is caused

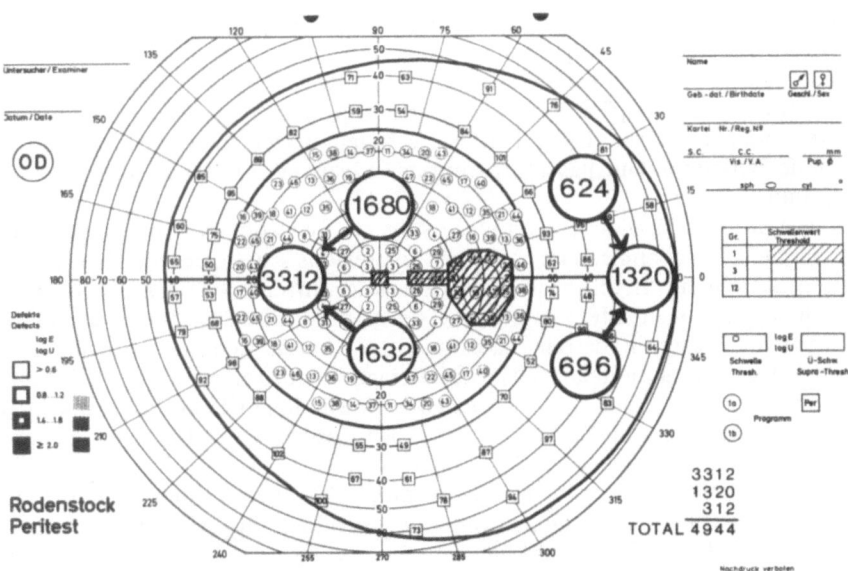

Fig. 4. Calculation of defect volume (DV) for several visual field areas (see text).

Table 4. Calculation of defect volume (DV) in the case shown in Fig. 2.

name: v.d. H.		total DV%: 35			
thr: 0.4	cent: 0.4		ceco: ∞	bl.sp.: 24	
DV 25° ↑	1308	DV P ↑	300	DV 25° + P↑	1608
↓	102	↓	0	↓	102
DV 25°↑↓	1410	DV P ↑↓	300	DV 25°+ P↑↓	1710
				TOTAL DV	1734

thr. = threshold, INSC
cent. = central threshold
ceco. = cecocentral area
bl. sp. = blind spot
DV 25° ↑ = defect volume in the upper half of the 25° visual field, etc.
DV P↑ = defect volume in the upper half of the peripheral visual field (outside 25°)

by cataract. We have shown earlier that the sensitivity of this threshold-related suprathreshold strategy is quite satisfactory (11). 70% of small early glaucomatous visual field defects, that were detected by high resolution, 1° classical meridional static perimetry, were detected by the Peritest. This means a 10% better detection rate than that of our own experimental automatic perimeter, the Scoperimeter, which was used with a lower resolution than that of the Peritest detection phase (10). The 6° resolution of the Scoperimeter is comparable to that of the Octopus programe 31 or 33. The detection percentage of the Peritest is much better than that of routine kinetic perimetry and has the additional advantage of standardization and reproducibility.

The printout provides a good idea of the configuration and intensity of the visual field defect and can be compared to previous kinetic perimetric examination quite easily if one realizes the essential differences between the two methods. Although interpolated grey scales may provide a somewhat more attractive picture in certain cases we feel that it does not provide any additional information and that the attraction does not outweigh the disadvantage of not being able to recognize the individual positions at which measurements have been made, as it is possible with the use of non-interpolated grey scales.

Because the influence of the examiner has been almost completely excluded in automatic examinations, the reproducibility of such methods is better than those of classical kinetic perimetry. Given this fact an automated visual field examination is in principle more suitable for follow-up examinations than manual kinetic perimetry. For this purpose the calculations of defect volume (DV) could be used. However one should not forget that even under the circumstances of standardized automated static perimetry fluctuations in relative defects may be in the order of 0.3 log unit (standard deviation). Therefore slight changes in the results of successive visual field examinations have to be interpreted with caution. It might be ideal to apply statistical programs to the results of automatic visual field examination as has been proposed by Fankhauser and co-workers (1,2). Repeated measurements are necessary for such programs. The DV calculation could then be presented with a standard deviation. Our own statistical programs are currently under investigation in our clinic.

REFERENCES

1. Bebie, H. and Fankhauser, F. Statistical programs for the analysis of perimetric data. Doc. Ophthalmol. Proc. Series 26 : 9 (1980).
2. Bebie, H. and Fankhauser, F. Ein statistisches Programm zur Beurteilung von Gesichtsfeldern. Klin. Mbl. Augenheilkd. 177:417 (1980)
3. De Boer, R. W., Van den Berg, T. J. T. P., Greve, E. L. and De Waal, B. J. Concepts for automatic perimetry, as applied to the Scoperimeter, an experimental automatic perimeter. Int. Ophthalmol. 5 :181 (1982).
4. Dannheim, F. Zur Anwender-Software für die neuen Rodenstock-Perimeter. B. Klinische Erfahrungen. Der Augenspiegel 28 : 604 (1982).
5. Dannheim, F. Clinical experiences with a new automated perimeter 'Peritest'. Doc. Ophthalmol. Proc. Series 35:309–312 (1983).
6. Greve, E. L. Single and multiple stimulus static perimetry in glaucoma: the two phases of visual field examination. Doc. Ophthalmol. 136 :1 (1973).
7. Greve, E. L. Some aspects of visual field examination related to strategies for detection and assessment phase. Doc. Ophthalmol. Proc. Series 22:15 (1980).
8. Greve, E. L. The Peritest. Doc. Ophthalmol. Proc. Series 22 : 71 (1980).
9. Greve, E. L. Visual fields, glaucoma and cataract. Doc. Ophthalmol. Proc. Series 22 : 79 (1980).
10. Greve, E. L., De Boer, R. W., Bakker, D. and Moed, J. L. Clinical evaluation of the Scoperimeter, an experimental automatic perimeter. Int. Ophthalmol. 5 :192 (1982).
11. Greve, E. L. and Dannheim, F. The Peritest, a new automatic and semi-automatic perimeter. Int. Ophthalmol. 5 : 201 (1982).

Authors' addresses:
Dr E. L. Greve
Glaucoma and Visual Field Dept.
Eye Clinic of the University of Amsterdam
Academic Medical Center
Meibergdreef 8, 1105 AZ Amsterdam
The Netherlands

Dr D. Bakker
Dept. of Ophthalmology
Sint Luras Hospital
Jan Tooropstraat 164, 1061 AE Amsterdam
The Netherlands

NEW PROGRAMS OF THE SCOPERIMETER

W. G. VAN VEENENDAAL, C. T. LANGERHORST,
T. J. T. P. VAN DEN BERG and E. L. GREVE
(Amsterdam, The Netherlands)

Key words. Visual field examination, automated perimetry, automation.

ABSTRACT

The Scoperimeter is an experimental automatic perimeter based on an oscillo-scope controlled by a micro-computer. This report describes the programs developed for various perimetric tests. The screening program does a quick detection and a limited assessment of defects. The threshold program measures thresholds with a resolution of six degrees. A further examination of parts of the visual field can be done in segments, in the central two degrees or along meridians. Also the concepts of a more statistical approach are discussed.

INTRODUCTION

An interesting possibility of computer-assisted perimetry is its programming potentiality. New strategies and new evaluation programs can be devised more readily than with fixed systems. For our experimental perimeter, named 'Scoperimeter' a number of programs have been developed. First of all there are 2 programs that examine the entire 25 degrees visual field. In addition programs are available that gather information about selected parts of the visual field. Furthermore programs are being developed to measure and to analyze the fluctuation of thresholds and evaluate the results of a visual field examination.

THE SCOPERIMETER HARDWARE

Our automatic perimeter ('Scoperimeter' (2)), uses an oscilloscope screen (ϕ 28 cm) for the generation of the stimuli. The stimuli have a useful lumi-nance range of circa 3 log units. The background illumination of the screen (circa 0.03 cd/m^2) is also generated by the oscilloscope beam. The distance

Greve, E. L., Heijl, A. (eds.) Fifth International Visual Field Symposium.
© *1983 Dr W. Junk Publishers, The Hague/Boston/Lancaster.*

between eye and screen is 30 cm so that the central field up to 25 degrees from fixation can be examined. The oscilloscope is interfaced with a small computer system (North Star). Communication with the perimetrist is via a graphics terminal on which also the progress of the examination can be monitored. When a stimulus is perceived the patient presses a button which is also interfaced with the computer. Parameters that are under the control of the software are: position and luminance of the stimulus and the fixation character (a '+' in the center for non-central measurements and an 'O' for measuring thresholds in the center of the field). The stimulus duration is also program-controlled but set at 100 msec for all the present programs.

GENERAL PROGRAM FEATURES

The major part of the computer software has been written in BASIC, an easy usable computer language. The program parts for entering patient data, for storing the results on floppy disc and for making copies of the screen are used by all programs. The perimetrist can operate the system by simply responding to the questions of the computer.

Fixation is checked by presentation of stimuli in the blind spot area. In case the fixation is correct these stimuli will not be perceived. The perimetrist is continuously informed how many of these stimuli are generated and how many are perceived. If necessary the patient can be reinstructed during the examination.

To test patient's reliability zero stimuli are interweaved between actual stimulus presentations. The numbers of presented and 'perceived' invisible stimuli are continuously displayed at the visual display unit.

In case three successive stimulus presentations are missed a stimulus with a high intensity that most probable will be seen is presented. This prevents that the so-called 'zero-fear' (3) occurs, i.e., a reaction of uncertainty from the patient in case no stimuli are visible for an extended period of time.

After the stimulus presentation has started the computer awaits a response of the patient. The waiting time is initially 1.5 sec but is adapted to the average reaction time of the patient. This is done by using the average of the last 5 response times plus 300 msec.

The perimetrist can interrupt an examination at any moment. After such an interruption the examination can be continued, restarted or ended. The patient can take a rest by keeping the response button pressed.

Every single step of the examination can be followed by the perimetrist on the screen of the visual display unit. When the examination has finished a copy of the screen can be made by the hard copy unit.

THE SCOPERIMETER SOFTWARE

a. The screening program

This examination starts with the measurement of the Individual Normal Sensitivity Curve (INSC). This INSC is determined from thresholds measured at 5 specific locations in the visual field. These locations are chosen in such a way that most likely at least 2 locations will not show a local reduction of sensitivity. This INSC is then corrected for the normal gradient of sensitivity to establish a normal value for every location. In the second phase 60 points in the visual field (for the distribution see Fig. 1) are tested at a 0.6 log unit suprathreshold (INSC) level. If the patient misses a stimulus it is presented once again. If the stimulus is missed again the location is tested in steps of 0.6 log units so that a classification of defects in 0.6 log unit classes is obtained. A third phase can be added in which 48 more locations are examined in the same way. This results in a resolution of circa 4.2 degrees. The classification of defects is indicated at the printout with non-interpolated grey scales, which makes the interpretation of the results quick and easy. The examination time is dependent on the number of defects and on the reaction time of the patient but is approximately 5 minutes for testing 108 positions.

b. The threshold program

This program is used when more accurate data are required. This can be necessary in case defects of slight intensity are expected. In the first phase thresholds are determined at 16 positions in the field using an iterative procedure (up and down method (1)). The remaining 44 points are then tested with a faster strategy (method of limits (1)), starting from the thresholds of neighbouring points. Thresholds are on the output indicated with tenths of log units (Fig. 2). 0 log unit is the maximum stimulus luminance. This program takes approximately 6 minutes.

Starting with the information obtained from the screening or the threshold program a more detailed examination of a restricted part of the visual field can be done. This may be necessary to obtain a better impression of the spatial and intensity distribution of the defect. This may be especially important for monitoring the defect in follow-up examinations.

c. The meridian program

This program examines points along a specific meridian in the 25 degrees visual field. Always two meridians in opposite visual field halves are measured using random presentations. Thresholds are determined with a 2 degrees resolution. This is done in two phases. Thresholds are first measured at positions 6 degrees apart using the up and down strategy. In the second phase the method of limits is used for the remaining points. The results of this program are presented as a section through the island of vision (Fig. 3). The examination time is approximately 2.5 minutes.

d. The center program

The central 2 degrees of the visual field can be examined more precisely with the center test. The fixation point is changed from the normal '+' into 'O', to permit stimulus presentation in the middle of the fixation character.

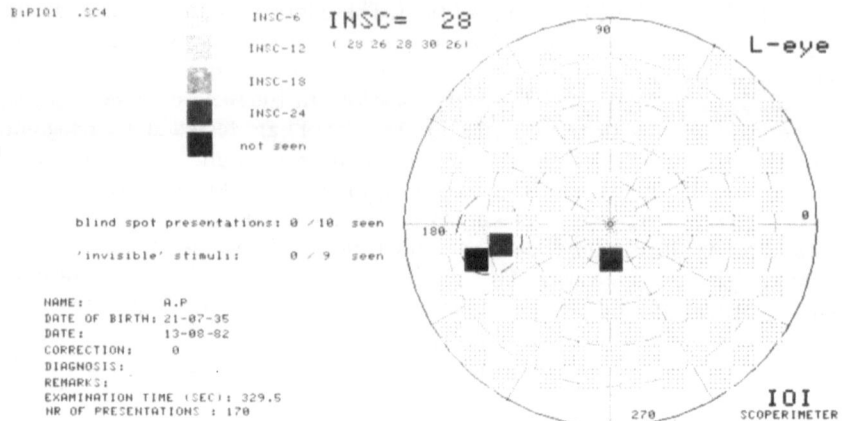

Fig. 1. An output of the screening program. The symbols represent intensities of defects relative to the patient's INSC.

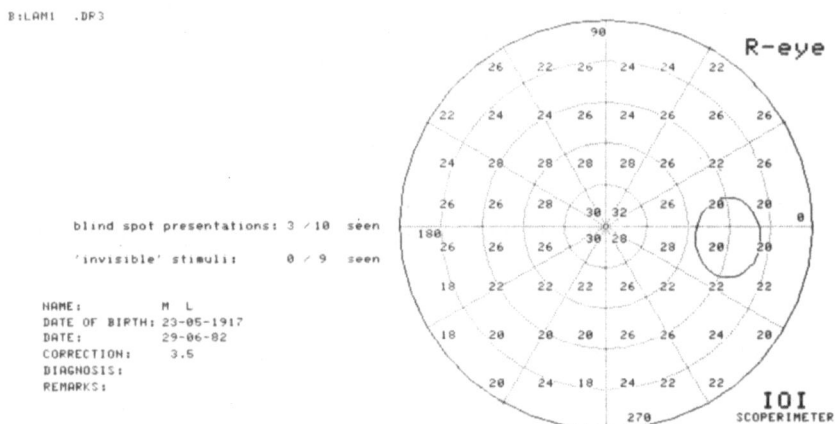

Fig. 2. A printout of the result of the threshold program. Thresholds are represented in tenths of log units. 0 log unit is the maximum stimulus luminance.

Threshold measurements are repeated four times. The result may be used in the determination of the INSC in the screening program. Threshold determination is also possible at 8 positions at 1 degree eccentricity. This program takes circa 1 minute. An output example is shown in Fig. 4.

e. *The segment program*

Thresholds can also be measured with a high resolution in a segment of the visual field. A rectangular 2 degrees grid is chosen, so the distribution of points is homogeneous for the entire segment. Two of these segments can be measured simultaneously, e.g. in opposite parts of the visual field. This

326

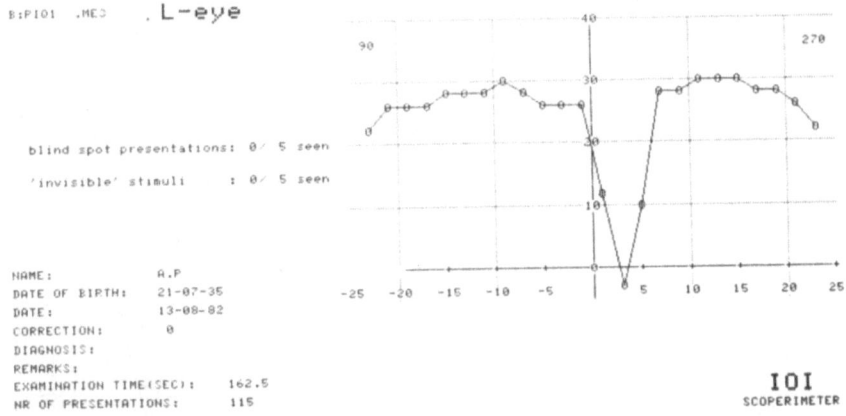

Fig. 3. The result of an examination by the meridian program. Units along the vertical axis are tenths of log units. In the graph is indicated (in degrees) which meridians are examined.

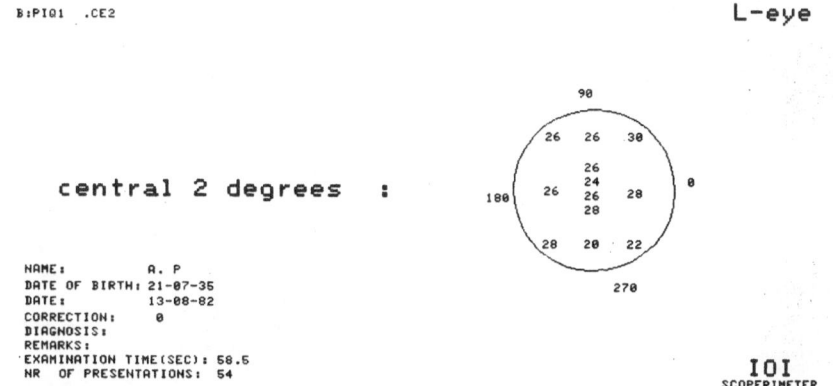

Fig. 4. The printout of the center program. Thresholds are indicated as in Fig. 2. The threshold determination is repeated four times.

procedure avoids improper fixation. To gain time this examination is also done in two phases, but still the examination time is between 12 and 15 minutes. An output example is shown in Fig. 5. As an alternative the meridian program can be used to obtain a high resolution. This can be done by measuring along 3 meridians close to each other. In that case however the resolution is higher in the center than in the periphery.

f. The statistical programs

Threshold measurements as used in the described programs will be hampered with statistical variation. This variation is inherent to physical measurements and will be dependent on the system that is being measured, in this case the

327

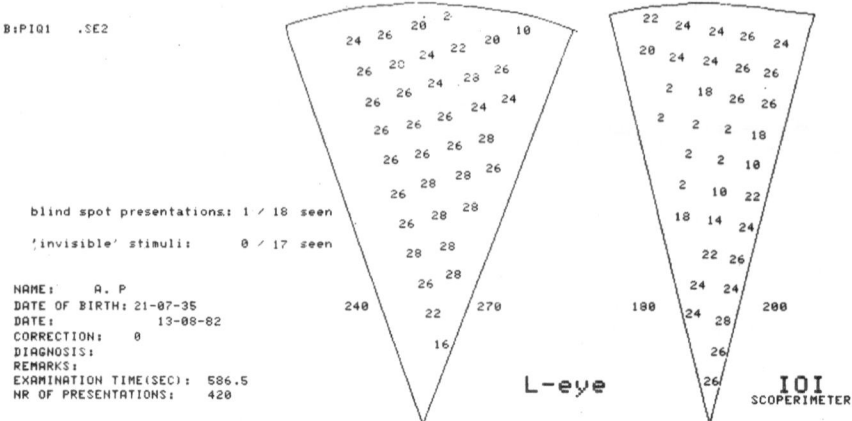

Fig. 5. The final result of the segment program. The thresholds are indicated as in Fig. 2. The meridians that border the segments are indicated.

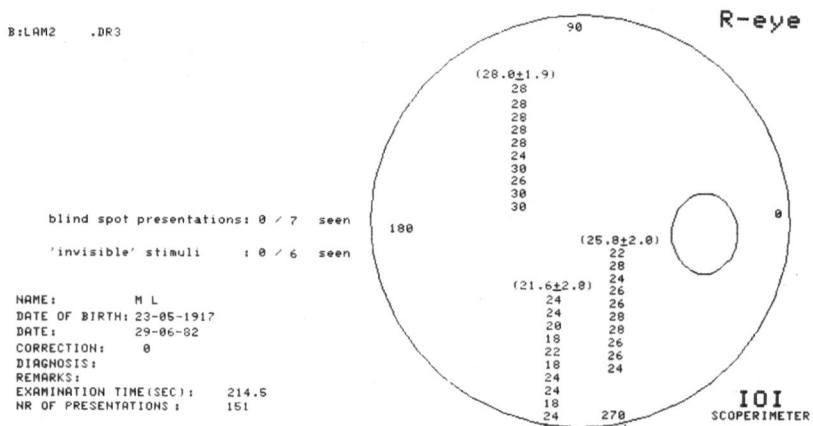

Fig. 6. The output of one of the statistical programs. Threshold determination is repeated ten times at the same location (the middle of the column). The computed mean and standard deviation are represented at the top of the column.

patient, and on the measuring instrument, the perimeter. In most cases the occurrence of the values that are obtained can be approximated with a Gaussian distribution which can be characterized by a mean and a standard deviation. The estimate of the real mean will improve by averaging more measured values. For the interpretations of the results of visual field examinations it is very important to know the variation because it determines the confidence intervals of the obtained values (e.g. 95% chance the threshold is between T1 and T2). Also the accuracy of derived measures as, e.g., the number of defect locations and the total defect volume is determined by the standard deviations of the individual thresholds. The confidence intervals

328

of these derived measures are of importance for the decision whether a visual field as a whole is defect or whether there is progression (or regression) of a visual field defect. These programs estimate the standard deviations of thresholds by repeated measurements. In one of the programs the perimetrist can select up to 7 positions where thresholds are measured 10 times in an identical way but in random order. From these 10 values an estimate of the mean and an estimate of the standard deviation is computed. By selecting normal and defective points a comparison between the standard deviations in these points can be made. An output example is shown in Fig. 6.

With this program we obtain information about the variation of thresholds on which decisions about significance of deviations of a visual field from normal or from a previous field can be based. Which measures and which criteria can be used is now under investigation.

REFERENCES

1. Bebie, H., Fankhauser, F. and Spahr, J. Static perimetry: strategies. Acta Ophthalmol. 54 : 325–338 (1976).
2. De Boer, R. W., Van den Berg, T. J. T. P., Greve, E. L. and De Waal, B. J. Concepts for automatic perimetry, as applied to the Scoperimeter, an experimental automatic perimeter. Int. Ophthalmol. 5 : 181–191 (1982).
3. Greve, E. L., Groothuyse, H. T. and Bakker, D. Simulated automatic perimetry. Doc. Ophthalmol. Proc. Series 14 : 23–29 (1977).

Authors' addresses:
W. G. van Veenendaal
Dr T. J. T. P. van den Berg
The Netherlands Ophthalmic Research Institute
P.O. Box 6411, 1005 EK Amsterdam
The Netherlands

C. T. Langerhorst
Dr E. L. Greve
Glaucoma and Visual Field Dept.
Eye Clinic of the University of Amsterdam
Academic Medical Center
Meibergdreef 8, 1105 AZ Amsterdam
The Netherlands

AUTOMATED PERIMETRY IN AVIATION MEDICINE
Visual field examination in 2500 flying personnel

J. T. W. VAN DALEN

(Soesterberg, The Netherlands)

Key words. Automated perimetry, aviation medicine.

ABSTRACT

Results of automated perimetry by means of the Fieldmaster-200 and Fieldmaster-225 in 2500 flying subjects are described. In 22 subjects (approx. 1%) a serious visual field defect was found. In 12 subjects aspecific defects were found. Since the visual field is of utmost importance in aviation, while mass conventional screening is not possible, it is suggested that use should be made of automated perimetry testing.

INTRODUCTION

In medical examinations of flight crews (military personnel and civilians) it has always been a disadvantage not to be able to assess the visual field adequately. In the large number of daily medical examinations at the National Aerospace Medical Center, only a manual method was used during ophthalmological examination. Only in selected cases was kinetic perimetry performed. In view of the great importance of intact visual fields in aviation, the significance of specific visual field defects for ophthalmological or neuro-ophthalmological diseases, the availability of improved testing devices and the increasingly favourable reports in the literature, we decided to undertake a further investigation of computer-aided perimetry.

On the basis of personal experience and literature research, a Fieldmaster — model 200 (Synemed Inc.) — was purchased. Later a Fieldmaster-225 became available.

This paper presents the results of visual field testing of 2500 subjects. Special emphasis was placed on visual field examination as a detection method for previously unsuspected ophthalmological or neuro-ophthalmological diseases, particularly in persons with supposedly normal eyes.

Greve, E. L., Heijl, A. (eds.) Fifth International Visual Field Symposium.
©1983 Dr W. Junk Publishers, The Hague/Boston/Lancaster.

SUBJECTS AND METHODS

Subjects

Two thousand five hundred subjects were examined, selected from military personnel, commercial aircrews and pilots. As a general rule the following subjects were examined: 1) all new applicants for a flight licence, 2) subjects over 40 years of age.

Methods

Most of the visual field examinations were performed by means of the Fieldmaster-200. Later the Fieldmaster-225 came into use. A full description of the examination methods will not be given here. A detailed description can be found elsewhere (1,6). However, we would like to make a few comments on the Fieldmaster-225. As the Fieldmaster-200, the Fieldmaster-225 is a fiber-optic perimeter. The Fieldmaster-225, however, is capable of performing contour perimetry; the level of intensity varies according to the location of the stimulus and its position relative to the center. Other important features of the Fieldmaster-225 are the possibilities of performing static perimetry (4 meridians) and the possibility of adding new functions and programs.

RESULTS

Significant visual field defects were found in 22 subjects (approx. 1%), indicative of an underlying disease. The classification of these diseases was as follows:

Glaucoma	: 7
Eye contusion	: 4
Neuro-ophthalmological diseases	: 3
Miscellaneous diseases	: 8

These miscellaneous diseases could be subdivided as follows:

Diabetes mellitus	: 2
Hypertension	: 2
Retinoschisis	: 1
Retinal vascular accident	: 2
Periphlebitis	: 1

In 13 subjects atypical visual field defects were found. Ophthalmological examination of these patients was entirely normal. The fact that the mean age of these patients was approximately 60 years is of interest. This, in combination with the kind of visual field defect (Bjerrum area and peripheral visual field), is compatible with the fact that the peripheral retina becomes less sensitive with increasing age. Several examples of visual field defects are given in Figs. 1–3.

332

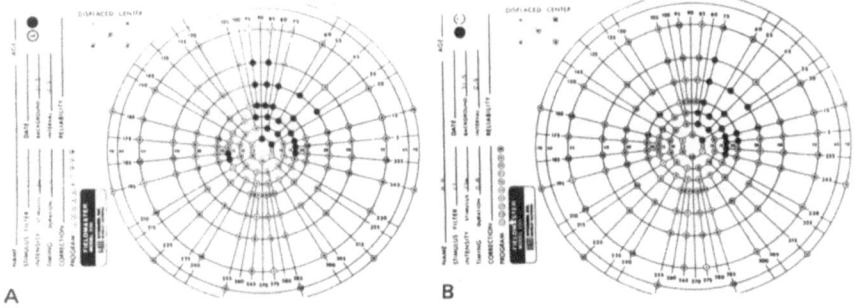

Fig. 1. (A–B) Right homonymous quadrant anopia due to a cerebro-vascular accident.

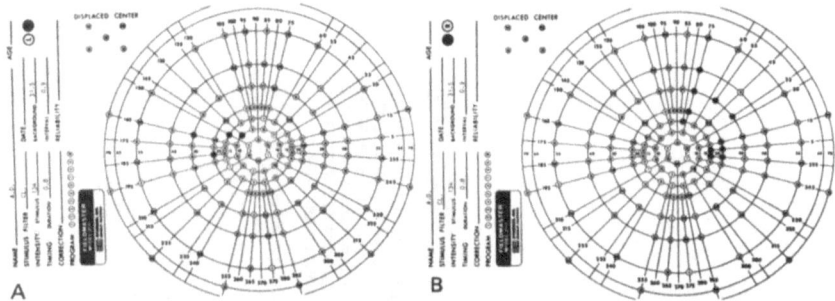

Fig. 2. (A–B) Visual fields of a now 36-year old patient, operated in 1978 for a pituitary adenoma. Visual fields, as assessed by the FM-200, showed a slight bitemporal central hemianopia, the kinetic perimetry (Goldmann perimeter) showing normal fields.

CONCLUSION AND DISCUSSION

Experience with visual field testing in 2500 subjects by means of automated perimetry indicates that this procedure is very useful for mass visual field examination.

In our series we found serious field defects in almost 1% of the tested flying population of the Netherlands. Literature data suggest visual field abnormality ranging from 1–9% in the normal population (2,3,8,10). The detection of 4 persons with glaucoma among our subjects was very important. As these glaucoma patients were in their initial stages, conservative treatment was still quite possible. Needless to say, a later discovery could have caused serious socio-psychological and socio-economical problems.

Since an intact visual field is of the utmost importance in aviation, we would suggest automated perimetry testing, as mass conventional visual field screening is not possible. Confrontation techniques do not seem to be of much use, nor does screening by means of the Friedmann visual field analyzer (VFA) (only central 30 degrees). What kind of apparatus is chosen is of secondary importance, provided the apparatus has a high detection rate and

333

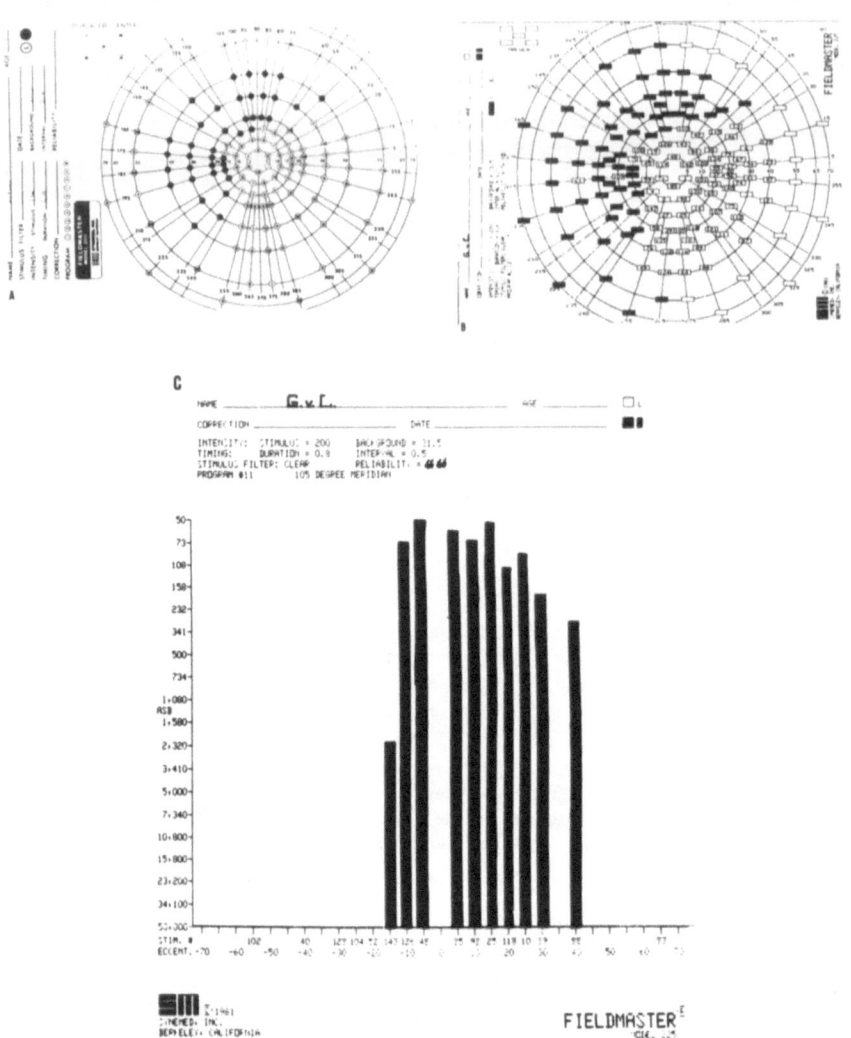

Fig. 3. (A–C) Visual fields, as assessed by the FM-200 (Fig. 3A) and the FM-225 (Fig. 3B) of a patient with retinoschisis of the left eye. Fig. 3C shows a static profile of the 105-285 degree meridian.

a low false—positive alarm rate. Very useful articles have been published recently concerning this matter.

ACKNOWLEDGEMENT

The author would like to thank J. C. Dejongh, J. H. Entrop, G. J. H. M. Faessen and J. W. Kappers for their help in preparing this manuscript.

REFERENCES

1. Dalen, J. T. W. van. Automated visual field screening in the flying Dutch population. Aviation, Space and Env. Med. 53(10):1006–1010 (1982).
2. Flocks, M., Rosenthal, A. R. and Hopkins, J. C. Mass visual screening via television. Ophthalmology 85:1141–1149 (1978).
3. Greve, E. L. and Verduin, W. M. Mass visual field investigation in 1834 persons with supposedly normal eyes. Albrecht von Graefes Arch. Clin. Exp. Ophthalmol. 183:286–293 (1972).
4. Johnson, C. A., Keltner, J. L. and Balestrery, F. G. Suprathreshold static perimetry in glaucoma and other optic nerve diseases. Ophthalmology 87:1278–1286 (1980).
5. Johnson, C. A. and Keltner, J. L. Automated suprathreshold static perimetry. Am. J. Ophthalmol. 89:731–741 (1980).
6. Johnson, C. A. and Keltner, J. L. Comparitive evaluation of the Autofield-I, CFA-120, Fieldmaster-101 PR, automated perimeters. Ophthalmology 87:777–784 (1980).
7. Keltner, J. L., Johnson, C. A. and Balestrery, F. G. Suprathreshold static perimetry. Initial clinical trials with the Fieldmaster automated perimeter. Arch. Ophthalmol. 97:260–272 (1979).
8. Keltner, J. L. and Johnson, C. A. Mass visual field screening in a driving population. Ophthalmol. 87:785–790 (1980).
9. Keltner, J. L. and Johnson, C. A. Automated perimetry I. A consumer's guide. Ann. Ophthalmol. 3:275–279 (1981).
10. Kuhn, H. S. Glaucoma detection in industry: multiple field pattern test. Ind. Med. Surg. 26:327–330 (1957).

Author's address:
Dr J. T. W. van Dalen
National Aerospace Medical Center
P.O. Box 22
3769 ZG Soesterberg
The Netherlands

335

ANGIOSCOTOMA: PRELIMINARY RESULTS USING THE NEW SPATIALLY ADAPTIVE PROGRAM SAPRO

H. HÄBERLIN, A. FUNKHOUSER and F. FANKHAUSER

(Bern, Switzerland)

Key words. Angioscotoma, spatially adaptive, automated perimetry.

ABSTRACT

The spatially adaptive program SAPRO, written for the Octopus 201, has been applied in a study of angioscotoma. A mosaic of the interpolated results of 34 separate examinations performed over a one-month period on angioscotoma within a normal visual field region subtending approximately $20°$ on both sides of the macula is shown. This is compared on the one hand with the fundus picture (inverted) of the same subject's eye. The agreement is remarkable. Also shown is a similar mosaic showing just the locations measured. The time saved by measuring with higher resolution only the areas of interest is apparent. Examples of program use as well as some of its features are also included.

INTRODUCTION

Preliminary versions of the SAPRO program have been described previously (2,3,4). Briefly, it is a program written to operate on the Octopus 201 automatic perimeter and it is spatially adaptive in that it is able to examine an area of the visual field with two or three levels of resolution depending on the situation it encounters as the field is quantitatively measured. There are two versions being prepared: a research variant which is extremely flexible and thus somewhat complicated to use, and a medical practice-oriented version which sacrifices some versatility in favor of application ease.

In the research version, the center, extent, initial resolution (measurement grid increments in x and y), as well as the sensitivity deviations away from the age-corrected normal values (norms) at which the higher resolutions begin to be used can be selected by the user. Various radii, corresponding to the central fixation control opening, the correction lens size, and the outer limit of the measurement area can be entered to configure the program for

Greve, E. L., Heijl, A. (eds.) Fifth International Visual Field Symposium.
©1983 Dr W. Junk Publishers, The Hague/Boston/Lancaster.

CIRCULAR

SAPRO

OCTOPUS SPATIALLY ADAPTIVE PROGRAM
                                          DATE: 4.8.1982
SELECT FUNCTION (M,P,S,D,E,?): M
  EX. TYPE: FIRST/SUPP/REP/TREND (F/S/R/T): F
  1 SURNAME,GIVEN NAMES: HAEBERLIN, HUGO
  2 DATE OF BIRTH: 15.4.1935
  4 EYE: R
  3 PATIENT NUMBER: H501.82R

  5 EXAMINATION TIME: 14.10
  6 CORRECTION (SPH., CYL., +AXIS): 0.0 0.0 0
  7 GEOMETRY TYPE (C OR R): C
  8 MINIMUM ECCENT.: 0   MAXIMUM ECCENT.: 30   QUADRANT (U,L,N,T,A): A
    (STIMULUS SIZE: 3   FINEST RESOLUTION STEP: 2.0 DEGREES)
  9 STRATEGY (C,F,S): S

    CHANGES (Y/N)?: N

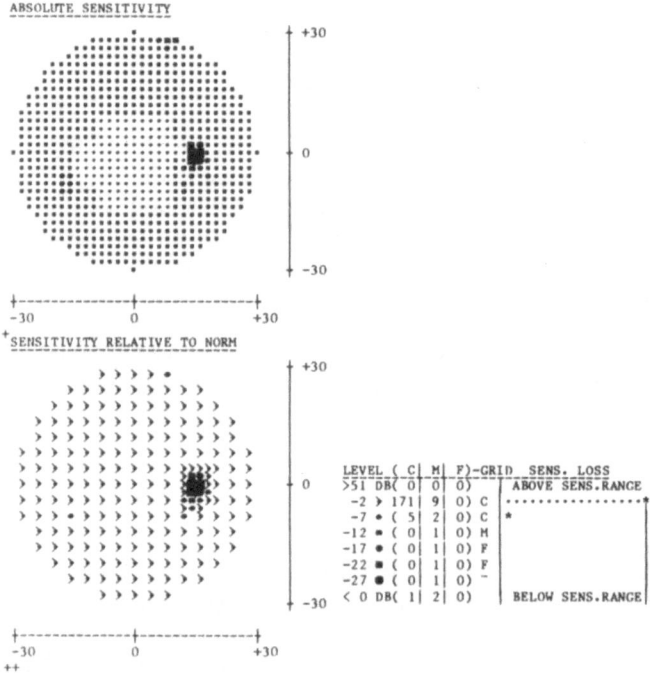

Fig. 1. Example of new SAPRO dialogue and printout modes (circular geometry).

non-standard conditions.* The initial stimulus luminance (as compared with the local norm) and the luminance step size are determined automatically and dynamically for each test location as the measurement proceeds. This was the version used for the angioscotoma investigation shown in Fig. 3, and it is

---

*In the Octopus 201, the Goldmann III stimulus should always remain at least 3° in eccentricity away from the central fixation control opening to prevent vignetting. For the same reason, it should not exceed 30° eccentricity so long as a correcting lens is in use. Standard measurement radii are 30°, 60° and 90° eccentricity.

RECTANGULAR

SAPRO

OCTOPUS SPATIALLY ADAPTIVE PROGRAM
                                            DATE: 10.8.1982
SELECT FUNCTION (M,P,S,D,E,?): M
  EX. TYPE: FIRST/SUPP/REP/TREND (F/S/R/T): S
  3 PATIENT NUMBER: F503.82R
  1 SURNAME,GIVEN NAMES: FUNKHOUSER ARTHUR
  2 DATE OF BIRTH: 3.09.1940
  4 EYE: RIGHT (OD)   PREVIOUS EXAMINATION DATE: 4.08.1982
  5 EXAMINATION TIME: 8.45
  6 CORRECTION (SPH., CYL., +AXIS): 0.5 1.25 30
  7 GEOMETRY TYPE (C OR R): R
  8 CENTER (X,Y): 15/0   EXTENT FROM CENTER (X,Y): 15/10
    (STIMULUS SIZE: 3   FINEST RESOLUTION STEP: 0.8 DEGREES)
  9 STRATEGY (C,F,S): C

                   CHANGES (Y/N)?: N

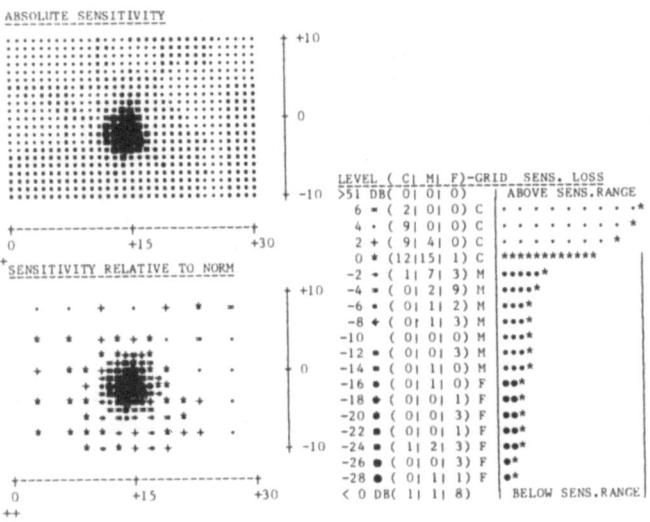

Fig. 2. Example of new SAPRO dialogue and printout modes (rectangular geometry).

currently undergoing clinical trials to determine which level settings seem to be most suitable for the various visual field conditions met in practice.

Two program dialogue examples shown in Fig. 1 and 2 illustrate the use of the simplified version. Here the dialogue is very similar to that found using the standard Octopus programs except that in place of choosing a program number, one is asked which measurement geometry is to be used, circular or rectangular. If circular is selected, the inner and outer eccentricities (to the nearest degree) can be entered, and the quadrant(s) to be investigated can be chosen (upper, lower, nasal, temporal, upper temporal, lower

339

nasal, . . . , or all 360 degrees). The center for this geometry is always at $0.0°$ (fixation point). If rectangular geometry is selected, the center and extent in x and y are to be given. In both cases, the program then determines automatically the optimum grid increment and the optimum stimulus size (Goldmann III, II, or I) for the increment to be used in order to provide the best resolution for the area size chosen without making the examination time inordinantly long.

Examples of results using the two geometry possibilities are shown in the lower parts of Figs. 1 and 2. Of the three figures in each case, the uppermost is an interpolated gray scale representation of the measured data, while the one below shows the test locations that were actually measured. The table to the right of the lower figure shows the loss increments (relative to norm) corresponding to the symbols used in the lower figure. It also shows a summation histogram of the loss distribution which gives an added indication of the extent and depth of any scotoma present.

Two other non-standard dialogue questions are immediately apparent. At the beginning, the user is asked to specify the type of examination (first, supplement, repetition, trend) to be performed. For a first examination a new patient file is opened for diskette storage. A supplementary examination, then, is any subsequent examination of that patient's eye which is not a repetition or a trend type. In the repetition, the operator is asked to specify a previous examination number and then this examination is repeated, taking over all the parameters that were specified at that time. However, the initial stimulus luminance values are taken over from the thresholds found previously in order to save examination time. Finally, a trend examination is similar to a repetition, except that it only examines with higher resolution those test locations which differ from those found in the reference examination. In the other three types, higher resolution examination occurs at deviations from the local norm value.

At the end of the dialogue, one can choose between three strategies: complete, fast, and search. Complete means that at each test location the contrast sensitivity threshold is fully determined using all three grids, if necessary. The fast strategy brackets only at those test locations whose thresholds lie below the local norm value. In the search mode, only two grids are applied and the coarser one set to have high resolution to increase the detection probability of small scotomas. Fast strategy quantitative bracketing is performed, and time is further saved in that the finest luminance interval is set to be 5 dB.

Examination type and strategy can be determined in the research version too, whereas in the simplified version all parameters other than those mentioned above are fixed. They will be set according to the values found to be the most useful in the clinical trials of the research version. It is thinkable that it may be necessary to have various parameter sets according to which disease entity (Glaucoma, retinopathy, etc.) is suspected to be present. It should be noted that this type of program represents a radical departure from normal Octopus system practice in that the visual field locations investigated are no longer standardized. This in turn makes longitudinal intercomparison of examination results more difficult.

340

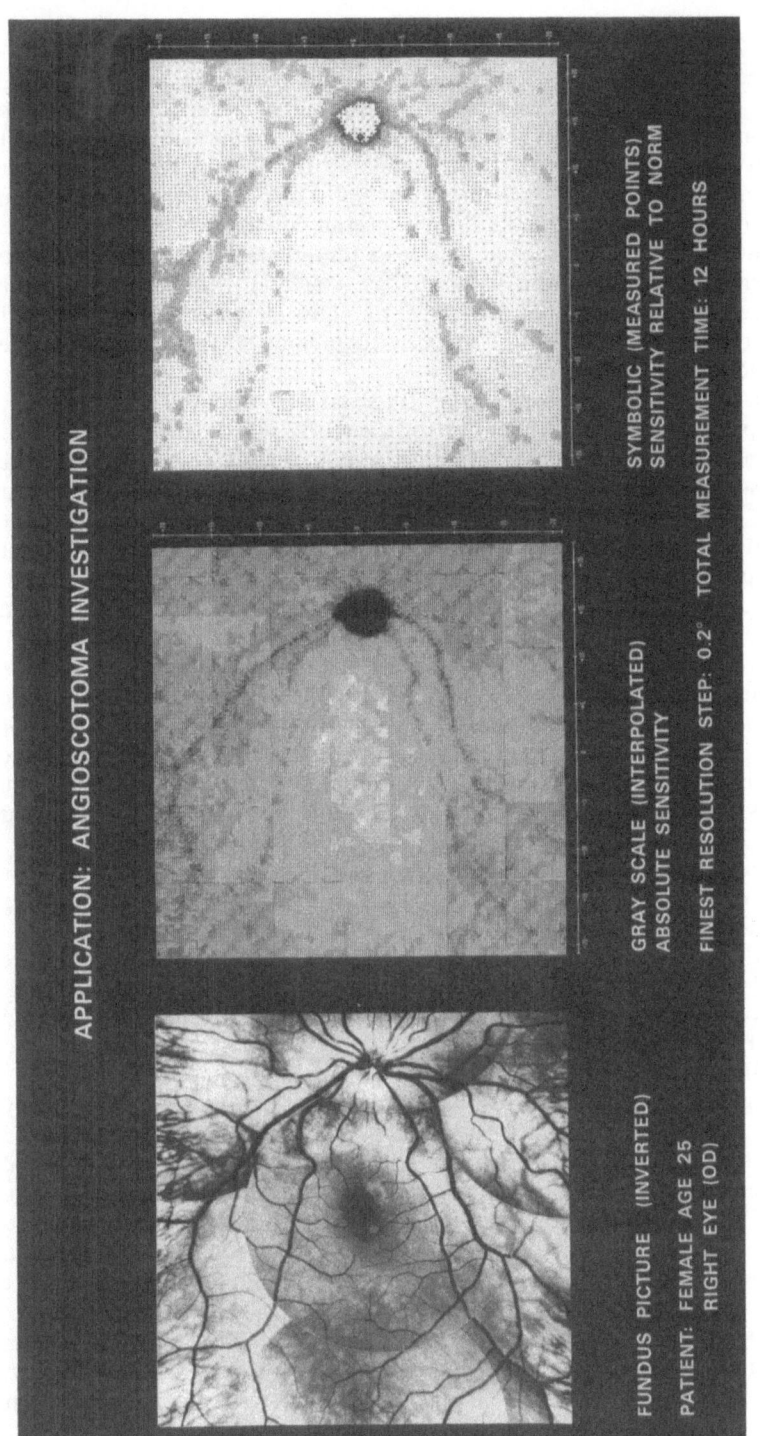

Fig. 3. Composite picture including the fundus picture (left), mosaic of interpolated SAPRO angioscotoma results (± 20°) (center), and mosaic of corresponding test locations measured (right).

The three pictures in Fig. 3 illustrate one possible use of the **SAPRO** program. The left-most photograph is the fundus picture (inverted top to bottom) of the right eye of a 25-year old woman with no apparent pathology. The next two are mosaics made up of 39 separate examinations carried out using the **SAPRO** program and using the highest resolution available on the Octopus 201 $(0.2°)$ with a stimulus size of Goldmann I. The central mosaic is the interpolated gray scale representation (corresponding to the upper figures in the lower parts of Figs. 1 and 2), while the one on the right shows the test locations that were actually measured. The agreement between the perimetrically-found angioscotoma and the vessels shown in the fundus picture is remarkable.

Comparing the two mosaics, the time savings achieved by using the **SAPRO** program become evident. Altogether, the mosaic took 12 hours of measurement time spread over a one-month period. If one examines the right-most mosaic, one sees that in areas lacking any scotoma, only the largest grid $(0.8°)$ was used. At the macula, only 4 minutes were necessary for the examination. On the other hand, at the arterial junction shown at the center of the upper row (and Fig. 4), 39 minutes of examination were required, since much more detail had to be resolved. Had one made this investigation using non-adaptive strategy (i.e. examining every point at high resolution), the time required would have been prohibitively long.

Another interesting feature of this program is seen when one looks at the blind spot in the right hand mosaic. The central region of the blind spot (with zero sensitivity) was examined only with the lowest resolution – the program is set to study with higher resolution only those regions where some sensitivity is present. Thus the border of the blind spot has been well resolved while the central region has been effectively ignored.

The widths of the angioscotomata have been here measured to be on the order of $0.6°$. It is doubtful, therefore, that instruments of lower resolving power will be able to resolve and map them adequately. In the right-hand mosaic, they appear wider, but that is because only the locations tested are displayed there, and given the resolution of the figure as here reproduced, it is no longer possible to distinguish which locations had a normal threshold and which below normal. (The angioscotoma loss in most places amounts to only 10 dB.)

As might be imagined, steady and repeatable fixation is also critically necessary for such fine resolution work. To this end, a specially constructed mirror attachment has been employed which splits the image of the fixated eye as seen on the Octopus monitor so that it includes half of the non-examined eye. When these two images are aligned (before the non-examined eye is occluded), one can be fairly confident that at least head rotation has been eliminated. Thanks to the graduated chin-rest system of the Octopus, vertical and horizontal positioning of the head can be reliably reproduced as well. The two pictures reproduced in Fig. 4 show a venous branching angioscotoma as measured on two occasions, one week apart. One sees that positioning and fixation accuracy was adequate and that

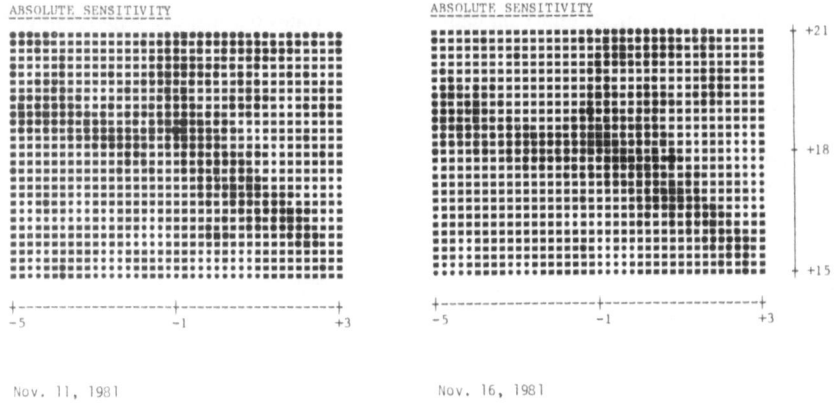

Fig. 4. Example of reproducibility of SAPRO angioscotoma examinations made one week apart.

measurement fluctuation, while present, does not obscure the angioscotoma observation.

Numerous workers have concerned themselves with angioscotomata in the past (e.g. 1). There would appear to be anomalous behaviour (i.e. widening under the influence of certain drugs, elevated intraocular pressure, etc.) which has yet to be adequately studied and may yield further information about metabolic and pathological processes in the human eye. While it most likely will not be necessary to repeat such an extensive mapping of the angioscotoma as was done here, now that we know the parameters necessary for their study, one can restrict oneself to a small region of the visual field (perhaps based on the fundus picture) and investigate pharmaceutical and other effects on scotoma (angio- as well as others) with greater ease than has been hitherto possible.

ACKNOWLEDGEMENTS

The authors would like to express their appreciation to H. Bebie and A. Jenni for many helpful discussions. We are also indebted to Mr Jenni for all his help in fabricating the poster. Finally, this work has been in part supported through generous donations from the Stanley Thomas Johnson Foundation.

REFERENCES

1. Evans, J. N. Introduction to Clinical Scotometry. New Haven, Yale University Press (1938).
2. Fankhauser, F., Häberlin, H. and Jenni, A. Octopus programs SAPRO and F. Albrecht von Graefes Arch. Klin. Exp. Ophthalmol. 216:155–165 (1981).
3. Häberlin, H. and Fankhauser, F. Adaptive programs for analysis of the visual field by automatic perimetry – basic problems and solutions. Doc. Ophthalmol. 50:123–141 (1980).

343

4. Häberlin, H., Jenni, A. and Fankhauser, F. Researches on adaptive high resolution programming for automatic perimeter. Int. Ophthalmol. 2:1−9 (1980).

Authors' address:
Eye Clinic
University of Bern
CH-3010 Bern
Switzerland

THE ACCURACY OF SCREENING PROGRAMS
A preliminary report on an on-going longitudinal investigation to ascertain the quantitativeness of qualitative 2-niveau-test procedures

A. FUNKHOUSER, N. WETTERWALD and F. FANKHAUSER

(Bern, Switzerland)

Key words. Screening, qualitative, quantitative, automatic perimetry.

ABSTRACT

Visual fields were first measured using qualitative screening strategy, then with a quantitative bracketing program, and finally with a screening program again. Agreement between the extent of defect as found by the screening program and that by quantitative bracketing is compared in order to ascertain the accuracy and reliability of the screening method. Reproducibility of the screening results as a function of quantitatively determined extent of defect was also measured. The probability of a test location being classified as normal, relative defect, or absolute defect as a function of quantitatively determined loss (deviation from local age-corrected normal value) is also presented.

INTRODUCTION

Many clinicians need to have a quick first look at a visual field which tells them in a yes–no fashion if pathology is present or not. For such purposes, the screening examinations 03 and 07 were created for the Octopus system (which normally utilizes quantitative methods). These two take little time to perform and provide visual field sensitivity information in terms of normal, relative defect (i.e. reduced sensitivity seems to be present at the tested location), and absolute defect. As a guarantee of result reliability, all results which are isolated are retested, as well as relative defects if they do not amount to more than 25% of the visual field results.

Unfortunately, there has been a tendency to rely too much on such tests, even in situations where it would be possible to make quantitative examinations. In particular, it seems that such screening results are sometimes used for follow-ups and changes in the visual field thus observed have been taken too seriously. In this investigation, we are gathering data in an attempt to ascertain just how far such screening results can be trusted — i.e. just how quantitative are they?

Greve, E. L., Heijl, A. (eds.) Fifth International Visual Field Symposium.
©1983 Dr W. Junk Publishers, The Hague/Boston/Lancaster.

INVESTIGATION METHOD

For 41 eyes thus far, contrast sensitivity has been first evaluated qualitatively using one of two special screening programs adjusted geometrically so that the test locations coincide with the standard Octopus programs 31, 32, 42, or 42. Next, the sensitivity thresholds have been determined quantitatively using the corresponding 31, 32, 41, or 42 program. Finally, the first evaluation has been repeated as a check on screening reproducibility. The strategy in the special screening programs is identical to that used in the standard Octopus programs 03 and 07. The examination strategy and retest logic of these programs are defined and described in detail in the Octopus System 201 operators manual (par. 4.3.4.1 and 4.9.4). Definitions of three terms as used in the figures:

1.   Extent of defect $= \dfrac{T-N}{T}$

where $N_{screening}$ = the average number of test locations whose sensitivity was classified as normal in one or the other screening evaluations.

$N_{quantitative}$ = the number of test locations whose measured sensitivity threshold lies above a boundary value which is 6 dB below the local norm value (see below). This boundary was chosen to correspond to the value of the initial stimulus shown at each test location in the screening tests.

T = the total number of test locations for a given examination (31, 32, 41, or 42).

2.   Reproducibility $= \dfrac{T-|\Delta N|}{T}$

where ΔN = the difference between the number of test locations classified as normal in the first screening evaluation and that of the second one.
T as above.

3.   Classification probabilities

$$P_N = \frac{N_i}{T_i} \qquad P_R = \frac{R_i}{T_i} \qquad P_A = \frac{A_i}{T_i}$$

where N_i = the average number of test locations (for all eyes in the study) which were classified by the screening evaluation to be normal for a given loss interval, i (4 dB wide). Only test locations whose norm value lay between 25 and 30 dB above zero were included.

R_i = the same as N_i except that it includes only those test locations classified as relatively defective.

346

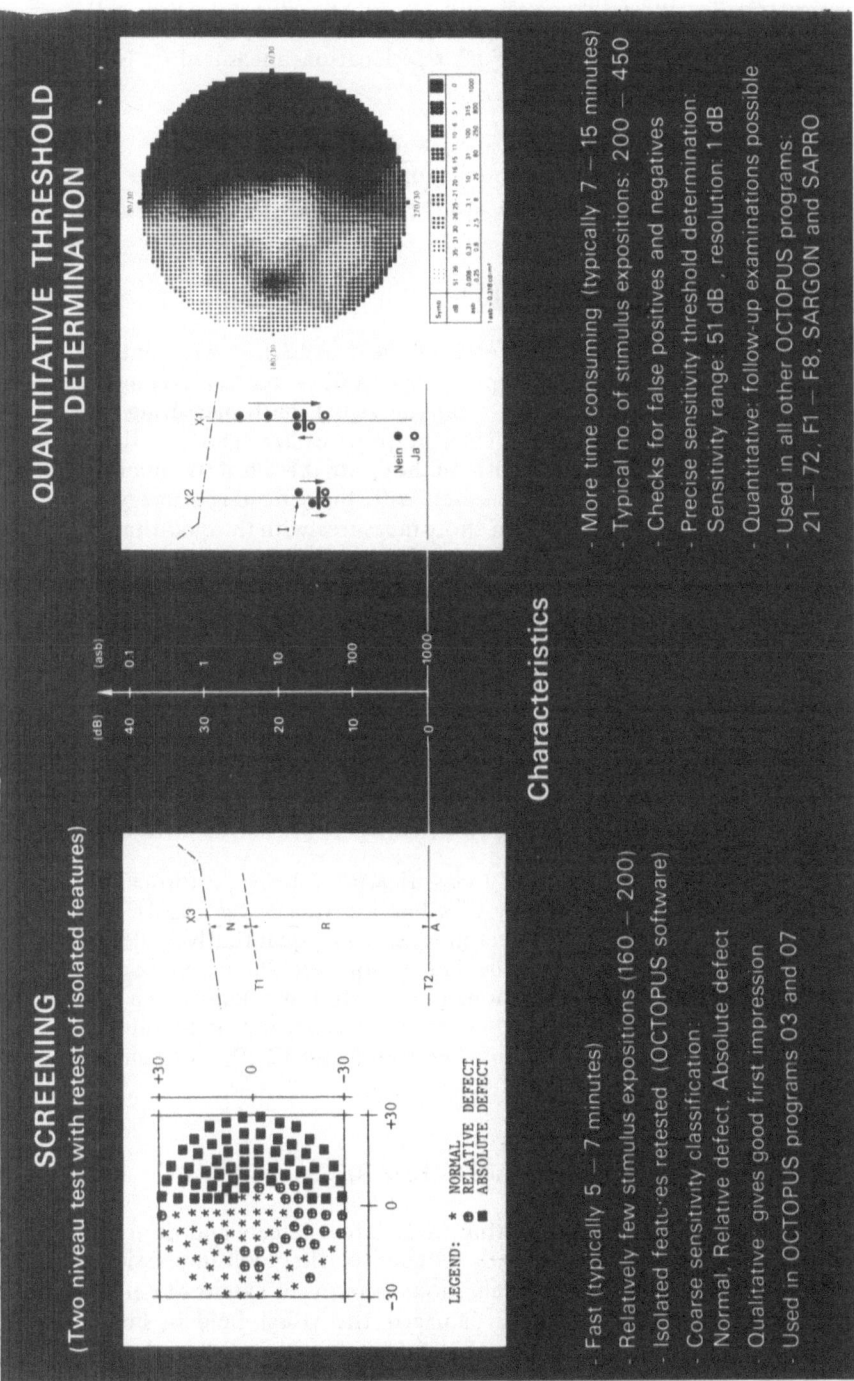

SCREENING
(Two niveau test with retest of isolated features)

QUANTITATIVE THRESHOLD DETERMINATION

LEGEND:
∗ NORMAL
⊙ RELATIVE DEFECT
■ ABSOLUTE DEFECT

(dB)	(asb)
40	0.1
30	1
20	10
10	100
0	1000

Characteristics

- Fast (typically 5 – 7 minutes)
- Relatively few stimulus expositions (160 – 200)
- Isolated features retested (OCTOPUS software)
- Coarse sensitivity classification:
  Normal. Relative defect. Absolute defect
- Qualitative: gives good first impression
- Used in OCTOPUS programs 03 and 07

- More time consuming (typically 7 – 15 minutes)
- Typical no. of stimulus expositions: 200 – 450
- Checks for false positives and negatives
- Precise sensitivity threshold determination.
  Sensitivity range 51 dB. resolution 1 dB
- Quantitative: follow-up examinations possible
- Used in all other OCTOPUS programs.
  21 – 72. F1 – F8. SARGON and SAPRO

Fig. 1. An example of a visual field examined with both a qualitative screening examination (03) and a quantitative program (31). The indicated strategies are as follows: X1 represents the full, normal bracketing method. X2 is the fast strategy which begins bracketing only at 4 dB below (I) the local norm value (upper dashed line). In the screening strategy, X3, a stimulus is shown at 6 dB below the norm (niveau T1) and if the subject responds, that location is taken as normal (N). If there is no response, the program will show a stimulus with maximum luminance (1000 asb) (niveau T2) when it next comes to that location. If there is a response, that location is classified as relative defect (R). If none then as absolute defect (A). Isolated results are retested. Some of the characteristics of the two program types are also listed.

347

A_i = the same as N_i and R_i except only for absolutely defective classified test locations.

T_i = total number of all test locations measured ($= N_i + R_i + A_i$).

Norm = the local age-corrected normal value at each test location.

Loss = the local deviation from the corresponding norm value (when the measured threshold is below norm).

RESULTS

Figure 1 shows a typical instance of a visual field examined with both a qualitative screening examination (Octopus program 03 — on the left) and a quantitative examination (program 31 — on the right), both measuring the central visual field from 0° to 30°. Their respective strategies are there indicated and some characteristics of both methods are there briefly summarized. Once again, the test locations measured with the screening strategy in this study were adjusted to coincide with those measured with the quantitative programs and thus did not occur at the locations shown in the 03 example.

Three plots (shown in the next three figures) summarize some of the empirical results which have been obtained to date in this study. Figure 2 shows the agreement between the extent of defect as determined by the screening examination and that found quantitatively. Correlation is good (92%), yet there is noticeable scatter present.

Figure 3 shows the reproducibility of the screening examinations as a function of extent of defect. As one might expect, the results of such examinations are more repeatable when the visual field is nearly normal and also when it is severely disturbed (i.e. almost no visual sensitivity). One sees that it rarely is worse than 80%.

As a further check on how accurately classification is being performed by the screening procedure, the probability of a test location being classified as normal, relative defect, or absolute defect in terms of its quantitatively determined threshold value was investigated. The results are shown in Fig. 4. Theoretically, if there were no fluctuations present, test locations with a loss greater than 6 dB should all be classified as being relatively or absolutely defective. We found, however, that for loss between 8 and 12 dB, for example, there was still a 40% chance to be classified as normal.

CONCLUSIONS AND REMARKS

Octopus screening strategy (with retesting of isolated defects and normals) produces fairly reliable results which are suitable for first-look impressions. They correlate well with quantitative evaluations in terms of extent of defect. Their reproducibility depends on how damaged the visual field is, but is almost always better than 80%. Even with extensive and well-thought-out retesting, though, fluctuations are still present. These limit the extent with

348

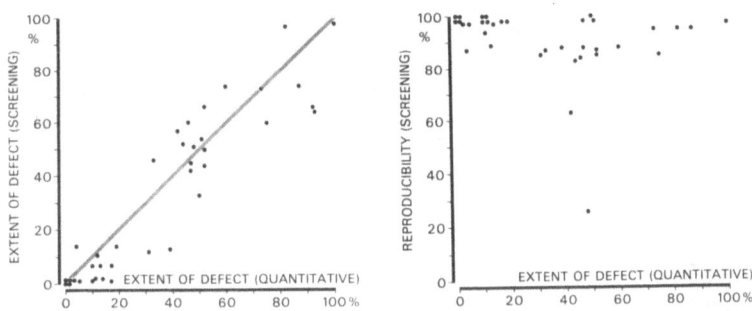

Fig. 2. Agreement between extent of defect as determined by the screening examinations and the quantitative programs.

Fig. 3. Reproducibility of successive screening examinations as a function of extent of defect (as determined quantitatively).

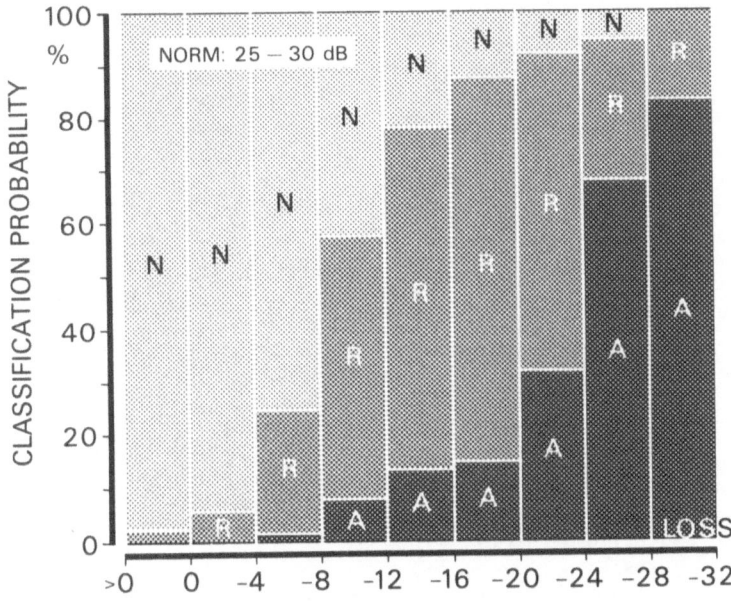

Fig. 4. Probability (as measured empirically) of a test location being classified as normal, relative defect, or absolute defect as a function of quantitatively measured loss increment. Only test locations having a norm between 25 and 30 dB were used in compiling this figure.

which such examinations can be relied upon. Were the retesting to be omitted, the situation would be even worse. If follow-up is contemplated in an individual case, a wide selection of quantitative programs and a statistical analysis package are available on the Octopus system and these should be utilized whenever one is interested in following changes that may or may not be occurring in the visual field under study.

ACKNOWLEDGEMENTS

This work is based on data produced by programs developed by H. Bebie and A. Jenni. They and J. Flammer have contributed many useful ideas in the writing of this paper. Mr Jenni is also to be thanked for his poster expertise.

Authors' address:
Eye Clinic
University of Bern
CH-3010 Bern
Switzerland

350

SPECIAL OCTOPUS SOFTWARE FOR CLINICAL INVESTIGATION

A. JENNI, J. FLAMMER, A. FUNKHOUSER and F. FANKHAUSER

(Bern, Switzerland)

Key words. Computerized perimetry, special examination, statistical analysis, JO, STATJO.

ABSTRACT

The development of new instrumentation has provided renewed stimulation for investigations of the visual field. Such studies can be given important support through goal-oriented, user-specified Octopus software programs. In some cases, the studies become possible only through the availability of such program supplements.

Utilizing a few examples, typical measurement procedures and statistical evaluation of the measurement results using the Octopus computer will be described.

INTRODUCTION

When he evaluates a visual field, the clinician is primarily concerned whether it differs from a normal one, and, if so, where, how deep, and how extended the defect is. He also wants to know if there are differences between some previous examination and any subsequent ones.

For such questions, the Octopus automatic perimeter system has available a number of routine programs for determining the state of a given visual field. As an aid for evaluation, the DELTA program is now also available which can perform several statistical analyses on data arising from the use of examination programs 31 to 44. Research-oriented clinicians often have special requirements for the examination program they wish to use. For this reason, the program SARGON was created which makes it possible for the user to fashion interactively his own program and store it permanently for subsequent applications.

It can also happen, though, in purely scientific investigations, that additional questions are asked which in daily clinical operation are of negligible importance. An example could be the classification of fluctuations of the differential threshold in various regions of the measured field or as a function of the disturbance depth. In addition, the researcher would like to have the measurement results presented in a form which permits simple and rapid further statistical evaluation.

It was due to such special requirements that a program package for clinical research has been developed. It consists of an examination program (JO) and an analysis program, STATJO. The ophthalmological background for such a program is given elsewhere (2). We shall limit ourselves here, therefore, to the technical aspects of this program package.

THE EXAMINATION PROGRAM JO

The examination is concerned with measuring 49 test locations which extend out to ±21 degrees horizontally and ±15 degrees veritcally. The grid interval is 6 degrees and the blind spot is omitted. In addition, the fixation point and four pericentral test locations with an eccentricity of 2 degrees are included.

The threshold determination is carried out using the normal Octopus strategy, but using half the standard intensity step size (1, 6). Thus the threshold is initially located using steps of 2 dB and checked in steps of 1 dB (1 dB = 0.1 log unit). The examination consists of two identical phases. This is to increase local threshold determination accuracy and to provide information concerning measurement reproducibility. In each phase, the threshold at each test location is measured. However, for the two test points designated as O and P in Fig. 1, the threshold is determined 5 times in each phase. The intent is to obtain information about measurement scatter in the center and periphery.

A further feature of this examination program is that the average reaction time of the patient is established and stored. As each phase proceeds, this is carried out 3 times, each time when a third of the determinations have been completed.

THE EXAMINATION PROCEDURE

In order to get near the true sensitivity threshold in a pathological visual field without a lot of wasted time, a special method which uses the age-corrected normal values is employed to measure one test point in each quadrant. The value which is found is then used to stipulate the initial intensity for the neighboring points within the same quadrant.

Next, the rest of the threshold determinations are carried out using the double bracketing procedure mentioned above. In addition, the two special test points, O and P, are tested 5 times.

At the end of the first phase, the operator is free to insert a pause, according to how tired the patient is, or to continue the examination. When the examination is taken up again, phase two is carried out exactly like the first one. That is, at every test location, the threshold is measured a second time, or five more times, if it is one of the two special points.

With every 'yes' answer, the patient signals that he saw the stimulus light and the apparatus retains and stores the time which elapses between the

352

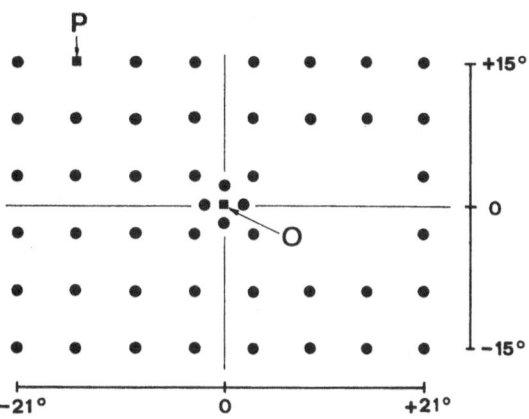

Fig. 1. Test locations in Octopus examination program JO. O, P: these points are determined ten times, providing information about the local fluctuation in the center and also peripheral.

stimulus and receiving the response. When each third of the phase is completed (i.e. 1/3, 2/3 and 3/3), the mean value of the last eight reaction times stored in a temporary buffer is computed and stored. These are then available later for the analysis program to use.

In contrast to the standard Octopus programs, at the end of the examination, the sex of the patient, the diagnosis, and the therapy utilized during the study are requested.

The examination results are displayed as shown in Fig. 3. Each doublet corresponds to one test location. The upper value gives the measurement result from the first phase and the lower that from the second one. The individual measured values for the test points which were determined five times during each phase are presented at the bottom of the printout form ordered left to right according to their time of measurement.

ANALYSIS USING THE STATJO PROGRAM

In order to make a judgement based on the numbers produced by the printout of the results, a relatively great amount of time must be taken to carry out the required computations. This time investment could be reduced only through the creation of a program such as the evaluation program STATJO. It performs a data reduction on the examination results and prints finally the calculated values in a table.

Mainly, the mean value and scatter for certain areas, test locations, phases, and reaction times are computed and displayed (see Table 1).

Explanation for the lines 1—18 in Table 1:

Lines 1—3 refer to the entire measured visual field array, while lines 4—14 are in accordance with the regions shown in Fig. 2. The first column shows the local mean or the mean value for the area of the measured thresholds. In the last column, the fluctuations are given. Of these, the standard deviation of

353

Table 1. Means and deviations calculated by STATJO from examinations measured with program JO.

			mean		fluctuation
		Surname, given name:	Xxxx Xxxxxxxx		
		Patient number / eye:	GO21.82L	1 : Examination number	
1		Overall mean: Phases 1+2	15.4 dB	R.M.S.	3.4 dB
2		Phase 1	16.2 dB		
3		Phase 2	14.6 dB		
4	P	Mean X -15 deg./ Y 15 deg.: Phases 1+2	8.5 dB	S.D.	3.4 dB
5		Phase 1	8.8 dB	S.D.	2.0 dB
6		Phase 2	8.2 dB	S.D.	4.4 dB
7		Mean center: Phases 1+2	21.2 dB	S.D.	1.3 dB
8	O	Phase 1	20.6 dB	S.D.	0.9 dB
9		Phase 2	22.8 dB	S.D.	1.4 dB
10	a	Midperipheral: Mean	15.2 dB	R.M.S.	3.5 dB
11	b	Pericentral: Mean	19.1 dB	R.M.S.	3.3 dB
12	c	Paracentral: Mean	19.4 dB	R.M.S.	3.4 dB
13	u	Upper half: Mean	16.1 dB	R.M.S.	2.4 dB
14	l	Lower half: Mean	16.7 dB	R.M.S.	4.6 dB
15	Nu No	Nasal step: Mean	- 1.7 dB	Confidence limit	1.7 dB
16		Reaction time mean: Phases 1+2	0.52 s	S.D.	0.12 s
17		Difference: Phase 1 - 2	0.08 s		

Deviation from expected values:

	Deviation	R.M.S.	Number of points
18	<= 4 dB	2.4 dB	6
	> 4 <= 10 dB	3.9 dB	35
	> 10 <= 16 dB	4.1 dB	6
	> 16 <= 20 dB	3.1 dB	2
	> 20 dB	-.-	

— Same range as in Fig. 2

— For explanation of numbered lines, see text.

the distribution of the respective ten local results are shown in lines 4–9, while on the rest of the lines, the root-mean square fluctuations for the local standard deviations are given.

Line 15 shows in the first column the difference between the threshold mean values from the 4 nasal superior test points and the 4 nasal inferior. In each case the combined results of both phases are given. The standard error of the difference is presented in the last column.

Line 16: here the mean reaction time, averaged over the two phases is displayed in the first column, while the second shows the associated standard deviation.

354

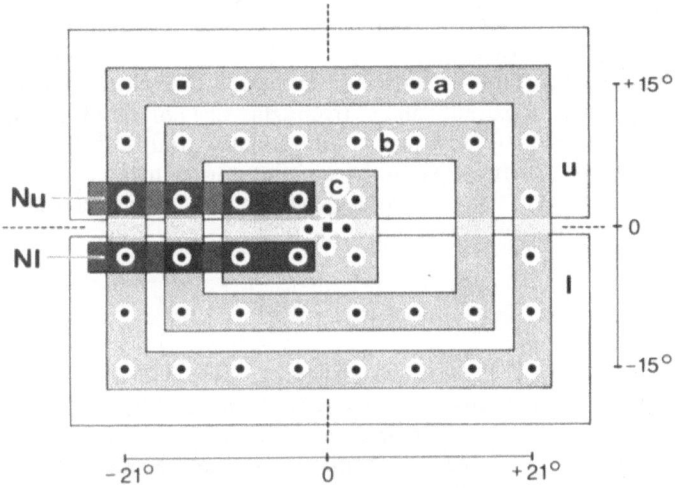

Fig. 2. The grouping of the test points as used by the STATJO program. a, b, c: eccentricity areas; Nu: nasal upper; Nl: nasal lower; u: upper half; l: lower half.

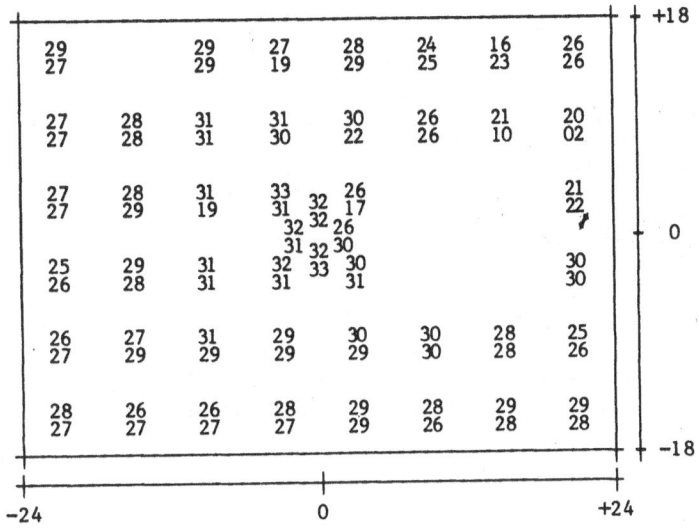

MULTIPLE DETERMINATIONS

	COORD. X = −15	/ Y = 15			
PHASE 1:	27	26	27	27	24
PHASE 2:	28	22	27	22	26

	COORD. X = 0	/ Y = 0			
PHASE 1:	33	33	32	33	32
PHASE 2:	34	33	34	33	34

Fig. 3. Example of printout: results as measured by program JO.

355

Line 17 gives the difference between the average reaction time from phase one and that of phase two.

Line 18 is responsible for showing how much the scatter depends on the deviation of the measured values from the age-corrected normal values (norms). To this end, the test points are put into groups. In the first column stands the amount of the deviation from the norm; in the second, the standard deviation within the associated group; while the last column gives the number of test points for this group.

DISCUSSION

With the JO program, the clinical researcher is provided a program which delivers information about the differential thresholds, their scatter, the reaction time, and false positive and negative answers of the patient. By the supplementary storage of such information as the diagnosis and medication code, and through the statistical processing of the results using the STATJO program, the evaluation during a study is far easier. A trial version of the program package described here has already been used in some studies (3, 4, 5).

REFERENCES

1. Bebie, H., Fankhauser, F. and Spahr, J. Static perimetry: strategies. Acta Ophthalmol. 54:325 (1976).
2. Flammer, J., Drance, S. M., Jenni, A. and Bebie, H. The Octopus program JO and STATJO — a special program for clinical investigation of the visual field. Can. J. Ophthalmol. (in press).
3. Flammer, J. and Drance, S. M. Reversibility of glaucomatous visual field defect after acetazolamide therapy. Can. J. Ophthalmol. (in press).
4. Flammer, J. and Drance, S. M. The effect of a number of glaucoma medications on the differential light threshold. Doc. Ophthalmol. Proc. Series 35:145–148 (1983).
5. Flammer, J., Drance, S. M. and Schulzer, M. The estimation and testing of the components of long-term fluctuation of the differential light threshold. Doc. Ophthalmol. Proc. Series 35:383–389 (1983).
6. Octopus Manual, Chapter 4.9. Interzeag AG, Rietbachstrasse 5, 8952 Schlieren, Switzerland.

Authors' address:
Eye Clinic
University of Bern
CH 3010 Bern
Switzerland

DISCUSSION

Discussion on 'Special Octopus software for clinical investigation', by A. Jenni, J. Flammer, A. Funkhouser and F. Fankhauser.

C. A. Johnson: I was wondering if I could get a point of clarification. On the bottom columns of the last slide (Table 1) we had deviation from expected value. Is that based upon the normal values, the age-matched mass normal values and such?

J. Flammer: It is indeed the deviation from our stock normal values. I can add something to this and that is that we have now controlled several hundred normal fields and we found the same normal values there.

C. A. Johnson: As a follow-up to that it is somewhat curious to me why there are two points that differ from the normals by a factor of almost 100. They are almost 2 log units different. What is the standard deviation of the dB variation and how does it change with age?

J. Flammer: The deviation that we have there which we call the short-term fluctuation is not age-related if we take out all the other factors in multiple regression analyses. It is much more dependent on the size of the sensitivity and this is quite typical. The more we go into a relative scotoma the higher the scatter becomes. If you come closer to an absolute defect the scatter is getting smaller. But you see if you have only two points the error of the estimation of the scatter is also high. We have just shown a calculated mean and we do not give confidence limits for the errors themselves. So it is quite possible if you are in a relative scotoma and you repeat the point twice, that you get quite a big difference. The reason for this may also be a tiring effect and so on.

A. Heijl: I think it is important that those perimeters that are custom programmable be used in ventures like this in the future.

OPTIMIZATION OF COMPUTER-ASSISTED PERIMETRY

J. R. CHARLIER, L. MOUSSU and J. C. HACHE

(Lille, France)

Key words. Automated perimetry, examinations strategies.

ABSTRACT

The overall features of optimal examination strategies applied to computer-assisted perimetry are described. Emphasis is placed on the concepts of specificity and adaptivity which result from the necessity to obtain the greatest information gain within the amount of time available to the clinical examination. Implications for computer hardware and software are derived, including the programmability and interactive control of examination protocols.

INTRODUCTION

Computer-assisted perimetry has now proved its capability in providing useful information in the ophthalmologist's everyday's practice and is expected to give a new impetus to an examination which is often regarded as cumbersome and unreliable. The present automated perimeters can be considered as an alternative to conventional manual equipment with such interesting features as the standardization and reproducibility of examination procedures as well as the decrease of the results dependence upon the perimetrist's skill. However, the first clinical reports on automated perimeters outlined their lack of flexibility as an important limitation to the assessment and quantitative evaluation of visual field defects (13, 17, 18).

Much is expected from future developments of automated perimetry and it is widely believed that the optimization of examination procedures will improve the present state of affairs (6, 7, 15).

The aim of the present study is to give a rigorous statement of the goals and constraints of visual field examination and to analyze their consequences for computer hardware and software involved in computer-assisted perimetry.

VISUAL FIELD EXAMINATION – GOALS AND CONSTRAINTS

The visual field examination consists of a series of psychophysical measurements of light perception. Its goal is to obtain new reliable information which,

Greve, E. L., Heijl, A. (eds.) Fifth International Visual Field Symposium.
©1983 Dr W. Junk Publishers, The Hague/Boston/Lancaster.

correlated with other signs and symptoms of disease, allow the formulation of a diagnosis. We would like to point out that this does not imply an accurate and detailed mapping of the luminance difference threshold. Simple characteristic features of alterations such as a stepped nasal margin or an enlarged blind spot provide important clues for a diagnosis and in many circumstances, a complete mapping of visual field defects does not supply further information.

Variability and fluctuation of responses

One first problem in visual field examination is the variation or fluctuation of responses with parameters difficult to measure or to keep under control. Each individual response involves three major elements.

First is the visual stimulation. The light distribution over the retina is determined by the stimulus generation system as well as the optical status of the eye. Nowadays, most instruments rely upon the projection onto a screen of stimuli of controlled luminance, size, position, velocity, duration, color, etc. However, the optics of the eye introduce many variations to what is received by the retina. The pupillary size and the opacity of the ocular media affect the intensity and sharpness of the retinal image. The morphology of the orbit and the eyelids limit the extent of the peripheral visual field. The eye orientation controls the stimulus position and the eye refraction its sharpness.

The second element involved in the responses is the processing of the visual stimuli through normal or pathological structures of the visual system.

Third are functions irrelevant to the visual system but which are still implied in the responses. These functions include central decision processes which are affected by the psychological status of the patient: his ability to concentrate on the task, his degree of suggestibility, his understanding of the test, his general fatigue, etc. Effector functions are also involved which can be affected by age or disease.

Time limitations

A second problem in visual field examination is time limitation. Due to the increase of fatigue, threshold responses and discrepancies augment with examination duration. Otherwise, equipment and clinical staff availability does not allow for time-consuming examinations. 10 to 12 minutes is generally considered as a reasonable limit (11) but this value will vary depending on the psychological status of the patient, his age, etc.

OPTIMIZATION OF EXAMINATION PROCEDURES

Examination strategies aim at the greatest gain of reliable information with a minimum amount of tests. The repertoire of available stimulations should include the tests most suitable for the detection and analysis of deficits (10). Consequently, a perimeter should permit the exploration of the visual functions under a variety of different techniques. Suprathreshold, static and kinetic perimetry are now recognized standards. However, other approaches such as combined scotopic, mesopic and photopic evaluation (12), multi-variable perimetry (4) and even objective perimetry might be worthwhile to develop.

The proper choice of tests should take into account all sources of information made available prior and during the examination. Flexibility and adaptation are the keys to optimal examination strategies. These features are compatible with the standardization and reproducibility required in daily office practice (14). This is true as far as we are not interested in obtaining a precise mapping of the visual field but rather in identifying characteristic features of alterations.

The initial knowledge of the patient's disease will direct the choice of a specific protocol. This protocol will be adapted to the patient's age, refraction and pupil size, i.e. information which is collected during the clinical investigation.

During the examination process, further adaptation will be introduced from the findings made from the analysis of responses. This adaptation will be based on two different criteria: one is to validate the responses, the other to identify specific features of the alterations.

Validation of responses

Each individual response is weighed according to its reliability.

External monitoring systems allow the rejection of unreliable responses. Such systems have already been developed for monitoring fixation steadiness from optical properties of the eye. Similar developments might be thought of for controlling other parameters which affect the results such as the patient's vigilance.

Another complementary approach is to test the responses according to specific properties of the visual field (9). The likelihood control consists of comparing the responses to normal values. It allows the detection of fixation unsteadiness by the presentation of stimuli within the blind spot area. It permits an evaluation of the patient's level of cooperation by testing his reaction to unseen stimuli. The control of adjacency is based upon the spatial continuity of the 'island of vision'. The sensitivity variation between neighbouring responses should be within a given interval depending upon the type of pathology involved. The control of coherence consists in comparing measurements obtained with different techniques as, for instance, static and kinetic perimetry.

Finally, averaging techniques can be applied in order to improve the 'signal to noise ratio' of responses (1).

Analysis of visual field defects

This analysis aims at the classification of visual field defects through the identification of specific features of the alterations. The degree of evidence of a given defect can be used to determine the orientation of the examination protocol. It necessitates a precise knowledge of the action of diseases as well

361

as a model for the resulting alterations and their evolution. Such work has already been carried out for the macular alterations (8), allowing the identification of foveolar, perifoveolar or macular impairments. Similar approaches could be made for other types of deficits. The diagnostic process would terminate when the likelihood of identity between one of the models and the collected responses would exceed a given threshold.

IMPLEMENTATION ON COMPUTERIZED SYSTEMS

The optimization rules which have been described previously can easily be applied on manual perimeters. Ther implementation on a computerized system is subjected to two major requirements: programmability and interactivity.

Programmability

Medicine is essentially an art and this is specifically true of visual field examinations (10). It is difficult to realize an agreement on the best decisions to be made at each examination step as long as a precise, mathematical statement of the problem is not available. The present situation will undoubtedly remain the same for quite a long time.

Another approach is to allow skilled perimetrists who have gained extensive clinical experience to program their own examination protocols. A major barrier to this development is programming. Programmability is not only the possibility to develop automated sequences of stimulations. It should allow the practician to cope easily with a repertoire of actions, storage facilities and computational capabilities which are not familiar to the clinical world. A serious difficulty is to express clinical concepts in terms of numerical data that can be processed by a computer. Specific programming functions are needed for the generation of visual stimuli and recording of responses. Other programming functions should be provided for the analysis of responses and the detection of such features as an enlarged blind spot or an arcuate defect. Such programming functions can be combined with linear programming techniques to develop examination protocols. They make up a 'language of perimetry' which allows a precise formalization of examination protocols and could benefit the exchange of methodologies between practicians dealing with the optimization of examination protocols.

Interactivity

Interactivity is needed to supply the examination protocol with data not directly accessible to the computer. This task might be reduced in future developments with the integration of the different examination tools within one computer network (2). Another purpose of interactivity is to cope with situations not expected in examination protocols. The operator must be provided with a direct, real time control of the examination including information on the ongoing procedure, on the acquired responses and on the present interpretation of the results performed by the computer.

He must also be able to act rapidly and accurately on the examination process. These features are made possible by the recent technological developments in display devices, light pens and time-sharing processing. The use of graphic displays seems to be an absolute necessity given the large amount of information to be transmitted. Combining color and graphics would further enhance data comprehension, reduce the operator's fatigue and allow higher data throughout. The operator should be able to select the mode of display most suitable for the interpretation of data (5): topographic representations of the 'island of vision' such as equisensitivity curves (isopters), grey density and color maps, profile displays and numerical tables.

A difficult problem to solve is the allocation of tasks between the computer and the operator. Different solutions can be proposed (16), depending upon the operator's expertise. One option is to give the operator no role except for surveying the examination and entering requested data. The other extreme option would give the operator a leading part and let the computer execute commands. In clinical situations, a compromise has to be found between these two extremes. Some tasks may be entirely automated and others left to the operator.

CONCLUSION

The rules described in this paper have been implemented or are under development on the automated perimeter 'perimatic' which is presently used in routine clinical work at Lille medical center.

A surprising fact is that the examination strategies which have been implemented are not quite different from those applied by skilled and experienced perimetrists on manual instruments. This can be explained by the use of inference and deductive rules. Future developments might include probabilistic deicison-making schemes which, combined with categorical reasoning, would exhibit medical expertise (19).

ACKNOWLEDGEMENT

This work was supported by grants from the French DGRST, INSERM and Fondation pour la recherche médicale.

REFERENCES

1. Bebie, H., Fankhauser, F. and Spahr, J. Static perimetry, accuracy and fluctuations. Acta Ophthalmol. 54:339−348 (1976).
2. Bechetoile, A. L'avenir de la périmétrie. In: Le glaucome primitif à angle ouvert. Simep. Bruxelles 11:133−136 (1981).
3. Charlier, J. R. and Hache, J. C. New instrument for monitoring eye fixation and pupil size during the visual field examination. Med. Biol. Eng. Comput. 2:23−28 (1982).
4. Dubois-Poulsen, A. Le champ visuel. Masson, Paris (1954).

5. Fankhauser, F. Problems related to the design of automated perimeters. Doc. Ophthalmol. 47(1):89–138 (1979).
6. Greve, E. L. Automatic and non-automatic perimetry. Int. Ophthalmol. 2(1):19–22 (1980).
7. Häberlin, H., Jenni, A. and Fankhauser, F. Researches on adaptive high resolution programming for automatic perimeters. Principles and preliminary results. Int. Ophthalmol. 2(1):1–9 (1980).
8. Hache, J. C., Francois, P., Limosin, J. J. and Toulotte, J. M. Méthode et intérêt de la simulation des affections maculaires sur ordinateur. Colloque IRIA Informatique médicale, Toulouse (1973).
9. Hache, J. C., Francois, P. and Charlier, J. R. La scotométrie en neuroophtalmologie. Intérêt d'un instrument de mesure automatique du champ visuel. Bulletins et mémoires de la Société Française d'ophtalmologie 7:125–129 (1980).
10. Harrington, D. The art of perimetry. Am. J. Ophthalmol. 80:414–417 (1975).
11. Heijl, A. Time changes of contrast thresholds during automatic perimetry. Acta Ophthalmol. 55:2–14 (1977).
12. Jayle, G. E. Bases physiologiques et valeur clinique de la périmétrie quantitative. Le check up périmétrique et l'explorateur universel du sens lumineux de Jayle et Blet. Arch. Ophthalmol. 20:685–705 (1960).
13. Keltner, J. L., Johnson, C. A. and Balestrery, F. G. Suprathreshold static perimetry. Initial trial with the Fieldmaster automatic perimeter. Arch. Ophthalmol. 97:260–272 (1979).
14. Keltner, J. L. and Johnson, C. A. Automated perimetry. A consumer guide. Ann. Ophthalmol. 275–279 (1981).
15. Krakau, C. E. T. A feasible development of computerized perimetry. Acta Ophthalmol. 59:485–494 (1981).
16. Michard, A. Task allocation between man and computer for an electronic appointment book. Rapport de recherche INRIA no. 85 (1981).
17. Portney, G. L. and Krohn, M. A. Automatic perimetry: background instruments and methods. Surv. Ophthalmol. 22:271–278 (1978).
18. Potts, D. Computers in ophthalmology. IEEE Press (1978).
19. Szolovits, P. and Pauker, S. G. Categorical and probabilistic reasoning in medical diagnosis. Artificial Intelligence 11:115–144 (1978).

Authors' addresses:
J. R. Charlier
Centre de Technologie Biomédicale INSERM
13 à 17 rue Camille Guérin
59800 Lille
France

L. Moussu, J. C. Hache
C.H.R. de Lille
Place de Verdun
59800 Lille
France

AUTOMATION OF THE GOLDMANN PERIMETER*

M. ZINGIRIAN, E. GANDOLFO and M. ORCIUOLO

(Genoa, Italy)

Key words. Perimetry, automation, standardization, Goldmann perimeter.

ABSTRACT

Automated perimeters of both lower and higher complexity have achieved limited diffusion due to poor standardization, difficulty in interpreting computerized test results and in comparing them with those of traditional perimetry. As a consequence, our present concept concerning automation of perimetry is not to build new computerized perimeters, but to provide automation for perimeters already well standardized and widely used. Therefore, we have devised a computerized unit adapted for the Goldmann perimeter. This unit automatically executes the traditional perimetric operations, without excluding manual use. Both kinetic and static procedures are carried out. In addition target surface and luminance selection, fixation control, data storage and representation of results are performed by the program. Standard, oriented and special programs available for visual field examination are described. The main advantages of the 'Automated Goldmann Perimeter' are: good level of standardization, easy interpretation of results and low cost.

A CRITICAL MOMENT FOR AUTOMATED PERIMETRY

Present-day automated perimetry is going through a critical phase.
— Computerized suprathreshold screening programs have poor reliability (high percentage of false negative responses) (1, 2, 3).
— Automated threshold measuring procedures produce static results difficult to interpret and to compare with those of traditional perimetry (4). In fact the average ophthalmologist is still conditioned towards an isopteric concept of the visual field.
— Lack of standardization affects present automated perimetry.

*Requests for offprints should be addressed to Miss Vanna Re, Librarian of the University Eye Clinic, Viale Benedetto XV, 16132, Genoa, Italy.

Greve, E. L., Heijl, A. (eds.) Fifth International Visual Field Symposium.
©*1983 Dr W. Junk Publishers, The Hague/Boston/Lancaster.*
ISBN 90 6193 731 0. Printed in the Netherlands.

365

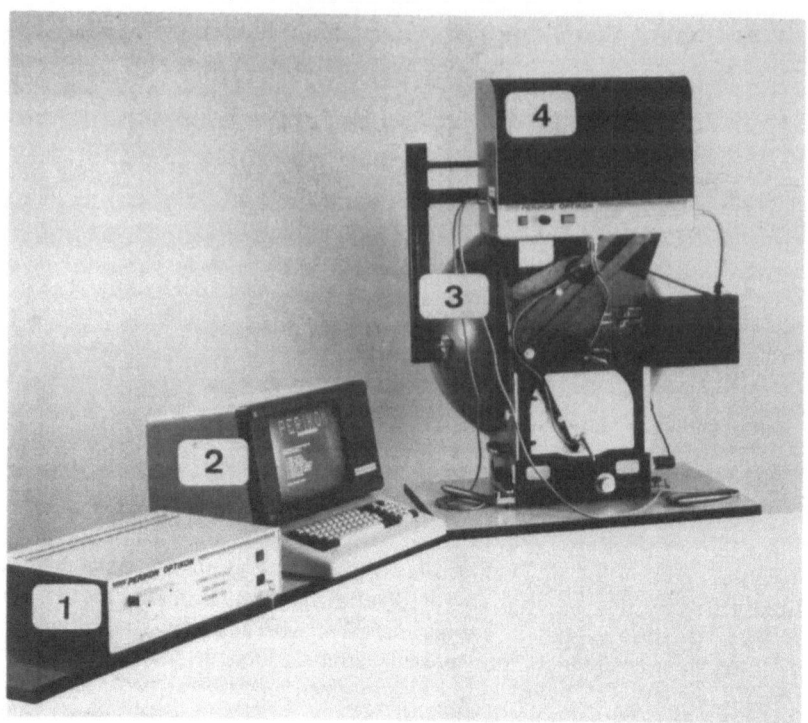

Fig. 1. The automated Goldmann perimeter; (1) central process unit; (2) monitor and keyboard; (3) Goldmann perimeter; (4) servo-mechanisms unit.

Therefore our present approach to automated perimetry is to limit development of new computerized prototypes and to promote automation of pre-existing, well-standardized and extensively used perimetric equipment.

As a consequence we have built a 'Computerized unit for Automation of any Goldmann or Goldmann-like Perimeter'. We have also provided this unit with a standard interface IEEE 488.

TECHNICAL DATA

The apparatus (Fig. 1) is composed of a traditional Goldmann perimeter in which the following functions are automatically controlled by a micro-computerized system (Z 80 based):

1. Target movement

A step motor provides angular movement (resolution 0.2°), while a d.c. motor provides radial movement (resolution 0.5°). Combining both movements allows an actual spatial resolution of the system corresponding to 32,400 different possible positions of the target on the screen. The maximum

366

velocity achieved is 10°/sec for angular movements and 20°/sec for radial movements.

2. Insertion of filters and diaphragms

D.c. motors with position control command the levers that modify target luminance and surface.

3. Fixation control

A proper ocular permits both visual and automatic fixation control. This device employs 3 phototransistors which send a signal to the central process unit in case of fixation loss. The sensitivity of the device can be regulated according to operator preference.

4. Target shutter control

This operation is provided by a two-position d.c. motor, acoustically isolated so as not to influence perception during static presentation. During kinetic examination the shutter automatically closes when the target is perceived and changes trajectory. In this manner unwanted stimulations are avoided.

5. Machine–operator interrelationship

The operator manages the entire perimetric examination through an alpha-numerical keyboard and checks test progress on a TV monitor. A simple perimetric language is used for listing the operations to be selected. In case of mishap that forces interruption of the program, the reason for the stop is indicated on the TV screen and an alarm is set off. The operator can interrupt the examination at any moment and review on the monitor the results obtained up to that time.

6. Representation of results

At the end of each examination the perimetric results are numerically displayed on a monitor or printed out. Isopter plotting is automatically carried out on the chart by a plotter, which connects the threshold points corresponding to every stimulus used.

7. Data storage

The device can be supplied with a dual standard 8″ floppy disc. This optional memory, due to its widespread capability, can store not only perimetric data, but also additional information regarding patients.

8. Programs available

Standard, oriented and special programs are normally supplied.

Standard kinetic program includes the following subroutines:
— automated selection of four targets;
— randomized kinetic presentation of each target and determination of 68 threshold points;
— display of results and plotting of four isopters;
— delineation of the blind spot with 8 coecofugal presentations.

Standard static meridian program consists of the following procedures:
— selection of the meridian to be explored;
— measurement of the liminance threshold at 47 points, spaced close together in the central area;
— an ascending strategy with a double resolution is employed to measure the threshold at every tested single point;
— the results of each examination are displayed on the monitor or plotted.

Oriented programs include, at the present time, only a procedure for the screening of glaucoma defects, according to the Armaly-Drance method.

Special programs:
— kinetic and static programs with a higher spatial resolution in a limited area of the visual field can be carried out;
— static circular perimetry on every parallel can be performed with any spatial resolution preselected by the operator;
— a shortened kinetic procedure for rapid screening purposes is also available;
— finally, a special program has been studied for the accurate examination of the blind spot area.

PERSPECTIVES IN PROGRAMMING

Since an IEEE 488 standard interface allows the perimeter to be connected to a more complex computer system, the operator will be able to implement also *individual programs* using the keyboard and 'Basic' language.

A program for the assessment of disturbed areas and for retesting with improved spatial resolution and a more adequate strategy is now in the implementation phase.

Programs for statistical comparison between results obtained from the same eye during two successive examinations will also be provided in the near future.

CONCLUSIONS

The automation of the Goldmann perimeter offers some advantages:
— use of the same instrument for both automatic and manual perimetry (kinetic and static) with similar procedures;
— comparability of test results with those of traditional perimetry;
— high spatial resolution available;

368

- possibility to connect the perimeter, as a peripheral unit, with a large computer in a more complex system for the implementation of individual (e.g. research) perimetric programs;
- possibility to obtain a sophisticated, fairly well standardized automated perimeter at a relatively low cost.

The disadvantages of this apparatus are mainly due to inertia in the projecting arm, that produces:
- difficulty in rapid target movement;
- time consumption during kinetic procedures.

A more definitive assessment of the validity of this computerized unit will only be obtained through more extensive clinical experimentation.

ACKNOWLEDGEMENT

This study was supported by a grant from the Consiglio Nazionale delle Ricerche, Rome, Italy.

REFERENCES

1. Greve, E. L. Automatic and non-automatic perimetry. Int. Ophthalmol. 2:19–22 (1980).
2. Greve, E. L. Some comments related to the article 'Use of Fieldmaster Automated Perimeter for the detection of early visual field changes in glaucoma' by C. Hong, Y. Kitazawa and S. Shirato. Int. Ophthalmol. 4:157 (1981).
3. Keltner, J. L. and Johnson, C. A. Capabilities and limitation of automated suprathreshold static perimetry. Doc. Ophthalmol. Proc. Series 26:49–55 (1980).
4. Zingirian, M., Gandolfo, E., Tagliasco, V. and Spinelli, G. A standardization-oriented approach to automated perimetry. Computers in Ophthalmology. Washington University, St. Louis (1979).

Authors' address:
University Eye Clinic
Viale Benedetto XV, 5
16132 Genoa
Italy

PRELIMINARY EXAMINATION OF THE SQUID AUTOMATED PERIMETER

JOHN L. KELTNER* and CHRIS A. JOHNSON

(Davis, California, U.S.A.)

key words. Automated perimetry.

ABSTRACT

The Squid is a new automated visual field device manufactured by Synemed, Inc., consisting of a projection perimeter controlled by an LSI-11/23 microprocessor. A variety of test programs are available to perform threshold evaluation of the visual field according to grid, meridional, radial and other target patterns. In addition to the standard test programs, special routines are available for data base management of patient records, storage and analysis of perimetry results, and the design and implementation of customized test procedures. The controllers for various stimulus attributes (luminance, duration, target position, etc.) are also accessible through FORTRAN callable subroutines. Test results can be saved on disk storage media (both a 20 Mbyte Winchester drive and two dual-sided, dual-density floppy disks are provided. A high resolution thermal printer proves a hard copy of test results according to several formats (grey scale density plot, static profiles or numerical threshold data). This paper describes the general operating principles and features of the Squid.

INTRODUCTION

A large selection of automated and semi-automated perimeters is currently available from various manufacturers. Many of them have been shown to be clinically useful for detection of visual field abnormalities (1, 3–6) with several of the more sophisticated devices exhibiting additional capabilities for detailed quantitative evaluation of the visual field. For general patient testing, such devices have been quite acceptable. However, a persistent problem with all automated perimeters to date has been their limited flexibility and adaptability for specific needs and their inability to incorporate new advances in perimetric testing (obsolescence). The examiner is able to vary

*To whom requests for offprints should be addressed.

Greve, E. L., Heijl, A. (eds.) Fifth International Visual Field Symposium.
©*1983 Dr W. Junk Publishers, The Hague/Boston/Lancaster.*

certain aspects of the procedure (e.g., target parameters, selection of test programs, etc.), but is not able to modify any of the basic test strategies or other key aspects of the examination process. This means that the examiner must adapt existing visual field requirements to meet the capabilities and limitations of the automated perimeter, rather than modifying the device to best satisfy his or her needs. An adversary relationship can thereby be established between the perimeter and the practitioner, with the perimeter allowing little room for compromise. In other words, many automated perimeters are not 'user friendly'.

We feel that the Squid model 300 (Synemed, Inc., Berkeley, California) represents a departure from this trend. In addition to providing a large array of standard tests, the Squid also has programs that allow the user to design and create custom test patterns. These tests are added to the existing library of test programs for future use. In addition, if the user wishes to completely revise the test strategies and operating characteristics of the Squid, he or she can write programs in FORTRAN that will control all aspects of the perimeter in any desired manner. The system can also be used as a general purpose laboratory computer, since it is supplied with a standard LSI-11 operating system (RT-11), FORTRAN language and all necessary peripheral devices. In this paper, we present a brief overview of the Squid's features and capabilities.

HARDWARE

The Squid has two main components, consisting of a projection perimeter and an operator's console that contains the microcomputer system (see Fig. 1). A white hemispherical bowl (1/2 meter radius) serves as the background field of the perimeter, with two diffused light sources at the top of the bowl providing a uniform background luminance. Accurate control of background luminance (adjustable from 4 to 300 asb) is maintained by a calibrated photocell that monitors the light reflected from the bowl surface.

The target is projected onto the background by means of a motor-driven mirror located in front of the patient's forehead. Target size (Goldmann sizes 0 through V), luminance (0.1 to 5,000 asb), color (white, red, yellow, green, blue), duration (0.4 seconds minimum), average interval between stimuli (0.4 seconds minimum), target location (static and kinetic testing) and rate of movement (kinetic testing) are all under computer control. The examiner can use the standard default values of these test parameters, or set them to any desired values within the range of the instrument. Target luminance is monitored by means of a calibrated photocell.

Fixation targets are presented by means of an additional projector at the top of the perimeter bowl. Three fixation targets are available: 1) a single red fixation point (15 min of arc diameter), 2) a 5 degree diamond pattern of four red targets surrounding fixation, and 3) a 10 degree diamond pattern of four red targets surrounding fixation.

The patient is seated in a movable chair that also incorporates the head and chin rest assembly, translucent occluders (for the non-tested eye) and

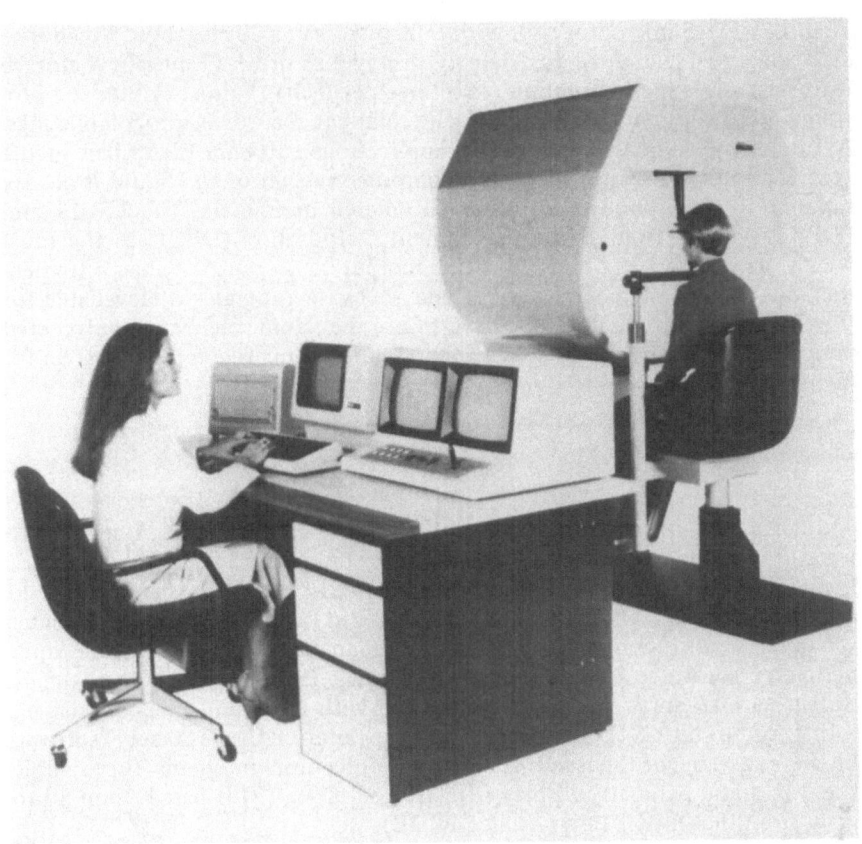

Fig. 1. Photo of the Squid automated perimeter.

lens holder. Alignment of the patient is accomplished by rotation and translation of the chair assembly (under motorized control) while observing the patient's eye in the television monitor. Eye movements are also monitored by the infrared television camera focused on the patient's eye. The camera views the patient's eye through a 33 mm diameter hole located in the region occupied by the blind spot. Objective monitoring of fixation is achieved by projecting the infrared reflections from the patient's eye onto a quadrant photodetector-like matrix, which is sensitive to changes in reflections produced by eye or head movements. The sensitivity of the eye monitor is adjustable, and a video display at the operator's console allows subjective monitoring of the patient's eye by the examiner. Controls at the operator's console allow the patient's pupil size to be measured directly from the video display. The operator's console also has a video monitor for viewing the target pattern and the progress of the test procedure, a video terminal (DEC VT-100) for communicating with the computer, and a joystick control for manipulating the target during computer-assisted kinetic testing.

The microcomputer system is housed in the operator console, and consists of an LSI-11/23 microprocessor with 64K memory, a 20 megabyte Winchester disk drive, two dual-sided dual-density floppy disk drives (1 megabyte storage for each) and a high resolution (150 lines per inch) thermal printer for providing 'hard copy' output of test results, patient records or program listings. A full compliment of systems and applications software (described in the next section) is also provided. The computer system of the Squid is clearly superior to that found in all other automated perimeters. The LSI-11 and PDP-11 systems from Digital Equipment Corporation (DEC) are the most widely used laboratory and industrial computers. Because of this, a tremendous number of peripheral devices and software programs are available for the LSI-11. Thus, one does not have to use the Squid solely as an automated perimeter. It can also be used as a general purpose microcomputer system for many applications.

SOFTWARE

Although the hardware components of the Squid are impressive, it is the software that provides most of the Squid's truly unique and powerful attributes. Included with the Squid is a full set of DEC LSI-11 systems software (RT-11 operating system, FORTRAN compiler, MACRO assembler and other related software), a DBL compiler (a COBOL-like language) and the custom Squid perimetry software. A word processing package (SATURN) is also available. Because a DEC software license is included with the Squid, the user also has access to the DECUS (Digital Equipment Corporation User's Society) software library consisting of thousands of software applications programs (for example, the 3-D static perimetry display of Hart and Hartz (2) is based upon a program from the DECUS library called HIDE).

The custom Squid software has six primary subsections (patient record management, test generation and management, static test administration, kinetic test administration, report generation, and test result comparison), as shown in Fig. 2. Each of these subsections also has a series of procedures that can be implemented for specific purposes. The Squid executive program is a menu-driven, modular system that allows the user to easily perform a variety of tasks. The patient record management section permits the user to add, delete and modify patient records and perimetric test results. Additional commands also allow the user to print individual patient records and make backup copies of patient records.

The static test administration subsection performs static threshold testing of the visual field. A total of 15 standard test programs (briefly described in Table 1) are available for static testing, as well as any custom-designed tests developed by the user. Standard stimulus and background values may be used, or individual settings may be changed (target luminance, size, duration, etc.).

Computer-assisted kinetic perimetry can be accomplished by the kinetic test administration subsection of the Squid executive program. The user is able to specify any stimulus or background parameter, or use the standard default settings. The target is moved by manipulating the joystick on the operator's console.

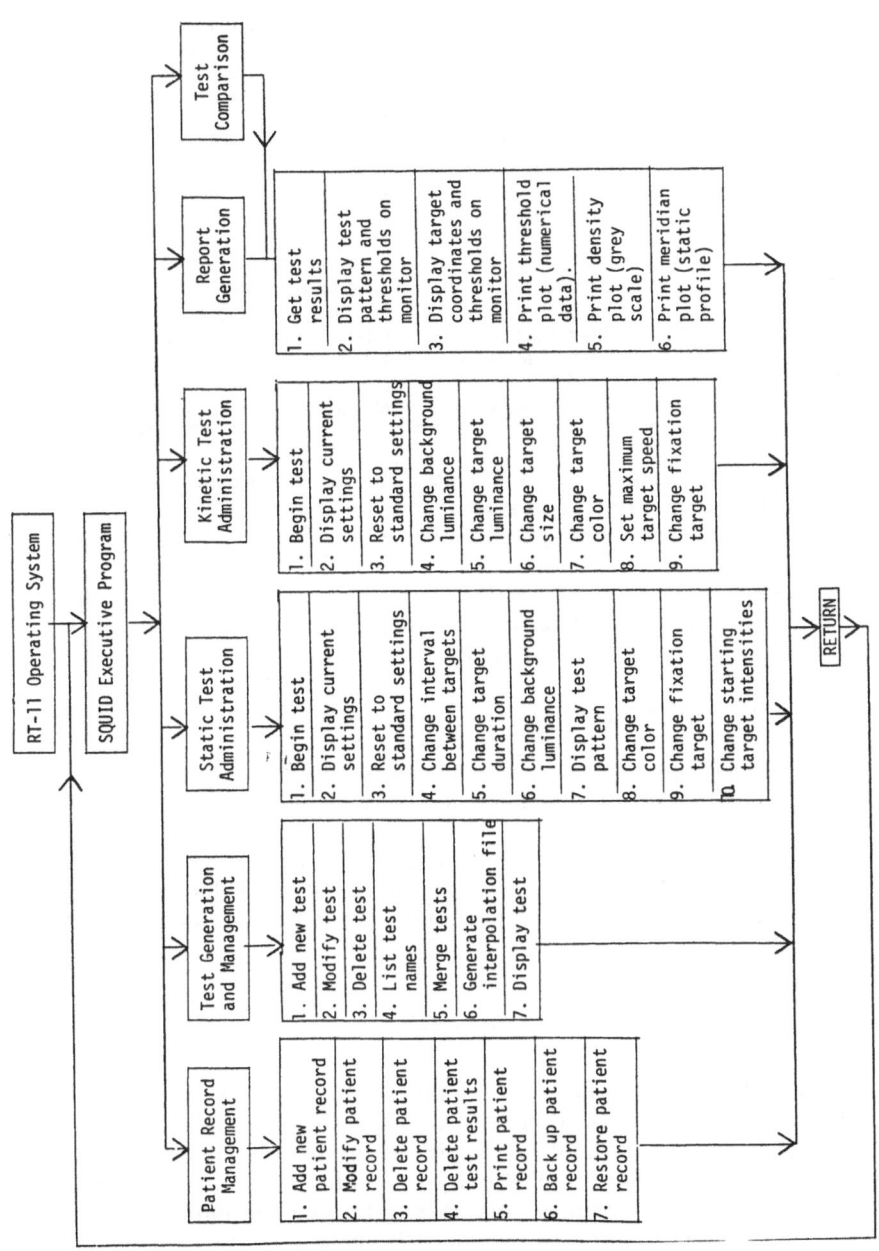

Fig. 2. Flow chart of programs and testing routines currently available for the Squid.

375

Table 1. Standard test programs for the Squid.

Program	No. of targets	Location	Description
STD110	9	Central 5 deg	Grid pattern, 3 deg spacing
STD150	57	Blind spot	Grid pattern, 1.5 deg spacing
STD160	16	Blind spot	Grid pattern, 3 deg spacing
STD170	57	Aphakic blind spot	Grid pattern, 1.5 deg spacing
STD180	16	Aphakic blind spot	Grid pattern, 3 deg spacing
STD210	66	Central 30 deg and horizontal meridian	Meridional pattern, glaucoma screen
STD220	83	Central 30 deg and horizontal meridian	Armaly/Drance screening pattern
STD230	54	Central 30 deg	Meridional pattern, glaucoma screen
STD 310	81	Central 30 deg	Grid pattern, 6 deg spacing
STD 320	80	Central 30 deg	Grid pattern, 6 deg spacing
STD410	65	30–60 deg	Grid pattern, 12 deg spacing
STD420	65	30–60 deg	Grid pattern, 12 deg spacing
STD710	54	Vertical meridian	Meridional pattern, neuro-op screen
STD720	54	Vertical meridian	Meridional pattern, neuro-op screen
STD730	54	Vertical meridian	Meridional pattern, neuro-op screen

The report generation subsection allows the user to direct the display of the test results to the printer (for a 'hard copy' of the results) or to the video monitor (for immediate viewing). The data is interpolated and is then presented according to a grey scale format, a meridional sensitivity profile format, or a numerical sensitivity value format. The test comparison routine computes the differences in threshold values between tests performed at two different times. The resulting difference file can then be displayed by the report generation section.

Perhaps the most intriguing portion of the Squid executive program is the test generation and management subsection. In this section, the user can custom-design and generate new test programs, modify existing test programs, merge two tests together, or delete old test programs. All of this can be quickly and easily accomplished by the user, even if he or she has no prior computer experience or knowledge of computer programming. In fact, the test generation section is so fast and simple to use, it is possible to construct a specialized test for an individual patient while the patient is seated at the instrument.

SUMMARY

We feel that the Squid Model 300 is a powerful automated perimetric test device. Our preliminary experience with the Squid has been most impressive. The major advances of the Squid over previous automated perimeters include user friendliness, flexibility, compatibility with other computer systems and peripherals, enhanced capabilities, simple modification and initiation of test programs, and resistance to obsolescence. It is our opinion that the Squid is a well-designed instrument from all standpoints.

ACKNOWLEDGEMENT

This study was supported in part by National Eye Institute Grant No. EY-03424 (to C. A. J.).

REFERENCES

1. Fankhauser, F., Spahr, J. and Bebie, H. Three years of experience with the Octopus automatic perimeter. Doc. Ophthalmol. Proc. Series 14:7–15 (1977).
2. Hart, W. M. and Hartz, R. K. Computer generated display for three dimensional static perimetry. Arch. Ophthalmol. 100:312–318 (1982).
3. Heijl, A., Drance, S. M. and Douglas, G. R. The value of an automatic perimeter (Competer) in detecting early glaucomatous field defects. Arch. Ophthalmol. 95:1560–1563 (1980).
4. Heijl, A. and Krakau, C. E. T. An automatic perimeter for glaucoma visual field screening and control: Construction and clinical cases. Albrecht von Graefes ARch. Klin. Exp. Ophthalmol. 197:12–23 (1975).
5. Johnson, C. A. and Keltner, J. L. Automated suprathreshold static perimetry. Am. J. Ophthalmol. 89:731–741 (1980).
6. Johnson, C. A., Keltner, J. L. and Balestrery, F. G. Suprathreshold static perimetry in glaucoma and other optic nerve disease. Ophthalmology 86:1278–1286 (1979).

Author's address:
Dr J. L. Keltner
Depts. Of Ophthalmology, Neurology and Neurological Surgery
University of California
Davis, CA 95616
U.S.A.

AN EVALUATION OF THE BAYLOR SEMI-AUTOMATED DEVICE

V. J. MARMION

(Bristol, U.K.)

Key words. Perimetry, Friedmann Mark II, Baylor adaptation.

ABSTRACT

The Baylor semi-automated device for the Goldmann perimeter was compared with standard routine using the Goldmann perimeter and the Friedmann Analyser Mark II. It was assessed on the basis of: 1) applicability; 2) standardisation; 3) compliance; and 4) perimetrist acceptability. It was found to compare reasonably on 1 and 2 but failed on the 3rd and 4th criteria.

INTRODUCTION

The Baylor semi-automated system (Fig. 1) offers the possibility of a rapid screening device which could be of great benefit in routine clinical perimetry. A visual screening device which has good clinical applicability would have to conform to four requirements: applicability to disease processes; standardisation and cross-correlation with other instruments; compliance with the patients' abilities; acceptability by the operator. In any clinical situation the economic viability of the instrument is an additional factor that will come into consideration in a substantial number of departments. The Baylor device was evaluated on the basis of the above criteria.

MATERIALS AND METHODS

Fifty patients who had chronic open angle glaucoma were examined using the instrument. It was felt that a minimum of fifty were required to ensure that the operator was familiar with the instrument. The results obtained were then compared with the Friedmann Mark II using a maximum sensitivity technique and the Goldmann perimeter using 112e/3e isopters.

Greve, E. L., Heijl, A. (eds.) Fifth International Visual Field Symposium.
©*1983 Dr W. Junk Publishers, The Hague/Boston/Lancaster.*

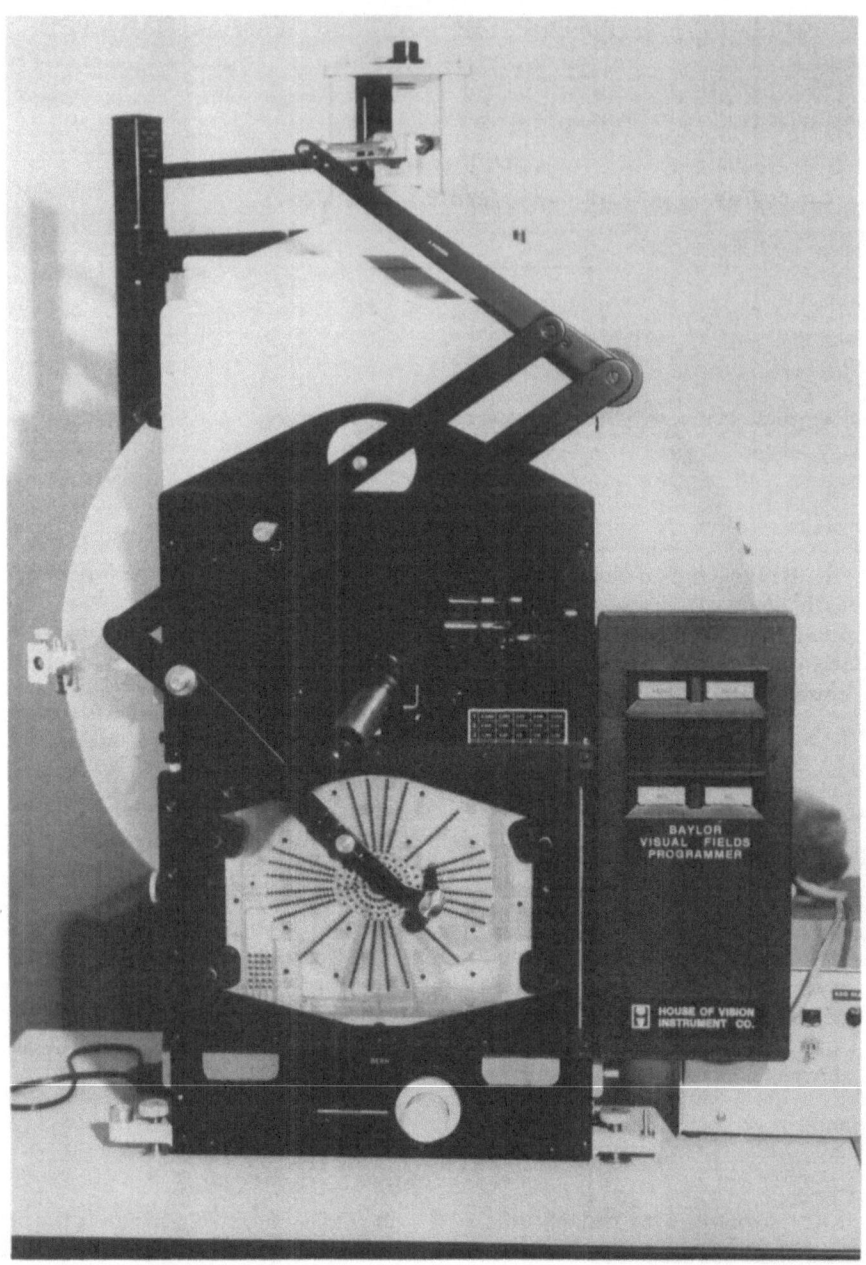

Fig. 1. Baylor semi-automated device.

RESULTS

In 43 cases the disease process was so advanced that there was no definitive advantage from using the Baylor perimeter. In 4 cases, all early glaucomas, the Baylor detected small defects which were not picked up by the routine Goldmann perimetry and in which the results on the Friedmann analyser were equivocal. All were nasal steps. There were three cases in which the Baylor failed to detect changes which has previously been discovered by the Friedmann analyser.

Examination of the central field was good. A better system of recording to show thresholds in more detail would help. The reaction of the patients to the Baylor techniques revealed a considerable degree of variability. Lack of adaptability in the programme meant that repeat examinations of areas were not possible once that area had been completed and the programme had moved on to the next section. The operator, an experience perimetrist, felt continually frustrated by the device. Internal malfunction occurred necessitating re-examination in twelve cases.

DISCUSSION

The Baylor semi-automated system has been used for a period of four months as a routine method of examination. During the period it has been shown to be a moderately satisfactory method of examination. Patient compliance with the method was not particularly good. The elderly especially did not adapt to the time sequence. This is a serious deficiency as a substantial proportion of perimetry is likely to be concerned with the elderly. It is preferable that a system which is used for glaucoma screening should be adaptable for routine follow-up where patient compliance is essential. The time schedule for examination was rarely achieved which presents problems in a busy clinic. The inability to re-check areas randomly was a serious drawback during routine perimetry as was malfunction of the instrument. These latter factors gave rise, not only to low patient acceptability but also were serious disadvantages to the operator.

Examinations with the Friedmann Mark II Analyser had better patient and operator compliance especially in the more elderly patients and were usually accomplished in under fifteen minutes per eye.

Author's address:
Dr V. J. Marmion
73 Pembroke Road
Clifton, Bristol BS8 3DW
U.K.

THE ESTIMATION AND TESTING OF THE COMPONENTS OF LONG-TERM FLUCTUATION OF THE DIFFERENTIAL LIGHT THRESHOLD

JOSEF FLAMMER, STEPHEN M. DRANCE* and MICHAEL SCHULZER

(Vancouver, British Columbia, Canada)

Key words. Scatter, long-term fluctuation, quantitative perimetry, automatic perimetry, glaucoma.

ABSTRACT

In the follow-up of patients with chronic open angle glaucoma, a quantitative comparison of visual fields is important. In order to make such comparisons, a knowledge of the short-term and long-term fluctuation of the differential light threshold is necessary. This study describes a method for evaluating the individual components of variance of the retinal sensitivity. The components have been weighted and statistically tested. The studies were carried out, predominantly in patients with glaucoma and glaucoma suspects, and the long-term fluctuation was highly significant in these groups. The long-term fluctuation was predominantly homogeneous in all test locations tested which means that the long-term fluctuation of the individual test locations, in contrast to short-term fluctuations, is usually of equal size and in the same direction.

INTRODUCTION

The clinical evaluation of the patient with chronic open angle glaucoma as well as scientific investigation of the status of the disease is often made by comparing two or more visual fields. Such comparisons are usually qualitative and their value therefore depends on the experience of the person who makes them. Visual fields can also be quantitatively compared but in order to quantitate the entire visual field, a process of data reduction becomes necessary. This is achieved in kinetic perimetry by planimetrizing the areas enclosed by isopters (3), and in static perimetry through the summation or the calculation of the mean of local retinal light thresholds (6). The introduction of the computerized perimeters has allowed such data reduction to be made automatically (2, 4, 7).

*To whom requests for offprints should be addressed.

Greve, E. L., Heijl, A. (eds.) Fifth International Visual Field Symposium.
©1983 Dr W. Junk Publishers, The Hague/Boston/Lancaster.

The individual retinal differential light thresholds, and any of the mathematical functions such as their summations or means, are statistical values which are subject to scatter. A knowledge of scatter is essential in order to form the judgement that a significant change has taken place. Scatter must therefore be taken into account in such studies. It has previously been shown that a localized increase in scatter has a predictive value for subsequent development of localized visual field defects (9).

The scatter in an individual patient has the following components:

1. *The testing conditions.* They can change during testing or between two tests. The introduction of automatic perimetry has greatly reduced this component but has not eliminated it entirely.

2. *The learning effect.* When two examinations take place within a matter of days or weeks, the mean values of retinal sensitivity at the second examination is usually higher than the first.

3. *The age effect.* Comparing visual fields taken years apart, the later field examination, even in healthy people, shows on average a small deterioration in the differential threshold (3).

4. *Short-term fluctuation (SF).* Every measurement of a psychophysical threshold has a scatter. We define the differential threshold as the difference (in logarithmic terms), or the quotient (in absolute terms) of the light stimulus from its background which has a chance of being seen 50% of the time (1). By definition, therefore, the scatter, although dependent on the patient and the test conditions, can never be zero. Any scatter which occurs during a visual field examination of approximately 20 minutes duration, is termed short-term fluctuation.

5. *Long-term fluctuation (LF).* During a period of hours and days, the retinal threshold shows variations which cannot be explained by any of the above factors and therefore a further component is added to the fluctuation, which Bebie and his co-workers (1) have called the long-term fluctuation. The LF therefore consists of changes in retinal sensitivity which are not explained by the learning process or by the SF. The LF is the net variation in the readings over time when the variation due to replicated measurements at a given time has been removed. In view of the fact that the various retinal locations tested can show a uniform (homogeneous) change in the sensitivity as well as a heterogeneous change (different changes in different locations), the long-term fluctuation has two components. The first is the homogeneous component LF (HO) and the second is the heterogeneous component LF (HE). The purpose of this study was to estimate and test the significance of these two components. This study will not consider the effect of various disease states and other factors on the long-term fluctuation. These problems will be dealt with in subsequent communications.

PATIENTS AND METHODS

Thirty-one eyes of 31 patients were examined. Six were ophthalmologically normal, fifteen had elevated intraocular pressures without visual field defects and the remaining nine had nerve fiber bundle defects. The age ranged from 27 to 77 years (a mean of 56 ± 16). All patients included were admitted to hospital for glaucoma evalution and repeated visual field examinations could be carried out. This selection of patients will have influenced the results and no generalization should be made from the results. For this reason, the analysis of variance employed the so-called fixed as opposed to randomized models.

The visual field was examined with Program JO on the Octopus perimeter, which was fully described elsewhere (4, 8). Forty-nine test locations each had two threshold determinations in two time phases. Every patient has had five visual field examinations within three days at constant times of the day. The first field was excluded from analysis in order to minimize the learning effects.

METHODS OF ANALYSIS AND THEIR RESULTS

1. A comparison of two visual fields of the same patient

Two visual fields plotted by the Program JO on a patient can be compared by an analysis of variance using the following model:

$$Y_{jkl} = \mu + L_j + V_k + LV_{jk} + E_{jkl} \tag{1}$$

Y is the individual threshold determination, μ the overall mean value, V is the effect of the individual visual field examination, L is the effect of the test locations, and E is the experimental error evaluated on the basis of the two replications. In this example, V is mainly due to the LE(HO) but in comparing results from a single individual, systematic trends cannot be mathematically separated. A confounding problem is therefore introduced. The learning effect can be diminished by removing the first examination. The interaction LV, represents the heterogeneous component of the LF and the experimental error E is the short-term fluctuation. The numerical grids of the 2 visual field examinations, performed on a 70-year old glaucoma suspect are shown in Fig. 1. The question which we want to answer using the above model is 'has there been a statistically significant change in the visual field?'. Table 1 shows the results of the analysis of variance. The retinal sensitivity in this patient has shown a statistically significant homogeneous change in all test locations. The mean sensitivity dropped from 25.8 to 25.3 dB. No significant heterogeneous changes have occurred. It should be stressed that we are dealing with a statistically significant change, and are not suggesting a clinical relevance of such reversible changes of the retinal threshold.

2. Analysis of multiple visual field examinations of many patients utilizing the average differential threshold over 49 test locations in the visual field

By using many visual fields (in this study 4) of many patients, (in this study 31), the long-term fluctuation of the entire group can be tested and evaluated. Any systematic trends of the group can be separated from the homogeneous component of the long-term fluctuation. In this example, the analysis does

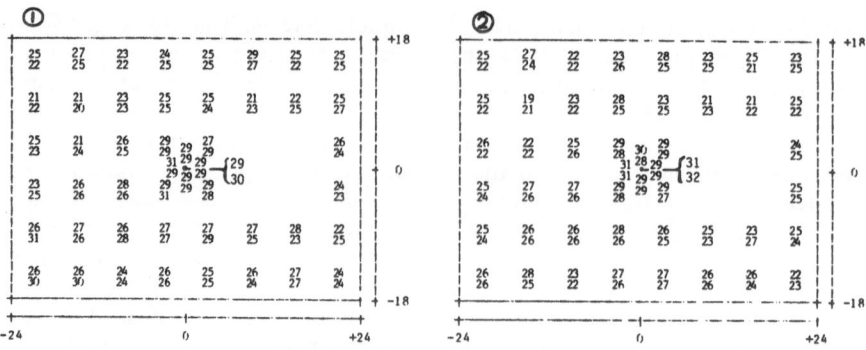

Fig. 1. The numerical grids of two visual field examinations performed in a 70-year old glaucoma suspect at two-hour intervals.

Table 1. Comparison of the two visual field presentations in Fig. 1, with an analysis of variance using Model 1.

Source of variation		Sum of squares	DF	Mean square	F	Significance of F
Test locations (L)		1045.387	48	21.779	11.445	0.000
LF (HO)	(V)	7.760	1	7.760	4.078	0.046
LF (HE)	(L–V interaction)	90.490	48	1.885	0.991	0.503
SF	(E)	186.481	98	1.903		

not take into account the differential threshold of individual test locations but the overall means of the visual field which results in a loss of information about the heterogeneous component of the long-term fluctuation. The following statistical model was used:

$$Y_{ikl} = \mu + P_i + V_k + PV_{ik} + E_{ikl} \tag{2}$$

Y is the mean differential threshold of the entire visual field in a single phase, μ is the overall mean of the entire group, P represents the patient effect and V is the effect of the individual visual field measurements. Because the homogeneous component of the long-term fluctuation is a random variable, its value, providing the sample size is large enough, is now included in the interaction PV. V shows the systematic trend of the whole group. The error term E in this model is not the short-term fluctuation but the scatter of the means of the two phases. The results of the analysis of variance of this model are shown in Table 2. Because of the heterogeneous population which was studied, it is not surprising that the patient effect is large. The systematic trend is low but the homogeneous long-term fluctuation is highly significant ($p < 0.001$).

3. Analysis of multiple fields of many patients utilizing the differential thresholds from the individual locations

If data reduction is not undertaken an additional source of variance is added due to the variation of the differential threshold of individual test locations. The theoretical model for this analysis is as follows:

386

Table 2. Analysis of variance taking the overall mean for each phase as the dependent variable and the patients and the visual fields as the independent factors.

Source of variation	Sum of square	DF	Mean square	F	Significance of F
Patients (P)	3250.691	30	108.356		
Systematic trend (V)	3.764	3	1.255		
LF (HO) (P−V interaction)	270.769	90	3.009	6.131	0.000
(E)	60.844	124	0.491		

Table 3. Mean of 31 analyses of variance (for each individual patient), including 4 visual fields and 49 test locations (Model 1).

Source of variation	Sum of squares	DF	Mean square	F	Significance of F
Test locations (L)	7476.240	48	115.755		
LF (HO) (V)	433.944	3	144.648	32.425	0.000
LF (HE) (L−V interaction)	812.016	144	5.639	1.264	0.056
SF (E)	874.356	196	4.461		

$$Y_{ijkl} = \mu + P_i + L_j + V_k + PV_{jk} + PL_{ij} + LV_{jk}$$
$$+ PLV_{ijk} + E_{ijkl} \tag{3}$$

In this study the number of cells was 6,760 which would have exceeded the capacity of the software package used in the analysis. Model 1 was therefore used for each individual patient utilizing the individual thresholds of the 4 visual fields. For the F tests, the group mean of the means of squares was used. The results are presented in Table 3. The factor 'patient' does not appear as the analysis was done for each individual patient.

The homogeneous component of the LF is highly significant ($p < 0.001$), whereas the heterogeneous component just failed to achieve significance.

4. Estimation of the components of variance

So far, the significance of individual factors has been considered but we also intended to estimate the contribution of the factors to the total variation.

The individual components are presented in Table 4. We obtained two estimations for the homogeneous component of the LF, one from Model 1 and the other from Model 2. Both estimates were fairly similar. The probable reason for the small difference is due on the one hand to the removal of the systematic trend in Model 2, and on the other hand, Model 1 includes the scatter of the individual threshold determinations, Model 2 the scatter of the means in the error term. The relatively large part played by the component 'patient' and test location is due to the inclusion of some of the glaucomatous visual field defects. The systematic trend is small. The homogeneous component of the long-term fluctuation in our patient group is between 1.1 and 1.2 dB, and contributed a definite component to the total variance. The SF is 2.1 dB, which is relatively large. This is also due to the inclusion of the pathological visual field defects.

387

Table 4. Estimation of component of variance.

Source	Sigma	Calculation from Table No.	Factor in the model
Patients	3.6719	2	P
Test locations	3.7298	3	L
Systematic trend	0.1110	2	V
LF (HO)	1.1221	2	P · V
	1.1960	3	V
LF (HE)	0.7676	3	L · V
SF	2.1121	3	E

DISCUSSION

We defined at the outset, the long-term fluctuation (LF) as that reversible scatter of the retinal sensitivity, which is not due to the learning effects, age effects, or the short-term scatter. The first two factors were largely excluded by the design of the study, the exclusion of the first visual field examination and the measurement of all visual fields of each patient in the same week, whereas the removal of the short-term fluctuation was accomplished in the analysis of variance. The analysis was based on more than 13,000 individual differential threshold measurements of 31 patients, predominantly suffering from glaucoma or glaucoma suspects. The homogeneous component of the long-term fluctuations LF (HO) was statistically highly significant ($p < 0.001$) and its component Sigma LF (HO) was between 1.1 and 1.2 dB. The heterogeneous component of the long-term fluctuation LF (HE) was not significant and its component Sigma LF (HE) was approximately 0.8 dB. This means that the heterogeneous fluctuations are in large part, a consequence of short-term fluctuation (SF).

Bebie and his co-workers (1), found a homogeneous component of 1.0 (which he called synchronous component) and a heterogeneous component (which he called uncorrelated component) of 1.3 dB. The differences between his results and ours is probably due to the different patient populations examined. Most of our patients had glaucoma field defects, or were glaucoma suspects. It is possible that in glaucoma patients, variations are more homogeneous than in other diseases. The importance of the two components of the long-term fluctuation are currently being investigated. The results presented show that when one compares visual fields quantitatively, the long-term fluctuation has to be taken into account. One has to look at a general trend over a number of visual fields and avoid forming judgements on the basis of small changes in two successive field examinations. This may explain, to some degree, the variations of results presented in clinical studies (5).

ACKNOWLEDGEMENTS

This study was supported in part by the E. A. Baker Foundation and the Medical Research Council of Canada; also supported in part by the Verrey Foundation and the Swiss National Fund (to J.F.).

388

REFERENCES

1. Bebie, H., Fankhauser, F. and Spahr, J. Static perimetry: accuracy and fluctuations. Acta Ophthalmol. 54:339–348 (1976).
2. Bebie, H. and Fankhauser, F. Program Delta. Interzeag AG, Rietbachstr. 5 CH-8952, Schlieren (1981).
3. Drance, S. M., Berry, V. and Hughes, A. Studies of the effects of age on the central and peripheral isopters of the visual field in normal subjects. Am. J. Ophthalmol. 63:1667–1672 (1976).
4. Flammer, J., Drance S. M., Jenni, A. and Bebie, H. The Octopus program JO and STATJO, a special program for clinical investigation of the visual field. Can. J. Ophthalmol. 18:115–118 (1983)
5. Flammer, J. and Drance, S. M. The effect of a number of glaucoma medications on the differential light threshold (to be published).
6. Heilmann, K. Augendruck, Blutdruck und Glaukomschaden. Buecherei des Augenarztes, Vol. 61, 72 Stuttgart, Ferdinand Enke (1972).
7. Holmin, C. and Krakau, C. E. T. Automatic perimetry in the control of glaucoma. Glaucoma 3:154–159 (1981).
8. Jenni, A., Flammer, J., Funkhouser, A. and Fankhauser, F. Special Octopus software for clinical investigation. Doc. Ophthalmol. Proc. Series 35:351–356 (1983).
9. Werner, E. B. and Drance, S. M. Early visual field disturbances in glaucoma. Arch. Ophthalmol. 95:1173–1175 (1977).

Authors' address:

Dept. of Ophthalmology
University of British Columbia
2550 Willow Street
Vancouver, B.C.
Canada V5Z 3N9

LATERAL INHIBITION IN THE FOVEA AND PARAFOVEAL REGIONS

KAZUTAKA KANI*, TOSHIO INUI, RYUGO HARUTA
and OSAMU MIMURA
(Nishinomiya, Japan)

Key words. Lateral inhibition, fundus controlled perimetry, spatial summation, receptive field, human vision.

ABSTRACT

Lateral inhibition in the light sense was investigated by using a fundus controlled perimeter to monitor simultaneously the fundus picture and stimulus location on the retina in four subjects.

The diameter of the inhibitory field becomes continuously larger from fovea to periphery. The diameter of the inhibitory field and the rate of its change with eccentricity, however, were generally smaller in our experiments than in those of several previous investigations using letter recognition (1, 2, 3).

These results suggest that lateral inhibition in the light sense may be organized at the retinal level.

INTRODUCTION

Lateral inhibition is an inhibitory interaction between signals from neighbouring neurones, and one of the basic mechanisms of sensory neural systems. This effect is well known in visual pathways. In ophthalmology, it is suggested that the functional amblyopia is accompanied by immaturity or insufficiency of this effect.

In this article, a new procedure to examine lateral inhibition effects using infrared television fundus camera (fundus controlled perimetry) is shown and these effects in the fovea and parafoveal regions are presented in normal subjects.

MATERIALS AND METHODS

1. Apparatus

Experiments were conducted with a modified fundus controlled perimeter which was originally designed by Kani and Ogita (6). The block diagram is

*To whom requests for offprints should be addressed.

Greve, E. L., Heijl, A. (eds.) Fifth International Visual Field Symposium.
©1983 Dr W. Junk Publishers, The Hague/Boston/Lancaster.

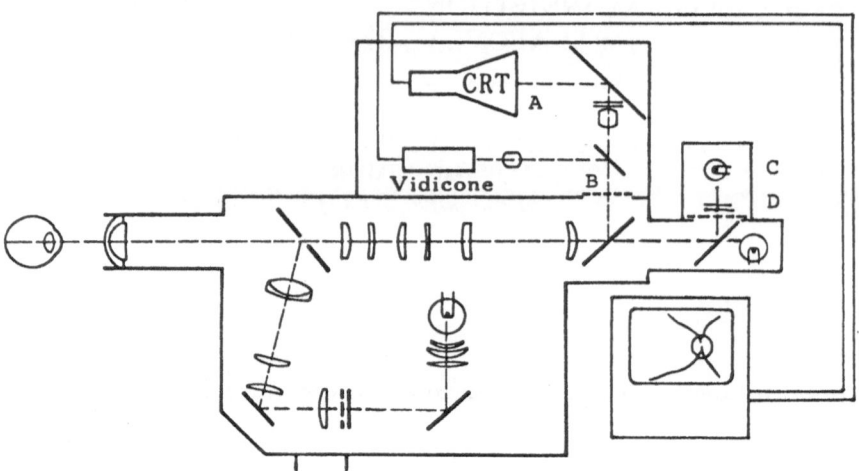

Fig. 1. Block diagram of the fundus controlled perimeter in this experiment. The fundus, the vidicone tube and the CRT were set at conjugate positions. Furthermore, the fundus images were focused on planes B and D.

shown in Fig. 1. The fundus images were focused on plane B and D. An aluminium plate was placed in plane D, and two parallel slits were made in the plate with a Nd:YAG laser processing device. The light emitted by the light source C passed through these two slits and were projected on the retina as inhibitory stimuli. An infrared Wratten filter was placed in plane B, and a pinhole was made in the filter by the laser. The light projected from the CRT (A) passed through this pinhole and illuminated the retina as a test stimulus. Stimulus light and background light beams were set up in a Maxwellian view arrangement. Details of the fundus controlled perimeter have been reported elsewhere (5, 6).

The fixation point was a black dot, 20 minutes in diameter. The background was illuminated by a single tungsten lamp powered by a stabilized DC power supply, and a light-balancing filter was used to raise the color temperature of the projected light to 6000°K. The circular background subtended 30 degrees in diameter, and the luminance was 10 apostilbs (5.6 trolands). Inhibitory stimuli and the test stimulus were illuminated by a single tungsten lamp and a CRT, respectively, and the colour temperature was the same as that of the background. The intensity of the stimuli could be changed with neutral density filters (Kodak Wratten No. 96) in steps of 0.1 log unit. The diameter of the test stimulus was 2.7 minutes and the inhibitory stimuli consisted of two rectangular slits 2.2 minutes wide and 16.2 minutes long (Fig. 2). The exposure duration of the test stimulus was controlled by an electro-mechanical shutter. The principal experimental variables were the retinal location of the stimuli and the distance between inhibitory stimuli. The distance between two slits used here were 4.2, 6.0, 10.2, 12.0, 17.5, 19.2, 24.6, 27.3, 33.8, 37.8 and 45.2 minutes. Lateral inhibition determinations were made at the retinal eccentricities, 0, 6 and 9 degrees in the horizontal meridian of the temporal part of the subject's retina.

392

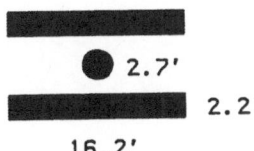

Fig. 2. Arrangement of the test stimulus and inhibitory stimulus. Test stimulus was a white spot placed at the center of the inhibitory stimuli (two slit lights).

2. Procedure

The subject's pupil was dilated with a mydriatic, 0.5% tropicamide. The subject was allowed approximately twenty minutes for background adaptation. In the initial experiment, the increment threshold of two parallel lines and test stimulus were determined, respectively. To obtain the following experimental data, the inhibitory stimuli were set 1.0 log unit above the threshold, 158 apostilbs. At the start of the experiment, the subject was instructed to press the key in his right hand if the test stimulus was seen independently and do nothing otherwise. The subject was told to be sure that the fixation point was in good focus before initiating each session. Throughout each session, the stimuli were monitored to make sure that they were not falling on a blood vessel.

The subjects participated in three experimental sessions, each of which corresponded to one of the retinal loci. Each session was conducted varying the distances between inhibitory stimuli randomly selected. First, the inhibitory stimuli were presented independently. Then the test stimulus was presented at the center of the inhibitory stimuli with an interval of one second. The exposure duration of the test stimulus was 200 ms and the inhibitory stimuli turned off simultaneously. Increment threshold of the test stimulus was obtained by the constant method.

3. Subjects

Two female subjects, K.T. (22-years old) and M.Y. (22 years old), and two male subjects, R.H. (25 years old) and K.K. (41 years old), participated in this experiment. Their visual acuity was > 1.0 in both eyes.

RESULTS

The results of these experiments are illustrated in Figs. 3 and 4. Figure 3 shows the inhibitory effects on the increment threshold at the fovea, 6 and 9 degrees in subject K.T. The abscissa shows the distance between the inhibitory stimuli, and the ordinate is the threshold elevation after presentation of the inhibitory stimuli. The distance between the inhibitory stimuli which gave a threshold elevation of 0.1 log unit was called 'the inhibitory field diameter'. Figure 4 shows the diameter of the inhibitory field plotted against the eccentricity from the fovea. The diameter of this field increased monotonically with eccentricity. This relation exhibits quite similar properties for the other three subjects.

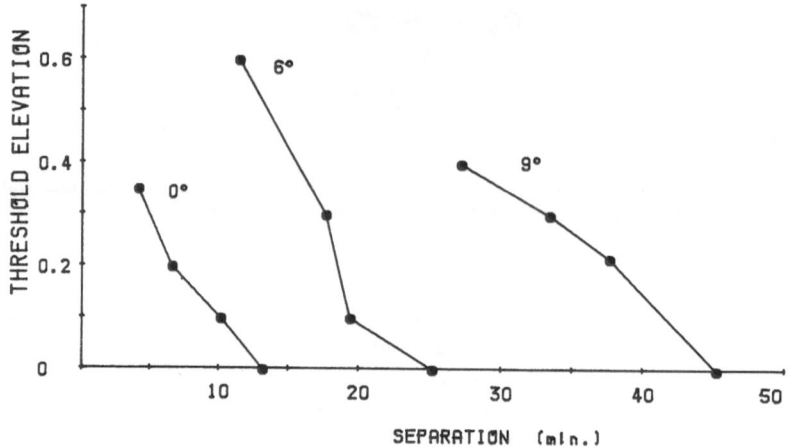

Fig. 3. Inhibitory effects on the increment threshold at several retinal loci. As the data showed no important differences among subjects, the data were pooled together and analyzed. The abscissa means the distance of the inhibitory stimuli, and the ordinate means the threshold elevation after presentation of the inhibitory stimuli.

DISCUSSION

Throughout the visual system, the neighbouring group of the neurones respond to information from neighbouring areas on the retinal surface. Typical modes of the interaction between neighbouring neurones are spatial summation and lateral inhibition. These functions have been investigated in electro-physiology and psychophysics with several procedures. These procedures, however, are so delicate and complicated that they are not suitable for clinical applications. Therefore, we developed a new method using a fundus controlled perimeter for studying the spatial summation in human vision (5, 7). In this study, the effects of lateral inhibition were studied using this fundus controlled perimeter. We measured the increment threshold for a test stimulus flanked on both sides at various distance by lines with supraliminal luminance.

The increment threshold increased after presentation of the inhibitory stimuli. The diameter of the inhibitory field was about 10 minutes at the fovea, 19 minutes at 6 degrees and 40 minutes at 9 degrees. It increased monotonically with increasing distance from the fovea. The results presented above generally agree with previous studies using interaction between letters or line segments (1, 2, 3). However, our results differ from previous results in the following respects: first, the size of the inhibitory field was constantly smaller than previously published. For example, the diameter at 6 degrees in our experiment was about 19 minutes, while earlier results varied between 1.3 and 4.2 degrees. Secondly, the change with eccentricity in our results was smaller than those of previous studies (1, 2, 3).

Interaction effects in letter recognition or between line segments might be organized at the cortical level. This is also suggested by the fact that the

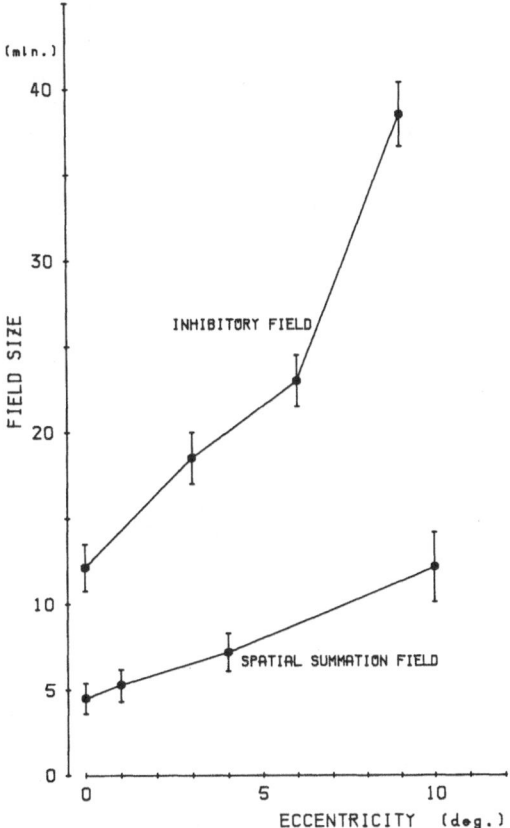

Fig. 4. The diameter of the inhibitory field plotted against the eccentricity from the fovea.

ratio of change with eccentricity in letter recognition is similar to that of the cortical magnification factors using intra-skull electrodes placed on the occipital lobe (4). On the other hand, our previous reports (5, 7) revealed that spatial summation effects of the light sense might be organized at the retinal level. In the present experiment, the diameter of the inhibitory field was about 2.9 times as large as the diameter of the critical area in which the energy of light stimulus was summated. Thus, this also strongly suggests that inhibitory interaction of light sense might be organized at the retinal level.

REFERENCES

1. Andriessen, J. J. and Bouma, H. Eccentric vision: adverse interactions between line segments. Vision Res. 16: 71–78 (1976).
2. Banks, W. P., Bachrach, K. M. and Larson, D. W. The asymmetry of lateral interference in visual letter recognition. Perception & Psychophysics 22:232–240 (1977).
3. Bouma, H. Interaction effects in parafoveal letter recognition. Nature 226:177–178 (1970).

4. Brindley, G. S. and Lewin, W. S. The sensations produced by electrical stimulation of the visual cortex. J. Physiol. 196:479–493 (1968).
5. Inui, T., Mimura, O. and Kani, K. Retinal sensitivity and spatial summation in the foveal and parafoveal regions. J. Opt. Soc. Am. 71:151–154 (1981).
6. Kani, K. and Ogita, Y. Fundus controlled perimetry – the relation between the position of a lesion in the fundus and in the visual field. Doc. Ophthalmol. Proc. Series 19:341–350 (1979).
7. Mimura, O., Kani, K. and Inui, T. Spatial summation in the foveal and parafoveal region. Doc. Ophthalmol. Proc. Series 26:139–146 (1981).

Author's address:
Dr K. Kani
Dept. of Ophthalmology
Hyogo College of Medicine
1-1, Mukogawa-cho, Nishinomiya
663 Japan

EXTRAFOVEAL STILES' π MECHANISMS

KENJI KITAHARA, RYUTARO TAMAKI, JUN NOJI,
ATSUSHI KANDATSU and HIROSHI MATSUZAKI

(Tokyo, Japan)

Key words. Stiles' π mechanism, extrafoveal color vision, threshold versus intensity (t.v.i.) curve.

ABSTRACT

A study was made on the increment threshold versus intensity (t.v.i.) curves for a blue (480 nm) test on a yellow (590 nm) background at retinal eccentricities up to $10°$ on two normal observers. The observed t.v.i. curves at the extrafovea yielded four branches, i.e., for rods or $\pi_{0(\mu)}$, the medium-wave sensitive mechanism or $\pi_{4(\mu)}$, and the short-wave sensitive mechanisms or $\pi_{1(\mu)}$ and $\pi_{3(\mu)}$ respectively.

It was found that the $\pi_{0(\mu)}$ branch of the t.v.i. curve tended to become more prominent, while the branch for $\pi_{4(\mu)}$ became less marked as they moved toward the periphery. The gradient of the branch for $\pi_{1(\mu)}$ decreased with an increase in eccentricity. Differences between the absolute thresholds for π_1 and π_3 tended to decrease toward the periphery, until they became difficult to differentiate.

INTRODUCTION

In order to make use of color perimetry clinically, it is necessary to obtain accurate knowledge of extrafoveal color mechanisms. In a previous paper (1) we studied the increment threshold versus intensity (t.v.i.) curves and the field sensitivity of Stiles long-wave sensitive mechanism or $\pi_{5(\mu)}$ at the fovea and at $10°$ and $20°$ extrafoveally.

Stiles (2) found that the t.v.i. curve obtained for a blue test light on a yellow background consists of three branches each separated by a 'change in law', i.e., the lowermost branch is attributed to the medium-wave sensitive mechanism (π_4), while the upper two define two short-wave sensitive mechanisms (π_1 and π_3). In this experiment, the first step in investigating the medium-wave sensitive mechanism and short-wave sensitive mechanism was to measure the t.v.i. curves with this test-background combination at different eccentricities up to $10°$ from the fixation point.

METHOD

A two-channel Maxwellian view optical system was used in this study. The light source was a 150 W xenon arc with a suitable stable power supply. A $1°$ diameter circular test (480 nm) was superimposed in the center of a $10°$ circular background (590 nm) field. The test field was exposed for 200 msec every two seconds. Narrow-band (10 nm half-band width) interference filters were used for the test and the background lights. The observers' fixation was controlled by a small red light from an accessory system. The biting board was adjusted at each eccentric position in order to allow the test flash and the background light to pass directly through the center of the pupil.

Measurements were made on the right eye of two normal male trichromats. Their pupils were dilated with 1% tropicamide. Prior to a series of measurements the observers were dark-adapted for one hour; they were adapted to each background for at least 2 min plus whatever additional time was needed for the measured results to become stable. For a measurement, the intensity of the test flash was adjusted by the subjects and test thresholds were measured at least five times for each background condition by the method of adjustment. The radiances of the test flash and the background light were determined with a Calibrated PIN-10 silicon photodiode (United-Detector Technology).

RESULTS

The t.v.i. curves were measured for a 480 nm test on a 590 nm background along the horizontal meridian in the temporal retina out to $10°$. Figure 1 shows the t.v.i. curves measured at the fovea for observers J.N. and K.K. The ordinate gives the log test intensity (log photons (480 nm) sec^{-1} deg^{-2}) while the abscissa specifies the background radiance (log photons (590 nm) sec^{-1} deg^{-2}). The curve for observer K.K. is transposed horizontally by 1 log unit in order to make the spacing more convenient. Both the solid line and the dotted line indicate the standard increment threshold function of Stiles (3). The t.v.i. curves for both observers consisted of three branches, which have the same results Stiles found (2), i.e., the lowermost curve corresponds to the medium-wave sensitive mechanism ($\pi_{4(\mu)}$) while the upper two define two short-wave mechanisms ($\pi_{1(\mu)}$ and $\pi_{3(\mu)}$). These three branches of both observers were found to fit very well the Stiles' template curve. The absolute thresholds for the π_4 mechanism of observers K.K. and J.N. were the same level. On the other hand, the difference between the absolute threshold for the π_3 mechanism was 0.4 log units.

The t.v.i. curves obtained at $3°$ temporal location from the fixation point for observers J.N. and K.K. are illustrated in Fig. 2. The ordinate and the abscissa are the same as in Fig. 1. The curve for observer K.K. is displaced horizontally by 1 log unit. The t.v.i. curves consisted of four parts, i.e., the lowermost branch corresponding to rods or $\pi_{o(\mu)}$, the second one corresponding to medium-wave sensitive mechanism or $\pi_{4(\mu)}$ and the upper two corresponding to short-wave sensitive mechanisms or $\pi_{1(\mu)}$ and $\pi_{3(\mu)}$

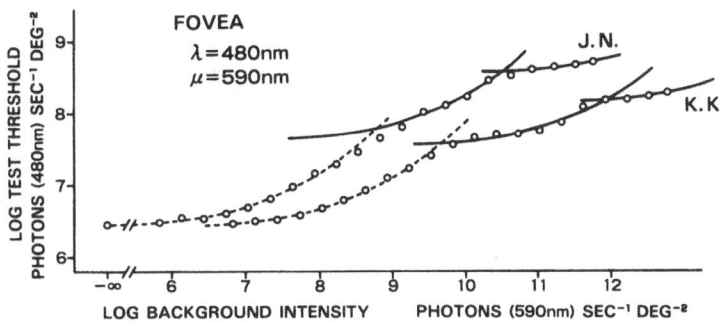

Fig. 1. The increment threshold versus intensity (t.v.i.) curves at the fovea for observers J.N. and K.K. The curve for observer K.K. has been transposed horizontally by 1 log unit. Both the solid line and the dotted line indicate the standard increment threshold function of Stiles.

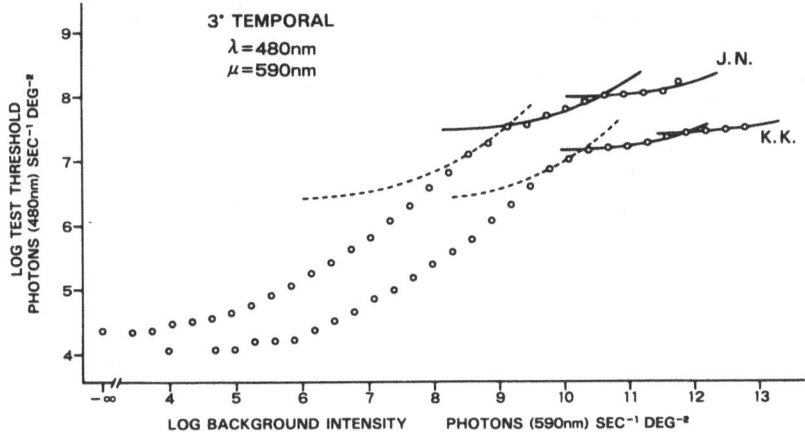

Fig. 2. The t.v.i. curves at 3° temporal location for observers J.N. and K.K. The curve for observer K.K. is displaced horizontally by 1 log unit.

respectively. The dotted line for π_4 and the solid lines for π_1 and π_3 indicate the Stiles' template curve. The absolute threshold for π_4 mechanism was determined by measuring the dark adaptation curve for a 480 nm test flash. The $\pi_{0(\mu)}$ branch of the t.v.i. curve appeared very prominent while the $\pi_{4(\mu)}$ branch was less marked. Similar results have been reported by Cabello and Stiles (4). The differences in the absolute threshold between π_0 and π_4 observers J.N. and K.K. were 2.1 and 2.4 log units respectively. The t.v.i. curves obtained at 10° temporal location for observers J.N. and K.K. are illustrated in Fig. 3. The curve for K.K. is displaced along the abscissa axis by 1 log unit. The t.v.i. curves can be divided into four parts, i.e., for $\pi_{0(\mu)}$, $\pi_{4(\mu)}$, $\pi_{1(\mu)}$ and $\pi_{3(\mu)}$ beginning with the lowermost one. The $\pi_{0(\mu)}$ branch became more prominent and the difference between the absolute thresholds for π_0 and π_4 was approximately 3.0 log units for both observers. The dotted line representing $\pi_{4(\mu)}$ in Fig. 3 is shown at the lowest possible field sensitivity.

399

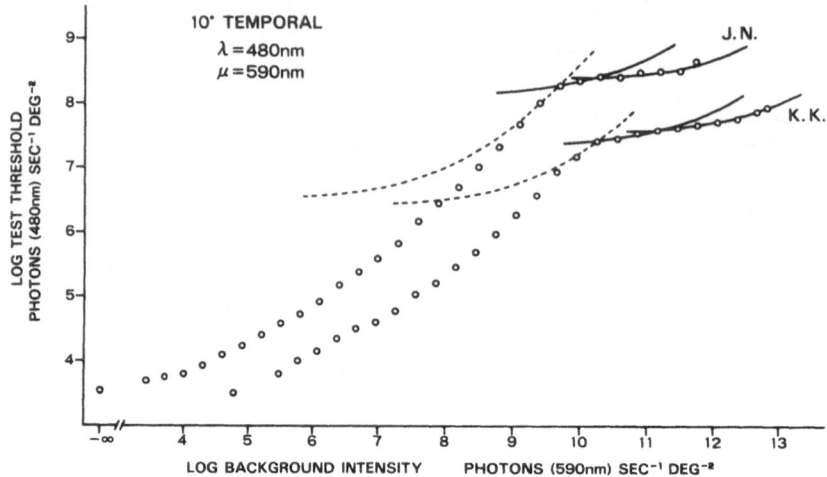

Fig. 3. The t.v.i. curves at 10° temporal location for observers J.N. and K.K. The curve for observer K.K. is displaced horizontally by 1 log unit.

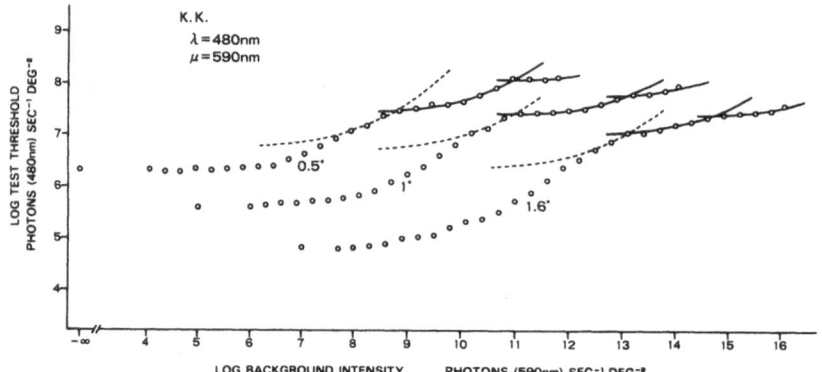

Fig. 4. The set of t.v.i. curves for observer K.K. at 0.5°, 1° and 1.6° temporal locations. The data for 1° temporal location has been displaced by 2 log units and the data for 1.6° temporal location has been displaced by 4 log units along the abscissa axis.

Since the $\pi_{1(\mu)}$ branch became shallow and the difference between the absolute thresholds for π_1 and π_3 decreased, they became difficult to distinguish. The absolute thresholds for the π_0 and π_4 mechanisms of observers K.K. and J.N. were almost the same level. On the other hand, the difference between the absolute threshold for the short-wave sensitive mechanisms (both π_1 and π_3) was approximately 0.8 log units.

The set of t.v.i. curves for observer K.K. at 0.5°, 1° and 1.6° temporal locations are illustrated in Fig. 4 and at 2°, 5° and 8° temporal locations are shown in Fig. 5. It is important to note that in Figs. 4 and 5 the data for 1° and 5° temporal locations have been displaced by 2 log units and the data for 1.6° and 8° temporal locations have been displaced by 4 log units along the abscissa axis. The absolute threshold for π_0 showed a marked decline while

400

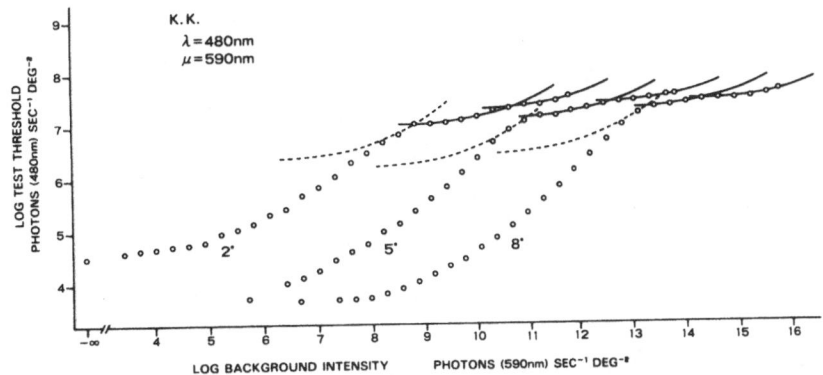

Fig. 5. The set of t.v.i. curves for observer K.K. at 2°, 5° and 8° temporal locations. The data for 5° and 8° temporal locations have been displaced horizontally by 2 and 4 log units respectively.

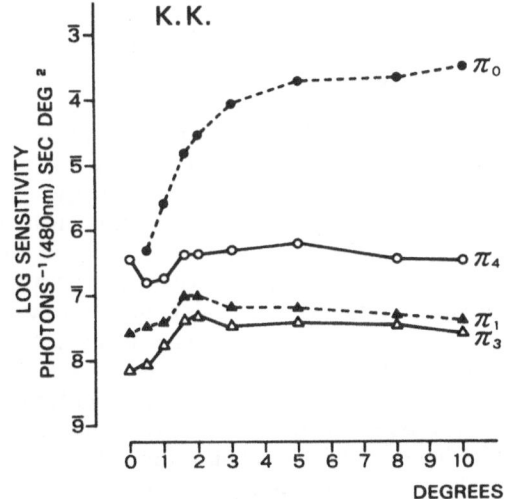

Fig. 6. The absolute sensitivity gradients for each mechanism for 480 nm test for observer K.K.

its branch became more prominent with an increase in eccentricity. The absolute threshold for π_4 showed no significant chang, while its branch became less prominent in the extrafoveal locations. The gradient of the $\pi_{1(\mu)}$ branch decreased with an increase in eccentricity and the difference between the absolute threshold for π_1 and π_3 tended to decrease toward the periphery. Therefore, they became difficult to distinguish there.

DISCUSSION

The absolute sensitivities for each mechanism for the 480 nm test (log photons sec^{-1} deg^2) obtained from the t.v.i. curves at retinal eccentricities up to 10° for observer K.K. are plotted as a function of degrees in eccentricity in Fig. 6.

401

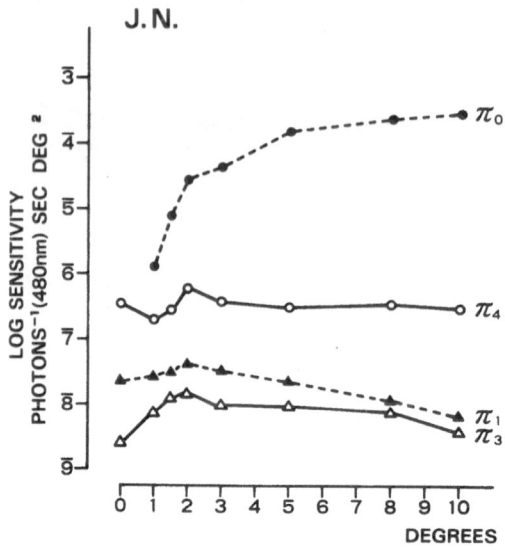

Fig. 7. The absolute sensitivity gradients for each mechanism for J.N.

The absolute sensitivity gradient for the π_0 mechanism ($\bullet$) showed a marked decline toward the fovea. The sensitivity gradient for π_4 ($\circ$) was approximately the same level up to $10°$ from the center of the fovea with a slight decline at $0.5°$ and $1°$ temporal locations. While, the sensitivity gradients for the $\pi_{1(\blacktriangle)}$ and the $\pi_{3(\triangle)}$ mechanisms showed a decline toward the fovea particularly the π_3 and the maximum sensitivity was observed at $2°$ temporal, from which the curve had a tendency to fall gradually toward the periphery. To evaluate these sensitivity gradients we have to consider the prereceptor losses within the eye, particularly the loss in the macular pigment. The density of the macular pigment at the fovea at 480 nm for observer K.K. was obtained in a different experiment. This observer's macular pigment density at 480 nm was 0.83 log units which is approximately 2 times that normally found in the occidental population (3). After correcting for the loss of macular pigment the difference between the π_4 test sensitivity at 480 nm at the fovea and at $10°$ temporal side was 0.83 log units. This difference showed the same trend that was found for π_5 in the previous experiment (1). The distribution of the density of the macular pigment in the retina remains uncertain. The sensitivity gradients for each mechanism for J.N. are plotted in Fig. 7.

Several important trends that have to be considered in order to make clinical use of color perimetry are found in this study. When the results from both observers were compared, it was found that the sensitivity gradients for π_0 and π_4 resembled each other both in their trends and in the value of absolute threshold. On the other hand, it was found that the sensitivity gradients for π_1 and π_3 differed both in their trends and the value of absolute threshold especially with an increase in eccentricity. This suggests a normal variation between cone mechanisms with an increase in eccentricity. The π_0

branch of the t.v.i. curve became more prominent outside the fovea while the π_4 branch became less marked. Therefore, it was found to be very difficult to detect the π_4 mechanism using the method of test threshold measurement with this combination of test light and background light. In order to detect the short-wave sensitive mechanisms, particularly the π_3 mechanism, we need a very high intensity of background light, e.g., more than 4.0 log photopic trolands were needed as a background intensity for K.K. to detect the π_3 mechanism at $10°$ from the center of the fovea.

REFERENCES

1. Kitahara, H., Kitahara, K., Irie, J., Shirakawa, A. and Matsuzaki, H. Extrafoveal Stiles' π_5-mechanism. Doc. Ophthalmol. Proc. Series 26:185–191 (1980).
2. Stiles, W. S. Further studies of visual mechanisms by the two-color threshold method. In: Coloquio sobre problemas ópticos de la visión (Madrid), Vol I: 65–103 (1953).
3. Wyszecki, G. W. and Stiles, W. S. Color science: concepts and methods, quantitative data and formulas. New York, Wiley (1967).
4. Cabello, J. and Stiles, W. S. Sensibilidad de bastogues y conos en la parafovea. An. Soc. Real. Esp. Física y Quim. A 46:251–282 (1950).

Authors' address:
Dept. of Ophthalmology
The Jikei University School of Medicine
19–18 Nishi-Shinbashi 3-chome, Minato-ku
Tokyo
Japan

LOSS OF INHIBITORY MECHANISMS AS A MEASURE OF CONE IMPAIRMENT: A METHOD APPLIED IN STATIC COLOUR PERIMETRY

EGILL HANSEN and THORSTEIN SEIM

(Oslo, Norway)

Key words. Static perimetry, inhibitory mechanisms, transient tritanopia, cone dystrophies.

ABSTRACT

Delayed recovery of blue light sensitivity after exposure to a bright yellow light is characteristically found in normal eyes due to inhibitory influence between retinal receptor mechanisms. Acting alone, the rods have a great ability for fast recovery. In rod monochromats as well as in progressive cone dystrophies, static perimetry performed immediately after extinction of a yellow adapting light, demonstrates a particularly high rod sensitivity. Normal individuals on the contrary, demonstrate clearly raised thresholds (transient tritanopia). Subdued or insignificant increases of threshold, intermediate to the above, is found in juvenile macular degeneration. The ability to recover after light exposure as can be shown by this kind of static perimetry, is an indirect, but significant indication of cone function.

INTRODUCTION

Perimetry, which essentially is a systematic registration of light thresholds in the visual field, is usually carried out with the eye adapted to a constant background illumination. Rapid changes of the adapting light bring forward other qualities of visual perception than those being tested under ordinary conditions. Particularly interesting is the decreased sensitivity to short wavelength lights that can be recorded during the early phase of dark adaptation after extinction of a bright yellow light, i.e., the phenomenon known as transient tritanopia (5, 6, 7). Changes of adaptation thus disclose strong inhibitory effects between different classes of receptors. The inhibitory action between receptor mechanisms is a characteristic of normal vision. Selective loss or damage of cone receptors in disease may not only imply damage of the receptor functions in question, but also a loss of inhibitory action upon other mechanisms. Registration of improved sensitivity in early dark adaptation may therefore serve to indicate damage of the cone mechanisms. By recording the threshold sensitivity to a short wavelength stimulus at defined intervals after extinction of a strong background light, a perimetric method has been developed for measuring the influence of inhibitory action in the visual field. It is the purpose of the present work to report some results with this type of perimetry.

MATERIAL AND METHODS

Examinations were carried out on three patients:

Patient 1, a female 19 years old with progressive cone dystrophy, was followed from the age of 11. There had been gradually reduced vision together with complete loss of colour vision. Her cone dystrophy appeared to be part of a hereditary systemic disorder affecting several organs (case 3 in an earlier report (3)). At the time of examination her visual acuity was 6/60 on each eye. The F D-15 test performed correctly at the age of 11 years, now showed completely confused pattern. She had good visual fields with big targets, but greatly restricted with small targets.

Patient 2, a female 22 years old with juvenile macular degeneration of the Stargardt type, had visual acuity 5/60 on the right eye and 6/60 on the left with a correction −1.5. She performed the F D-15 test with confusion along the red−green axes. In the Nagel anomaloscope she accepted settings in a broad range with deviation in the direction of protanomaly (40−60 as compared to a norm of 40).

Patient 3, a male 38 years old, a typical rod monochromat, had visual acuity 6/36 on each eye with a correction +2 cyl. 90°. The patient was case 6 in an earlier report (2). There was moderate photophobia, but no nystagmus. Spectral sensitivity curves and ERG with flicker stimuli showed a rod pattern. Confusion existed along the scotopic axis with the F D-15 test. He had typical achromatic settings with the anomaloscope.

The persons taking part in the examinations were all trained in static perimetry and maintained a good fixation (which was occasionally controlled). Two normal persons were used as reference, both of which had normal visual acuity and colour vision.

The spatial arrangement of the stimuli is shown in Fig. 1, upper part. The circular, yellow adapting field (A) is projected on a white screen coated with $BaSO_4$. The blue test field (C) is presented in the center of the adapting field. Two modified tungsten-halogen projectors (Prado Universal) were used as light sources. The projectors were equipped with electromechanical shutters, controlled by an electronic timing device. The optics of the two projectors was modified to obtain high field luminances. The light levels (cd/m^2) were measured by a Pritchard spotmeter, Model 1980A-P1, in the direction of the observer's eye. The yellow field was produced by a Wratten filter No. 21 (Figs. 2 and 3) or No. 22 (Fig.s 4−6). The blue test field was produced by a Balzer narrow-band interference filter having maximum transmission at

406

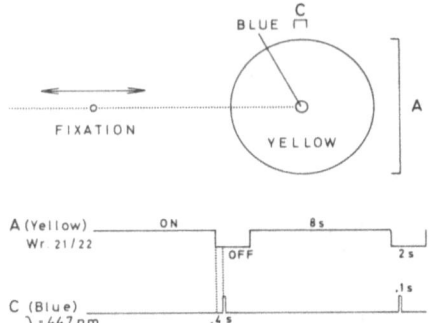

Fig. 1. The spatial arrangement and the temporal sequence of the test stimulus and background light.

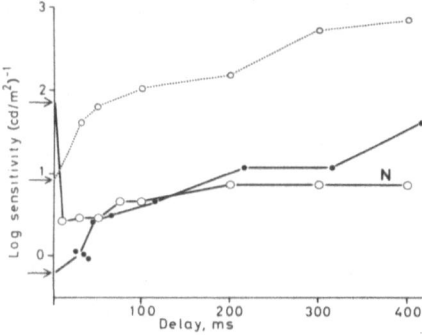

Fig. 2. Threshold sensitivity to a blue stimulus in a patient with progressive cone dystrophy (dark circles) and a normal person (N) at varying intervals after extinction of the adapting field. The stimulus was seen 6.5° peripherally in the upper field. $I_A = 125$ cd/m^2, $\phi_A = 13.5°$, $\phi_C = 1.3°$. The stippled line indicates the response of a normal person with greatly reduced intensity of the adapting light; registration made 50° peripherally. $I_A = 5.2$ cd/m^2, $\phi_A = 15.5°$, $\phi_C = 2.3°$. The arrows indicate the sensitivity level during yellow illumination.

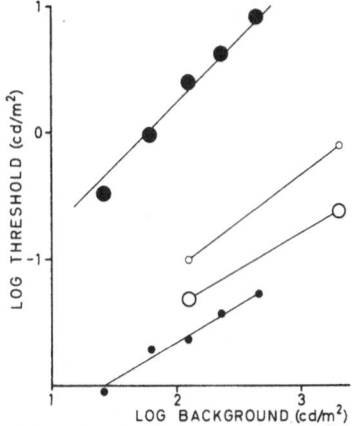

Fig. 3. Thresholds of a blue stimulus registered on a yellow field of varying intensity (great circles) and the thresholds registered 400 ms after extinction of the adapting field (small circles). Dark circles indicate the response of a patient with progressive cone dystrophy and open circles that of a normal person. The stimulus presentation was 6.5° peripherally in the upper field. $\phi_A = 13.5°$, $\phi_C = 1.4°$.

407

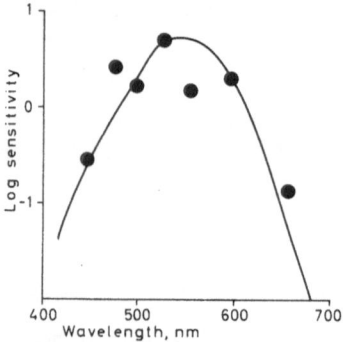

Fig. 4. Spectral sensitivity of a normal person registered during the dark phase at a 10° perimetric angle. The stimuli were near monochromatic and were presented 400 ms after extinction of the adapting yellow field. $I_A = 820$ cd/m². The graph indicates the green primary of Walraven (8).

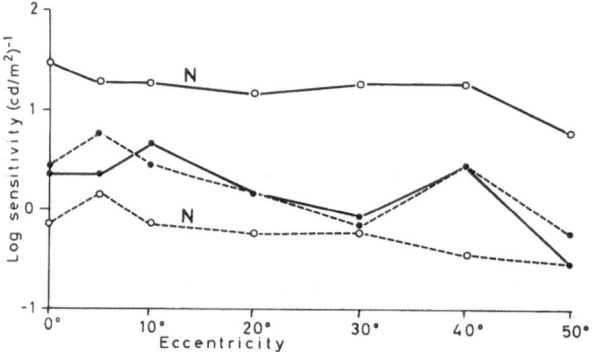

Fig. 5. Static perimetry by use of a blue stimulus light against a yellow surface (full lines) and the threshold sensitivity to the same stimulus recorded in the dark phase (broken lines). Black symbols indicate the response of a patient with juvenile macular degeneration and open symbols that of a normal person. $I_A = 2500$ cd/m², $\phi_A = 17°$, $\phi_C = 1.6°$.

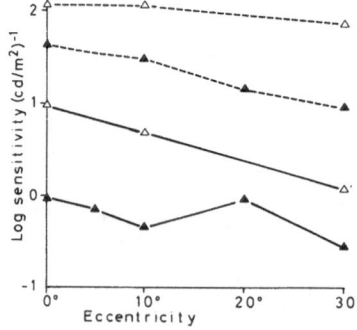

Fig. 6. The same registration as in Fig. 5 obtained on a rod monochromat at two levels of intensity of the yellow field. Dark symbols indicate the response at moderately high intensity, $I_A = 925$ cd/m², and open symbols that at reduced intensity, $I_A = 120$ cd/m². $\phi_A = 17°$, $\phi_C = 1.6°$.

408

$\lambda = 447$ nm. Light intensity was regulated by the use of Balzer metal-coated grey filters. The diameter, ϕ_A. of the adapting field varied between 13.5° and 17° and that of the blue test field, ϕ_C, between 1.3° and 2.3°.

Two registrations of the blue stimulus thresholds were made: a) against a constant yellow background and b) in the dark phase 400 ms after extinction of the yellow field. Normally the duration of the adapting light was 8 seconds (except for the experiment shown in Fig. 3 where a 15 seconds duration was used) and that of the dark phase 2 seconds. The duration of the blue test flash was 100 ms. The temporal sequence of the stimuli is shown in Fig. 1, lower part.

RESULTS

Figure 2 shows the threshold sensitivity to a blue stimulus light recorded at different intervals after extinction of an adapting yellow light. Two completely different response patterns were found. In the normal observer there was a considerable decrease of threshold sensitivity, starting immediately after extinction of the field and still lasting after 400 ms. In a patient with cone dystrophy, on the other hand, there was a sensitivity increase, starting immediately after extinction and falling further off throughout the 400 ms period, by the end of which time her sensitivity level was even higher than for the normal observer. Thus, in this patient with presumably no cone vision a considerable recovery of sensitivity to blue light was demonstrated. Increasing sensitivity could also be shown for the normal observer in the periphery by use of an adapting field of low intensity ($I_A = 5.2$ cd/m^2). The response curve here reflects rod activity and is quite similar to that of the cone dystrophy patient. How the recovering of light sensitivity is influenced by the intensity of the adapting light, is shown in Fig. 3. In our patient with progressive cone dystrophy there was a decrease of thresholds of about 2 log units after extinction of the adapting light, this being more pronounced at greater intensity. In the normal observer, on the contrary, there was a threshold *increase* of nearly 0.5 log unit, i.e., a transient tritanopia response.

The transient tritanopia in the normal was clearly manifest and quite constant across the visual field as is seen in Fig. 5. The clear and marked transient tritanopia could be shown at moderate adapting light level as well as with a high intensity field (Fig. 5). The reduction of threshold sensitivity was about 1.5 log units. Registration of spectral sensitivity during the dark phase shows a relatively good fit to the green primary (Fig. 4).

In a patient with juvenile macular degeneration (Fig. 5) the static perimetry curve indicates a moderate reduction of threshold sensitivity in the light phase, while the sensitivity level registered during the dark phase is raised compared with that of the normal observer. The curves obtained in the two phases are close to each other. This means that in our patient where red and green sensitive receptors were chiefly affected, the transient tritanopia phenomenon was subdued or lacking.

A particularly low sensitivity to the blue stimulus light was found in a rod monochromat by registration against a stready yellow background (Fig. 6).

409

On the other hand this patient showed a very high sensitivity increase after extinction of the adapting light, making a difference of about 1.5 log units between the perimetric curves in the two phases. Instead of a transient tritanopia effect this patient without functioning cones, demonstrated a fast recovery of light sensitivity which is essentially different from the response of the normal observer. It is interesting that even with strong adapting light the threshold sensitivity in the dark phase was still at a level more than 1 log unit above that of the normal observer. On reducing the intensity of the adapting light there was a further increase of threshold sensitivity during the dark phase.

DISCUSSION

The idea behind this form of static perimetry is to evaluate the functional activity of the long wavelength receptors by measuring the change of threshold response of the short wave receptors. The double registration of thresholds to the blue stimulus, a) on field and b) after extinction of the field, gives a good estimate of the strength of the interactions between the receptor systems. The normal suppressing activity is dependent on functioning cones. Recovering red and green cone mechanisms are supposed to inhibit or otherwise suppress the blue cone signal during early dark adaptation (5). We may differentiate between the typical transient tritanopia found in normals and the *reduction* or lack of this phenomenon in patients with ocular pathology. Transient tritanopia is clearly manifest in normals and amounts to approximately the same degree in central and peripheral areas indicating that the degree of inhibition is nearly constant. Mollon and Polden (4) found that the green mechanism accounted for the thresholds in the dark phase, which is also confirmed in Fig. 4.

The activity of the cone receptors implies a suppression effect upon the rod mechanism which may be considerable. It is only with a lack of cone function or in extensive damage of cone receptors that full rod sensitivity may be measured in the dark phase. Such a response could be demonstrated in our paitents with progressive cone dystrophy and congenital rod monochromacy. A great increase of light sensitivity was shown immediately after extinction of the adapting field, as distinct from the equally rapid *decrease* of sensitivity recorded in the normal observer. What is involved here, is a rod response function apparently uninfluenced by other receptor activities. In Fig. 2 a similar type of response was registered in a normal observer using an adapting field of very low intensity where the normal cone activity was substantially reduced.

In cases with incomplete damage of cone functions, as in our patient with juvenile macular degeneration, a minimal or no reduction of the sensitivity level was registered in the dark phase. This indicates that the blue receptor mechanism is functioning without noticeable inhibition from the long wavelength receptors. Those patients characteristically have a red—green colour vision defect due to reduced sensitivity of the red and green cones and a relatively better preserved blue mechanism (1). The weakly manifest or

410

insignificant transient tritanopia in our patient resembles the lack of transient tritanopia found in blue cone monochromacy (4).

By this method of static perimetry a good indication may be obtained of the inhibitory influence of the long wavelength receptors within localized areas of the visual field. It may therefore, although indirectly, give a significant measure of the functional capacity of those receptors. Registration of a reduced sensitivity to the blue stimulus light in the dark phase is consistent with well-functioning red or green cones, while an increased sensitivity indicates a functional defect of the red and green mechanisms.

REFERENCES

1. Hansen, E. The photoreceptors in cone dystrophies. Mod. Probl. Ophthalmol. (Basel) 13: 318−327 (1974).
2. Hansen, E. Typical and atypical monochromacy studied by specific quantitative perimetry. Acta Ophthalmol. (Kbh.) 57: 211−224 (1979).
3. Hansen, E., Frøyshov Larsen, I. and Berg, K. A familial syndrome of progressive cone dystrophy, degenerative liver disease, endocrine dysfunction and hearing defect. I. Ophthalmological findings. Acta Ophthalmol. (Kbh.) 54:129−144 (1976).
4. Hansen, E., Seim, T. and Olsen, B. T. Transient tritanopia experiment in blue cone monochromacy. Nature (London) 276:390−391 (1978).
5. Mollon, J. D. and Polden, P. G. Colour illusion and evidence for interaction between cone mechanisms. Nature (London) 258:421−422 (1975).
6. Mollon, J. D. and Polden, P. G. Absence of transient tritanopia after adaptation to very intense yellow light. Nature (London) 259:570−571 (1976).
7. Stiles, W. S. Increment thresholds and the mechanisms of colour vision. Doc. Ophthalmol. 3:138−165 (1949); In: Mechanisms of Colour Vision. Academic, New York (1978).
8. Walraven, P. L. A closer look at the tritanopic convergence point. Vision Res. 14:1339−1343 (1974).

Authors' address:
Dept. of Ophthalmology
State Hospital and Institute of Physics
University of Oslo
Oslo,
Norway

PERIMETRIC TECHNIQUES USED TO ASSESS RETINAL STRAIN DURING ACCOMMODATION

JAY M. ENOCH, ROBERT A. MOSES,
ROLF W. NYGAARD and DALE ALLEN
(Berkeley, California/Saint Louis, Missouri, U.S.A.)

Key words. Accommodation, retinal stretch, myodiopter.

ABSTRACT

Two modified permetric techniques have been employed to allow quantifi-cation of retinal strain or stretch during accommodation. Maximum retinal displacement occurs at the ora serrata. One technique provides a measure of the anterior functional boundary of the temporal retina (nasal field) by transcleral (diascleral) illumination. The second method makes available infor-mation on the displacement of the point of fixation relative to the blind spot. The two measures are independent and complementary. These are difficult techniques.

INTRODUCTION

Previous studies have suggested that a result of ocular accommodation for near is increased traction by the ciliary musculature on the choroid and hence on the overlying retina. Animal studies (16) have shown that there is motion across the entire choroid from posterior pole to equator. There is actually a gradient of movement which approaches zero near the optic nerve head (11). Depending on the subject or eyeball tested, human psychophysical measures of visual field bisection (5, 7, 13), suggest that retinal stretch accompanies accommodative effort and might not be uniform (linear) across the retina (5). Ciliary muscle myograms (1, 4) and psychophysical work using Haidinger's brushes (2), transcleral illumination of the ora serrate (12), and Badal system perimetry (9) suggest that retinal strain accompanies accommodative effort. It is desirable to enhance quantification of this effect. Two perimetric methods are described.

This study investigates retinal stretch during accommodative strain by the techniques of transcleral or diascleral illumination of the functional leading edge of the temporal retina (really a form of perimetry), and a visual field test technique similar to that used by Hollins (9) to measure the angle from the center of the blind spot to the point of fixation. The transcleral technique is

Table 1. Transcleral illumination experiment data.

Subject	Age	Transcleral illumination experiment	Contact lens refraction
TF	25	−0.070 mm/D	−4.00 D
DA	28	−0.038	−1.25
RN	34	−0.070	−4.50
MF[a]	21	−0.050	No R_x

[a]Reported by Moses, 1970; different method.

an attempt to verify earlier findings by Moses (12) obtained by slit-lamp observation of the transilluminated ora serrata during patient accommodation. Moses suggested an average anterior retinal movement of 0.05 mm per diopter of accommodation at the ora in a young (21-year old) observer (see also Table 1).

Our blind spot measurement technique allows assessment of retinal stretch occurring at the posterior pole in response to accommodative strain (5, 7, 9). A correction was made for magnification effects.

METHODS

The fixation target and blind-spot stimulus were mounted on a 3-dimensionally adjustable lathe bed riding on a modified Thompson rail. Targets used contained fine detail and included a central fixation spot that subtended 3′ of visual arc regardless of test distance from the observer.

During diascleral laser illumination (Fig. 1), the observer's temporal sclera was illuminated with a steady state 3 mm × 15 mm projected horizontal strip of white light. This provided an essentially equal-luminance background onto which the laser spot was projected, reduced spurious signals, and provided sufficient illumination to monitor the position of the observer's corneal apex (by auxilliary telescope and cross hair). An optical system directed a red laser beam (632.8 nm at 0.5 mW) through a 2 Hz rotating sectored disk, an attenuating filter, and a right angle deflecting prism mounted on a movable micrometer stage. A vernier dial permitted 0.002 mm resolution of the horizontal movement of the laser beam. A spotting telescope was used to fix the image of the observer's corneal apex on a fine cross-hair reticule. Change in the observer's eye position was recorded on a dial indicator unit with readout resolution finer than 0.01 mm.

The blind-spot stimulus consisted of a yellow LED (Stanley ESBY5501) square-wave flickering at 3 Hz and apertured through a set of pinholes that always subtended 2′ of visual arc regardless of the accommodative distance (see Fig. 2). The stimulus itself was driven by a stepping motor (Bodine Electric 34T1) and moved linearly across the temporal hemifield of the target plane on a 1/4-40 lead screw slide. A microprocessor maintained the stimulus at a fixed retinal illuminance and at a constant rate of motion, 1° per second, regardless of test distance. Using the target in Fig. 1 for this test resulted in small cyclotorsional eye movements in young observers. To minimize this, the target shown in Fig. 2 was substituted.

414

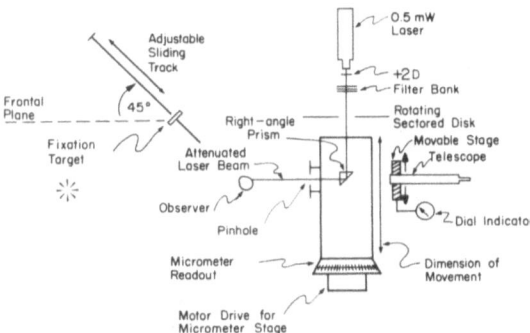

Fig. 1. Schematic drawing of the apparatus used for transcleral determination of the position of the anterior functional retinal boundary. The fixation target used is included as an insert.

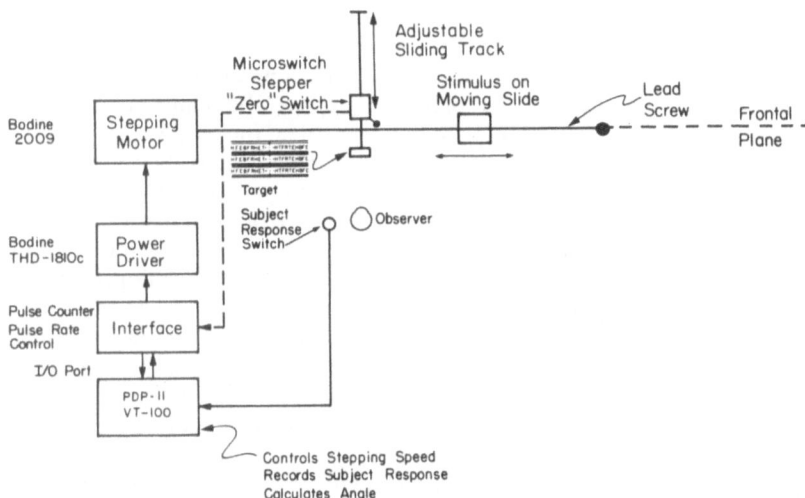

Fig. 2. Schematic drawing of the apparatus used to measure the inner and outer bounds of the blind spot. By switching fixation from the top center (see inset), to the middle center, to the bottom center level of the fixation target different levels of the blind spot could be sampled.

Procedurally, the observer was placed in a highly secure bite-bar appratus with multiple forehead and occipital restraints. The observer's left eye was occluded (both experiments), and his right eye was aligned with the center of a detailed illuminated, fixation target by adjusting the lathe bed stage while centering the target through a multiple (aligned) pinhole sighting device. This procedure was repeated for all target-distance settings. The procedure ensured

415

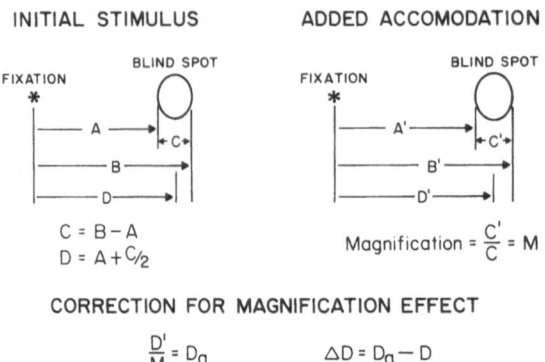

INITIAL STIMULUS ADDED ACCOMODATION

$$C = B - A$$
$$D = A + C/2$$

$$\text{Magnification} = \frac{C'}{C} = M$$

CORRECTION FOR MAGNIFICATION EFFECT

$$\frac{D'}{M} = D_a \qquad \Delta D = D_a - D$$

Fig. 3. Scheme for correcting data for magnification effects caused by accommodation in the blind spot measurement experiment.

maintenance of the fixation point on the same axis as the centrum of the accommodated target. The retinal illuminance of the white portion of the target was set at 5000 trolands in order to optimize stready fixation (3) and to permit testing within the Weber portion of the increment luminance sensitivity function.

In the experiment using transcleral illumination, the target was displaced nasally 45° to the mid-sagittal plane to expose the temporal sclera. The observer responded to the first appearance of a flickering spot in the far nasal visual field. Threshold corresponded to the *functional* leading edge of the temporal retina. Both the method of adjustment (motorized movement of the laser spot at 0.01 mm/sec under the control of the observer) and a staircase method (response key controlled by the observer) were employed. Data from one observer (DA: age 28) were collected in one diopter steps per session, in the order from 2D to 7D of accommodation. All three observers (TF: age 25; DA: age 28; RN: age 34) also yielded data on only two different diopter settings per session, the first setting always being 2D of accommodation. This procedure reduced fatigue and allowed for data normalization. Six pulses were delivered per trial (at least 4 of which had to be detected for a positive response) with 10-minute rest periods between accommodative steps. Each of the observers wore a well-centered contact lens corrected for infinity in all experiments.

In the blind spot perimetry experiment, the observer was again placed in the secure bite-bar, head-clamp stage. He responded to the disappearance and reappearance of a flickering stimulus as it moved in alternate directions across his blind spot (points A and B in Fig. 3). The distance of the midpoint (D) from the point of fixation defined the angular position of blind-spot center. Data were collected in an illuminated room following careful target alignment. The fixation targets were vertically tripartite (Fig. 2) to enable sampling of the blind spot at selected parallel displacements relative to the horizontal meridian (Fig. 3). In this way, possible eye rotation (torsion) could be monitored. That is, the relative width of the blind spot would change for the different fixation positions if the eye executed a cyclorotation. Two drops of

416

2.5% phenylephrine hydrochloride were instilled for the blind-spot experiment to minimize alteration of retinal illuminance with accommodation. A simple finger lift signaled the visual angle position of the medial and temporal margins of the blind spot with respect to the point of accommodative fixation as the LED illuminated stimulus slowly moved laterally or medially across the visual field meridian. Data were collected either in order of increasing accommodative effort or by using two different test distances as discussed in the first experiment.

RESULTS

Data obtained in three subjects for transcleral determinations of the leading functional edge of the temporal retina (nasal field) are shown in Fig. 4. Linear determinations (essentially tangential to the sclera) of position of the laser beam were measured. The 2D points from the 3 data sets are approximately superimposed to facilitate comparison of displacement rate (slope). These data are presented in this form for ease in comparison with the earlier measurements of Moses (12) using transcleral shadowing of the ora serrata. Representative slopes of the individual sets of data from this experiment are compared to Moses' data in Table 1. The two methods show retinal displacement of the same order of magnitude. Clearly, it is premature to compare slope across age, or any other parameter.

It is possible to translate position on the sclera into projected visual field angle measure at the entrance pupil of the eye. This can be done if one uses an established schematic eye (8, 14, 15). We plan to execute such an analysis in the near future.

In the second experiment, a series of problems were encountered. Figure 5 (upper part) shows uncorrected data on two of our subjects compared to those presented by Hollins (9). In both instances D' was determined from the blind spot measurements (Fig. 3). Clearly, the measurement trend is different in both sets of data. The cause is not clear. Our measurements are truncated in a dioptic range because we encountered small cyclorotational movements when we measured relative blind-spot width for horizontal passes just above $(1°-2°)$ or just below the horizontal meridian for different accommodative amplitudes. Data presented were not confounded in this manner.

Assuming that the actual width of the blind spot (C) is *not altered* by accommodation, magnification can be factored out. In Fig. 5 (lower part), we correct for magnification as shown in Fig. 3; i.e., D_a is plotted as a function of amplitude of accommodative stimulus. The resultant angular shifts are large, i.e., one degree in the entrance pupil should translate into roughly 0.3 mm on the retina near the posterior pole (8). If the translation at the functional edge of the retina or the ora serrata approximates 0.5 mm to 0.7 mm for ten diopters of accommodation in young observers, one does not expect the size translation recorded at fixation relative to the blind spot to be of the same magnitude. Nevertheless, magnification cannot be overlooked. If Hollins' data are corrected for magnification effects as defined, a non-rational result occurs. Even without correction for magnification, Hollins (9)

417

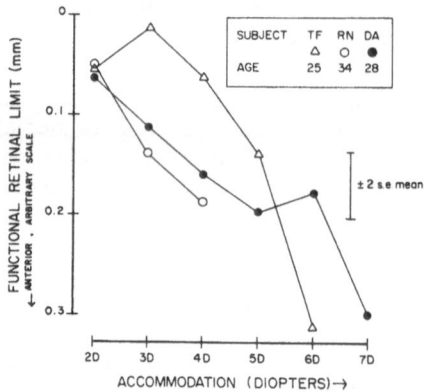

Fig. 4. Data on the three subjects (ages in box) obtained during the transcleral illumination experiment. The ordinate scales linear position of the functional retinal limit in a plane parallel to the mid-sagittal plane and approximately tangent to the subject's globe.

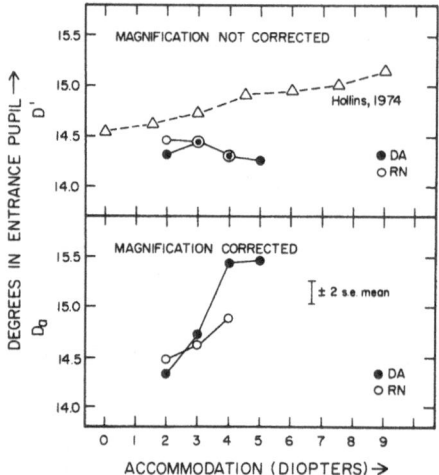

Fig. 5. Upper part: data on two subjects obtained from the blind spot experiment. Data uncorrected for magnification are shown alongside similar (uncorrected) data obtained by Hollins (9). D' has been computed in this figure (see Fig. 3). Lower part: the two-subject data shown in the upper part corrected for magnification effects. D_a is plotted here (see Fig. 3).

also showed surprisingly large measured changes. Obviously, these questions need to be pursued in an orderly manner in the future.

DISCUSSION AND CONCLUSIONS

The forward advance of the retina with the choroid during accommodation is a well-established physiological change. This is not a small change, i.e., several years ago, Enoch (6) showed that the actual area of an average retina

418

increased by a total of 30 mm^2 (a 2.4% increase in retinal surface) with 0.5 mm advance of the ora serrata (12). Furthermore, it has been shown that there are characteristic tears of the retina associated with marked accommodative strain, usually induced by pharmeceutical action (10).

It is important to look at these effects of accommodation. Here, two perimetric techniques are used which allow estimation of the forward movement of the retina: 1) at the temporal retinal functional boundary, using the transcleral illumination method; and 2) at the fovea, using the blind-spot plotting technique. Our second method is similar to that of Hollins (9), except that we use the natural pupil and do not use a Badal system, and we consider magnification and cyclotorsional confounds. We also used a high-intensity background and test fields (as did Hollins) and a modest mydriatic to minimize effects of pupil size change.

These are difficult experiments. There are some extremely important questions which need to be asked in an orderly way. First, what is the effect of age on the resultant strain on the retina for a given accommodative stimulus? That is, we do know that the eye lens hardens and becomes less flexible with age. We do not know whether an equivalent amount of ciliary body contraction is needed for one diopter of accommodation, e.g., at forty or fifty years of age, as compared to a teenager. These techniques may improve our estimate of the so-called myodiopter, i.e., to enable us to see if the retinal translation for a given visual stimulus is equal at different ages.

There are other questions of interest, such as: what is the effect of accommodative strain in a rather hyperopic individual, or a very myopic person? Furthermore, are there individuals who exhibit large amounts of retinal strain associated with accommodation, and what are their characteristics? Are these properties found in those predisposed towards retinal detachment or other retinal anomaly? In short, many aspects of the accommodative mechanism have not been studied, and certainly require more attention than they have received in the past. We hope to improve our techniques and pursue these questions.

ACKNOWLEDGEMENTS

We wish to thank Professor Oleg Pomerantzeff of the Retina Foundation, Boston, for assistance in analysis of data as it relates to the schematic eye. Christa Niemeyer of the Johannes Gutenberg University, Mainz, DFR assisted us in certain places of this project.

This research was supported in part by N.E.I. Research Grants EY-03674 (to J.M.E.) and EY-00256 (to R.A.M.), and Training Grant EY-07076 (to J.M.E.), N.I.H., Bethesda, Maryland, U.S.A.

REFERENCES

1. Adel, N. L. Role of the ciliary musculature in accommodation and myopia. Opt. J. and Rev. Optom. 100:23–26 (1963).

2. Adel, N. L. Electromyographic and entoptic studies suggesting a theory of action of the ciliary muscle in accommodation for near and its influence on the development of myopia. Am. J. Optom. and Arch. Am. Acad. Optom. 43:27–28 (1966).
3. Alpern, M. Variability of acommodation during steady fixation at various levels of illuminance. J. Opt. Soc. Am. 48:193–197 (1958).
4. Alpern, M., Ellen, P. and Goldsmith, R. I. The electrical response of the human eye in far-to-near accommodation. A.M.A. Arch. Ophthalmol. 60:592–602 (1958).
5. Blank, K. and Enoch, J. M. Monocular spatial distortions induced by marked accommodation. Science 182:393–395 (1973).
6. Enoch, J. M. Effect of substantial accommodation on total retinal area. J. Opt. Soc. Am. 63:899 (1973).
7. Enoch, J. M. Marked accommodation, retinal stretch, monocular space perception and retinal receptor orientation. Am. J. Optom. and Physiol. Opt. 52:375–392 (1975).
8. Enoch, J. M. and Laties, A. An analysis of retinal receptor orientation: II. Predictions for psychophysical tests. Invest. Ophthalmol. 10:959–970 (1971).
9. Hollins, M. Does the central human retina stretch during accommodation? Nature 251:729–730 (1974).
10. Lemcke, H. H. and Pischel, D. K. Retinal detachments after the use of phospholine iodide. Trans. Pac. Coast Otoophthalmol. Soc. Annu. Meet. 47:153–157 (1966).
11. Luedde, W. H. Hensen and Voelcker's experiments on the mechanism of accommodation: an interpretation. Trans. Am Ophthalmol. Soc. 25:250 (1927).
12. Moses, R. A. Accommodation. In: Adler's Physiology of the Eye. Clinical Applications, R. A. Moses (ed.), C. V. Mosby and Co., St. Louis (1970).
13. Ogle, K. N. Researches in Binocular Vision. Hafner, New York (1964).
14. Pomerantzeff, O., Fish, H., Govignon, J. and Schepens, C. Wide angle optical model of the human eye. Ann. Ophthalmol. 3:815–819 (1971).
15. Pomerantzeff, O. Personal communication (1982).
16. Van Alphen, G. W. H. M. On emmetropia and ametropia. Acta Ophthalmol. Suppl. 142:44 (1961).

Authors' addresses:
Drs J. M. Enoch, R. W. Nygaard and D. Allen
School of Optometry
University of California, Berkeley
Berkeley, CA 94720
U.S.A.

Dr R. A. Moses
Dept. of Ophthalmology
Washington University School of Medicine
Saint Louis, MO 63110
U.S.A.

STATIC FUNDUS PERIMETRY IN AMBLYOPIA:
COMPARISON WITH JUVENILE MACULAR DEGENERATION

S. G. JACOBSON, M. A. SANDBERG and E. L. BERSON

(Boston, Massachusetts, U.S.A.)

Key words. Amblyopia, strabismus, juvenile macular degeneration, perimetry, threshold, fovea.

ABSTRACT

Cone increment thresholds were measured in 18 patients with strabismic amblyopia using a hand-held stimulator ophthalmoscope that allowed the examiner to visualize the stimulus on the fundus and test known retinal loci. With this technique of static fundus perimetry, all patients with amblyopia showed small to moderate elevations in threshold at the foveola and 50% had a nasal-temporal asymmetry in thresholds. Nasal retinal thresholds were elevated in patients with esotropia while temporal retinal thresholds were elevated in patients with exotropia. In contrast, patients with juvenile macular degeneration showed profound threshold elevations at the foveola with symmetrical elevations of threshold at paracentral retinal loci.

INTRODUCTION

When the amblyopic eyes of patients with strabismic amblyopia have been evaluated with monocular static perimetry, different patterns of central visual loss have been described. For example, some studies describe marked crater-like depressions in sensitivity centered at the fovea (5, 6), while others have demonstrated relatively small sensitivity losses at the foveola (2, 10). Generalized sensitivity loss across the whole central visual field (1, 12) and even paracentral scotomas deeper than the central scotoma (6, 10) have been reported. All previous studies have used static perimetry techniques in which the test lights are projected into the visual field.

A major difficulty encountered in previous investigations and a possible reason for some of the conflicting findings has been the unstable fixation of the amblyopic eye (4). We have minimized this problem in the present study by performing monocular static perimetry using a hand-held stimulator ophthalmoscope (13). This instrument allows the examiner to visualize the stimulus on the fundus and measure cone increment thresholds at known retinal loci. With this technique of fundus perimetry we evaluated patients with amblyopia and compared the results to those of patients with juvenile macular degeneration.

SUBJECTS AND METHODS

Among the 20 adult patients with amblyopia in this study, there were 18 patients with strabismic amblyopia, 1 patient with anisometropic amblyopia and 1 patient with strabismus and anisometropia. All of these patients had visual acuity of 6/60 or worse in the amblyopic eye and 6/6–6/9 in the fellow eye. Also tested were 3 patients with alternating strabismus and no amblyopia (6/6 in both eyes), 1 patient with a paralytic strabismus (6/6 in both eyes) and 6 patients with juvenile hereditary macular degeneration (6/60 in both eyes). Details of the method for measuring cone increment thresholds using a hand-held dual-beam Maxwellian view stimulator ophthalmoscope and certain results from a series of 41 normal subjects have been previously reported (14). In the present study, monocular thresholds were measured at 4 retinal loci – 0°, anatomical foveola; 10° temporal, 10° nasal, and 20° nasal to the foveola. The white targets (6, 12, 30 and 60 min in diameter) were flashed at 5 Hz (20 msec duration) and superimposed on a 10° steady white background (5 log photopic trolands), which is above rod saturation. Thresholds were determined by a method of limits in steps of 0.1 neutral density.

RESULTS

Figure 1 shows representative increment thresholds at 4 retinal loci in both eyes of a normal subject (A), 3 patients with strabismic amblyopia (B–D), and a patient with juvenile macular degeneration (E). Figure 1A demonstrates the well-known features of the normal threshold versus area (tva) function. Threshold falls with increasing stimulus area and the slope of the function becomes steeper with increasing eccentricity from the foveola (16). Normal subjects showed comparable thresholds for corresponding retinal locations in the 2 eyes ($\not> 0.2$ log unit difference) and symmetry was consistently observed between the 10° nasal and temporal loci in each eye ($\not> 0.2$ log unit difference).

In all 18 patients with strabismic amblyopia, the thresholds at the foveola in the amblyopic eye were higher than in the fellow eye. For the 6 min diameter stimulus, for example, the interocular difference in threshold ranged from 0.3 to 1.0 log unit, with a mean of 0.6 log unit. Nine of the patients, 7 esotropic and 2 exotropic, showed only this elevation of threshold at the amblyopic foveola; 10° nasal and 10° temporal retinal thresholds were normal and symmetrical and 20° nasal thresholds were normal (Fig. 1B). In 7 of the remaining patients, however, there were threshold elevations not only at the foveola but also at the 10° nasal retinal locus of the amblyopic eye (Fig. 1C); thresholds at the 10° temporal and 20° nasal loci in amblyopic

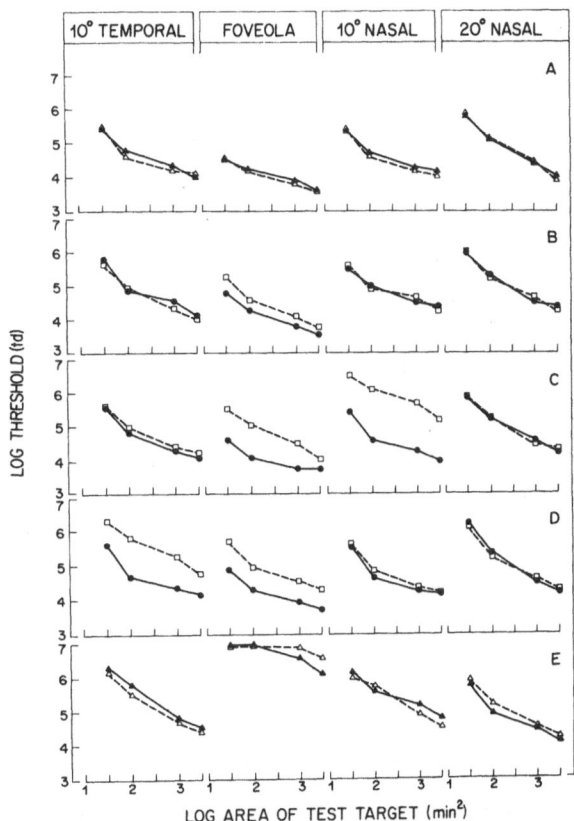

Fig. 1. Increment thresholds at 4 retinal loci in (A) a normal subject; (B and C) 2 patients with left esotropia and amblyopia; (D) a patient with right exotropia and amblyopia; and (E) a patient with juvenile macular degeneration. (B–D) filled circles, amblyopic eye; open squares, fellow eye; (A, E) filled triangles, right eye; open triangles, left eye.

and fellow eyes were similar and normal. Six of these 7 patients were esotropic or had a history of esotropia in childhood and one patient, whose early history was not known, was orthotropic after recent surgery for exotropia. The 2 remaining patients, both with long-standing exotropia, also demonstrated a nasal-temporal asymmetry in the amblyopic eye but the abnormally high threshold was at 10° in the temporal retina (Fig. 1D). The 10° and 20° nasal loci were normal in both eyes. Patients with juvenile macular degeneration showed a very different pattern of results (Fig. 1E). Thresholds in both eyes were profoundly elevated at the foveola, abnormally high but symmetrical at 10° nasal and 10° temporal and normal at 20° nasal.

The patient with anisometropic amblyopia had elevated thresholds only at the foveola of the amblyopic eye. The esotropic, amblyopic eye of another patient with significant anisometropia showed not only elevated foveolar thresholds but also a high nasal retinal threshold. An adult patient with paralytic strabismus of 5 years duration due to a unilateral abducens nerve

423

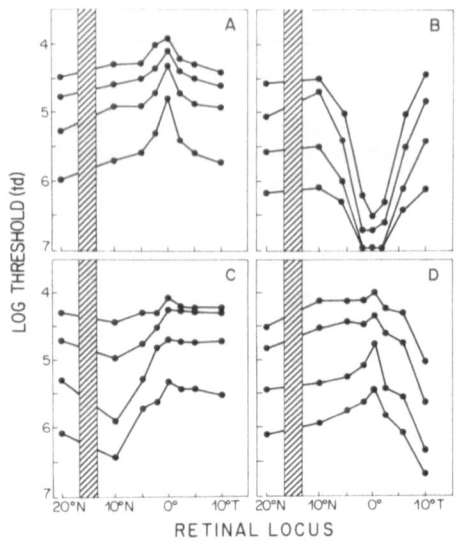

Fig. 2. Increment thresholds at 8 retinal loci in (A) a normal subject; (B) a patient with juvenile macular degeneration; (C) the amblyopic eye of a patient with esotropia; and (D) the amblyopic eye of a patient with exotropia. The 4 retinal sensitivity profiles for each subject represent results from the 4 target sizes (from top to bottom: 60, 30, 12 and 6 min diameter). Shaded area represents the optic nerve head.

palsy showed normal and symmetrical thresholds in both eyes. The 3 patients with alternating strabismus and no amblyopia also had entirely normal profiles.

To further characterize the nasal-temporal asymmetries found in amblyopic eyes, we measured cone increment thresholds with the stimulator ophthalmoscope at 8 rather than 4 retinal loci in 2 patients with strabismic amblyopia and compared these results to those from a normal subject and a patient with juvenile macular degeneration (Fig. 2). Figure 2A shows the normal retinal sensitivity profile tested with the 4 targets of diminishing size (top to bottom). Sensitivity is maximum at the foveola and falls off symmetrically with increasing eccentricity. Figure 2B is the sensitivity profile from the patient with juvenile macular degeneration and shows a deep central scotoma with all target sizes and a symmetrical sensitivity loss extending 10° nasal and temporal from the foveola. The sensitivity profiles in Figs. 2C and 2D highlight the afore-mentioned finding in amblyopic eyes of reduced foveolar sensitivity and asymmetric paracentral sensitivity loss. Whereas the esotropic patient in Fig. 2C shows a nasal retinal impairment of sensitivity, the exotropic patient in Fig. 2D has impaired temporal retinal sensitivity.

Figure 3 is a comparison of cone increment thresholds in 2 groups of patients with the same Snellen acuity of 6/60. In Fig. 3A are measurements from the foveola of the amblyopic eyes of 8 patients with strabismic amblyopia and unsteady central fixation. In Fig. 3B are results from both eyes of 4 patients with juvenile macular degeneration tested at their preferred eccentric locus of fixation (between 5 and 10 degrees superior and/or nasal to the

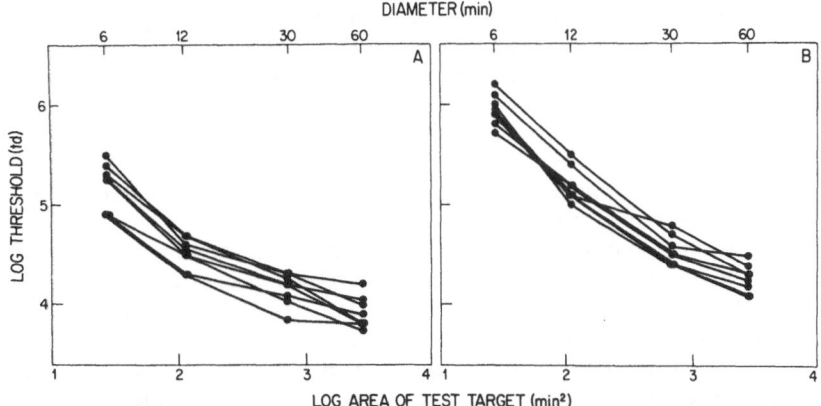

Fig. 3. (A) Foveolar increment thresholds for the amblyopic eyes of 8 patients with strabismic amblyopia, central fixation and visual acuity of 6/60; (B) increment thresholds at the preferred eccentric fixation locus in both eyes of 4 patients with juvenile macular degeneration and visual acuity of 6/60.

foveola). The tva functions from these 2 groups of patients showed marked differences. Thresholds for all target sizes were less elevated in the patients with amblyopia than in the patients with juvenile macular degeneration. The slopes of the tva functions (based on the 6- and 60-minute diameter targets) for amblyopic eyes (mean, 0.62), although abnormally high compared to those from the foveola of the fellow eye of these same patients (mean, 0.47), were much lower than those of patients with juvenile macular degeneration (mean, 0.86).

DISCUSSION

With a technique of static fundus perimetry we found that patients with severely reduced visual acuity due to strabismic amblyopia had small to moderate sensitivity loss at the anatomical foveola of the amblyopic eye. Whether these abnormal foveolar thresholds in amblyopia represent the bottom of a small crater was not determined in most cases because our sampling interval across the central retina was 10°. In the few patients that we did test at 2–5° intervals, no crater-like defects were found, thus demonstrating that the foveola in strabismic amblyopia retains higher sensitivity than surrounding retinal areas.

A relationship between increment thresholds and visual acuity is said to occur in organic macular disease but not in amblyopia (2). The results of our comparison of the tva functions from the fixation loci of patients with amblyopia and patients with juvenile macular degeneration support this notion. For example, thresholds for the 6-min target at the foveola of amblyopic eyes with central fixation are what would be predicted, based on cone spatial density (14), for a visual acuity of 6/12 rather than 6/60, the actual visual acuity reported by these patients. Patients with juvenile macular

425

degeneration fixated at eccentric retinal loci where visual acuity would normally be between 6/15 and 6/30 (3, 9). Thresholds for the 6-min target at these loci were elevated by about 0.5 log unit above the expected norms for this area. Predicted visual acuity based on this threshold elevation (14) would be 6/30 to 6/60, which corresponds well with the actual visual acuity of 6/60 in these patients. This comparison with juvenile macular degeneration suggests that the deficit in amblyopia does not behave as if due to a decrease in the density of functioning cone photoreceptors (8).

An interesting and unexpected finding in the present study was the nasal-temporal asymmetry in the amblyopic eye under monocular viewing conditions. Marked threshold elevations at the 10° nasal or 10° temporal retinal loci occurred in 50% of eyes with strabismic amblyopia tested. Nasal-temporal asymmetries are a well-known finding in such patients when testing is performed with binocular perimetric techniques. These 'hemi-retinal suppression scotomas', however, are said to disappear with monocular testing (11). Our findings confirm those previous studies that described deep paracentral scotomas in many amblyopic subjects with monocular testing (6, 10).

A question that must be considered is whether there is any relationship between the type of strabismus, i.e., esotropia or exotropia, and the hemi-retinal area where there is sensitivity loss. In our series of patients, those with nasal retinal sensitivity loss were, except one, esotropic or had a history of esotropia. The only patients with a temporal retinal sensitivity loss had long-standing exotropia. This suggests that in some patients with strabismic amblyopia, the retinal region most likely to have 'inhibition' under binocular viewing conditions, i.e., nasal retina in esotropia and temporal retina in exotropia, can have sensitivity loss under monocular conditions. A similar interpretation has been given for nasal-temporal asymmetries found on a visual two-point discrimination task in exotropes (11) and on a visual acuity task in esotropes (15).

We also have attempted to answer certain other questions about the nasal-temporal asymmetry, albeit in a limited way. To determine if the asymmetry was exclusive to strabismic amblyopia, we tested 2 patients with anisometropia and amblyopia. The patient without strabismus had no asymmetry, while the patient with an esotropia showed a nasal retinal threshold elevation. To decide if any paracentral asymmetry could occur independent of a foveolar sensitivity loss, we tested 3 patients with alternating strabismus and normal visual acuities. No asymmetries were detected in these patients. A patient with adult onset paralytic esotropia also had normal results. The monocular paracentral sensitivity loss in strabismic amblyopia may therefore only occur, like the central visual loss, if a constant and comitant strabismus is present possibly during a susceptible period of visual development (7).

ACKNOWLEDGEMENT

This work was performed in the Berman-Gund Laboratory for the Study of Retinal Degenerations, Harvard Medical School, Massachusetts Eye and Ear Infirmary, Boston, Massachusetts, U.S.A. Support was provided in part by

Specialized Research Center Grant P50EY-02014 from the National Eye Institute and in part by the Retinitis Pigmentosa Foundation (Baltimore, Maryland) and the George Gund Foundation (Cleveland, Ohio). We are grateful to Mr A. H. Hanson for his help in testing some of the patients.

REFERENCES

1. Aggarwal, D. P. and Verma, G. Static perimetry in the study of amblyopic scotomata. Br. J. Ophthalmol. 64:713–716 (1980).
2. Aulhorn, E. Die gegenseitige Beeinflussung abbildungsgleicher Netzhautstellen bei normalem und gestörtem Binocularsehen. Doc. Ophthalmol. 33:26–61 (1967).
3. Aulhorn, E. and Harms, H. Visual perimetry. In: Handbook of Sensory Physiology, Vol. VII/4, Jameson, D. and Hurvich, L. (eds.). Springer, Berlin (1972).
4. Burian, H. M. and von Noorden, G. K. Binocular Vision and Ocular Motility. Mosby, St. Louis, 243 (1974).
5. Flynn, J. T. Spatial summation in amblyopia. Arch. Ophthalmol. 78:470–474 (1967).
6. Francois, J., Verriest, G. and Verluyten, P. Comparison of the results of static and kinetic perimetry in the central region of the visual field of the amblyopic eye. Strabismus Symp. Giessen Karger, Basel/New York, 45–50 (1966).
7. Jacobson, S. G., Mohindra, I. and Held, R. Age of onset of amblyopia in infants with esotropia. Doc. Ophthalmol. Proc. Series 30:210–216 (1981).
8. Jacobson, S. G., Sandberg, M. A., Effron, M. H. and Berson, E. L. Foveal cone electroretinograms in strabismic amblyopia: comparison with juvenile macular degeneration, macular scars and optic atrophy. Trans. Ophthalmol. Soc. U.K. 99:353–356 (1980).
9. Kirschen, D. G. and Flom, M. C. Visual acuity at different retinal loci of eccentrically fixating functional amblyopes. Am. J. Optom. & Physiol. Optics 55:144–150 (1978).
10. Mackensen, G. Monoculare und binoculare statische Perimetrie zur Untersuchung der Hemmungsvorgänge beim Schielen. Albrecht von Graefes Archiv für Ophthalmol. 160:573–587 (1959).
11. Nawratzki, I. and Jampolsky, A. A regional hemiretinal difference in amblyopia. Am. J. Ophthalmol. 46:339–344 (1958).
12. Pasino, L. and Maraini, G. Le champ visuel central en vision monoculaire dans l'amblyopie. Annal. Oculistique 196:563–569 (1963).
13. Sandberg, M. A. and Ariel, M. A hand-held two channel stimulator ophthalmoscope. Arch. Ophthalmol. 95:1881–1882 (1977).
14. Sandberg, M. A. and Berson, E. L. Visual acuity and cone spatial density in retinitis pigmentosa (submitted).
15. Sireteaunu, R. and Fronius, M. Naso-temporal asymmetries in human amblyopia: consequence of long-term interocular suppression. Vision Res. 21:1055–1063 (1981).
16. Sloan, L. L. and Brown, D. J. Area and luminance of test object as variables in projection perimetry. Vision Res. 2:527–541 (1962).

Authors' address:
Berman-Gund Laboratory
Massachusetts Eye and Ear Infirmary
243 Charles Street
Boston, MA 02114
U.S.A.

THE VISUAL FIELD IN ALTERNATING HYPERPHORIA

ROSA FUSCO, MIRIA D'AIETTI and GUY VERRIEST

(Naples, Italy/Ghent, Belgium)

Key words. Alternating hyperphoria, photopic, mesopic and scotopic profile, perimetry, Keiner's theory.

ABSTRACT

Photopic, mesopic and scotopic static sensitivities were measured along the principal oblique meridians in 14 subjects with alternating hyperphoria and in 12 normal subjects. Significantly depressed sensitivities in the lower nasal quadrant were characteristic for the former group.

INTRODUCTION

Alternating hyperphoria or dissociated vertical deviation may be defined as the clinical condition in which, by interrupting fusion by means of a screen, the occluded eye is noticeably deviated upwards (with excycloduction). It can occur as an isolated clinical phenomenon, but in a more or less complete dissociated vertical deviation syndrome, it is often associated with squint (esotropia or exotropia), with (usually latent) nystagmus, with anomalies of binocular vision, and with torticollis towards the shoulder on the side of the fixating eye.

Although alternating hyperphoria is frequent its mechanism is still debated. Some authors think that the condition is merely due to some neurological or muscular anomaly such as supranuclear anomaly (1, 5, 10), disturbance in the innervation of the oblique muscles (9), change in extraocular muscle tonus (7) or paresis of depressor muscles (8). Others think that the muscular imbalance could be owed to some sensory factor. Chavasse and Worth (2) considered the upwards movement of the occluded eye as a return to a complete rest position, due to an insufficient retinal stimulation. Extending Keiner's (6) theory on esotropia, Crone (3) assumed that alternating hyperphoria could be explained by the hypothesis that the motor impulses from the lower nasal quadrant are deficient.

Accordingly it was interesting to verify if the presumed oculomotor inferiority of the nasal inferior quadrant could be proved simply by comparing its threshold sensitivities to that of the other quadrants.

Greve, E. L., Heijl, A. (eds.) Fifth International Visual Field Symposium.
©1983 Dr W. Junk Publishers, The Hague/Boston/Lancaster.

SUBJECTS AND METHODS OF EXAMINATION

We examined a) 14 subjects presenting a more or less complete dissociated vertical deviation syndrome (6 males and 8 females of ages ranging between 12 and 35 years, mean 18.6 years, the visual acuity of all examined eyes was $\geqslant 0.8$); b) 12 normal controls (4 males and 8 females of ages ranging between 15 and 24 years, mean 19.1 years, the visual acuity of all examined eyes was $\geqslant 0.9$). Correction was worn during the experiment if it improved visual acuity.

We performed, in monocular vision, profile static sensitivity measurements along the two principal oblique meridians ($225°-45°$ and $315-135°$) in one eye of each of these subjects using the $30'$ white target of the Tübingen perimeter and the fixation device consisting of 4 red points. Each threshold value was determined from 3 measurements and these were made from $30°$ eccentricity on one side through the fixation point to $30°$ eccentricity at the other side at each 2 or $3°$. In order to avoid local adaptation the examination was frequently interrupted while the patient was asked to close his eye for a few seconds.

A first series of measurements was made at a photopic background luminance of 3.18 cd.m^{-2} (nominally 10 asb), a second one at a mesopic background luminance of 0.0764 cd.m^{-1} (0.24 asb), and a third one at a scotopic backgound luminance of 0.00637 cd.m^{-2} (0.02 asb). Between series the patient rested during 20 min adapting his eye to the lower background luminance.

RESULTS

For each of the two groups of eyes we calculated for given eccentricities in the visual field the arithmetical mean of the thresholds in $\log_{10}$ cd.m^{-2} and the corresponding standard deviation. We also calculated, by means of Student's t test, the significance of the difference between each pair of means.

All these results are presented in Fig. 1. This shows very clearly that, as expected, the group of hyperphoric eyes is less sensitive than the control group in the nasal inferior quadrant, although sensitivities of the pathologic group are normal or even better than normal in other sectors. As a consequence, the temporal superior—nasal inferior profile is asymmetrical in the hyperphoric eye, while it is symmetrical in the normal eye. The relative defect increases markedly towards the periphery, where the significance of the difference from the normal mean is very high ($p < 0.001$) at all three levels of adaptation. However, the relative defect is most obvious with the mesopic background luminance.

Some other significant differences seem to indicate a reduced mean sensitivity of the hyperphoric eyes in the nasal superior quadrant during photopic conditions and, on the contrary, a greater mean sensitivity of the hyperphoric eyes in the temporal superior quandrant in photopic conditions and in the temporal inferior quadrant in mesopic conditions. The significance level of such differences compared to the normal mean is never high ($p < 0.01$).

430

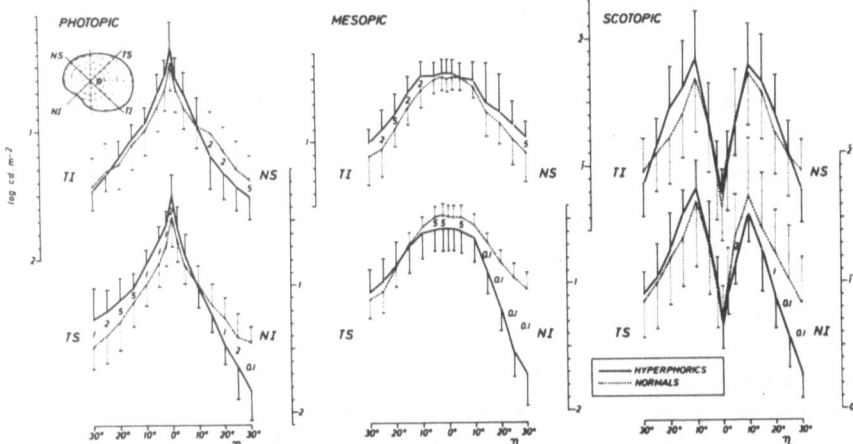

Fig. 1. Mean log relative increment sensitivities and standard deviations for a 30' white target along the two principal oblique meridians and for three background luminances (photopic: 3.18 cd.m^{-2}; mesopic: 0.0764 cd.m^{-2}; scotopic: 0.00637 cd.m^{-2}) in a group of 14 eyes suffering from alternating hyperphoria and in a group of 12 normal control eyes. The significances of the differences between the pairs of means is indicated by numerals (no figure: $p > 0.05$; 5: $0.05 > p > 0.02$; 2: $0.02 > p > 0.01$; 1: $0.01 > p > 0.001$; 0.1: $0.001 > p$).

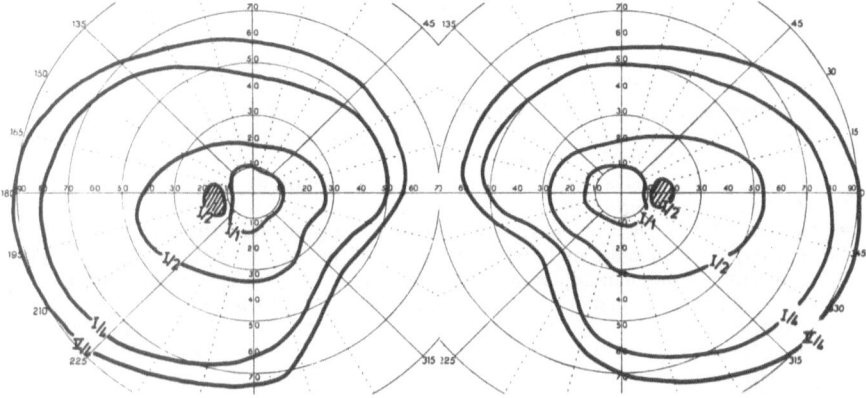

Fig. 2. Result of standard kinetic photopic visual field measurement by means of the Goldmann perimeter in a 12-year old girl suffering from alternating hyperphoria.

DISCUSSION

Our experiment demonstrates very clearly a relative sensitivity defect in the nasal inferior quadrant of the hyperphoric eyes and shows that mesopic static perimetry is the most useful method to demonstrate such a defect (because of a weaker gradient). Standard photopic kinetic perimetry, performed in 2 cases, confirms that the sensitivity decrement exists in both eyes and is greater peripherally. Moreover it discloses that it is greatest along

431

the principal oblique meridian bisecting the right angle between the horizontal and vertical meridians (Fig. 2).

The shown sensitivity loss is a proof of Crone's hypothesis according to which alternating hyperphoria is due to a deficiency of the motor impulses from the nasal inferior quadrant (3).

More precisely, such a defect causes dorsumduction, incycloduction and adduction of the fixating eye. In order for this eye not to perform the corresponding movement but maintain fixation it is necessary that the supranuclear centers send a supplementary impulse to the elevators. Even if the synergism-antagonism scheme of Hering's law is possibly weakened in alternating hyperphoria, it can be assumed that the supplementary rising impulse is also sent to the covered eye and that this actually rises because of the lack of fusion.

In fact, Crone postulated only an abnormality in the afferent way of the oculomotor impulses (3) and did not expect a nasal inferior perimetric sensitivity defect (4). It has also to be mentioned that the role of retinal stimulation is confirmed by the Bielschowsky phenomenon, in which the non-fixating eye deviates downwards (even to below the horizontal) when a neutral filter is placed in front of the fixing eye.

The mild abnormalities stated along other meridians are not convincing because of the lower significance of the differences with the control group and especially because they were not present at all three adaptation levels. Enhanced sensitivity could be due to weaker inhibition.

REFERENCES

1. Bielschowsky, A. Ueber angeborene und erworbene Blickfelderweiterungen. Ber. Dtsch. Ophthalmol. Ges. 37:192–197 (1911).
2. Chavasse, B. and Worth, C. Squint, 7th ed. Blackston, Philadelphia (1939).
3. Crone, R. A. Alternating hyperphoria. Br. J. Ophthalmol. 38:591–604 (1954).
4. Crone, R. A. Personal communication (1982).
5. Hugonnier, R. and Hugonnier, S. Strabisme, hétérophories, paralysies oculomotrices, 4th ed. Masson, Paris (1981).
6. Keiner, G. B. J. New viewpoints on the origin of squint. Nijhoff, The Hague (1951).
7. Posner, A. Noncomitant hyperphorias, considered as aberrations of the postural tonus of the muscular apparatus. Am. J. Ophthalmol. 27:1275–1279 (1944).
8. Scobee, R. G. The oculorotary muscles, 2nd ed. C. V. Mosby, St. Louis (1952).
9. Verhoeff, F. H. Occlusion hypertropia. Arch. Ophthalmol. 25:780–795 (1941).
10. Von Noorden, G. K. In: Burian H. and Von Noorden, G. K., Binocular Vision and Ocular Motility, 2nd ed. C. V. Mosby, St. Louis (1980).

Authors' addresses:
R. Fusco and M. d'Aietti
Cattedra di Ottica Fisiologica
IIa Facultà di Medicina e Chirurgia,
Università degli Studi,
Nuovo Policlinico,
Cappella dei Cangiani, I-80131 Naples
Italy

Dr G. Verriest
Oogheelkunde
Akademisch Ziekenhuis
De Pintelaan 185
B-9000 Ghent
Belgium

TEMPORAL RESOLUTION IN THE PERIPHERAL VISUAL FIELD

PATRICE M. DUNN and ROBERT W. MASSOF

(Baltimore, Maryland, U.S.A.)

Key words. Flicker perimetry, temporal summation, temporal contrast sensitivity.

ABSTRACT

Despite considerable interest in the development of flicker perimetry, little work has been reported on the basic temporal response characteristics of vision across the normal visual field. Those few studies that have addressed this problem have been restricted to the determination of the critical duration for Bloch's law of complete temporal summation or to the determination of critical flicker fusion frequency. In the present study, the entire temporal summation and temporal contrast sensitivity (TCS) functions were determined at the fovea and at 10, 20, 40 and 50 degrees in the temporal field. A single-channel Maxwellian-view optical system was used which allowed exact superposition of stimulus and adaptation fields, each of which subtended 5.15° of visual angle. Temporal summation functions (Experiment I) were obtained by pulsing square-wave stimuli upon the adaptation field of 500 trolands, for durations from 1 to 999 msec. TCS functions (Experiment II) were obtained by sinusoidal modulation about a mean luminance of 500 trolands, at frequencies from 0.5 to 50 Hz. In both experiments an ascending method of limits was used, with stimulus luminance (Experiment I) or sine-wave amplitude (Experiment II) increased until a threshold response was obtained. Data were obtained from 3 normal observers. The results indicated that neither temporal summation nor TCS functions changed with eccentricity.

INTRODUCTION

Flicker perimetry has been advocated as a clinical tool for the investigation of ocular pathologies (10). Foveal, and in some cases peripheral abnormalities of the temporal contrast sensitivity (TCS) function have been reported in amblyopia (22), rod monochromacy (19), ocular hypertension (21), and retinitis pigmentosa (8, 13). However, little work has been reported on the normal temporal response characteristics of vision as a function of eccentricity.

Greve, E. L., Heijl, A. (eds.) Fifth International Visual Field Symposium.
©1983 Dr W. Junk Publishers, The Hague/Boston/Lancaster.

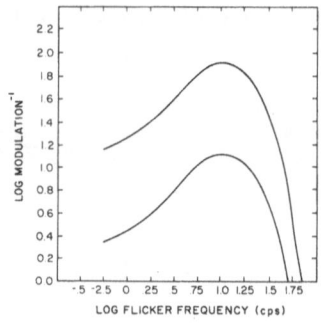

Fig. 1. A constant sensitivity loss at all temporal frequencies would simply translate the temporal contrast sensitivity function down on the ordinate, with no change in the shape of the function. Because contrast physically cannot exceed a value of 1.0 (0.0 log modulation), the effect of vertically translating the curve is to change the cut-off frequency (i.e. the frequency requiring 0.0 log modulation for flicker detection). The cut-off frequency corresponds to the traditionally measured critical flicker fusion frequency, i.e. CFF. Thus, among other explanations, a change in CFF with eccentricity could reflect the change in sensitivity with eccentricity.

While it is clearly important to understand temporal summation and temporal resolution across the visual field, certain aspects of earlier studies have led to some confusion.

A relationship between critical duration (T_c) for complete temporal summation and critical flicker fusion frequency (CFF) has been described by a number of investigators (14—18). However, interpretation of this relationship is confounded by the fact that CFF depends on both stimulus size (Granit-Harper Law) and adaptation luminance (Ferry-Porter Law) (12), as does T_c (1, 3). Changes in the value of CFF or T_c may therefore reflect changes in retinal sensitivity or spatial processing rather than reflecting changes in temporal processing *per se*. Since the CFF and T_c represent cut-off points on the TCS and temporal summation functions respectively, a change of luminance or spatial parameters — which would produce a vertical shift of the function — would in the case of the TCS function yield a change in CFF, reflecting a shift in sensitivity rather than reflecting a change in the temporal response (Fig. 1). Such confounding effects of spatial and luminance parameters are responsible for some of the discrepancies between the CFF literature and the complete TCS functions as determined by De Lange (4, 5, 6) and others.

Both temporal summation and temporal contrast sensitivity are determined by the impulse response function, assuming linear behavior of the visual system (2, 12, 17); derivation of these functions and the relationship between them have been formally discussed elsewhere (2). Both the temporal summation and the TCS functions are therefore expected to bear the same relationship to eccentricity. Ronchi and Molesini (16) showed that the impulse response function, as reflected in the TCS function, did not change with eccentricity over a range of luminances from 0.5 to 500 cd.m^{-2}. These authors further demonstrated that interpretation of the behavior of temporal summation with respect to eccentricity, based on T_c, can vary depending on how T_c is defined. This further emphasizes the need for the determination of the entire temporal summation function.

A study of the visual temporal response characteristics across the visual field should involve determination of the entire temporal summation and TCS functions, rather than the cut-off values — i.e. T_c and CFF — to provide a complete description of the impulse response function. The confounding effects of borders can be avoided by the use of spatially-contiguous stimulus and adaptation fields. Finally, since spatial resolution is known to change with eccentricity (11), the stimulus size chosen should be large enough to avoid confounding spatial summation effects at the adaptation luminance used. The present study was designed according to those requirements to yield temporal summation and TCS functions across the temporal visual field for three normal observers.

METHOD

A single-channel Maxwellian-view optical system was used for both experiments; a light-emitting diode (LED) with peak output at 575 nm and half-band width of 50 nm provided both stimulus and adaptation fields. The image which represented both stimulus and adaptation field subtended 5.15° of visual angle. Stimulation of various retinal locations was achieved by rotating the observer while maintaining Maxwellian view; measurements were made at the fovea and 10, 20, 40 and 50° on the temporal field meridian. For the determination of the temporal summation functions (Experiment I), the LED provided a continuous adaptation luminance (L) of 500 photopic trolands, upon which square-wave stimuli of variable luminance ΔL were superimposed by pulsing the LED output from L to $L + \Delta L$ for a duration t. At 13 values of t from 1 to 999 msec. the threshold value of ΔL required for stimulus detection was determined using an ascending method of limits. At each location 5 measurements were made for each duration t. In Experiment II the TCS functions were obtained by modulating the LED output sinusoidally about a mean luminance (L) of 500 photopic trolands and determining the percent modulation required for detection of flicker at 14 frequencies from 0.5 to 50 Hz. An ascending method of limits was again used, and 5 measurements during each of 4 trials were obtained at each field location. Thus in both experiments the same adaptation luminance, field locations, and stimulus and adaptation size and spectral distribution were used. No spatial or border cues were available to the observer, so that responses were dependent only on temporal changes in the stimulus. The left eyes of 3 ophthalmologically-normal observers, aged 17, 29 and 33 years, were assessed, The relatively large size of the stimulus made it unnecessary to correct for refractive error (11, 20).

RESULTS

Data for 2 of the 3 observers are presented here; those obtained for the 3rd observer, while showing the same effects as those presented, were incomplete.

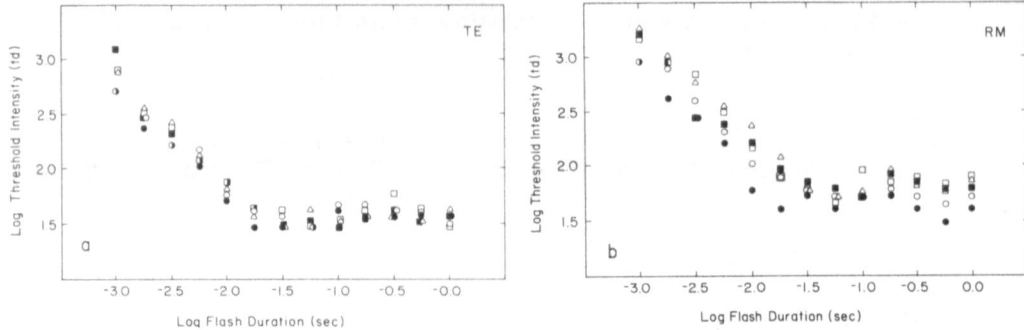

Fig. 2. Temporal summation functions for observers TE (a) and RM (b) plotted as log threshold intensity (trolands) as a function of log flash duration. Each symbol represents the mean values for different positions along the horizontal temporal meridian of the visual field: fovea (filled circles), 10° (open circles), 20° (open squares), 40° (filled squares), and 50° (open triangles). None of the data have been translated along the ordinate.

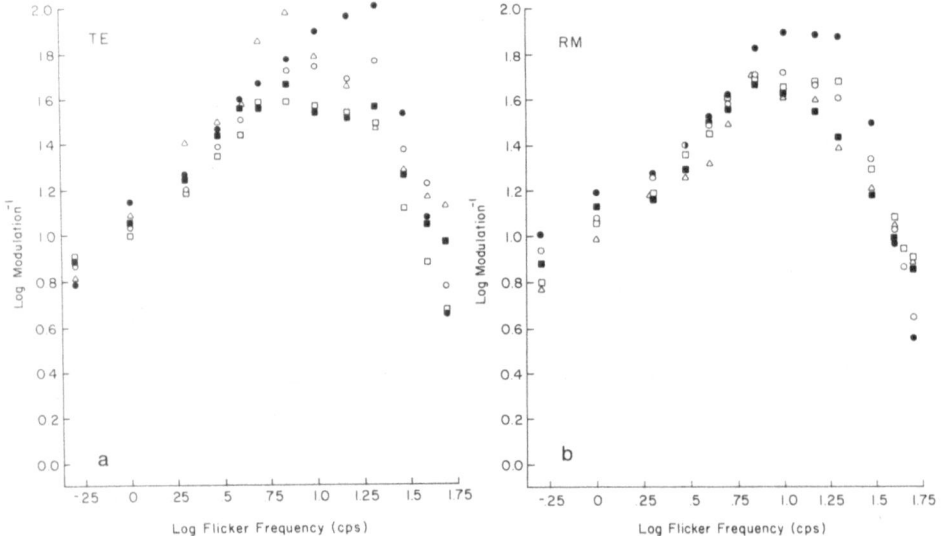

Fig. 3. Temporal contrast sensitivity functions for observers TE (a) and RM (b) plotted as log reciprocal modulation (sensitivity) as a function of log flicker frequency. The interpretation of the symbols is the same as that for Fig. 2. None of the data have been translated along the ordinate.

Temporal summation functions obtained at all 5 field locations are plotted together for each observer in Fig. 2 (a and b). The temporal summation functions for different eccentricities are superimposable without either vertical or horizontal translations, and they show no departures at any eccentricity from the basic form of the function. The lack of a vertical shift, implying constancy of the Weber fraction across the visual field tested, may be attributed to the large stimulus size; the peripheral increase in this fraction decreases as stimulus size increases (7, 9). The lack of a horizontal shift in the function with eccentricity corresponds to a constancy of the critical duration T_c, and

436

implies more generally that under the present conditions temporal summation does not vary with eccentricity.

TCS functions obtained at all 5 field locations are plotted together for each observer in Fig. 3 (a and b). Plotted values represent the means of 5 medians obtained from 5 trials at the given temporal frequency and visual field location. The TCS functions are basically the same shape and at the same level for all eccentricities, although there is some suggestion of a possible discrepancy between the central and eccentric TCS functions, especially at the higher frequencies. To the extent that these TCS functions are similar, they indicate that under the conditions of the present study temporal resolution does not vary with eccentricity.

DISCUSSION

The results of the present study indicate that neither the temporal summation function nor the temporal contrast sensitivity function varies with visual field location. Determinations of the entire functions, as opposed to the cut-off values T_c and CFF, provide more complete descriptions of the temporal response characteristics of the visual system. The finding that both functions bear the same relationship to eccentricity was predicted from the fact that both derive from the impulse response function; their invariance across the visual field, in agreement with Ronchi and Molesini's data (16), suggest that under the conditions of the present study the impluse response function itself does not change with retinal locale. This finding is at variance with that of Tyler (21), who found that the normal TCS function obtained at the fovea differed from that obtained peripherally ($20°$ superior-temporal). Tyler's stimulus, although of similar subtense to ours, was surrounded by a dark border and his adaptation luminance was lower ($40\,cd.m^{-2}$); further, there was no control for pupil size in his study. Whether these methodological differences can account for the discrepancy between the 2 sets of data is unclear. It is interesting to note that although his data for normals clearly differ between the fovea and the periphery, for the ocular hypertensives the central and peripheral data can be superimposed by shifting the curves vertically, thus indicating only a change in sensitivity rather than in temporal processing.

In conclusion, the present study has demonstrated that the impulse response function of the visual system, as reflected in both the temporal summation and temporal contrast sensitivity fucntions, does not vary across the normal visual field. These derived functions provide a more complete description of the temporal aspects of the normal visual system than do the cut-off values of these functions — critical duration or CFF — which have traditionally been reported.

ACKNOWLEDGEMENT

This study was supported by a research grant from the National Eye Institute (EY-02952).

437

REFERENCES

1. Baumgardt, E. Threshold quantal problems. In: D. Jameson and L. M. Hurvich (eds.), Visual Psychophysics, Vol. VII/4, Handbook of Sensory Physiology. New York, Springer-Verlag (1972).
2. Bird, J. F. and Massof, R. W. A general zone theory of color and brightness vision. II. The space—time field. J.O.S.A. 68:1471—1481 (1978).
3. Dannheim, F. and Drance, S. M. Studies of temporal summation of central retinal areas in normal people of all ages. Ophthalmol. Res. 2:295—303 (1971).
4. DeLange, H. Relationship between critical flicker frequency and a set of low-frequency characteristics of the eye. J.O.S.A. 44:380—389 (1954).
5. DeLange, H. Attenuation characteristics and phase-shift characteristics of the human fovea-cortex systems in relation to flicker fusion phenomena. Doctoral Dissertation, Technical University, Delft (1957).
6. DeLange, H. Research into the dynamic nature of the human fovea-cortex system with intermittent and modulated light II. Phase shift in brightness and delay in color perception. J.O.S.A. 48:784—789 (1958).
7. Dunn, P. M. and Lakowski, R. Fully-photopic and -scotopic spatial summation in chromatic perimetry. Doc. Ophthalmol. Proc. Series 26:199—205 (1981).
8. Ernst, W., Clover, G. and Faulkner, D. J. X-linked retinitis pigmentosa: reduced rod flicker sensitivity in heterogenous fundus. Invest. Ophthalmol. & Vis. Sci. 20:812—816 (1981).
9. Fankhauser, F. and Schmidt, T. Die Untersuchung der raumlichen Summation mit stehender und bewegter Reismarke nach der Methode der quantitativen Lichtsinn-perimetrie. Ophthalmologica 135:660—666 (1958).
10. Harrington, D. O. The visual fields: a textbook and atlas of clinical perimetry, pp. 53—55. C. V. Mosby, St. Louis (1981).
11. Johnson, M. A. Spatial properties of chromatic mechanisms in the peripheral retina. Thesis, Johns Hopkins University (1982).
12. Kelly, D. H., Jameson, D. and Hurvich, L. M. (eds.), Visual Psychophysics, Vol. VII/4, Handbook of Sensory Physiology. New York, Springer-Verlag (1972).
13. Massof, R. W., Fitzke, F. W. and Finkelstein, D. Foveal temporal resolution in retinitis pigmentosa. (Abstr.) Invest. Ophthalmol. & Vis. Sci., Suppl. 210 (1980).
14. Matin, L. Critical duration, the differential luminance threshold, critical flicker frequency and visual adaptation: a theoretical treatment. J.O.S.A. 58:404—415 (1968).
15. Pieron, H. Vision in intermittent light. In: Neff, W. D. (ed.), Contributions to Sensory Psychology, Vol. I. Academic Press, New York (1965).
16. Ronchi, L. and Molesini, G. Time resolution at extremely low scotopic luminances. J.O.S.A. 64: 887—889 (1974).
17. Roufs, J. A. J. Dynamic properties of vision I. Experimental relationship between flicker and flash thresholds. Vis. Res. 12:261—278 (1972).
18. Roufs, J. A. J. Dynamic properties of vision II. Theoretical relationships between flicker and flash thresholds. Vis. Res. 22:279—292 (1972).
19. Skottun, B. C., Nordby, K. and Rosness, R. Temporal summation in a rod mono-chromat. Vis. Res. 22:491—493 (1982).
20. Sloan, L. L. Area and luminance of test object as variables in the examination of the visual field by projection perimetry. Vis. Res. 1:121—138 (1961).
21. Tyler, C. Flicker sensitivity losses in glaucoma. Invest. Ophthalmol. & Vis. Sci. 20: 204—121 (1981).
22. Wesson, M. D. and Loop, M. S. Temporal contrast sensitivity in amblyopia. Invest. Ophthalmol. & Vis. Sci. 22:98—102 (1982).

Authors' address:
Wilmer Ophthalmological Institute
The Johns Hopkins University School of Medicine
Baltimore, MD 21205
U.S.A.

TEMPORAL RESOLUTION AND STIMULUS INTENSITY IN THE CENTRAL VISUAL FIELD

P. ROSSI*, G. CIURLO, C. BURTOLO and G. CALABRIA

(Genoa, Italy)

Key words. Flicker fusion, temporal resolution.

ABSTRACT

The authors have investigated the relationship between stimulus luminance and FFF in the central visual field. A logarithmic relationship was found.

INTRODUCTION

Flicker fusion frequencies (FFF) are strictly related to the visual field area tested and to the photometrical features of the stimulus.

This work is intended to report the standards of FFF within the central visual field and to discuss the changes of FFF caused by increasing test luminances.

MATERIAL AND METHODS

Three normal emmetropic individuals were studied. The threshold luminances for targets of 1/4 and 4 mm diameter were measured at the fixation point and at 5° and 10° nasally.

The threshold luminances were increased by 0.4 log units, as described in a previous paper (2), and FFF's were tested using a rotating sector device mounted on a Goldmann perimeter (1).

A descending technique was used, each measurement being repeated 8 times. The target luminance was then progressively increased in 0.3 log unit steps and the corresponding FFF's assessed as above.

The mean value and the standard deviation of each set of measurements were calculated. The correlation coefficient between series of FFF's corresponding to increasing levels of luminance was calculated to compare the FFF increase rate with the size or location of the target.

*To whom requests for offprints should be addressed.

Greve, E. L., Heijl, A. (eds.) Fifth International Visual Field Symposium.
©1983 Dr W. Junk Publishers, The Hague/Boston/Lancaster.

Tables 1–3. Mean and standard deviation of FFF in different visual field areas (target diameter 1/4 mm; values within brackets, target diameter 4 mm).

Patient 1

	0	5°	10°
Threshold	5.6 ± 2.07 (18.25 ± 0.5)	7.25 ± 0.5 (18.75 ± 0.75)	10.25 ± 0.5 (20.75 ± 0.5)
Threshold + 0.3 l.u.	11 ± 0.81) (21 ± 0.81)	17 ± 0.81 (22.25 ± 0.5)	12.25 ± 1.25 (25.75 ± 0.5)
Threshold + 0.6 l.u.	17.5 ± 0.57 (24.6 ± 0.54)	19.25 ± 0.95 (26.75 ± 0.5)	18.33 ± 0.57 (26.75 ± 0.57)
Threshold + 0.9 l.u.	20.25 ± 0.5 (26.25 ± 2.83)	20.75 ± 0.5 (30.25 ± 0.5)	22.5 ± 1 (30.25 ± 0.5)

Patient 2

	0	5°	10°
Threshold	18.5 ± 3.69 (20.25 ± 0.95)	18.5 ± 0.81 (21 ± 0.81)	16.75 ± 0.95 (22 ± 0.81)
Threshold + 0.3 l.u.	23.75 ± 0.95 (24 ± 1.38)	22.25 ± 0.95 (23 ± 0.81)	17.5 ± 1 (24.75 ± 0.5)
Threshold + 0.6 l.u.	25.5 ± 0.57 (26.5 ± 2.38)	24 ± 0.81 (25 ± 0.81)	22.75 ± 0.95 (26 ± 3.36)
Threshold + 0.9 l.u.	27.5 ± 0.57 (31.25 ± 0.95)	25.5 ± 3.69 (26.5 ± 0.95)	25.25 ± 2.87 (27.5 ± 3.10)

Patient 3

	0	5°	10°
Threshold	8.5 ± 1.29 (17 ± 0.81)	8.33 ± 0.57 (18 ± 0.81)	10 ± 0.82 (16.25 ± 0.5)
Threshold + 0.3 l.u.	13 ± 0.81 (17.75 ± 0.5)	10.5 ± 0.57 (21 ± 0.5)	10.25 ± 0.5 (20 ± 0.81)
Threshold + 0.6 l.u.	16.25 ± 0.5 (20.2 ± 1.09)	14.25 ± 0.5 (23 ± 0.81)	12.25 ± 1.25 (21 ± 0.81)
Threshold + 0.9 l.u.	18.5 ± 0.57 (27 ± 1.41)	16.25 ± 0.5 (25 ± 0.5)	18.25 ± 1.25 (22.5 ± 0.57)

RESULTS

Tables 1 to 3 show the mean values and the standard deviation of FFF measurements at different levels of luminance in three patients.

In each patient, the correlation coefficients between sets of measurements with different target sizes or visual field area were never lower than 0.85; the great majority ranging between 0.95 and 0.98.

COMMENT

The previous measurements allow the following considerations:

1. Flicker perimetry using threshold stimuli and a descending technique is a very reliable method.
2. FFF's do not change significantly when threshold stimuli of the same size are used to test different areas of the central visual field.
3. Threshold stimuli are fused at frequencies that widely vary among different individuals.
4. FFF's directly increase with target luminance: the photometric standards of the Goldmann perimeter fall into the first, straight part of the Ferry-Porter diagram, where a logarithmic relationship is found between FFF's and target luminance.
5. The previous relationships hold both when targets of different sizes are presented in the same area of the visual field and when the same target is presented in different areas of the central visual field.

CONCLUSIONS

The previous investigation suggests that the relationship between FFF's and target luminance within the central visual field is a steady logarithmic one, and that it does not change with either target size or location.

REFERENCES

1. Ciurlo, G., Rossi, P. and Suetta, G. Nuovo apparecchio per la flicker-perimetria. Min. Oftal. 20:61–68 (1978).
2. Zingirian, M., Ciurlo, G., Rossi, P. and Burtolo, C. Flicker fusion and spatial summation. Doc. Ophthalmol. Proc. Series 26:127–130 (1981).

Author's address:
Dr. P. Rossi
University Eye Clinic
Viale Benedetto XV, 5
16132 Genoa
Italy

DIABETIC RETINOPATHY: PERIMETRIC FINDINGS

E. GANDOLFO, M. ZINGIRIAN, G. CORRALLO and
F. CARDILLO PICCOLINO
(Genoa, Italy)

Key words. Diabetic retinopathy, kinetic perimetry, static perimetry, visual field defects.

ABSTRACT

Perimetry of diabetic retinal lesions permits us to demonstrate interesting and sometimes surprising findings. Retinal hemorrhages generate visual field (VF) defects of not absolute depth. Exudates cause a well-detectable VF defect when they are grouped together in large spots. In this case a relative scotoma is found. Exudative maculopathy generates a 'plateau' in the central sensitivity' so that the defect can be well detected only by static analysis. Only if maculopathy is present for a long time, a central scotoma detectable by kinetic perimetry can arise. Macular cystoid edema generates characteristic local depressions in central static profile. But this finding is temporary because afterwards the function falls in the form of a deep central scotoma. Ischemic areas either peripheral or central cause a fall in the sensitivity of 0.5–1 l.u. in comparison with corresponding well-perfused areas. At the border between normal and ischemic territories the fall in sensitivity is sudden. Usually, dramatic and wide diabetic alterations do not completely destroy retinal function: this fact suggests maximum caution during laser or xenon therapy. Absolute VF defects are present in cases of proliferative retinopathy and when different types of lesions are grouped together in the same area.

INTRODUCTION

The perimetric examination is extremely useful in the functional evaluation of eyes affected by diabetic retinopathy (d.r.) because perimetry supplies precise quantitative information on the damage.

However, the attempts made to follow the development of d.r. with traditional perimetric criteria have often been frustrated by serious difficulties (1–3).

Analyzing the perimetric damage produced by typical d.r. lesions, the reason for the discrepancy that exists between the great analytical power of perimetry and its apparent clinical limitations in the follow-up of d.r. is easily understood. D.r. is characterized, in fact, by the polymorphism of its

Greve, E. L., Heijl, A. (eds.) Fifth International Visual Field Symposium.
©*1983 Dr W. Junk Publishers, The Hague/Boston/Lancaster.*

lesions and this is reflected in perimetric examination results. Besides, the same retinal area is very often the site of lesions of varied nature and seriousness: hemorrhages, exudates, edema, ischemia.

Such a situation makes it difficult to evaluate the origin of visual field damage. In a similar fashion, it is difficult to understand the reason for an eventual variation in perimetric results.

The aim of our research was to individualize the type of perimetric damage derived from singular lesions typical of d.r. in an effort to delineate valid perimetric criteria in the follow-up of patients.

MATERIALS AND METHODS

In order to reach our goal, a large number of subjects with d.r. underwent detailed perimetric examination using a Goldmann apparatus. We centered our attention on those anatomically well-preserved retinal areas in which fairly large lesions, that could cause an appreciable perimetric defect, and also sufficiently isolated lesions to exclude the possible influence of nearby lesions of a different origin, were observed.

An accurate fluorangiographic study allowed us to leave out those cases in which evident ischemia could worsen the perimetric damage due to the lesions studied, and analogously to point out pure ischemic lesions to study their effect on retinal sensitivity, without the aggravating influence of other factors such as hemorrhages, exudates, etc.

A total of 85 eyes affected by d.r. (mostly of simple type or in a pre-proliferative stage) and never treated by laser were examined.

For the most part, the patients were young (max. age 56, min. age 19, average age 37) and cooperative during the perimetric examination.

A fluorangiographic map of the ocular fundus was made for all the patients to show those retinal areas of greatest interest for our research.

All eyes underwent standard kinetic perimetry (4 isopters: 1 peripheral with absolute stimulus, 2 intermediate passing the parallels of 45° and 30° in the temporal field, and 1 central that would exclude the blind spot), followed by a static and kinetic scotometric examination with numerous targets directed towards pre-chosen areas.

RESULTS

Some typical lesions of d.r. are not perimetrically appreciable: microaneurisms, small exudates, pinpoint hemorrhages do not produce noticeable defects. Only if these lesions are close together they can disturb isopteric regularity and produce localized sensitivity reductions detectable by static examination.

Retinal and pre-retinal hemorrhages of a certain size (at least 3—4° in diameter) generate noticeable kinetic defects like isopteric depressions. Static perimetry demonstrates that one is always dealing with relative defects.

Exudates cause perimetric defects evident only when grouped together in large plaques. In such a case the presence of a relative scotoma in which sensitivity decreases from the periphery towards the center is noted.

Exudative maculopathy is accompanied by a reduction in central sensitivity.

444

Such damage can rarely be shown with kinetic perimetry. In these cases static exploration is fundamental: it allows us to profile the sensitivity in the central area that appears lower than normal and irregularly flattened in a more or less saw-tooth-like shape (Figs. 1A, B). Only in some cases where plaques of hard exudates localized in the fovea exist, we can observe a funnel-like depression of central sensitivity and a central scotoma detectable by kinetic perimetry.

In cystoid edema of the macula, static exploration demonstrates at first an irregularity of the pericentral threshold with cuneiform depressions of the profile.

Central sensitivity remains discrete and above all maintains its normal cusp-like shape (Figs. 2A, B). In the more evolved phases of central edema the situation inverts: central sensitivity falls dramatically, the profile shows a deep indentation in the central tract, the defect is easily shown with the scotometric kinetic method.

The ischemic areas in d.r. represent the field of major perimetric interest.

Upon kinetic exploration, the presence of ischemic areas, involving practically all of the retinal periphery, produces a constriction of the external isopter of the visual field that reproduces the morphology of non-perfused territories. The large peripheral ischemic areas are the only hypoxic territories in which absolute damage of retinal sensitivity is noted. Usually the fall in sensitivity is not that serious and is limited to about 1 l.u. with respect to the normal. Sensitivity fall occurs suddenly on passing from perfused to hypoxic zones: normally within the span of $1-3°$ the maximum depression linked to ischemia is reached.

The mid-peripheral ischemic areas cause the onset of an indentation in the intermediate isopters upon kinetic examination of the VF. A detailed scotometric analysis permits delineation of the defect. The morphology of the scotoma follows that of the hypoxic focus shown by fluorangiography. Static examination reveals a sensitivity depression between 0.5 and 1 l.u. with a rather steep gradient in the transition zone between healthy and hypoxic tissue.

Analysis of the central-paracentral ischemic areas is often difficult since one deals with minimally extended lesions. Sometimes small isopteric indentations can be observed. Accurate scotometry can delineate a small relative scotoma when the hypoxic zone has a diameter of at least $3-4°$. The depth of this defect in static examination is about 0.5 l.u. with respect to the surrounding areas. A rather steep gradient is found at the margins.

The perimetric damage provoked by fibro-vascular proliferation remains to be considered. Our attention was limited to proliferation on the retinal plane, since endovitreal invasion causes anomalous perimetric situations that unfavorably influence result reliability. Even with such limitation, perimetry of proliferative lesions is difficult to evaluate and of little significance. Vessel proliferation on the retina produces a sensitivity disturbance proportional to the intensity of hyperpermeability.

The fibrous cords on the retina cause sharper defects that are often absolute.

It should not be forgotten that the defect caused by retinal proliferation almost never reflects the isolated damage of that lesion, because it is often included in a larger and more widespread damage due to ischemia, edema, and metabolic disturbances of the underlying retina.

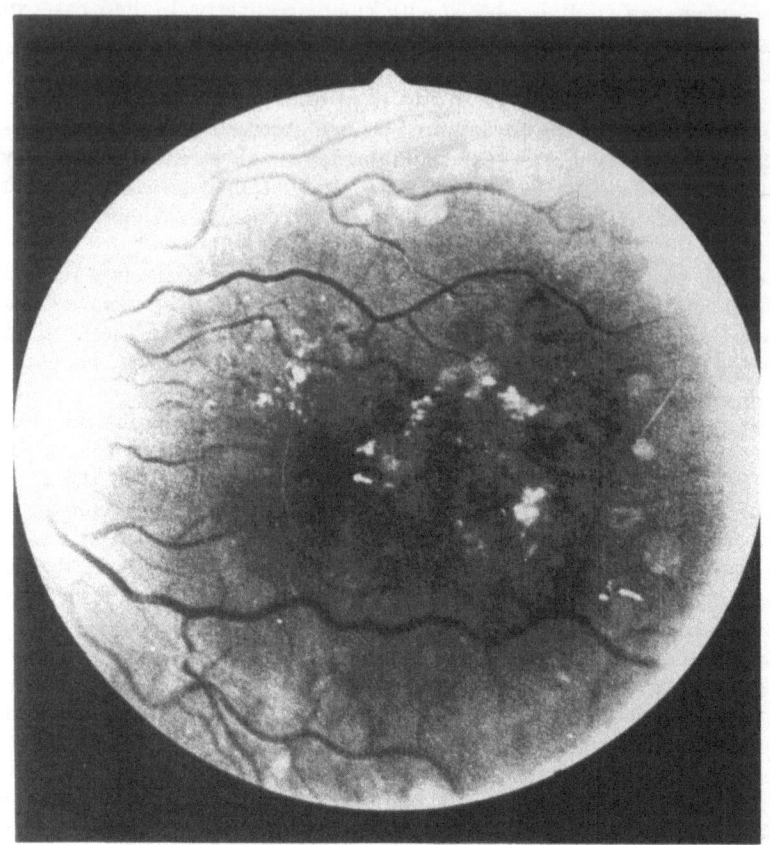

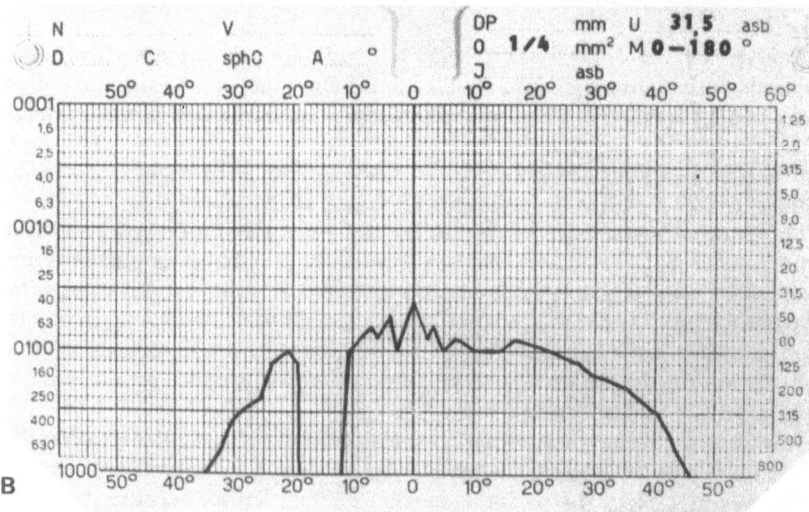

Fig. 1. (A) Exudative maculopathy. (B) Static profile in the illustrated case.

446

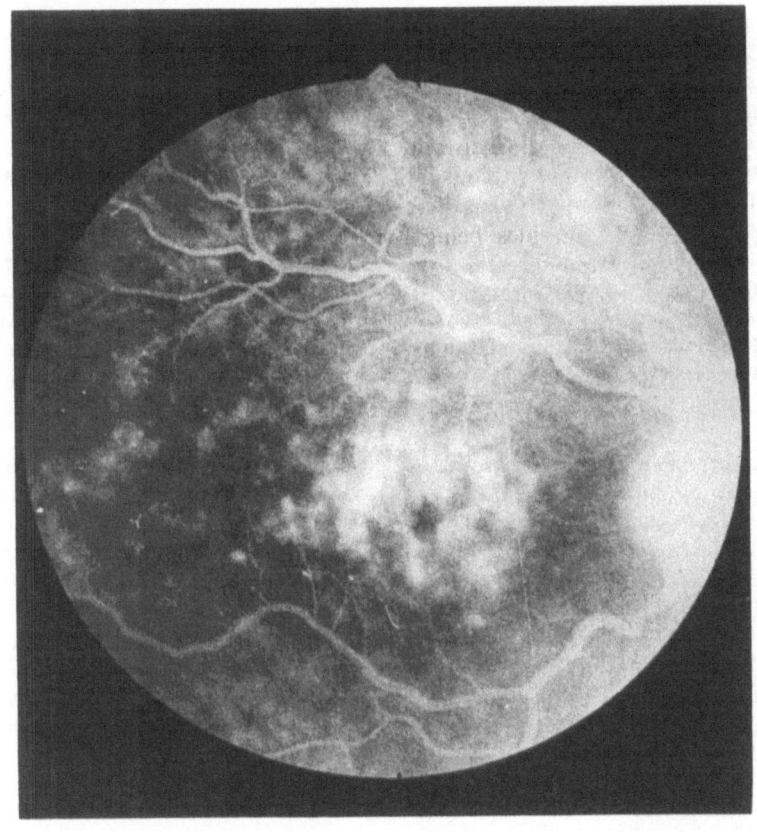

A

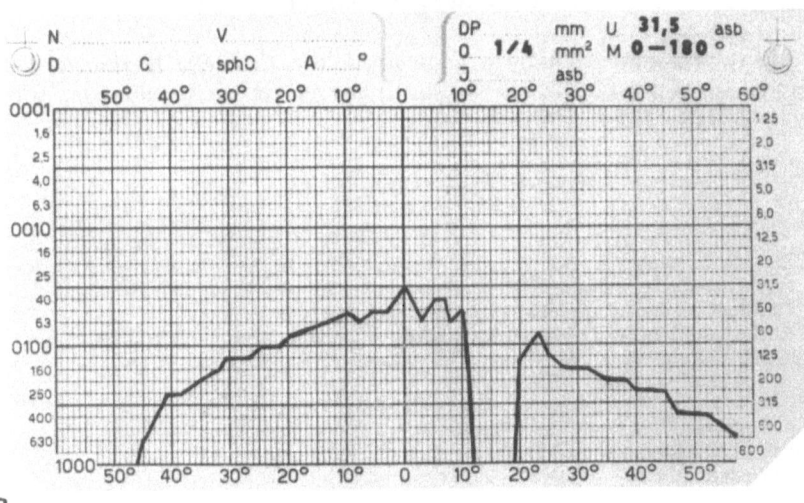

B

Fig. 2. (A) Cystoid edema (fluorangiography). (B) Static profile in the illustrated case.

COMMENT

Perimetry shows that damage provoked by most of the studied lesions is relative and permits the maintaining of discrete residual function. If there is functional exclusion of a retinal territory, it is because processes overlap at a certain point in the same district, or because complications arise, like endovitreal hemorrhage and vitreous-retinal fibrosis.

Therefore perimetry has practical value in the evaluation of only non-proliferative d.r. Besides being limited to non-proliferative d.r., perimetric exploration must be directed towards single retinal territories, angiographically well defined, in which morphological alteration requires functional evaluation.

If the fluorangiographic examination reveals cystoid edema of the macula, it will be the repeated static exploration, more than visus behaviour or the repetition of angiography to give us information on the evoluation of macular damage.

The presence of ischemic areas suggests the possibility of slowing d.r.'s evolution by means of photocoagulation. A good perimetric examination, however, usually tells us that the areas we intend to destroy are not retinal territories already functionally excluded but areas still possessing some sensitivity. This knowledge asks for extreme caution and the need to limit retinal photocoagulation as much as possible.

In those cases in which ischemic damage has produced an absolute defect (one deals for the most part with cases in which there is also an occlusion of a large branch of the central vein of the retina), photocoagulative treatment could be more intense and extend up until the confines of the functionally excluded area shown by perimetric examination.

ACKNOWLEDGEMENT

This study was supported by a grant from the Consiglio Nazionale delle Ricerche, Progetto Finalizzato Medicina Preventiva e Riabilitativa, sotto Progetto Malattie Degenerative, Rome, Italy.

REFERENCES

1. Bloom, A., Heath, A., Kelsey, J. H., Hunger, P. R. and Brigden, W. D. The use of the Roth-Keeler central field scotometer in the study of diabetic retinopathy. Ophthalmol. Res. 3:166 (1972).
2. Roth, J. A. Central visual field in diabetes. Br. J. Ophthalmol. 53:16 (1969).
3. Wisznia, K. I. et al. Visual fields in diabetic retinopathy. Br. J. Ophthalmol. 55: 183—188 (1971).

Authors' address:
University Eye Clinic
Viale Benedetto XV, 5
16132 Genoa
Italy

STATIC PERIMETRY IN CENTRAL SEROUS RETINOCHOROIDOPATHY (MASUDA'S TYPE) USING A FUNDUS PHOTO-PERIMETER

MASAAKI TOMONAGA, TADASHI MIYAMOTO,
HIROTAKA SUZUMURA and YASUO OHTA

(Tokyo, Japan)

Key words. Central serous retinochoroidopathy, fundus photo-perimeter, static color perimetry.

ABSTRACT

We measured the visual field within 16° from the fovea quantitatively and statically in patients with central serous retinochoroidopathy using a fundus photo-perimeter.

Perimetry was performed in two meridians, 45° to 225° and 135° to 315°, at 2° intervals.

The maximum luminance of the stimuli was 271 cd/m² and the background luminance was 0.15 cd/m². The size of the stimuli was 6 minutes. Three different stimuli; white, red (λ max 620 nm) and blue (λ max 450 nm) were used.

We evaluated changes in retinal sensitivity in localized lesions under these circumstances and obtained the following results: a uniform, gentle gradient in the decrease in retinal sensitivities in accordance with the localized lesions was not obtained; rather, there was a scattering in the decrease of retinal sensitivity according to site. This was marked in cases with blue stimuli, and less so with red and white stimuli. Decreased sensitivity was most pronounced in areas with leakage in the fluorescein fundus angiographs.

INTRODUCTION

We measured the central quantitative static visual field with a fundus photo-perimeter to determine changes in the sensitivity of localized lesions in central serous retinochoroidopathy and compared the results with the central visual field of healthy persons and fluorescence fundus photographs.

MATERIALS AND METHODS

We measured the visual field of five eyes of five students with normal visual acuity (> 1.0) and of four eyes in four patients with central serous retino-

Greve, E. L., Heijl, A. (eds.) Fifth International Visual Field Symposium.
©1983 Dr W. Junk Publishers, The Hague/Boston/Lancaster.

450

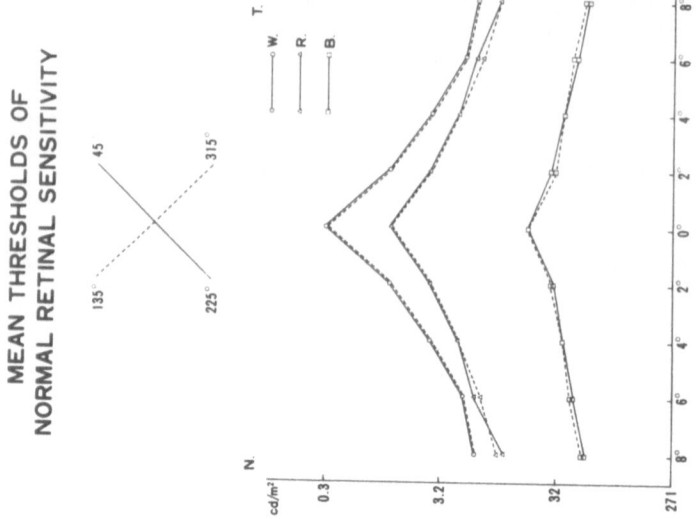

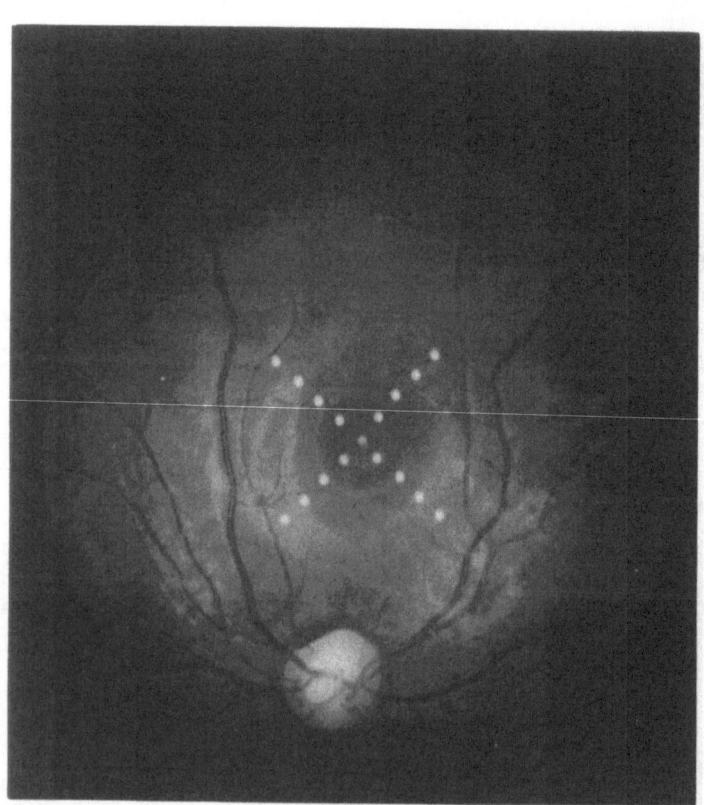

Fig. 1. Left: fundus photograph of a normal eye and detection point; right: normal retinal sensitivity.

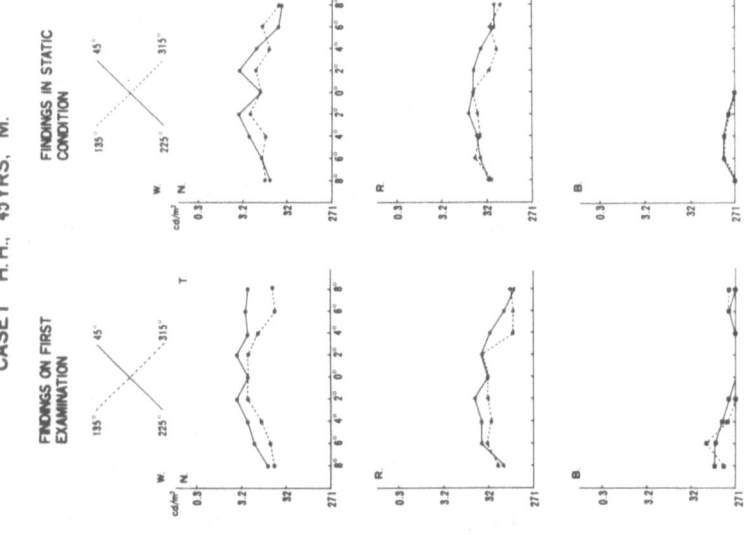

CASE 1   H.H., 45YRS,   M.

FINDINGS ON FIRST
EXAMINATION

FINDINGS IN STATIC
CONDITION

Fig. 2. Fluorescence fundus photograph and results of static perimetry.

451

choroidopathy in the first examination and static condition stages and compared the results. Fluorescein fundus photographs were taken in all the patients and were compared with the visual fields.

The quantitative static visual field was measured with a fundus photoperimeter along two meridians, i.e., 45° through 225° and 135° through 315°, at two-degree intervals within the central 16 degrees of the field in order to determine the field in three dimensions. We used three kinds of stimuli, i.e., white, red (dominant wavelength: 620 nm) and blue (dominant wavelength: 450 nm). The size of the stimuli was 6 minutes. Maximum stimulus luminance was 271 cd/m^2, and background luminance was 0.15 cd/m^2.

RESULTS

The right side of Fig. 1 shows the mean threshold of the retinal sensitivity for each stimulus in five persons with a normal visual acuity of more than 1.0. The solid line in the figure represents the 45°−225° meridian, and the dotted line represents the 135°−315° meridian. The following figures are arranged in the same manner. The sensitivity threshold decreases in the order of white, red, and blue stimuli. The patterns of the sensitivity along the two meridians are almost the same, indicating the island of the central visual field sloping gently upward. The left side of Fig. 1 shows a fundus photograph of a normal eye and the detection points.

Figure 2 shows case No. 1, a 45-year old man. The left is a fluorescence fundus photograph, and the right shows the results of perimetry. The following figures are arranged in the same manner. The fluorescence fundus photograph shows evidence of fluorescein leakage in the temporal area of the fovea.

The results of perimetry at the first examination showed variation in the sensitivity along the meridians 45° through 225° and 135° through 315° and a decrease in the threshold of the foveal sensitivity consistent with retinal edema. In addition, there is a marked decrease in sensitivity toward the fluorescein leakage site. Examination of the visual field in the static stage, when retinal edema was considered to have disappeared ophthalmoscopically, also revealed a decrease in sensitivity toward the fluorescein leakage site and, in particular, a visual field defect in the temporal area for the blue stimulus. In this patient, light coagulation was performed at the site of fluorescein leakage twice, six days and one month after the first examination.

Figure 3 shows case No. 2, a 43-year old man. There is evidence of fluorescein leakage in the superior temporal area of the fovea. The patient recovered after light coagulation but relapsed two months later with evidence of fluorescein leakage in the superior nasal area of the fovea. A second light coagulation procedure was not performed, and the course during drug treatment was observed. There was a decrease in the foveal threshold and a depression in the superior nasal area for the blue stimuli at the first examination. In the static stage, the threshold of foveal sensitivity returned to almost normal for all of the white, red, and blue stimuli, but a depression in the superior nasal area for the blue stimulus was observed.

Case No. 3, shown in Fig. 4, is a 49-year old man showing evidence of

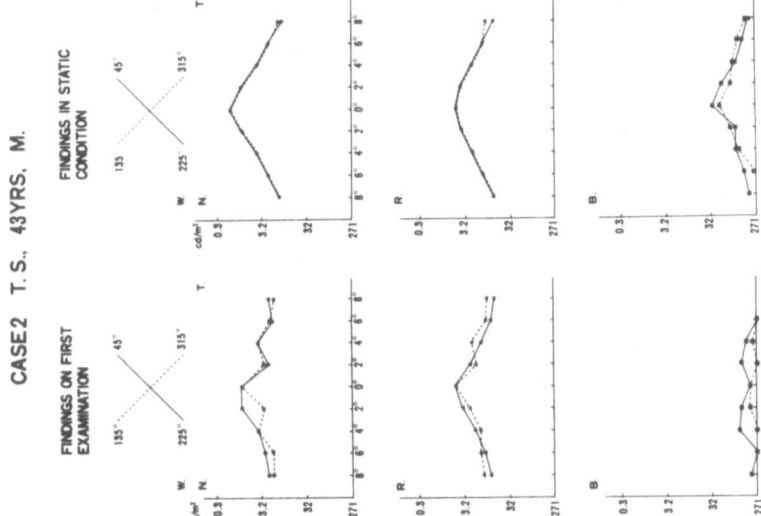

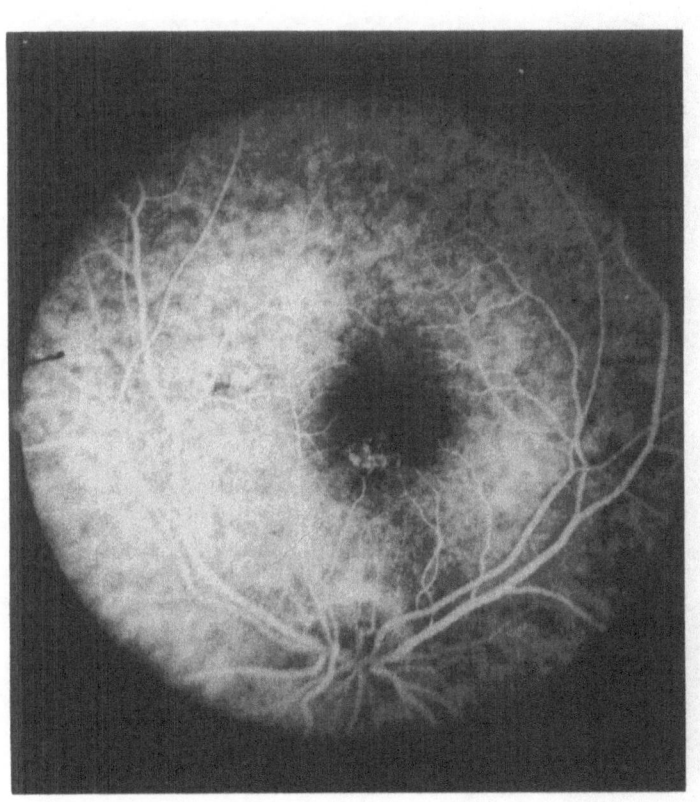

Fig. 3. Fluorescence fundus photograph and results of static perimetry.

453

454

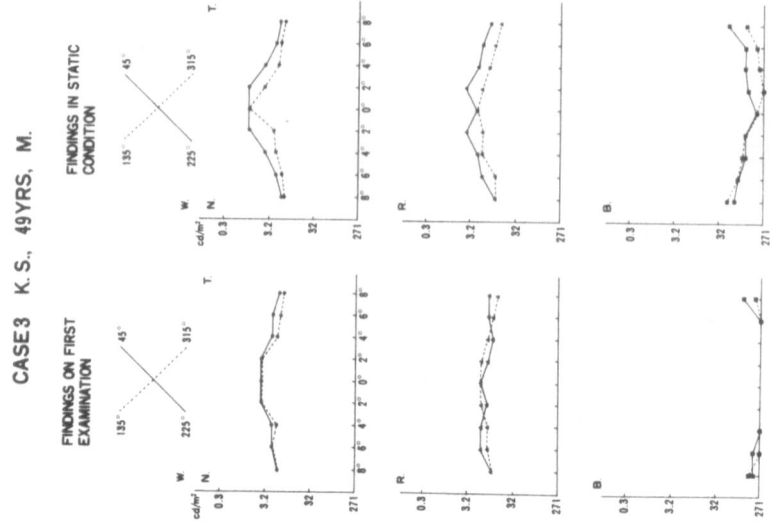

CASE 3   K. S., 49 YRS, M.

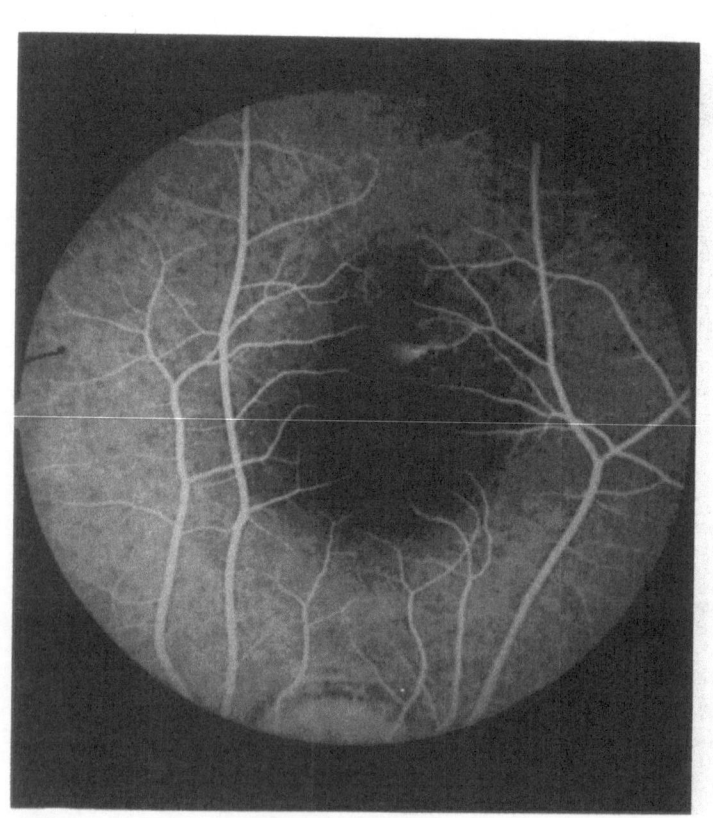

Fig. 4. Fluorescence fundus photograph and results of static perimetry.

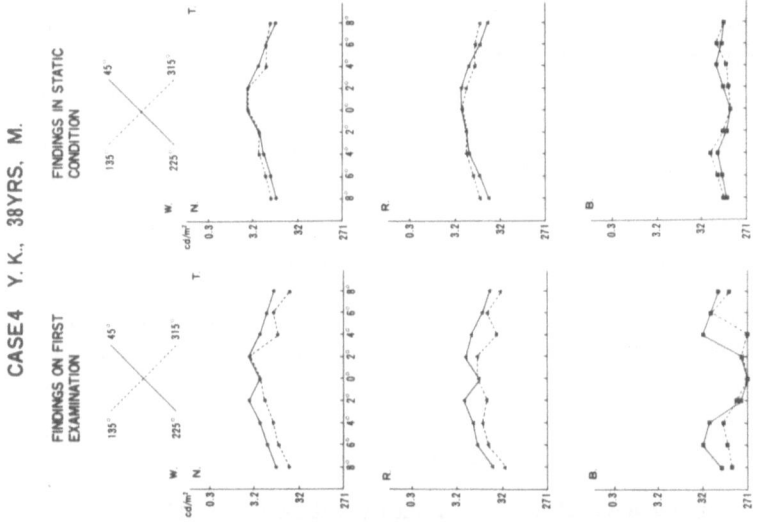

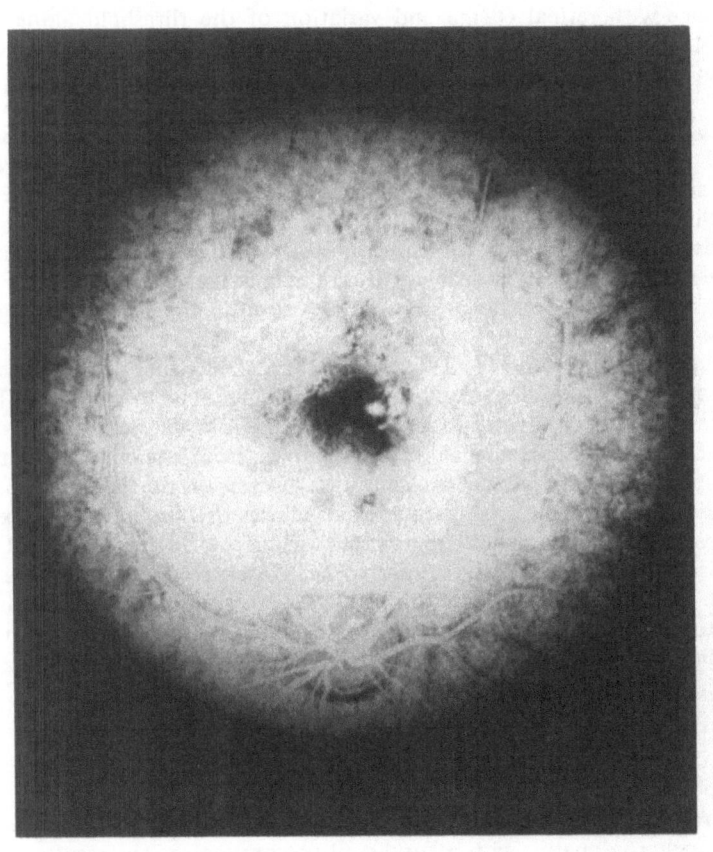

Fig. 5. Fluorescence fundus photograph and results of static perimetry.

455

fluorescein leakage in the inferior temporal part of the fovea. Light coagulation was performed six days after the first examination. A depression within the central four degrees of the field for all stimuli (white, red and blue) was observed at the first examination. The depression for the blue stimulus was particularly marked. In addition, there was a slight depression in the inferior temporal area for all stimuli. In the static stage, a recovery of the depression for each stimulus was observed, but there still remained a depression in the inferior temporal area for blue.

Case No. 4 in Fig. 5 is a 38-year old man showing evidence of fluorescein leakage directly under the fovea. The first examination revealed a marked depression within the central two degrees for all of the stimuli. In the static stage, recovery was observed for white and red stimuli, but the depression for blue stimuli still remained.

DISCUSSION

Cases of central serous retinochoroidopathy within one week from the onset showed a decrease in the retinal sensitivity for the white, red, and blue stimuli in accordance with retinal edema and variation of the threshold along the meridians 45°–225° and 135°–315°. A decrease in the retinal sensitivity was observed in the central part and in the direction corresponding to the site of fluorescein leakage. A decrease in the sensitivity for the blue stimulus was particularly marked. In patients in the static stage, when retinal edema was considered to have disappeared ophthalmoscopically, the course of recovery was unfavorable in regard to the blue stimulus with a remaining decrease in the sensitivity in a direction corresponding with the site of fluorescein leakage, although there was recovery in the threshold of sensitivity for the white and red stimuli. However when the site of fluorescein leakage was very close to the fovea, for example in case 4, only a depression in the sensitivity in the foveal region was observed.

Amsler, Matsuo and Endo (1, 2) reported qualitative visual field studies in central serous retinochoroidopathy using Amsler charts. The present study has significance in quantitatively supporting the qualitative visual field findings.

Ohta (3, 4, 5) has reported that the ability to discriminate color along the blue—yellow axis is markedly decreased in this disease, on the basis of experiments on hue and brightness, and stated that he uses this finding as an auxiliary diagnostic parameter in judging therapeutic effects in this disease. Our findings also show that when the course of the onset, recovery, and cure of this disease and the site of fluorescein leakage were studied from the standpoint of retinal sensitivity, blue stimuli are considered to be the most sensitive for detecting functional disturbances in the central area of the retina and also to be the most suitable for determining prognosis.

CONCLUSION

We measured the central quantitative static visual field in cases of central serous retinochoroidopathy with a fundus photo-perimeter. The results show that the retinal sensitivity does not have a constant gentle slope consistent with retinal edema and that there is variation of the sensitivity along the meridians tested. Blue stimuli are considered to be the most sensitive for detecting functional disturbances in the central area of the retina and to be the most suitable for determining the prognosis of central serous retinochoroidopathy.

REFERENCES

1. Amsler, M. Amsler charts manual — method of using the test charts of qualitative vision. Hamblin Instrument Ltd., London.
2. Matsuo, H. and Endo, N. Early diagnosis in macula diseases. Ophthalmology 10: 702–712 (1968).
3. Ohta, Y. Color confusion of the acquired anomalous color vision — relation between hue and luminosity. Acta Soc. Ophthalmol. Japan 65:1973–1982 (1961).
4. Ohta, Y., Miyamoto, T. and Harasawa, K. Experimental fundus photoperimeter and its application. Doc. Ophthalmol. Proc. Series 19:351–358 (1978).
5. Ohta, Y., Tomonaga, M., Miyamoto, T. and Harasawa, K. Visual field studies with fundus photoperimeter in postchiosmatic lesion. Doc. Ophthalmol. Proc. Series 26:119–126 (1981).

Authors' address:
Dept. of Ophthalmology
Tokyo Medical College Hospital
Kasumigaura Hospital
3920 Ami-cho, Inashiki-gun
Ibaragi-ken, 300-03
Japan

457

BOUNDARY CURVES FOR DIVIDING VISUAL FIELDS INTO SECTORS CORRESPONDING TO A RETINOTOPIC PROJECTION ONTO THE OPTIC DISC

JOHN F. HILLS, JONATHAN D. WIRTSCHAFTER*
and PAUL MAEDER

(Minneapolis, Minnesota, U.S.A.)

Key words. Analytic techniques, glaucoma, optic disc, perimetry.

ABSTRACT

Computer analysis of visual field data obtained from automated perimetry is increasingly employed for the detection of glaucomatous field defects. A family of curves has been calculated which describe the boundaries of arbitrarily defined visual field sectors. These boundaries have been chosen based on descriptions of typical glaucomatous field defects and histological examination of retinal nerve fiber pathways. The boundary curves are calculated by using either straight lines or elliptical and parabolic equations. Automated perimeters produced by various manufacturers or analysis programs developed by different investigators can use these equations to compute and define standardized boundaries. While we hope that other investigators will adopt these curves as a *de facto* standard, these expressions allow considerable flexibility for changing the boundaries to match desired field sectors. Examples of these equations and plots of the boundaries are given for areas of interest previously described. The simple expressions for these curves allow rapid computation of the region into which any visual field data point will fall. The data points may be predefined as in static perimetry or postdefined as in kinetic perimetry. Thus the computer can assign data points to specified areas based only upon x, y coordinates (in degrees) without further intervention by the perimetrist.

Glaucomatous visual field defects have been clinically observed to follow the general distribution of the nerve fibers. Wirtschafter et al. (5) have previously described a method of dividing fields into sectors for analysis and comparison. The current work represents an attempt to produce explicit algebraic formulas for the sector boundaries. Describing the borders in this manner allows simple computer algorithms to determine into which sector any specified point will fall.

Boundaries of the visual field sectors have been characterized using three general classes of curves — straight lines, parabolas, and ellipses. The blind

*To whom requests for offprints should be addressed.

Greve, E. L., Heijl, A. (eds.) Fifth International Visual Field Symposium.
©*1983 Dr W. Junk Publishers, The Hague/Boston/Lancaster.*

spot has been assumed to be centered 1.5 degrees inferior and 15.5 degrees temporal to the point of fixation. The dimensions of the blind spot may be chosen to be rather large, 9 degrees horizontally by 13 degrees vertically to accommodate variability in size and location of the blind spot and variations in fixation. The equation of the ellipse can be explicitly stated:

$$\frac{(Y + 1.5)^2}{(6.5)^2} + \frac{(X - 15.5)^2}{(4.5)^2} = 1.0$$

Or in general terms:

$$\frac{(Y - Y_0)^2}{(a)^2} + \frac{(X - X_0)^2}{(b)^2} = 1.0$$

where (X_0, Y_0) is the center point of the blind spot, a is 1/2 the vertical extent and b is 1/2 the horizontal extent of the blind spot. Solving the equation for Y in terms of X yields:

$$Y = -1.5 \pm 6.5 \sqrt{1 - \left(\frac{X - 15.5}{4.5}\right)^2}$$

This equation can only be solved for X with the range of 11 to 20 degrees. A peripapillary visual field sector can also be defined by using an ellipse of larger dimensions than those assigned for the blind spot. Morin (2) has stressed that enlargement of the blind spot deserves attention in patients with glaucoma. If a peripapillary sector is utilized it will be necessary to determine if each examined point is to be assigned exclusively to one sector (either the peripapillary sector or to one of the 15 nerve fiber bundle sectors designated on the basis of a presumed retinotopic projection onto the optic disc). The data points could also be used non-exclusively and assigned to both the peripapillary sector and a nerve fiber bundle sector. Based on no empirical data we would be inclined to think that the former approach is relatively cleaner than the latter. The dimensions of the peripapillary sector can be specified as desired. If it is specified as 4 degrees larger than the blind spot each direction, the peripapillary sector will extend within 7° of the foveal fixation point (Fig. 2). As the diameter of the perifoveal visual field sector is increased it has greatest proportional effect on the area of the visual field sector temporal to the fovea which is correspondingly decreased.

Straight lines have been chosen to represent the borders of the groups of fibers in the nasal retina which give rise to sectors of the visual fields (Fig. 1). These lines follow the simple expression:

$$Y = aX + b$$

By specifying two points on the line (X_0, Y_0) and (X_1, Y_1) the value of a can be calculated:

$$a = (Y_0 - Y_1)/(X_0 - X_1)$$

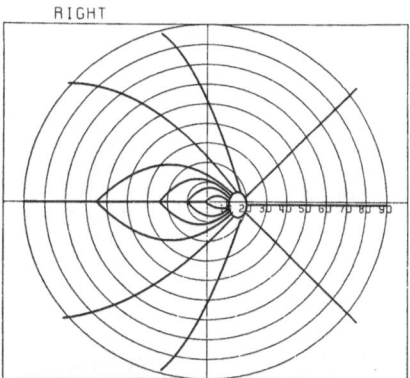

Fig. 1. Visual field sector boundaries for the full 90° radius visual field of the right eye as generated by a computer using the equations described in this paper. The borders are plotted for the blind spot as described in an ellipse, for the temporal sectors as straight lines, and for the nasal sectors as sections of parabolas. Note that the biggest variation from the anatomic course of the nerve fiber bundles occurs in the mid-peripheral nasal visual field along the horizontal meridian (corresponding to the horizontal raphe of the temporal retina). The effect of this variation may be mitigated by the large receptive fields of retinal ganglion cells in this region. The number or location of the curves can be easily manipulated by changing values shown in Table 1.

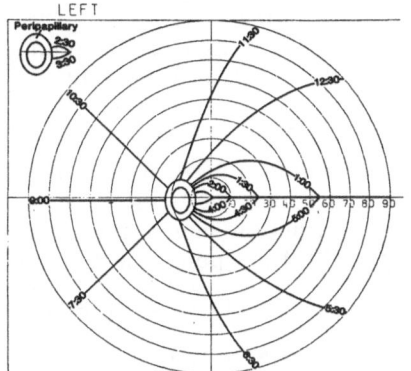

Fig. 2. Visual field sector boundaries for the full 90° radius visual field of the left eye including a 4° peripapillary sector. Some apparent discrepancy occurs because the boundary labels are derived from the point where each boundary projects to the border of the blind spot (not the outer border of the peripapillary sector).

Substituting this value for *a* into the general equation and solving for *b* yields:

$$b = Y_0 - aX_0$$

The borders are designated according to a 12-hour clock notation with regard to the margin of the blind spot. Calculated values for the lines plotted at 1:30, 3:00 and 4:30 in the visual field of the right eye are given in Table 1. Note that the 3:00 boundary, the horizontal line temporal to the center of the blind spot, is set at $Y = -1.5$ degrees because of the relative anatomic

461

Table 1. Values of coefficients for the general equation: $Y = a_0 + a_1X + a_2X^2$.

Border label	a_0	a_1	a_2
3:00	−1.5	0.0	0.0
4:30	14.0	−1.0	0.0
5:30	−52.0	2.073	2.687×10^{-2}
6:30	−21.12	0.9466	5.808×10^{-3}
7:00	−14.72	0.5276	1.446×10^{-2}
7:30	−11.0	0.2181	2.819×10^{-2}
8:00	−7.0	0.2146	4.854×10^{-2}
8:30	−0.7273	−0.6818	4.545×10^{-2}
9:30	0.9091	0.8273	-8.182×10^{-2}
10:00	7.0	0.15	-5.5×10^{-2}
10:30	11.0	−0.2887	-3.113×10^{-2}
11:00	13.64	−0.5460	-1.443×10^{-2}
11:30	23.0	−1.082	-7.855×10^{-3}
12:30	52.0	−2.206	-3.287×10^{-2}
1:30	−16.0	1.0	0.0

The borders are designated and the values of the coefficients are shown for the visual field of the right eye. For the visual field of the left eye, the sign of each coefficient in column a_1 is changed and the border labels are changed by folding the clock over the Y-axis.

relationships of the fovea and the optic disc. The horizontal boundary dividing the fields into upper and lower segments nasal to fixation is the trivial line: $Y = 0.0$ for X less than -1.0 degrees.

The curved borders designated from 5:30 around to 12:30 have been represented with sections of parabolas, general form:

$$Y = a_0 + a_1X + a_2X^2$$

The coefficients can be derived using a system of simultaneous equations based on three points taken from the border to be specified. For example, three points (X, Y) chosen from the plot of the 6:30 border are: $(11, -10)$, $(-10, -30)$, and $(-60, -57)$. These points yield the following equations:

$$-10 = a_0 + 11a_1 + (11)^2a_2 = a_0 + 11a_1 + 121a_2, \tag{1}$$

$$-30 = a_0 + (-10)a_1 + 100a_2 \tag{2}$$

$$-57 = a_0 + (-60)a_1 + 3600a_2 \tag{3}$$

Equation (1) minus equation (2) yields:

$$20 = 21a_1 + 21a_2 \tag{4}$$

Subtracting equation (3) from equation (2) yields:

$$27 = 50a_1 - 3500a_2 \tag{5}$$

Divide equation (4) by 21 (to isolate a_1) and multiply the result by 50, (to subtract from equation 5) gives:

$$20.619048 = 3550a_2 \tag{6}$$

$$a_2 = 20.619048/3550 = 5.8081824 \times 10^{-3} \tag{6a}$$

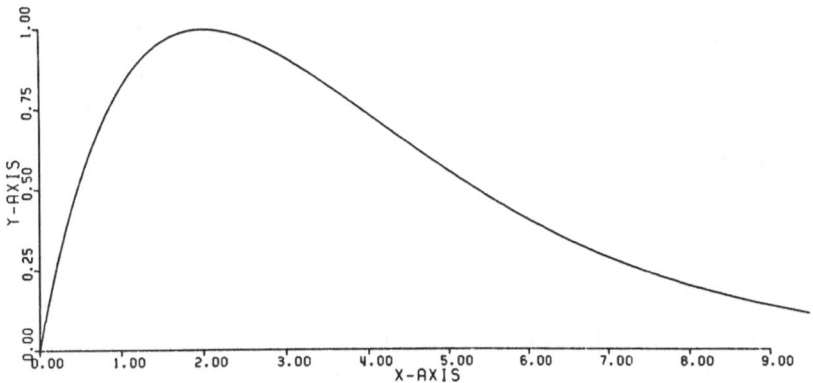

Fig. 3. Example of a boundary curve generated by an exponential equation ($Y = Xe^{-X}$) showing that it is possible to generate an inflection point in the curve. Inflections are not possible with parabolic equations so that parabolic equations are less able to represent the anatomic course of the retinal nerve fiber layer in the temporal retinal periphery. The disadvantages of using exponential equations are discussed in the text. Note that Y does not return to 0.

This result can be substituted into either equation (5) or (4) to calculate the value of a_1 (which works out to be 9.4657277×10^{-1}). These are then substituted into equations (1), (2), or (3) to yield a_0. The coefficients used in plots 1–4 are given in Table 1. Using this method to find the coefficients will always produce an equation for a curve which passes through the three points. Thus to assure smooth curvature along the entire border it is best to choose three widely separated points. For the plotted curves the points have generally been chosen at the margin of the blind spot, at the extreme periphery (or at the horizontal meridian for curves that do not extend to the periphery) and at a convenient midpoint between the other two.

Parabolic curves alone produce a slight error in representing the course of nerve fibers in the temporal retina (3, 4). In the visual field of the right eye the problem occurs at the 7:00, 7:30, 10:30 and 11:00 borders. An exponential curve (Fig. 3) might serve to overcome this error and we have done some initial calculations using the equation:

$$Y = Xe^{-X},$$

or more generally:

$$(Y - Y_0) = a_0 + a_1 (X - X_0) \exp(-a_2(X - X_0)).$$

This curve produces a tail which could approximate the path of nerve fibers as they approach the horizontal meridian. However, there does not appear to be a simple method for specifying points and solving to find the coefficients with this equation. Since the exponential equation does not return to $Y = 0$, it would be necessary to truncate the lower portion of the curve by the choice of the value of a_0. In order to be useful and adaptive to the needs of perimetrists, some relatively quick and easy method to manipulate the boundaries must be available. Investigation into the possible use of the

463

exponential equation is continuing but the parabolic expressions may prove to be sufficiently close to the observed field changes and are much easier to work with. Clinical experience may not support the expected need to closely mimic the retinal nerve fibers as they approach the horizontal meridian. It should be remembered that ganglion cell receptive fields become rather large in the peripheral retina.

We have met the objectives of this effort by providing explicit equations for use with computer programs to assign all tested points to the appropriate visual field sector. These points may be predefined as in static perimetry or postdefined as in kinetic perimetry. By expressing all of the curves in the form of Y as a function of X, whenever a point (X_1, Y_1) is selected, the computer can use the X_1 value and compute the Y locations of the sector borders. Y_1 can then be compared with the border values and the appropriate sector can be selected. All of the borders (ellipses, lines, and parabolas) are easily manipulated and new borders can be quickly calculated to define areas of interest.

ACKNOWLEDGEMENTS

Through the cooperation of William M. Hart, Jr., M.D., Ph.D. Figs. 2 and 3 were generated and plotted by the visual fields data-base system at the Department of Ophthalmology, Washington University School of Medicine, St. Louis, Missouri (1).

This study was supported in part by an unrestricted grant from Research to Prevent Blindness, Inc. to the University of Minnesota, and National Eye Institute Grant No. EY-02044 to Washington University School of Medicine, St. Louis, Missouri.

REFERENCES

1. Hart, W. M., Jr. and Hartz, R. K. Computer processing of visual field data: I. Recording, storage and retrieval. Arch. Ophthalmol. 99:128–132 (1981).
2. Morin, J. P. Changes in the visual fields in glaucoma: static and kinetic perimetry in 2,000 patients. Trans. Am. Ophthalmol. Soc. 77:622–642 (1979).
3. Polyak, S. The Vertebrate Visual System. University of Chicago Press, 277 (1957).
4. Vrabec, R. The temporal raphe of the human retina. Am. J. Ophthalmol. 62: 926–938 (1966).
5. Wirtschafter, J. D., Becker, W. L., Howe, J. B. and Younge, B. R. Glaucoma visual field analysis by computed profile of nerve fiber function in optic disc sectors. Ophthalmology 89:255–266 (1982).

Author's address:
Dr J.D. Wirtschafter
Depts. of Ophthalmology, Neurology and Neurosurgery
School of Medicine
University of Minnesota Hospital
Box 493, Minneapolis, MN 55455
U.S.A.

THE ROLE OF PERIMETRY IN RETINAL DETACHMENT*

E. GANDOLFO, M. ZINGIRIAN and P. CAPRIS

(Genoa, Italy)

Key words. Retinal detachment, kinetic and static perimetry, pre-operative phase, post-operative phase, surgery results.

ABSTRACT

The results of perimetry in diagnosis, analysis and follow-up of eyes suffering from retinal detachment (r.d.) are evaluated. Classic kinetic and static procedures with the Goldmann perimeter are utilized. An r.d. usually generates an absolute visual field (VF) defect that reproduces the topography of the detached retina. Only a very recently and slightly detached retina retains a certain sensitivity. Perimetry helps to determine the exact extent of the r.d. in doubtful cases. After surgery perimetry indicates the manner of the functional recovery, that is never complete. Usually, maximum recovery is reached within 3–4 weeks but a moderate improvement is still possible within the first 6 months. Perimetry indicates that better functional results are obtained when surgery is carried out in recent r.d. (max. 15 days). Fairly good results are present in 1–2 months old r.d. and progressively worse in older cases. The sensitivity improvement detected by perimetry in a reattached retina is also inversely proportional to the importance of the surgical insult. The results of perimetry in particular cases of r.d., such as retinoschisis, macular hole, relapse, etc., are also considered.

INTRODUCTION

Perimetry represents the most refined instrument for functionl evaluation of the eye and therefore is extremely important in an affliction like retinal detachment (r.d.) in which serious functional disturbances are observed both before and after surgery.

The role of perimetry differs substantially in the pre-operative and post-operative phase.

*Requests for offprints should be addressed to: Miss Vanna Re, Librarian of the University Eye Clinic, Viale Benedetto XV, 16132, Genoa Italy.

Greve, E. L., Heijl, A. (eds.) Fifth International Visual Field Symposium.
©*1983 Dr W. Junk Publishers, The Hague/Boston/Lancaster.*

Before surgery, visual field (VF) examination supplies additional information on the true extension of r.d., on the duration of the disease, and on the seriousness of degenerative phenomena that preceded and followed detachment.

In the post-operative phase, perimetry gives us information on the speed and extent of functional recovery, on the eventual presence of complications linked to the surgical method, on the possibility of relapses, and on the residual sensitivity deficit.

These notions are easily deducible examining the existing literature, yet, an accurate kinetic and static perimetric study carried out in a large number of patients over several years has helped us to develop some new and interesting notions.

MATERIALS AND METHODS

All the patients hospitalized in our clinic over the last 3 years suffering from r.d. underwent an accurate perimetry using a Goldmann apparatus. A complete kinetic and static examination (along the meridians considered most interesting) was carried out. VF examination was repeated on patient release and performed again 1 month, 3 months, and then every 6 months post release.

Of the 742 patients admitted to the study only 40% were considered valid. The cases excluded were those in which perimetric examination collaboration was not good, follow-up was below the minimum considered indispensable (18 months), visus was too low to guarantee fixation stability during the static examination, and surgery did not lead to reattachment.

An accurate map of the eye fundus was designed for all patients during the course of the study by means of indirect ophthalmoscopy according to Schepens.

Following retina reattachment, the map was remade for a precise evaluation of complications, residual alterations and factors that could disturb perimetric findings.

In a certain percentage of cases, we conducted more complete investigations including chromatic sense analysis, mesopic, static and flicker perimetry, fluorangiography and photographic controls of the fundus.

RESULTS

Pre-operative phase

In this phase, perimetry demonstrates quite clearly the depth and extension of the defect corresponding to the r.d. The defects extension is shown by kinetic examination.

In partial detachments without macular involvement, one notes that the line of demarcation between uninvolved and compromised areas of the VF does not exactly coincide with the line that divides the elevated retina from that adherent portion. The detached retina, in fact, maintains discrete function

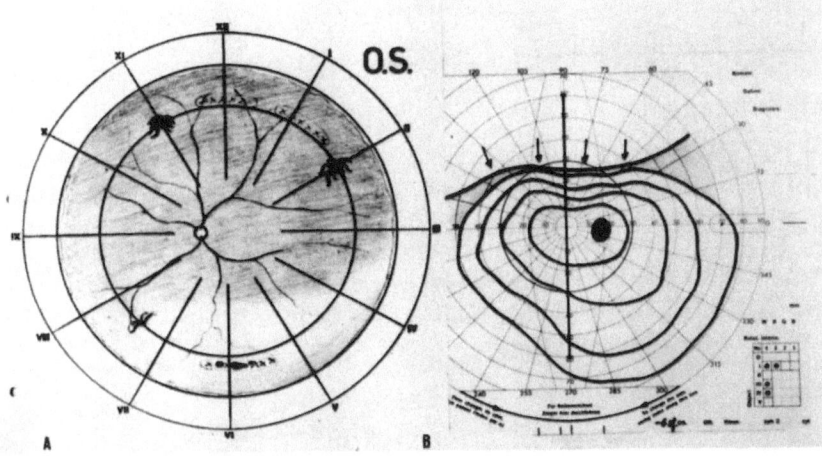

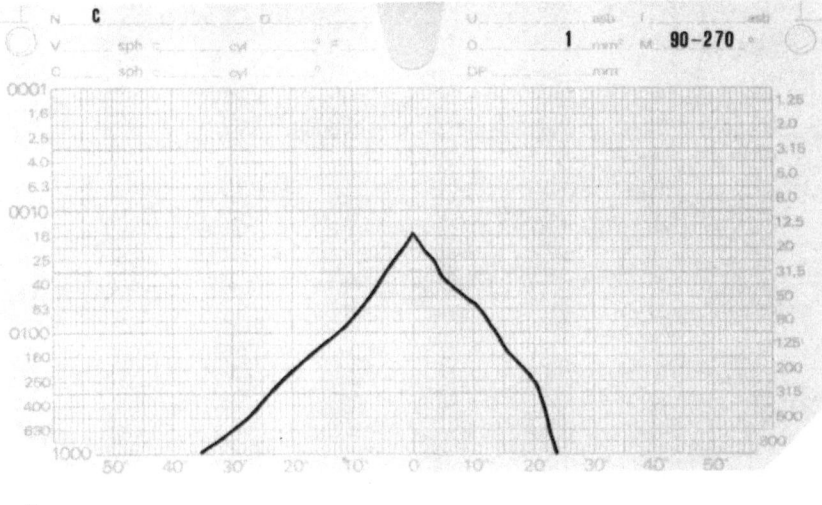

Fig. 1. (A) Retinal detachment with recent and slight swelling and without macular involvement; (B) perimetric findings in the same case; (C) the static profile.

if the swelling is both relatively recent and of modest proportions. Such sensitivity behavior is clear on static examination conducted along a trajectory perpendicular to the line of demarcation between detached and adherent portions of the retina (Figs. 1A, B, C).

The defect becomes absolute only when the retina forms large bumps or when the r.d. is present for a long time (2 months). In such cases the sensitivity gradient is very steep and the isopters tend to overlap. This behavior is also seen in cases of long-term self-contained r.d. (Figs. 2A, B, C).

467

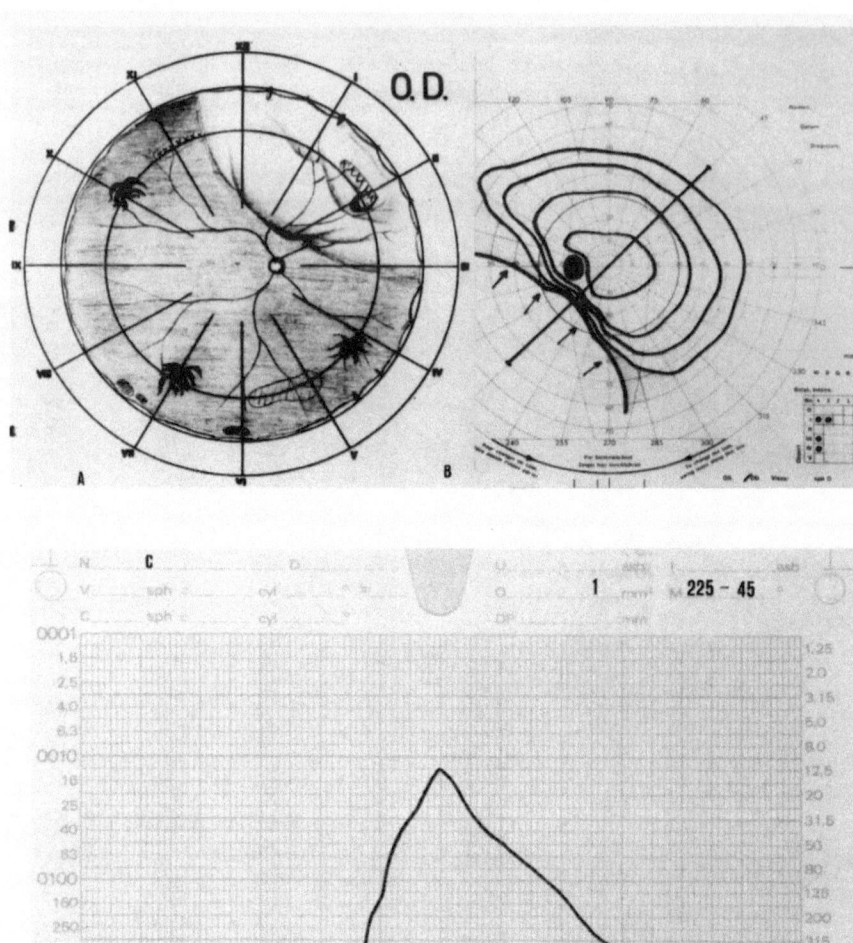

Fig. 2. (A) Retinal detachment with large bumps, without macular swelling; (B) perimetric findings; (C) the static profile.

In cases in which the macula is not involved, a depression in central sensitivity is still frequently noted (60%). In r.d. with macular swelling of recent occurrence, the presence of a central scotoma is characteristically noted. Static profile shows a central depression of about 0.3–0.6 l.u. This is because macular photoreceptors are more sensitive to metabolic disturbances due to the r.d. since they receive little nutrition from the retinal circulation depending above all on choroidal circulation. Three to four weeks after the onset of macular swelling such threshold behavior is no longer demonstrable.

In subtotal r.d., VF examination is more difficult but still permits, in the

468

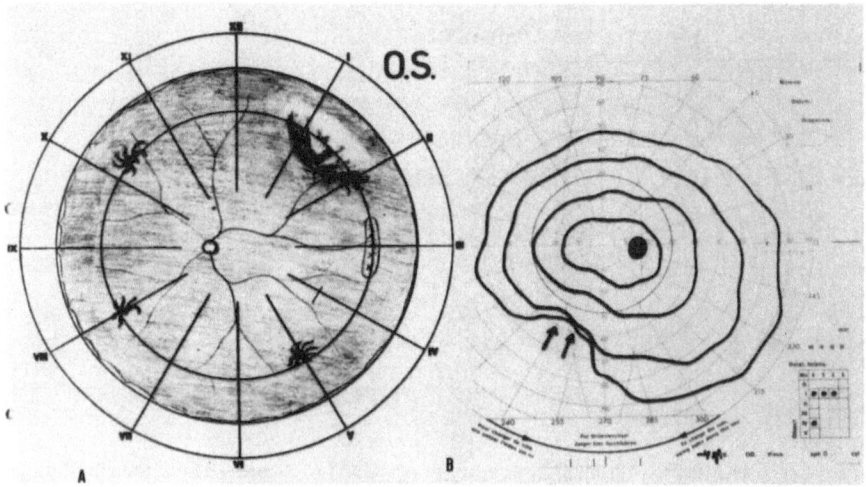

Fig. 3. (A) Reattached retina after localized surgery; (B) perimetric findings in the same case (macula was not involved).

case of recent and slight swelling, the construction of a good map of retinal sensitivity. The zones that conserve a certain function are those areas that detached last and this fact can supply useful information on the evolution of the r.d.

Perimetry helps to determine the exact extent of the r.d. in doubtful cases.

In the case of macular hole, the central defect is absolute and the gradient of the sensitivity between detached and adherent zones is usually not steep due to the serious degenerative phenomena present in the areas not involved in r.d.

In the case of retinoschisis the perimetric defect should in theory be absolute due to the interruption of inter-retinal neuronal connections. In reality this is not verified since the threshold behavior is similar to that of normal r.d. In these cases, perimetry can be very useful in discovering if the disease has an evolutive character.

For those eyes already operated on, the onset of alterations in VF often indicates the tendency to relapse with the presence of a very thin liquid layer not detectable by ophthalmoscopy.

Post-operative phase

After reattachment, the absolute peripheral limits of the VF enlarge, but they reach different extension relative to the surgical technique employed. If surgery is restricted to the area of breakage (scleroplasty with inclusion, localized folding or plombage) the VF limits reacquire normal extension except in the territory treated, where an incision of variable entity persists (Figs. 3A, B).

The perimetric defect only slightly exceeds the width of the treated zone. A much greater defect indicates an overdose of energy.

469

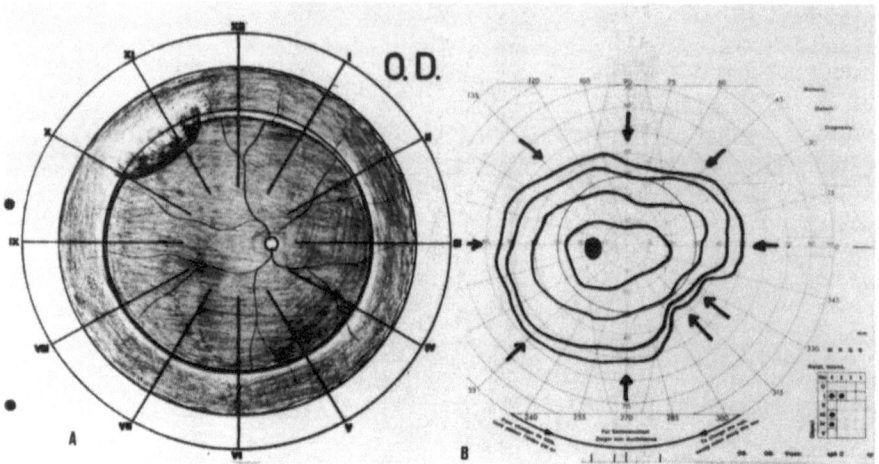

Fig. 4. (A) Reattached retina after equatorial cerclage procedure; (B) perimetric findings in the same case (macula was involved).

If the operation included equatorial cerclage, the absolute limits of the VF are permanently concentrically restricted. Such contraction is variable and seems to depend more on the force of constriction of the cerclage than on its site (Figs. 4A, B).

Static examination permits exact evaluation of central threshold recovery that is influenced by different factors. If there is no macular detachment and timely surgery is performed restoration of an almost normal central sensitivity occurs in 85% of the cases. By timely surgery, we mean those procedures carried out within 15 days after r.d. onset.

If there is macular involvement, early surgery is even more important in order to have good functional recovery. An operation carried out more than 15 days after the onset of macular swelling makes good central functional recovery extremely difficult. Functional improvement can still be discrete in r.d. of 4–6 weeks duration. In the case of disease present for more than 2 months, the threshold level obtained will always be very slight.

Sensitivity restoration is rather rapid following anatomical healing from r.d. Normally maximum recovery is reached within a month if media torbidity does not persist. Successively, only slight further improvements are noted in the span of 6 months.

The type of energy utilized to obtain retinopexy (dyathermy, cryothermy, photocoagulation, etc.) does not influence the functional result. Certainly an energy overdose will cause damage in the treated area and at the macular level. During the course of our study we noted that the phenomena of energy overdose were more frequent with the use of cryothermy, than with other methods.

In macular hole r.d., the extension of central damage is less if one obtains hole obliteration with a few spots of photocoagulation. This damage is greater with the use of dyathermy or cryothermy, especially if one performs a macula indentation technique.

470

In the cases in which we carried out a complete functional estimation including kinetic and static photopic perimetry, mesopic, scotopic and flicker perimetry, chromatic sense examination, etc., we noted that permanent damage of retinal function is more persistent if such function is analyzed with more sensitive methods. In fact, disturbances of the mesopic and scotopic results and of the FFF appear still present even years after surgery.

The presence of serious degenerative fenomena (high myopia, retinoschisis, atrophy, etc.) appears more important than the age of the patient in relation to the possibility for permanent functional damage.

CONCLUSIONS

The damage to retinal sensitivity provoked by r.d. is very serious, but successful surgery can restore good levels of light threshold.

A direct proportion exists between the earliness of surgery and the foveal threshold levels reached.

Not all retinal functions recover at the same time and some of these, such as FFF and scotopic and mesopic thresholds, remain permanently altered.

REFERENCES

1. Alexandridis, E. and Janzarik, B. I. Restitution of retinal sensitivity after cured retinal detachment. Doc. Ophthalmol. Proc. Series 14:281–284 (1977).
2. De Sanctis, G. Comportamento del campo visivo nel distacco di retina dopo intervento chirurgico. Rass. Ital. Ottalmol. 4:589–601 (1935).
3. Foulds, W. S., Reid, H. and Chisholm, I. A. Factors influencing visual recovery after retinal detachment surgery. Mod. Probl. Ophthalmol. 12:49–57 (1974).
4. Kreissig, I. Prognosis of return of macular function after retinal reattachment. Mod. Probl. Ophthalmol. 18:415–429 (1977).

Authors' address:
University Eye Clinic
Viale Benedetto XV, 5
16132 Genoa
Italy

COMPUTER ANALYSIS OF KINETIC FIELD DATA DETERMINED WITH A GOLDMANN PERIMETER

HIROSHI KOSAKI and HAJIME NAKATANI

(Osaka, Japan)

Key words. Glaucomatous visual field, Goldmann's kinetic perimetry, computer.

ABSTRACT

A personal computer (HP-85, YHP) was used to analyze kinetic fields determined with a Goldmann perimeter. Fifty cases of primary glaucoma were chosen for this study.

Reduced size copies of the field were made and a simplified profile of the visual island was drawn by the computer. Areas of each isopter were calculated and an attempt was made to evaluate the field changes compared with those of the normal field. Improvement or loss of field was also evaluated in terms of areas of isopters. Graphic presentation of changes in the areas of isopters was made and an adequate intraocular pressure level was estimated for each individual.

PURPOSE

In the diagnosis and treatment of glaucoma, Goldmann kinetic visual field topography is used at present only to give patterns, and is contributing usefully to medical practice. However, visual field topography contains more information. For example, if it is possible to measure the area of isopters or the volume of visual island from field topography, and these obtained values are then numerically processed, the data will contribute to a more detailed diagnosis and assessment of the progress in the clinical treatment of glaucoma. Furthermore, it will be very useful in deciding the therapeutic measures to be taken. Here, we present our processing method for the above by using a personal computer.

METHOD

Kinetic visual field topography obtained by a Goldmann perimeter was set on a graphic tablet (Model 9111A, YHP) (Fig. 1), and the data of the topography

Greve, E. L., Heijl, A. (eds.) Fifth International Visual Field Symposium.
©1983 Dr W. Junk Publishers, The Hague/Boston/Lancaster.

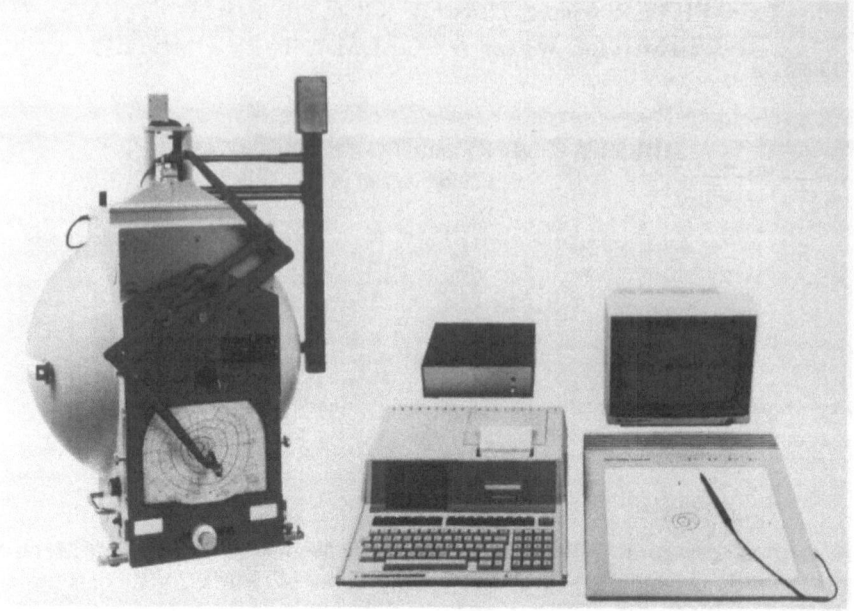

Fig. 1. Right: graphic tablet (Model 9111A, YHP); center: personal computer (Model HP-85, YHP); left: computer processing device set in Goldmann perimeter.

were put into a personal computer (model HP-85, YHP) (Fig. 1) by tracing over the isopter with a plotting pen. These data were stored on a cassette tape, and processed using different programs as necessary.

RESULTS

We were able to process the following items:
1. Reduced size of kinetic visual field topography (1/4 size).
2. Cross section of a visual island.
3. Assessment of abnormalities in the isopter areas and the visual island volumes (Fig. 2) abnormality, here, is expressed as a percentage, comparing the patient's reading with normal values of areas and volumes for the patient's age (1).
4. Assessment of the progress in isopter areas and visual island volumes (Fig. 3). Here, the present measured values are compared with those of the previous measurements, and the increase or decrease is represented as a percentage.
5. Graphic representation of the progress in isopter areas and visual island volumes (Fig. 4). Here, the movement in values of the two from the first examination to the present are shown on a graph, together with the movement in intraocular pressure.
6. Prognosis of visual field changes (Fig. 5). The relationship between progress

474

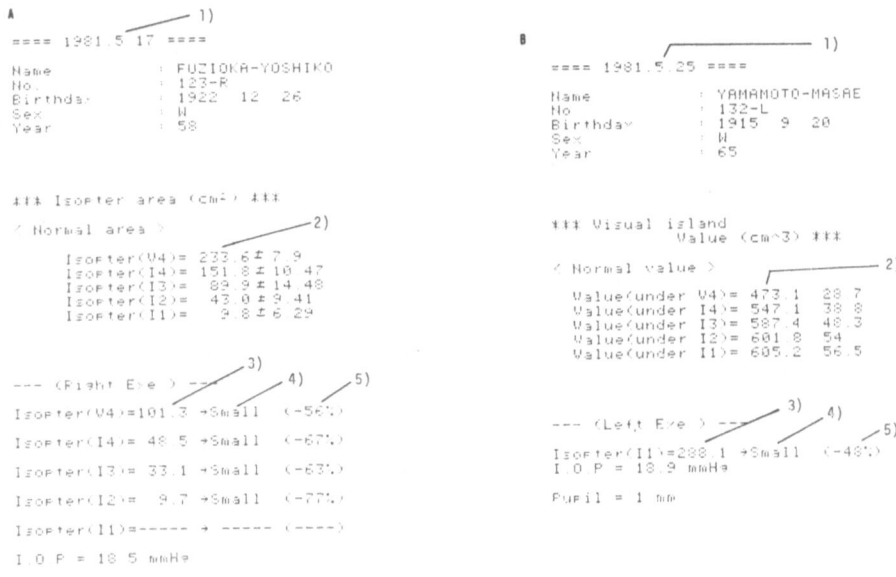

A
==== 1981.5.17 ====

Name   : FUZIOKA-YOSHIKO
No.   : 123-R
Birthday   : 1922 12 26
Sex   : W
Year   : 58

*** Isopter area (cm²) ***

< Normal area >

    Isopter(V4)= 233.6 ± 7.9
    Isopter(I4)= 151.8 ± 10.47
    Isopter(I3)= 89.9 ± 14.48
    Isopter(I2)= 43.0 ± 9.41
    Isopter(I1)=   9.8 ± 6.29

--- (Right Eye) ---

Isopter(V4)=101.3 →Small (-56%)

Isopter(I4)= 48.5 →Small (-67%)

Isopter(I3)= 33.1 →Small (-63%)

Isopter(I2)= 9.7 →Small (-77%)

Isopter(I1)=----- → ----- (----)

I.O.P = 18.5 mmHg

Pupil = 4.5 mm

B
==== 1981.5.25 ====

Name   : YAMAMOTO-MASAE
No   : 132-L
Birthday   : 1915 9 20
Sex   : W
Year   : 65

*** Visual island
              Value (cm³) ***

< Normal value >

    Value(under V4)= 473.1   28.7
    Value(under I4)= 547.1   38.8
    Value(under I3)= 587.4   48.3
    Value(under I2)= 601.8   54
    Value(under I1)= 605.2   56.5

--- (Left Eye) ---

Isopter(I1)=288.1 →Small (-48%)
I.O.P = 18.9 mmHg

Pupil = 1 mm

Fig. 2. Assessment of abnormalities in the isopter areas and the visual island volumes (with percentage); A) areas; B) volumes. 1 = date of examination; 2 = normal value areas (cm²) (A) and normal volumes (cm⁻³) (B) in different ages; 3 = actually measured values; 4 = assessment whether values are beyond normal limits; 5 = percentage presentation of abnormalities.

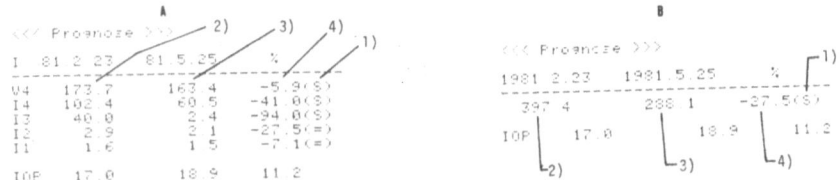

A
<<< Prognose >>>

     1981.2.23   1981.5.25   %
V4   173.7   163.4   -5.9(S)
I4   102.4   60.5   -41.0(S)
I3   40.0   2.4   -94.0(S)
I2   2.9   2.1   -27.5(=)
I1   1.6   1.5   -7.1(=)

IOP   17.0   18.9   11.2

B
<<< Prognose >>>

1981.2.23   1981.5.25   %

397.4   288.1   -27.5(S)

IOP   17.0   18.9   11.2

Fig. 3. Assessment of the progress in isopter areas and visual island volumes (with percentage); S shows decrease from previous values, and = shows same as previous values; A) areas; B) volumes. 1 = comparison with previous values; 2 = previous values; 3 = present values; 4 = progress (%).

of visual field changes and intraocular pressure are shown in Fig. 5A. When intraocular pressure is around 15 mm Hg or less, little changes in visual field are seen, while when intraocular pressure goes up to about 20 mm Hg for a long time, worsening of the visual field is seen. Figure 5B shows the correlation between field area and intraocular pressure. The straight line shows measured values and the dotted straight line is extrapolated from the straight line. The dotted curve shows 95% confidence limits. We can see here that at high intraocular pressure, the field area decreases.

7. Estimation of adequate intraocular pressure for individual patients in view

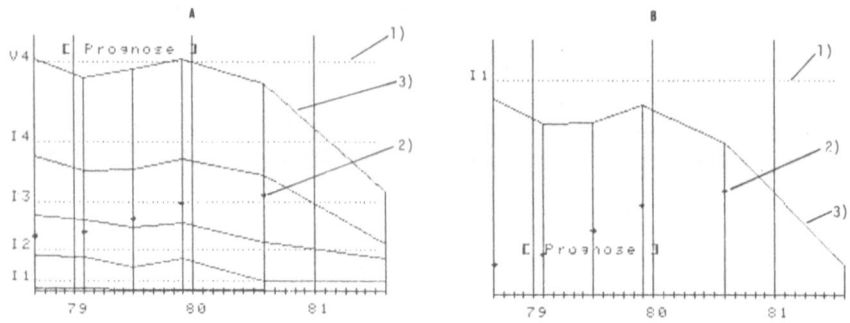

Fig. 4. Graphic representation of the progress in isopter areas and visual island volumes (with progress of IOP). The scale of the horizontal axis is in months; A) areas; B) volumes. 1 = normal values for age; 2 = IOP values; 3 = movement graph for the last 3 years.

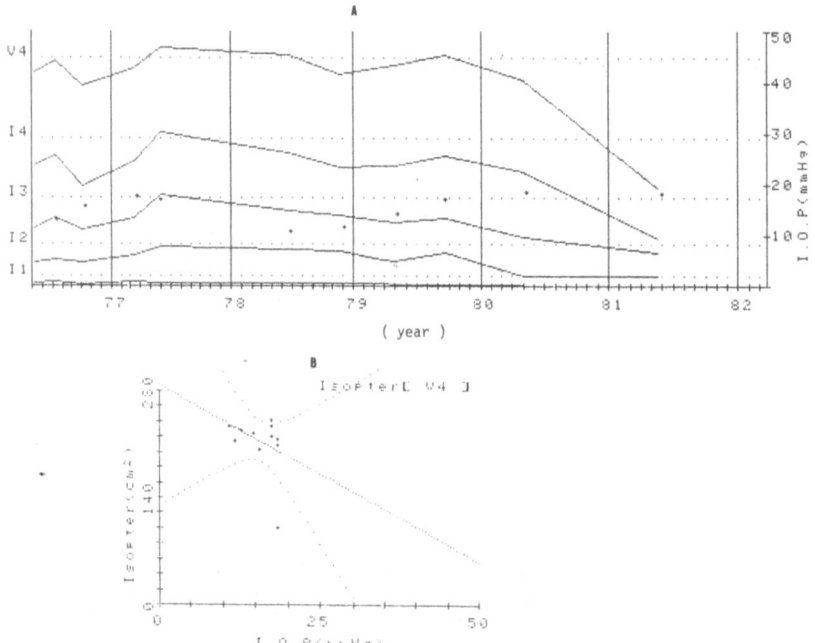

Fig. 5. Prognosis of visual field changes; A) progress of visual field changes and IOP; B) the correlation between field areas and IOP. (Figures for I4, I3, I2, I1 are abbreviated.)

of the progress in their visual field changes. Here, we deal with the relationship between progress in visual field changes and intraocular pressure. The example shows that the patient has been keeping IOP at around 12–13 mm Hg, while keeping good visual field progress during the period. (Figure is abbreviated.)

It has become possible to put visual field data obtained by a Goldmann

476

perimeter into a computer and to process that data together with other data which had already been stored in the computer. This has enabled us to provide a more simplified and more detailed assessment of the progress of glaucoma. It is more helpful in diagnosis and in making decisions on the therapeutic measures to be taken, than macroscopic assessment of data expressed in patterns.

REFERENCE

1. Kosaki, H. and Higashitarumizu, K. Normal kinetic visual field topography of the Japanese by Goldmann Perimeter. 1st Japanese Perimetric Society Symposium, Tokyo, 14 December, 1980.

Authors' address:
Dept. of Ophthalmology
Osaka University Medical School
Osaka
Japan

PERIMETRIC CHANGES CAUSED BY ETHYL ALCOHOL*

E. GANDOLFO

(Genoa, Italy)

Key words. Ethyl alcohol, kinetic perimetry, static perimetry (photopic and mesopic), flicker perimetry.

ABSTRACT

The author evaluates the effect of ethanol on the visual field (VF). The following perimetric tests are carried out: standard kinetic perimetry (3 isopters), photopic and mesopic static perimetry along the $0°-180°$ meridian and FFF (flicker fusion frequency) along the same meridian. All tests are performed first under normal conditions and afterwards on the same subjects (20 young men) having a blood alcohol level (b.a.l.) of 0.05%.

The ethanol, at the utilized doses, possesses only moderate effects, either positive or negative, on kinetic and static results. Positive effects are the increase of central sensitivity both in photopic and mesopic conditions and a slight global improvement of the mesopic static profile. Negative effects are the enlargement of the blind spot and angioscotomata, some irregularities of the threshold in the pericoecal area and a certain contraction of the periferal isopters. On the contrary the effects of the FFF are more evident and always negative. The possible causes of these behaviors are considered and discussed.

INTRODUCTION

Alcohol consumption is widespread and of major importance in industrialized countries. Excluding abuse, we believe that the majority of us, at least during certain hours of the day, carry out our normal daily activities with a blood alcohol level (b.a.l.) of 0.03—0.05%.

The principal pharmacological activity of ethanol is expressed at the level of the central nervous system. Only depressive effects at first involving cortical functions and successively vegetative functions are present.

*Requests for outprints should be addressed to: Miss Vanna Re, Librarian of the University Eye Clinic, Viale Benedetto XV, 16132, Genoa, Italy.

Alcohol effects involve the sense organs precociously and in particular the visual apparatus (5).

Alcohol influence on vision has been the object of numerous studies that have investigated on: IOP (7, 10, 12), extrinsic ocular motility (4, 5, 9, 11) pupil movements (3), visual acuity (2, 5), ERG-EOG-VEP (8, 14, 15), dark—light adaptation (1, 6), etc.

The effect of alcohol on the visual field (VF) has been studied, but that research is dated (5, 13), and perimetric assessment had not yet benefited from the more recent advances in ophthalmological semeiology.

The great increase in alcohol use, the lack of modern research and the increasing importance of a good VF in the dynamic life of today encouraged us to carry out the present study.

MATERIALS AND METHODS

The VF of 20 male subjects between 25 and 30 years of age, without any organic or ocular problems, was examined. The exam was carried out first under normal conditions (without alcohol ingestion for at least 12 hours) and successively after the consumption of alcohol in a sufficient quantity to cause a b.a.l. of 0.05%. With the ingestion of 100 ml of whisky (hydro-alcoholic solution containing 31.6% ethanol by weight) in 5 min the desired b.a.l. was reached. The b.a.l. so induced remained more or less constant throughout the test (40—50 min).

To assure the desired b.a.l. values, an apparatus to determine the ethanol content in expired air was used.

We used the 'Breathalyzer' made by Etzingler of Geneva that utilizes a spectrophotometric procedure based on the comparison of two solutions of sulphoric acid bichromate. A small amount of air expired was passed through one of these solutions.

In our experiments we checked the b.a.l. before starting perimetric examination (30 min after alcohol ingestion) and at the end of testing.

The perimetric tests performed were the following:
1. kinetic photopic perimetry: with 3 targets (VI/4; I/3; I/1) including a detailed study of the blind spot;
2. static photopic perimetry: along the 0—180° meridian, with threshold determinations at the following eccentricities: 2, 4, 6, 10, 15, 20, 30, 40, 50°, after the point 0°;
3. static mesopic perimetry: along the 0—180° meridian, with exploration of point 0° and the following eccentricities on both sides: 3, 6, 10, 20, 30, 50°. The background luminance was regulated to 0. 24 asb. and the target used was III. A dark adaptation of 15 min was induced before mesopic perimetry;
4. flicker perimetry: FFF was examined in photopic conditions along the temporal horizontal meridian at the following eccentricities: 0, 5, 20, 40°, according to the technique of Zingirian et al. (16).

480

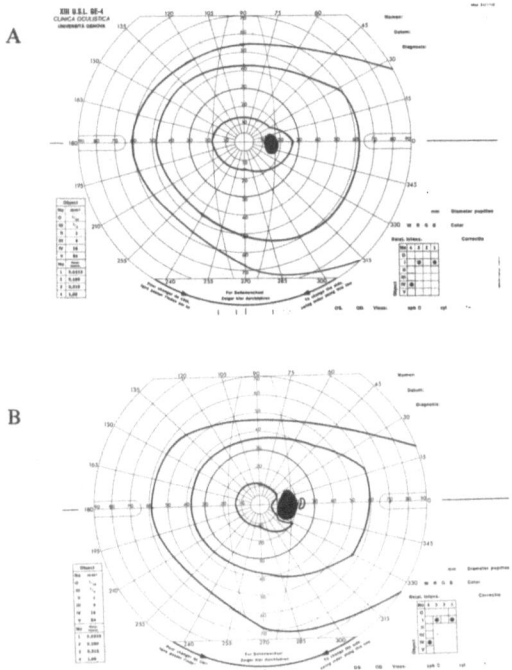

Fig. 1. (A) Kinetic photopic perimetry under normal conditions; (B) kinetic photopic perimetry after alcohol.

RESULTS

1. Kinetic photopic perimetry

Alcohol had little influence on the perimetric results. A contraction of the intermediate isopter more evident in the nasal sectors was consistently observed. Such contraction, usually limited to 4–8°, was noted in 75% of the cases (15 eyes).

The presence of a certain enlargement of the blind spot, especially in the horizontal diameter, was found less frequently (12 eyes: 60%). Other statistically significant findings included the contraction of the outer isopter in the upper sectors (5 cases: 25%) and contraction of the central isopter with exclusion of the blind spot (4 cases: 20%) (Figs. 1A, B).

2. Static photopic perimetry

A fairly constant and unexpected increase in central senstivity averaging 0.3 l.u. was found. A lowering of peripheral sensitivity beyond 20–30° of eccentricity was frequent (8 cases: 40%). In some cases then, in which kinetic

481

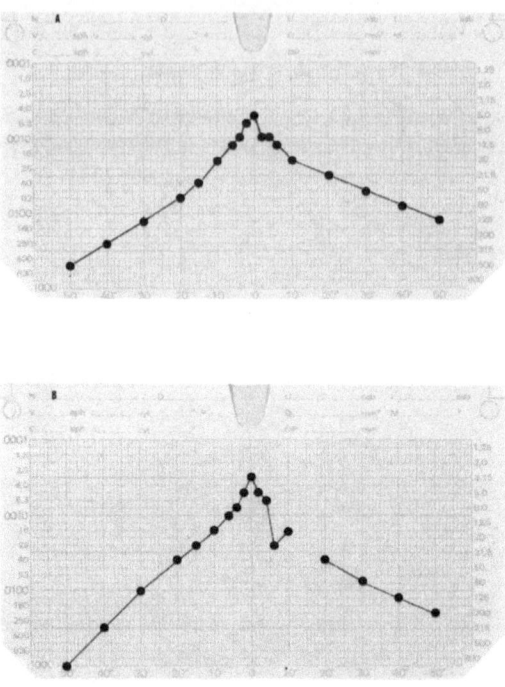

Fig. 2. (A) Static photopic profile under normal conditions; (B) static photopic profile after alcohol.

perimetry had shown enlargement of the blind spot, a widening of the coecal funnel, on static examination, was noted. A saw-tooth appearance of the static profile at he pericoecal level was evident in a couple of subjects (Figs. 2A, B).

3. Static mesopic perimetry

A certain overall improvement of the threshold was noted in the majority of cases following alcohol ingestion (13 eyes: 65%). This improvement was more evident at the central plateau and less evident in the periphery. In other subjects however appreciable differences in the curve before and after alcohol intake were not demonstrated. (Figs. 3A, B).

4. Flicker fusion frequency

In all the subjects examined, alcohol consumption caused deterioration of the FFF that, being of a modest entity at the level of the fixation point, becomes more evident when exploration is carried out more eccentrically. The lowering of the FFF was about 25% at the fovea level, increasing to 30–35% at 5°, to 40–50% at 20° and was above 65% at 40°.

482

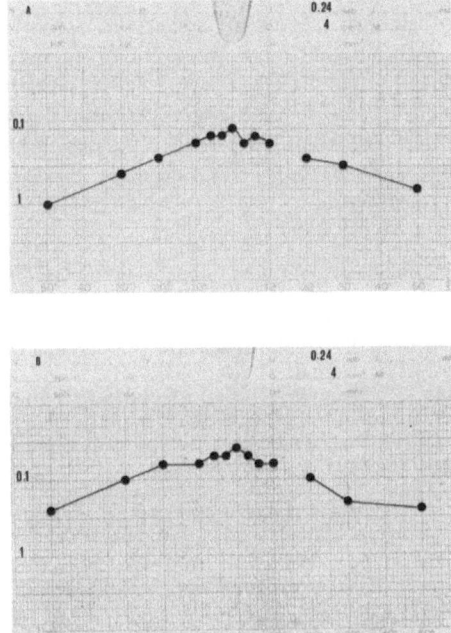

Fig. 3. (A) Static mesopic profile under normal conditions; (B) static mesopic profile after alcohol.

CONCLUSIONS

A b.a.l. of 0.05% has little influence on the perimetric performances of a normal eye in a young and healthy individual.

The influence of alcohol on the VF appears less serious and dangerous than that verified for binocular vision.

Our research has produced some interesting perimetric results: increase in central sensitivity both in photopic and mesopic conditions, enlargment of the blind spot, slight contraction of central and intermediate isopters and serious disturbance in the FFF.

The improvement in central sensitivity is probably linked to the vasodilating action of alcohol on the chorioretinal circulation. It is also possible that lowering of inhibitory control induced by alcohol can artificially improve threshold due to the greater ease with which the subject responds in the case of incertain perception.

The worsening of the coecal and pericoecal perimetric findings is connected to the dilation of the principal retinal vascular trunks that causes an increase in angioscotomas.

Variations in the intermediate and central isopters are linked to the increase in latency of psycho-physical response induced by ethanol.

The lowering of the peripheral isopter in the upper sectors results from a modest degree of ptosis produced by alcohol through relaxation of the eyelid musculature.

Overall analysis of the results obtained reveals a greater incidence of 'beneficial' effects of alcohol on retinal sensitivity when the b.a.l. is maintained under 0.05%. With a higher b.a.l. 'negative' effects seem to prevail.

The constant lowering of the FFF is testimony to the deleterious influence of alcohol on the functions that involve a more complex control mechanism.

As binocular vision is disturbed even with a modest b.a.l., so the complex interneuronal system that governs FFF appears compromised following limited consumption of alcohol.

REFERENCES

1. Adams, A. J. and Brown, B. Alcohol prolongs time course of glare. Nature 257: 481–483 (1975).
2. Adams, A. J., Brown, B., Flom, M. C. et al. Alcohol and marijuana effects on static visual acuity. Am. J. Optom. Physiol. Opt. 52:729–735 (1975).
3. Brown, B., Adams, A. J. et al. Pupil size after use of marijuana and alcohol. Am. J. Ophthalmol. 83:350–354 (1977).
4. Cohen, M. M. and Alpern, M. Vergence and accommodation, VI. The influence of ethanol on the AC/A ratio. Arch. Ophthalmol. 81:518–525 (1969).
5. Colson, Z. W. Effect of alcohol on vision. Exp. Invest. J. A. M. 115:1525–1527 (1940).
6. Forester, B. and Starck, H. Über die Hell- und Dunkeladaptation unter Alkoholeinfluss. Dtsch. Z. Ges. Gerichtl. Med. 49:66–69 (1959).
7. Houle, R. E. and Grant, W. M. Alcohol vasopressin and intraocular pressure. Invest. Ophthalmol 6:145–154 (1967).
8. Jacobson J. H., Hirose, T. and Stokes, P. E. Changes in human ERG induced by intravenous alcohol. Opthalmologica 158 Suppl.: 669–677 (1969).
9. Klein, S. and Klein, A. Räumliches Sehen und Farbensinn unter dem Einfluss von Alkohol. Dtsch. Gesundh. Wes. 29/37:1753–1756 (1974).
10. Leydhecker, W., Krieglstein, G. K. and Uhlich, E. Experimentelle Untersuchung zur Wirkungsweise alkoholischer Getränke auf den Augeneindruck. Klin. Mbl. Augenheilk. 173:75–79 (1978).
11. Lopez Marin, I., Jordano, J. et al. Modificaciones de la visión binocular con alcoholemias moderadas. Arch. Soc. Esp. Oftal. 40(7):733–739 (1980).
12. Peczon, J. D. and Grant, W. M. Glaucoma, alcohol and intraocular pressure. Arch. Ophthalmol. 73:495–501 (1965).
13. Sedan, J. Mon angioscotome. Revue Oto. N. Ophtal. 19:358–366 (1947).
14. Skoog, K. The C-wave of human D.C. registered ERG. Acta Ophthalmol. 52:913–923 (1974).
15. Skoog, K., Welinder, E. and Nilsson, S.E.G. The influence of ethyl alcohol on slow off-responses in the human D.C. registered ERG. Vision Res. 18:1041–1044 (1978).
16. Zingirian, M., Ciurlo, G., Rossi, P. and Burtolo, C. Flicker fusion and spatial summation. Doc. Ophthalmol. Proc. Series 26:127–130 (1980).

Author's address:
Dr E Gandolfo
University Eye Clinic
Viale Benedetto XV, 5
16132 Genoa
Italy

LEUKOCYTOCLASTIC VASCULITIS ASSOCIATED WITH BILATERAL CENTRAL FIELD LOSS; IMPROVEMENT ON CORTICOSTEROIDS AND MERCAPTOPURINE

D. W. ZAUEL, R. RANSBURG, M. GREIST
R. ARFFA and K. JULIAN
(Indianapolis, Indiana, U.S.A.)

Key words. Leukocytoclastic vasculitis, optic neuritis.

ABSTRACT

This is a case report — the first known to the authors — of a patient with optic neuritis associated with cutaneous leukocytoclastic vasculitis, which, together with the optic neuritis, improved following steroid and immuno-suppressive therapy.

INTRODUCTION

The varied nature of systemic vasculitis has been described by Sams (4). Moore and Fauci (3) reported on the neurologic manifestations of the disease in a recent article. While others have described optic neuritis in systemic connective tissue disease having, among other features, vascular inflammation, this is the first known report of optic neuritis associated with leukocytoclastic vasculitis.

Leukocytoclastic vasculitis is characterized by small erythematous maculo-papular skin lesions which are typically transient. Pathologically thickened vessel walls are infiltrated with neutrophilic leukocytes. Occasionally, a lesion will show only infiltration of lymphocytes. The vessel walls may be weakened, allowing red blood cells to leak into the tissue producing petechial hemor-rhages or purpuric spots. The cause of the disease is unknown. Some of the suspected etiologic agents are infection, drugs, chemicals, foreign proteins, immune mechanisms, and associated disease such as carcinoma.

CASE REPORT

A 16-year old right-handed, white, female described photopsia for three weeks and failing vision for two months. She gave a history of drug abuse but denied taking drugs by injection. The patient enumerated the drugs taken by mouth: amphetamines, some kind of laced 'punch' followed by visual

Greve, E. L., Heijl, A. (eds.) Fifth International Visual Field Symposium.
©1983 Dr W. Junk Publishers, The Hague/Boston/Lancaster.
ISBN 90 6193 731 0. Printed in the Netherlands.

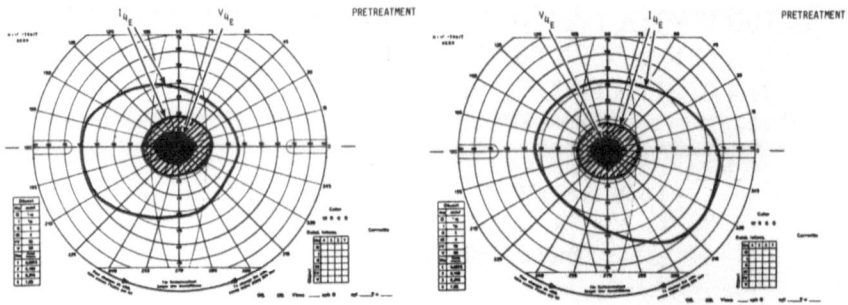

Fig. 1. Left: pretreatment; right: pretreatment.

hallucinations, and multiple unknown medications. The patient denied methanol ingestion.

Examination revealed dense central scotomas (Fig. 1), visual acuity 20/400 OU with eccentric fixation, depression of the pupillary light reflexes, and bilateral disc edema (Fig. 2); the diagnostic impression was bilateral optic neuritis.

General physical and pelvic examinations, as well as rheumatologic evaluation, were unremarkable, except for a few erythematous macular skin lesions (1–2 cm), some with central, punctate scars (1–2 mm), located on the anterior aspects of the lower legs. The history indicated that the skin lesions had begun with a few pruritic papules which resolved. Dermatologic consultation suggested that the findings on the legs were consistent with vasculitis. Biopsies of the lesions, however, initially were non-diagnostic, and specimens of skin in non-sun-exposed areas were reported normal and showed no immunofluorescent staining.

Laboratory findings: folate level 14.4; B12, 510; Westergren sedimentation rate, 3; collagen vascular survey, normal, with normal complement levels; RA slide test, negative; LE-prep, negative, ANA and DNA binding, negative; mild elevation of SGOT; SGPT, normal; FTA-Abs, nonreactive; Australian antigen and antibody, normal; cardiology consultation with echocardiogram, normal; angiotension converting enzyme, normal; and PPD and mumps skin tests were normal. Spinal tap and fluid, including gammaglobulin studies, were unremarkable; and cryoglobulins were normal.

X-ray studies, including CT scan of the head, sinus films, and chest X-ray, were unremarkable.

The patient was started on 100 mg of oral prednisone (Deltasone®) daily. The central scotomas became smaller and less dense over a period of several weeks (Fig. 3). New skin lesions did not appear. Oral prednisone therapy was continued with tapering dosages over a period of three months. As the prednisone was being tapered to 10 mg a day, new cutaneous lesions appeared (Fig. 4); biopsy now revealed leukocytoclastic vasculitis (Fig. 5). Prednisone was increased to 60 mg daily, and several months later, as the prednisone was tapered to 20 mg, the patient once again developed recurrent skin lesions. The prednisone was increased to 25 mg every morning; in addition, mercaptopurine (Purinethol®) 50 mg daily was prescribed. These medications were

486

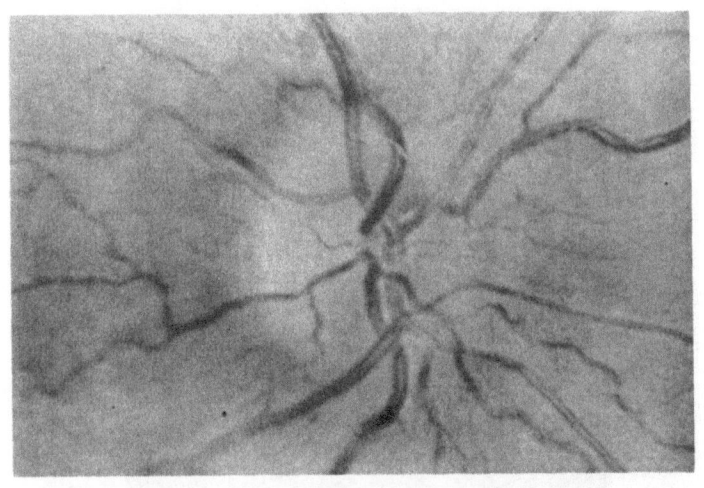

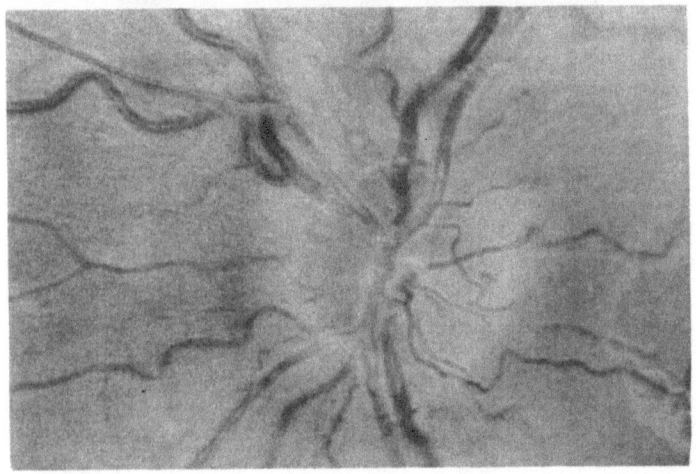

Fig. 2. Top: pretreatment OD; bottom: pretreatment OS.

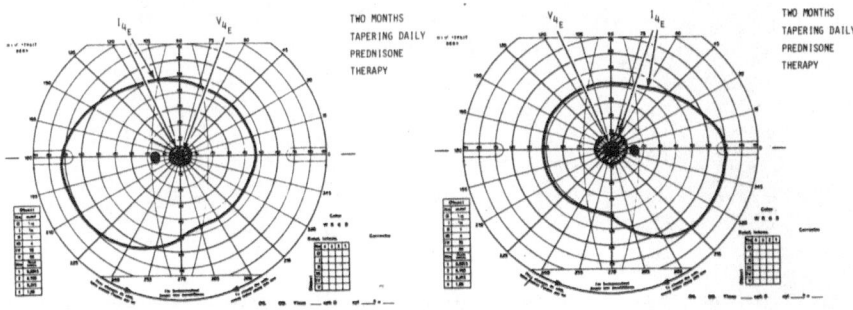

Fig. 3. Left: two months tapering daily prednisone therapy; right; two months tapering daily prednisone therapy.

487

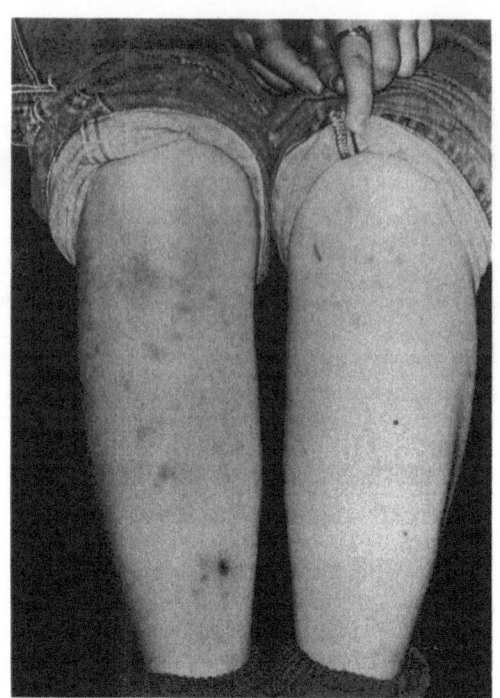

Fig. 4. Vasculitic skin lesions.

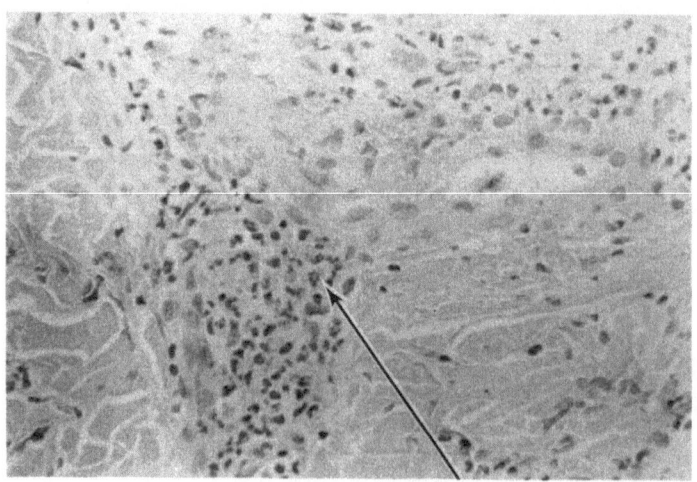

Fig. 5. Dermal blood vessels show infiltration with a mixed inflammatory infiltrate composed of lymphocytes and polymorphonuclear leukocytes. Nuclear dust (leukocytoclasia) is seen around the involved vessel wall (H & E 220X).

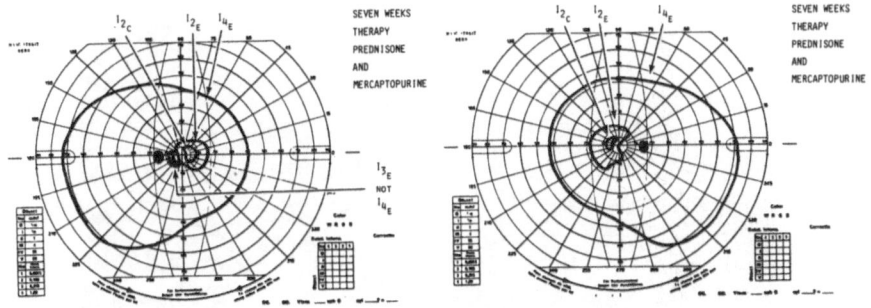

Fig. 6. Left: seven weeks therapy prednisone and mercaptopurine; right: idem.

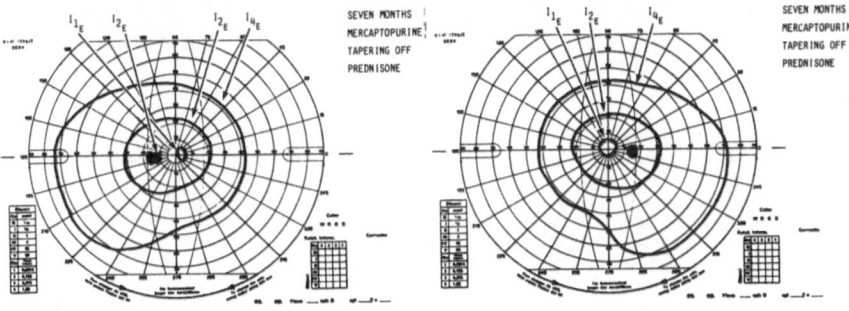

Fig. 7. Left: seven months mercaptopurine tapering off prednisone; right: idem.

tapered over a span of seven months to their present levels: 5 mg of prednisone daily and mercaptopurine 50 mg three days out of seven days. During this time, there was gradual improvement in the central scotomas (Figs. 6 & 7). The disc edema and hyperemia subsided, leaving atrophic-appearing nerve heads (Fig. 8); nevertheless, the visual acuity improved to 20/20 OD and 20/25 OS, and to date the patient has had no further recurrence of the cutaneous lesions. The reduced dosages of medications are being continued for the present.

DISCUSSION

The etiology of the vasculitis and associated optic neuritis in this case remains obscure. Clinically, the patient had dense central scotomas with bilateral disc edema. While the optic nerve heads were similar in appearance to acute Leber's disease, our patient had no family history of optic nerve disease, and the disease is rare in females. Optic neuritis occurs in connective tissue disorders (2); in this patient, however, there was no evidence, other than the skin lesions, of systemic connective tissue disease. Laboratory data, including spinal fluid evaluation, were unremarkable.

489

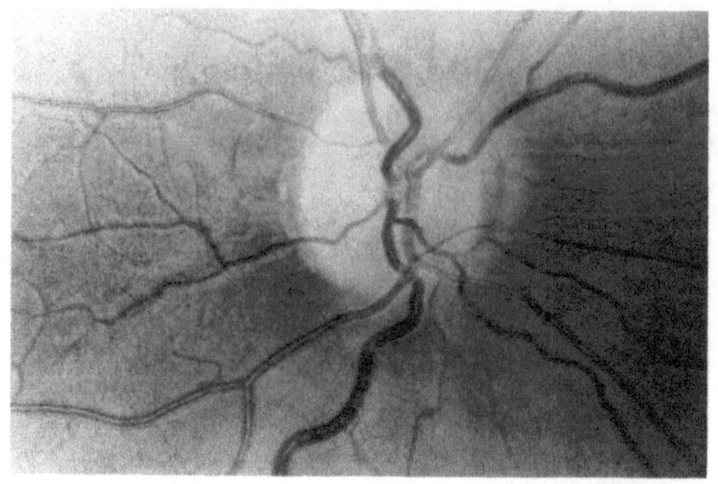

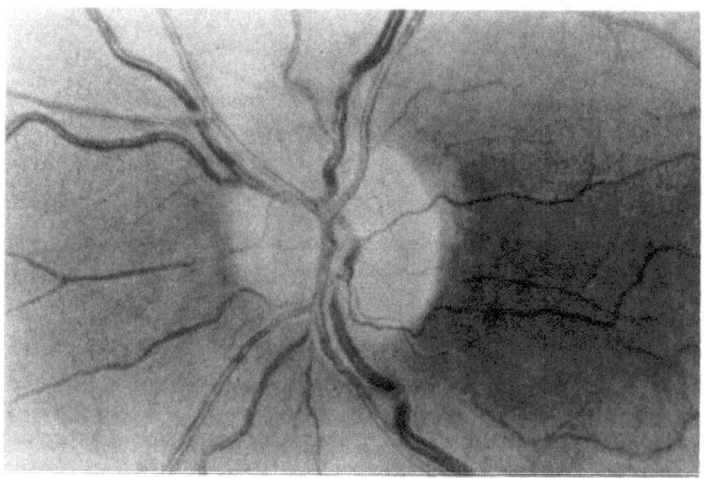

Fig. 8. Top: post-treatment OD; bottom: idem.

This patient gave a definite history of illicit medication usage. Whether the drugs she ingested could have been a factor in the development of cellular immune mechanisms within the walls of the affected blood vessels is unknown. This is an interesting speculation, however, as it is known that the intravascular deposition of immune complexes is associated with several types of vasculitis (1).

It has been reported that the use of immunosuppressive therapy and steroids resulted in the prompt remission of symptoms of systemic vasculitis and were effective in maintaining remissions (3). Our patient was treated with daily prednisone, alone, for 4—5 months; during this time, dosages were

490

reduced on two occasions with the subsequent development of recurrent skin lesions, and remission was incomplete. The patient was then started on mercaptopurine daily, together with prednisone, therapy; she responded with slow but continued improvement of the central scotomas and has had no further recurrence of the skin lesions. The present plan is for continued follow-up and a gradual reduction in medications, titrated to response.

SUMMARY

A 16-year old female presented with optic neuritis and pruritic skin lesions. The lesions were found pathologically to represent leukocytoclastic vasculitis. The patient had no other evidence of systemic connective tissue disease. Whether drug abuse may have been a factor in the etiology of the vasculitis is unknown.

Initially, the patient was treated with steroids alone, with definite but incomplete improvement; with the subsequent addition of mercaptopurine and continued steroid therapy, there has been remarkable improvement in the central scotomas and visual acuity, as well as resolution of the cutaneous lesions, without recurrence to date.

ACKNOWLEDGEMENT

This study was supported in part by Research to Prevent Blindness.

REFERENCES

1. Conn, D. L., McDuffie, F. C., Holley, K. E. and Schroeter, A. L. Immunologic mechanisms in systemic vasculitis. Proc. Mayo Clinic 51:511 (1976).
2. Dutton, J. J., Burder, R. M. and Klingele, T. G. Autoimmune retrobulbar optic neuritis. Am. J. Ophthalmol. 94:11–17 (1982).
3. Moore, P. M. and Fauci, A. S. Neurologic manifestations of systemic vasculitis. Am. J. Med. 71:517–524 (1981).
4. Sams, W. M. Jr. Continuing medical education, necrotizing vasculitis. J. Am. Acad. Dermatol. 3:1–13 (1980).

Authors' address:
Dept. of Ophthalmology
Indiana University Medical Center
Indianapolis, IN 46223
U.S.A.

THREE-DIMENSIONAL DISPLAY OF STATIC PERIMETRY

FUMIO MIZOGUCHI, YUJIN OWADA, SHIROAKI SHIRATO
and YOSHIAKI KITAZAWA

Key words. Visual field examination, three-dimensional representation.

ABSTRACT

A system for three-dimensional representation of the visual field was developed for displaying the results of static perimetric examinations. The strategy we adopted is to make use of webbing the three-dimensional space. The system has been implemented in a NEAC 50 in the interactive mode of graphic display and the three-dimensional representation was made on a Hewlett Packard plotter and a Tektronix 4301 graphics display.

Greve, E. L., Heijl, A. (eds.) Fifth International Visual Field Symposium.   493
©1983 Dr W. Junk Publishers, The Hague/Boston/Lancaster.

THE RELATIONSHIP BETWEEN VISUAL ACUITY, PUPILLARY DEFECT AND VISUAL FIELD LOSS

H. STANLEY THOMPSON, PAUL MONTAGUE, TERRY COX
and JAMES J. CORBETT

Key words. Visual acuity, visual field defects, pupil response

ABSTRACT

Loss of visual acuity, loss of visual field, and loss of pupillary function were compared in 64 patients with varied damage to the optic nerve. Loss of acuity depended on the location of the field defect but the pupil defect was proportional to the amount of visual field loss. Based on this information, a pattern of dots was constructed representing the retinal distribution of pupillomotor force (in log units). This pattern can be used to estimate the approximate amount of pupillary defect expected from a particular visual field defect.

Greve, E. L., Heijl, A. (eds.) Fifth International Visual Field Symposium.
©1983 Dr W. Junk Publishers, The Hague/Boston/Lancaster.

OPHTHALMOSCOPIC PERIMETRY

J. TERRY ERNEST and JOHN S. READ

Key words. Visual field examination, fundus perimetry, ophthalmoscopic perimetry.

ABSTRACT

We have constructed and tested a computer-assisted television ophthalmoscope for the examination of the visual field. The instrument is capable of both kinetic and static perimetry with direct visualization of test target position on the ocular fundus. The ocular fundus is viewed using modified Zeiss optics and a low-light-level television camera. The viewing (background) light source is a 500 Watt tungsten lamp furnishing either white or green (560 nm interference filter and a half band width of 10 nm) resulting in a retinal illuminance approximately equal to that from a Goldmann perimeter when the patient has an 8 mm pupil. The target is the end of a fiber optic placed in a plane conjugate with the retina. Its light source is a 150 Watt heat filtered Xenon arc lamp furnishing either white light or light of different colors. The colored targets are obtained with near-monochromatic light at 14 different wavelengths between 460 and 700 nm. The target light intensity can be rapidly varied under computer control in 0.03 log unit increments with a neutral density wedge. The target size is approximately 150 microns on the retina (about 0.5 degrees, or 9 mm at 1 meter). With each 1 second target presentation the images are scanned and digitized and when the patient indicates that the target has been seen the digitized image is stored. The visual fields are analyzed using semi-automatic programs under the control of the operator. The images (100–200) are aligned using an interactive image comparison program. The operator identifies both a vascular landmark and the target in each image and the computer generates either density or meridian plots superimposed on the image of the ocular fundus. Ophthalmoscopic perimetry eliminates fixation problems and makes possible precise retinal localization of defects in the visual system.

DISCUSSIONS

Discussion on 'Lateral inhibition in the fovea and parafoveal regions', by K. Kani, T. Inui, R. Haruta and O. Mimura.

C. A. Johnson: How do these values for summation and inhibition zones compare to those other studies such as those looking at Westheimer-type functions, such as Jay Enoch and others have examined?

K. Kani: Somewhat different, although the difference is smaller than that of other experiments.

W. M. Hart: Do you think that there would be an advantage of using concentric types of targets rather than lateral lines for measuring the inhibitory zone?

K. Kani: This is only a technical point. We used the parallel lines only because they are easy to make, while it is very difficult to make an annular target.

I. Bodis-Wollner: Was cycloplegia, an artificial pupil, used?

K. Kani: We used the fundus-controlled perimeter, which was made for an artificial pupil, 5 mm in diameter.

Discussion on 'Extrafoveal Stiles' π mechanisms', by K. Kitahara, R. Tamaki, J. Noji, A. Kandatsu and H. Matsuzaki.

C. A. Johnson: How were the curves plotted in terms of their absolute positions?

K. Kitahara: For π_4 mechanisms we measured the dark adaptation curve for 480 nm and we took the value of the cone threshold. For the π_1 and π_3 mechanisms we used the Stiles' temporal curve to fit — well, just by eyes.

Greve, E. L., Heijl, A. (eds.) Fifth International Visual Field Symposium.
©1983 Dr W. Junk Publishers, The Hague/Boston/Lancaster.

Discussion on 'Perimetric techniques used to assess retinal strain during accommodation', by J. M. Enoch et al.

C. A. Johnson: I would like to start out the discussion by saying that this is an ever-expanding field. There is work by Salladin and Stark (1) that seems to indicate that in presbyopia the lens is not resilient but the ciliary muscle effort remains present in older age groups. I was wondering if this might be a way of examining the magnification issue?

J. M. Enoch: Salladin and Stark's work and that of others is important. They had an impedance measuring device, and they were able to measure ciliary body activity separate from changes in the eye lens.

In our measure of retinal strain using the bisection technique, we demonstrated non-linear retinal stretch associated with accommodation (2). I, then in my mid-forties, showed these same changes. Hans Goldmann, then I guess in his late sixties or early seventies, said, 'Jay, I am getting some of the same changes'. It is clear that these retinal (stretching) strain effects are still present in older people and that it would be very nice to have a measure of these and to understand their significance.

J. D. Wirtschafter: The obstruction by balloon of carotid artery — cavernous sinus fistulas with subsequent decrease in ophthalmic and central retinal venous pressure allowed us to observe with serial photographs the displacement of the retinal vessels. Some of the movement occurred within the first day, but most of the changes occurred after the first day and before the ninth day. This retinal movement was most evident in the regions about $15-30°$ from the optic disc. This indicates another mechanism by which retinal displacement occurs.

J. M. Enoch: When DFP first came into use, characteristical peripheral retinal tears were recorded which were associated with, I assume, abnormally large ciliary muscle responses — either that or these were structurally weak retinas (3).

REFERENCES

1. Salladin, J. J. and Stark, L. W. Presbyopia: new evidence from impedance cyclography supporting the Hess-Gullstrand Theory. Vision Res. 15: 537–541 (1975).
2. Blank, K. and Enoch, J. M. Monocular spatial distortions induced by marked accommodation. Science 182:393–395 (1973).
3. Blank, K., Provine, R. R. and Enoch, J. M. Shift in the peak of the photopic Stiles-Crawford function with marked accommodation. Vision Res. 15:499–507 (1975).

Discussion on 'Static fundus perimetry in amblyopia: Comparison with juvenile macular degeneration', by S.G. Jacobson, M.A. Sandberg and E. L. Berson.

E. C. Campos: Can the sensitivity loss of the fovea found in amblyopia be equated to the sensitivity of a peripheral retinal location? In other words, does the fovea behave as an eccentric point?

S. G. Jacobson: The foveolar thresholds in amblyopic eyes are certainly less elevated than what would be predicted, based on cone spatial density, for an acuity of 6/60. In fact, the thresholds are more like those expected for a visual acuity of 6/12. As a contrast, thresholds at the fixation loci of patients with juvenile macular degeneration correspond well to their visual acuity of 6/60.

J. M. Enoch: What is the range of variability of the thresholds you measured?

S. G. Jacobson: When we tested patients repeatedly at the same session, at different sessions or with different examiners, there was never more than 0.2 log units measured variation in the thresholds.

Discussion on 'The visual field in alternating hyperphoria', by R. Fusco et al.

J. L. Keltner: The nasal inferior quadrant was the most affected area. Was it similar in other quadrants?

G. Verriest: The relative defect was present only in the nasal inferior quadrant but the determinations were made only along the four principal oblique meridians. The defect can be shown also with kinetic perimetry but then it is not very striking.

J. L. Keltner: This was done when the eye was non-hyperphoric — the eye was not up?

G. Verriest: Yes, it was made in monocular vision, the other eye being occluded.

J. L. Keltner: Could you explain why the other quadrants are not depressed, because when the eye drifts up they don't perceive diplopia so they are suppressing all visual signals? Sometimes with fatigue they will drift up. They may do that on their own and they don't perceive diplopia. I just wonder why it's only the inferior nasal quadrants?

G. Verriest: You speak again about binocular vision while our study was done in monocular vision. It was based on the theory of Crone, which was itself based on the theory of Keiner for esotropia.

E. C. Campos: One should test the eye which is deviated in patients with DVD, thus under binocular conditions and not monocularly.

498

G. Verriest: Surely, it should be very interesting to perform experiments on binocular vision, but it has not been done. The result was positive in monocular vision and thus I think that it would be still more positive under binocular conditions. This is something to do.

Discussion on 'Temporal resolution in the peripheral visual field', by P. M. Dunn and R. V. Massof.

A. Heijl: I think that it is important to have data for normals established before we try to collect data in pathology. We have no other papers in this symposium where the same functions have been studied. Nevertheless, I think, if I understand it correctly, that we have two related papers by Dr Calabria the results of which seem to fit very well with the results of Dr Dunn. I wonder if Dr Calabria would like to elaborate on that?

G. Calabria: It seems to me that our results are very close to the theoretical results of Dr Dunn. We made some investigations on the flicker fusion frequencies in glaucoma. The old results indicating that in glaucoma there is an impairment of the flicker fusion may be due to the fact that liminal targets were never used. Using a threshold target in glaucoma we always have the same results (flicker fusion frequencies). This I think agrees with the results of Dr Dunn.

S. M. Drance: I wonder if I could ask a question? It is said that the temporal contrast sensitivity function is one of the few psychophysical measurements that does not change with age. Did either of the authors say anything about this or have they looked at the question of age in normals?

C. A. Johnson: I was wondering regarding the temporal contrast sensitivities – in the fovea there are changes with background illumination – I wonder whether you have done this experiment with different background luminances?

P. M. Dunn: That is sort of the plan but it has not been done yet.

J. T. Ernest: Is the temporal contrast sensitivity affected by generalized retinal disease outside the tested areas?

P. M. Dunn: I don't know if that has ever been looked at. I assume if there was a contiguous area it might well. I expect that you would see that more with a smaller target than with the one we used.

Discussion on 'Diabetic retinopathy: Perimetric findings', by E. Gandolfo, M. Zingirian, G. Corallo and F. Cardillo Piccolino.

G. Spaeth: Along the lines of the previous paper, – have you made comparisons in patients after panretinal photocoagulation?

E. Gandolfo: We have studied, in a previous paper, the effect of photo-coagulation upon the sensitivity of the retina, but in this paper we have not studied the effect of the single lesions after photocoagulation. The effect of coagulation varies depending on the kind of treatment used, the kind of laser or Xenon lamp used, but in this paper we have not controlled the effect on these lesions.

J. T. Ernest: Diabetic retinal lesions are highly variable over time. Did the authors measure sequential changes.

E. Gandolfo: The results of perimetry of the lesions seem not to change with time. And only when different lesions occur in the same territories we can detect a decrease in the sensitivity.

Discussion on 'Static perimetry in central serous retinochoroidopathy (Masuda's type) using a fundus photo-perimeter', by M. Tomonaga, T. Miyamoto, H. Suzumura and Y. Ohta.

J. T. Ernest: Once the macular area fluid has gone, how long does it take for complete recovery of your static visual field measurement?

M. Tomonaga: About one month.

J. T. Ernest: I have asked that question because we worked with the Stiles-Crawford phenomenon and found that after the fluid disappears it took a very long time before that function came back to normal. I am much surprised, I thought it would be even longer before your function came back to normal.

M. Tomonaga: In our study, the static condition stage is when retinal edema has disappeared. In this stage we measured the visual field contrast sensitivity with the fundus photo-perimeter, and they were not completely back to normal.

A. Heijl: Could I then ask another question? We just heard that the Stiles-Crawford phenomenon was not normal until later than that. Would that explain the differences between blue and red or how do you think we should interpret the fact that blue is most affected? Is that due to a small edema that we cannot detect clinically or is it due to something that has to do with the blue cones?

M. Tomonaga: Yes, blue cones are weaker.

A. Heijl: And you mean that you could have a permanent impairment of the function of the blue cones in this area?

M. Tomonaga: Yes, blue cones are weaker than red and green, I think. We also observed the course of the retinal choroidopathy using the usual type I Nagel anomalyscope. We observed the so-called pseudo-protanomaly. For an observation period of a couple of years it never reached the normal range.

500

J. T. Ernest: But the circle of confusion was normal?

M. Tomonaga: Yes, that is right.

Discussion on 'Boundary curves for dividing visual fields into sectors corresponding to a retinotopic projection onto the optic disc', by J. F. Hills, J. D. Wirtschafter and P. Maeder.

G. Spaeth: You presented this idea last year. Do you have any results that you can give us on the use of this in analyzing fields?

J. D. Wirtschafter: In addition to the material I presented last year we had a chance to look now at just a few visual fields sequentially and I will tell you what I think is the most exciting kind of result that we are seeing. We have looked at patients who have undergone treatment for glaucoma, having begun at a different point. The average score in the clinical impression concerning their visual field was that overall they improved on the treatment, that is looking at the Octopus data as it originally came out of the machine. Scoring the data we found that those areas which normally don't have much glaucomatous field loss improved a great deal. The areas along the horizontal raphe were the same or got worse. That is a very informal and preliminary analysis of some data.

S. M. Drance: Independent of the therapy?

J. D. Wirtschafter: I am not in a position to say that but I can say that this method allows you to compare improvement in one area with another. I don't have the numbers to make any statement of the therapy. You were kind enough to send me some fields and I just haven't had the chance to look at those.

A. Heijl: I suppose that if we use the data of Dr Wirtschafter and program that into our automatic perimeters we could use your formulae to find areas of suspect pathology easier and then we could program the computer to search that area in some kind of adaptive way. Is that anything that you think could be worthwhile to try?

J. D. Wirtschafter: Yes, but I don't have the experience with it yet. This provides a format for of at least deciding where the money is, either in cases in general or in a particular case that comes up. One could decide on the basis of the initial examination that the subsequent examinations on a given patient would have twice as many points in certain designated areas and half as many points or just the basic examination in other areas, so to that extent you could use this as a way of saying, O.K. this is where we will invest the other points rather than try a geometric definition of other points which almost inevitably leads to some waste of data in locations that you would not necessarily want, because you could not allocate it to one of these areas that you were testing.

501